D1325329

Fourth Edition

Plastic Surgery

Lower Extremity, Trunk, and Burns

Volume Four

Content Strategist: Belinda Kuhn
Content Development Specialists: Louise Cook, Sam Crowe, Alexandra Mortimer
e-products, Content Development Specialist: Kim Benson
Project Managers: Anne Collett, Andrew Riley, Julie Taylor
Designer: Miles Hitchen
Illustration Managers: Karen Giacomucci, Amy Faith Heyden
Marketing Manager: Melissa Fogarty
Video Liaison: Will Schmitt

Fourth Edition

Plastic Surgery

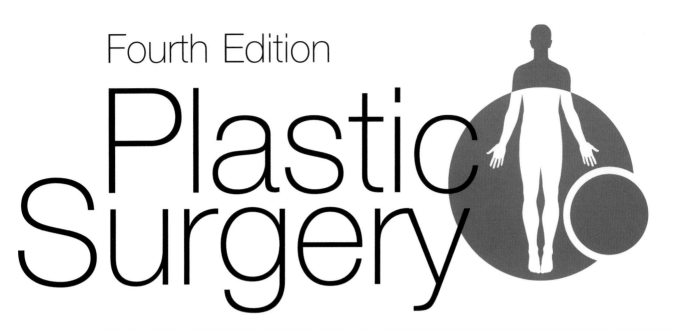

Lower Extremity, Trunk, and Burns

Volume Four

Volume Editor

David H. Song
MD, MBA, FACS
Regional Chief, MedStar Health
Plastic and Reconstructive Surgery
Professor and Chairman
Department of Plastic Surgery
Georgetown University School of Medicine
Washington, DC, USA

Editor-in-Chief

Peter C. Neligan
MB, FRCS(I), FRCSC, FACS
Professor of Surgery
Department of Surgery, Division of Plastic
Surgery
University of Washington
Seattle, WA, USA

Multimedia Editor

Daniel Z. Liu
MD
Plastic and Reconstructive Surgeon
Cancer Treatment Centers of America at
Midwestern Regional Medical Center
Zion, IL, USA

For additional online figures, videos and video lectures visit Expertconsult.com

ELSEVIER London, New York, Oxford, Philadelphia, St Louis, Sydney 2018

ELSEVIER

First edition 1990
Second edition 2006
Third edition 2013
Fourth edition 2018

Notices

Knowledge and best practice in this field are constantly changing. As new research and experience broaden our understanding, changes in research methods, professional practices, or medical treatment may become necessary.

Practitioners and researchers must always rely on their own experience and knowledge in evaluating and using any information, methods, compounds, or experiments described herein. In using such information or methods they should be mindful of their own safety and the safety of others, including parties for whom they have a professional responsibility.

With respect to any drug or pharmaceutical products identified, readers are advised to check the most current information provided (i) on procedures featured or (ii) by the manufacturer of each product to be administered, to verify the recommended dose or formula, the method and duration of administration, and contraindications. It is the responsibility of practitioners, relying on their own experience and knowledge of their patients, to make diagnoses, to determine dosages and the best treatment for each individual patient, and to take all appropriate safety precautions.

To the fullest extent of the law, neither the Publisher nor the authors, contributors, or editors, assume any liability for any injury and/or damage to persons or property as a matter of products liability, negligence or otherwise, or from any use or operation of any methods, products, instructions, or ideas contained in the material herein.

Volume 4 ISBN: 978-0-323-35706-7
Volume 4 Ebook ISBN: 978-0-323-35707-4
6 volume set ISBN: 978-0-323-35630-5

your source for books,
journals and multimedia
in the health sciences
www.elsevierhealth.com

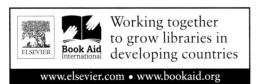

Working together
to grow libraries in
developing countries

www.elsevier.com • www.bookaid.org

The
publisher's
policy is to use
**paper manufactured
from sustainable forests**

Printed in Canada
Last digit is the print number: 9 8 7 6 5 4 3 2 1

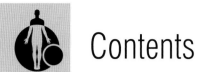

Contents

Volume Three: Craniofacial, Head and Neck Surgery, and Pediatric Plastic Surgery

Part 1: Head, neck, and craniofacial surgery: edited by Eduardo D. Rodriguez

Part 2: Pediatrics: edited by Joseph E. Losee

Section I: Clefts

Volume Four: Lower Extremity, Trunk, and Burns

edited by David H. Song

Volume Five: Breast

edited by Maurice Y. Nahabedian

Section I: Aesthetic Breast Surgery

Section II: Reconstructive Breast Surgery

Volume Six: Hand and Upper Extremity

edited by James Chang

Video Contents

Lecture Video Contents

Preface to the Fourth Edition

When I wrote the preface to the 3rd edition of this book, I remarked how honored and unexpectedly surprised I was to be the Editor of this great series. This time 'round, I'm equally grateful to carry this series forward. When Elsevier called me and suggested it was time to prepare the 4th edition, my initial reaction was that this was way too soon. What could possibly have changed in Plastic Surgery since the 3rd edition was launched in 2012? As it transpires, there have been many developments and I hope we have captured them in this edition.

We have an extraordinary specialty. A recent article by Chadra, Agarwal and Agarwal entitled "Redefining Plastic Surgery" appeared in *Plastic and Reconstructive Surgery—Global Open*. In it they gave the following definition: "Plastic surgery is a specialized branch of surgery, which deals with deformities, defects and abnormalities of the organs of perception, organs of action and the organs guarding the external passages, besides innovation, implantation, replantation and transplantation of tissues, and aims at restoring and improving their form, function and the esthetic appearances." This is an all-encompassing but very apt definition and captures the enormous scope of the specialty.[1]

In the 3rd edition, I introduced volume editors for each of the areas of the specialty because the truth is that one person can no longer be an expert in all areas of this diverse specialty, and I'm certainly not. I think this worked well because the volume editors not only had the expertise to present their area of subspecialty in the best light, but they were tuned in to what was new and who was doing it. We have continued this model in this new edition. Four of the seven volume editors from the previous edition have again helped to bring the latest and the best to this edition: Drs Gurtner, Song, Rodriguez, Losee, and Chang have revised and updated their respective volumes with some chapters remaining, some extensively revised, some added, and some deleted. Dr. Peter Rubin has replaced Dr. Rick Warren to compile the Aesthetic volume (Vol. 2). Dr. Warren did a wonderful job in corralling this somewhat disparate, yet vitally important, part of our specialty into the Aesthetic volume in the 3rd edition but felt that the task of doing it again, though a labor of love, was more than he wanted to take on. Similarly, Dr. Jim Grotting who did a masterful job in the last edition on the Breast volume, decided that doing a major revision should be undertaken by someone with a fresh perspective and Dr. Maurice Nahabedian stepped into that breach. I hope you will like the changes you see in both of these volumes.

Dr. Allen Van Beek was the video editor for the last edition and he compiled an impressive array of movies to complement the text. This time around, we wanted to go a step further and though we've considerably expanded the list of videos accompanying the text (there are over 170), we also added the idea of lectures accompanying selected chapters. What we've done here is to take selected key chapters and include the images from that chapter, photos and artwork, and create a narrated presentation that is available online; there are annotations in the text to alert the reader that this is available. Dr. Daniel Liu, who has taken over from Dr. Van Beek as multimedia editor (rather than video editor) has done an amazing job in making all of this happen. There are over 70 presentations of various key chapters online, making it as easy as possible for you, the reader, to get as much knowledge as you can, in the easiest way possible from this edition. Many of these presentations have been done by the authors of the chapters; the rest have been compiled by Dr. Liu and myself from the content of the individual chapters. I hope you find them useful.

The reader may wonder how this all works. To plan this edition, the Elsevier team, headed by Belinda Kuhn, and I, convened a face-to-face meeting in San Francisco. The volume editors, as well as the London based editorial team, were present. We went through the 3rd edition, volume by volume, chapter by chapter, over an entire weekend. We decided what needed to stay, what needed to be added, what needed to be revised, and what needed to be changed. We also decided who should write the various chapters, keeping many existing authors, replacing others, and adding some new ones; we did this so as to really reflect the changes occurring within the specialty. We also decided on practical changes that needed to be made. As an example, you will notice that we have omitted the complete index for the 6 Volume set from Volumes 2-6 and highlighted only the table of contents for that particular volume. The complete index is of course available in Volume 1 and fully searchable online. This allowed us to save several hundred pages per volume, reducing production costs and diverting those dollars to the production of the enhanced online content.

In my travels around the world since the 3rd edition was published, I've been struck by what an impact this publication has had on the specialty and, more particularly, on training. Everywhere I go, I'm told how the text is an important part of didactic teaching and a font of knowledge. It is gratifying to see that the 3rd edition has been translated into Portuguese, Spanish, and Chinese. This is enormously encouraging. I hope this 4th edition continues to contribute to the specialty, remains a resource for practicing surgeons, and continues to prepare our trainees for their future careers in Plastic Surgery.

Peter C. Neligan
Seattle, WA
September, 2017

[1] Chandra R, Agarwal R, Agarwal D. Redefining Plastic Surgery. *Plast Reconstr Surg Glob Open*. 2016;4(5):e706.

List of Editors

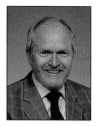

Editor-in-Chief
Peter C. Neligan, MB, FRCS(I), FRCSC, FACS
Professor of Surgery
Department of Surgery, Division of Plastic Surgery
University of Washington
Seattle, WA, USA

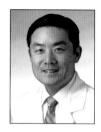

Volume 4: Lower Extremity, Trunk, and Burns
David H. Song, MD, MBA, FACS
Regional Chief, MedStar Health
Plastic and Reconstructive Surgery
Professor and Chairman
Department of Plastic Surgery
Georgetown University School of Medicine
Washington, DC, USA

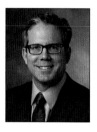

Volume 1: Principles
Geoffrey C. Gurtner, MD, FACS
Johnson and Johnson Distinguished Professor of
Surgery and Vice Chairman,
Department of Surgery (Plastic Surgery)
Stanford University
Stanford, CA, USA

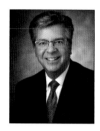

Volume 5: Breast
Maurice Y. Nahabedian, MD, FACS
Professor and Chief
Section of Plastic Surgery
MedStar Washington Hospital Center
Washington, DC, USA;
Vice Chairman
Department of Plastic Surgery
MedStar Georgetown University Hospital
Washington, DC, USA

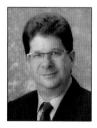

Volume 2: Aesthetic
J. Peter Rubin, MD, FACS
UPMC Professor of Plastic Surgery
Chair, Department of Plastic Surgery
Professor of Bioengineering
University of Pittsburgh
Pittsburgh, PA, USA

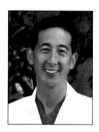

Volume 6: Hand and Upper Extremity
James Chang, MD
Johnson & Johnson Distinguished
Professor and Chief
Division of Plastic and Reconstructive Surgery
Stanford University Medical Center
Stanford, CA, USA

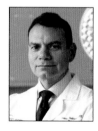

Volume 3: Craniofacial, Head and Neck Surgery
Eduardo D. Rodriguez, MD, DDS
Helen L. Kimmel Professor of Reconstructive
Plastic Surgery
Chair, Hansjörg Wyss Department of Plastic
Surgery
NYU School of Medicine
NYU Langone Medical Center
New York, NY, USA

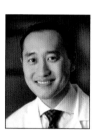

Multimedia editor
Daniel Z. Liu, MD
Plastic and Reconstructive Surgeon
Cancer Treatment Centers of America at Midwest-
ern Regional Medical Center
Zion, IL, USA

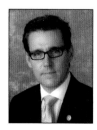

Volume 3: Pediatric Plastic Surgery
Joseph E. Losee, MD
Ross H. Musgrave Professor of Pediatric Plastic
Surgery
Department of Plastic Surgery
University of Pittsburgh Medical Center;
Chief Division of Pediatric Plastic Surgery
Children's Hospital of Pittsburgh
Pittsburgh, PA, USA

List of Contributors

The editors would like to acknowledge and offer grateful thanks for the input of all previous editions' contributors, without whom this new edition would not have been possible.

VOLUME ONE

Hatem Abou-Sayed, MD, MBA
Vice President
Physician Engagement
Interpreta, Inc.
San Diego, CA, USA

Paul N. Afrooz, MD
Resident
Plastic and Reconstructive Surgery
University of Pittsburgh Medical Center
Pittsburgh, PA, USA

Claudia R. Albornoz, MD, MSc
Research Fellow
Plastic and Reconstructive Surgery
Memorial Sloan Kettering Cancer Center
New York, NY, USA

Nidal F. Al Deek, MD
Doctor of Plastic and Reconstructive Surgery
Chang Gung Memorial Hospital
Taipei, Taiwan

Amy K. Alderman, MD, MPH
Private Practice
Atlanta, GA, USA

Louis C. Argenta, MD
Professor of Plastic and Reconstructive Surgery
Department of Plastic Surgery
Wake Forest Medical Center
Winston Salem, NC, USA

Stephan Ariyan, MD, MBA
Emeritus Frank F. Kanthak Professor of Surgery,
Plastic Surgery, Surgical Oncology,
Otolaryngology
Yale University School of Medicine;
Associate Chief
Department of Surgery;
Founding Director, Melanoma Program
Smilow Cancer Hospital, Yale Cancer Center
New Haven, CT, USA

Tomer Avraham, MD
Attending Plastic Surgeon
Mount Sinai Health System
Tufts University School of Medicine
New York, NY, USA

Aaron Berger, MD, PhD
Clinical Assistant Professor
Division of Plastic Surgery
Florida International University School of Medicine
Miami, FL, USA

Kirsty Usher Boyd, MD, FRCSC
Assistant Professor Surgery (Plastics)
Division of Plastic and Reconstructive Surgery
University of Ottawa
Ottawa, Ontario, Canada

Charles E. Butler, MD, FACS
Professor and Chairman
Department of Plastic Surgery
Charles B. Barker Endowed Chair in Surgery
The University of Texas MD Anderson Cancer Center
Houston, TX, USA

Peter E. M. Butler, MD, FRCSI, FRCS, FRCS(Plast)
Professor
Plastic and Reconstructive Surgery
University College and Royal Free London
London, UK

Yilin Cao, MD, PhD
Professor
Shanghai Ninth People's Hospital
Shanghai Jiao Tong University School of Medicine
Shanghai, China

Franklyn P. Cladis, MD, FAAP
Associate Professor of Anesthesiology
Department of Anesthesiology
The Children's Hospital of Pittsburgh of UPMC
Pittsburgh, PA, USA

Mark B. Constantian, MD
Private Practice
Surgery (Plastic Surgery)
St. Joseph Hospital
Nashua, NH, USA

Daniel A. Cuzzone, MD
Plastic Surgery Fellow
Hanjörg Wyss Department of Plastic Surgery
New York University Medical Center
New York, NY, USA

Gurleen Dhami, MD
Chief Resident
Department of Radiation Oncology
University of Washington
Seattle, WA, USA

Gayle Gordillo, MD
Associate Professor
Plastic Surgery
The Ohio State University
Columbus, OH, USA

Geoffrey C. Gurtner, MD, FACS
Johnson and Johnson Distinguished Professor
of Surgery and Vice Chairman,
Department of Surgery (Plastic Surgery)
Stanford University
Stanford, CA, USA

Phillip C. Haeck, MD
Surgeon
Plastic Surgery
The Polyclinic
Seattle, WA, USA

The late Bruce Halperin†, MD
Formerly Adjunct Associate Professor of Anesthesia
Department of Anesthesia
Stanford University
Stanford, CA, USA

Daniel E. Heath
Lecturer
School of Chemical and Biomedical Engineering
University of Melbourne
Parkville, Victoria, Australia

Joon Pio Hong, MD, PhD, MMM
Professor
Plastic Surgery
Asan Medical Center, University of Ulsan
Seoul, South Korea

Michael S. Hu, MD, MPH, MS
Postdoctoral Fellow
Division of Plastic Surgery
Department of Surgery
Stanford University School of Medicine
Stanford, CA, USA

C. Scott Hultman, MD, MBA
Professor and Chief
Division of Plastic and Reconstructive Surgery
University of North Carolina
Chapel Hill, NC, USA

Amir E. Ibrahim
Division of Plastic Surgery
Department of Surgery
American University of Beirut Medical Center
Beirut, Lebanon

Leila Jazayeri, MD
Microsurgery Fellow
Plastic and Reconstructive Surgery
Memorial Sloan Kettering Cancer Center
New York, NY, USA

Brian Jeffers
Student
Bioengineering
University of California Berkeley
Berkeley, CA USA

Lynn Jeffers, MD, FACS
Private Practice
Oxnard, CA, USA

Mohammed M. Al Kahtani, MD, FRCSC
Clinical Fellow
Division of Plastic Surgery
Department of Surgery
University of Alberta
Edmonton, Alberta, Canada

Gabrielle M. Kane, MB, BCh, EdD, FRCPC
Associate Professor
Radiation Oncology
University of Washington
Seattle, WA, USA

Raghu P. Kataru, PhD
Senior Research Scientist
Memorial Sloan-Kettering Cancer Center
New York, NY, USA

Carolyn L. Kerrigan, MD, MSc, MHCDS
Professor of Surgery
Surgery
Dartmouth–Hitchcock Medical Center
Lebanon, NH, USA

Timothy W. King, MD, PhD, FAAP, FACS
Associate Professor with Tenure
Departments of Surgery and Biomedical
Engineering;
Director of Research, Division of Plastic Surgery
University of Alabama at Birmingham (UAB)
Craniofacial and Pediatric Plastic Surgery
Children's of Alabama – Plastic Surgery;
Chief, Plastic Surgery Section
Birmingham VA Hospital
Birmingham, AL, USA

Brian M. Kinney, MD, FACS, MSME
Clinical Assistant Professor of Plastic Surgery
University of Southern California
School of Medicine
Los Angeles, CA, USA

W. P. Andrew Lee, MD
The Milton T. Edgerton MD, Professor and
Chairman
Department of Plastic and Reconstructive
Surgery
Johns Hopkins University School of Medicine
Baltimore, MD, USA

**Sherilyn Keng Lin Tay, MBChB, MSc,
FRCS(Plast)**
Consultant Plastic Surgeon
Canniesburn Plastic Surgery Unit
Glasgow Royal Infirmary
Glasgow, UK

Daniel Z. Liu, MD
Plastic and Reconstructive Surgeon
Cancer Treatment Centers of America at
Midwestern Regional Medical Center
Zion, IL, USA

Wei Liu, MD, PhD
Professor
Plastic and Reconstructive Surgery
Shanghai Ninth People's Hospital
Shanghai Jiao Tong University School of
Medicine
Shanghai, China

Michael T. Longaker, MD, MBA, FACS
Deane P. and Louise Mitchell Professor and Vice
Chair
Department of Surgery
Stanford University
Stanford, CA, USA

H. Peter Lorenz, MD
Service Chief and Professor, Plastic Surgery
Lucile Packard Children's Hospital
Stanford University School of Medicine
Stanford, CA, USA

Susan E. Mackinnon, MD
Sydney M. Shoenberg Jr. and Robert H.
Shoenberg Professor
Department of Surgery, Division of Plastic and
Reconstructive Surgery
Washington University School of Medicine
St. Louis, MO, USA

Malcolm W. Marks, MD
Professor and Chairman
Department of Plastic Surgery
Wake Forest University School of Medicine
Winston-Salem, NC, USA

Diego Marre, MD
Fellow
O'Brien Institute
Department of Plastic and Reconstructive
Surgery
St. Vincent's Hospital
Melbourne, Australia

David W. Mathes, MD
Professor and Chief of the Division of Plastic
and Reconstructive Surgery
University of Colorado
Aurora, CO, USA

Evan Matros MD, MMSc
Plastic Surgeon
Memorial Sloan-Kettering Cancer Center
New York, NY, USA

Isabella C. Mazzola, MD
Attending Plastic Surgeon
Klinik für Plastische und Ästhetische Chirurgie
Klinikum Landkreis Erding
Erding, Germany

Riccardo F. Mazzola, MD
Plastic Surgeon
Department of Specialistic Surgical Sciences
Fondazione Ospedale Maggiore Policlinico, Ca'
Granda IRCCS
Milano, Italy

Lindsay D. McHutchion, MS, BSc
Anaplastologist
Institute for Reconstructive Sciences in Medicine
Edmonton, Alberta, Canada

Babak J. Mehrara, MD, FACS
Associate Member, Associate Professor of
Surgery (Plastic)
Memorial Sloan Kettering Cancer Center
Weil Cornell University Medical Center
New York, NY, USA

Steven F. Morris, MD, MSc, FRCSC
Professor of Surgery
Department of Surgery
Dalhousie University
Halifax, Nova Scotia, Canada

Wayne A. Morrison, MBBS, MD, FRACS
Professorial Fellow
O'Brien Institute
Department of Surgery, University of Melbourne
Department of Plastic and Reconstructive
Surgery, St. Vincent's Hospital
Melbourne, Australia

**Peter C. Neligan, MB, FRCS(I), FRCSC,
FACS**
Professor of Surgery
Department of Surgery, Division of Plastic
Surgery
University of Washington
Seattle, WA, USA

Andrea J. O'Connor, BE(Hons), PhD
Associate Professor
Department of Chemical and Biomolecular
Engineering
University of Melbourne
Parkville, Victoria, Australia

Rei Ogawa, MD, PhD, FACS
Professor and Chief
Department of Plastic
Reconstructive and Aesthetic Surgery
Nippon Medical School
Tokyo, Japan

Dennis P. Orgill, MD, PhD
Professor of Surgery
Harvard Medical School
Medical Director, Wound Care Center;
Vice Chairman for Quality Improvement
Department of Surgery
Brigham and Women's Hospital
Boston, MA, USA

Cho Y. Pang, PhD
Senior Scientist
Research Institute
The Hospital for Sick Children;
Professor
Departments of Surgery/Physiology
University of Toronto
Toronto, Ontario, Canada

Ivo Alexander Pestana, MD, FACS
Associate Professor
Plastic and Reconstructive Surgery
Wake Forest University
Winston Salem, NC, USA

Giorgio Pietramaggior, MD, PhD
Swiss Nerve Institute
Clinique de La Source
Lausanne, Switzerland

Andrea L. Pusic, MD, MHS, FACS
Associate Professor
Plastic and Reconstructive Surgery
Memorial Sloan Kettering Cancer Center
New York, NY, USA

Russell R. Reid, MD, PhD
Associate Professor
Surgery/Section of Plastic and Reconstructive
Surgery
University of Chicago Medicine
Chicago, IL, USA

Neal R. Reisman, MD, JD
Chief
Plastic Surgery
Baylor St. Luke's Medical Center
Houston, TX, USA

Joseph M. Rosen, MD
Professor of Surgery
Plastic Surgery
Dartmouth–Hitchcock Medical Center
Lebanon, NH, USA

Sashwati Roy, MS, PhD
Associate Professor
Surgery, Center for Regenerative Medicine and
Cell based Therapies
The Ohio State University
Columbus, OH, USA

J. Peter Rubin, MD, FACS
UPMC Professor of Plastic Surgery
Chair, Department of Plastic Surgery
Professor of Bioengineering
University of Pittsburgh
Pittsburgh, PA, USA

Karim A. Sarhane, MD
Department of Surgery
University of Toledo Medical Center
Toledo, OH, USA

David B. Sarwer, PhD
Associate Professor of Psychology
Departments of Psychiatry and Surgery
University of Pennsylvania School of Medicine
Philadelphia, PA, USA

Saja S. Scherer-Pietramaggiori, MD
Plastic and Reconstructive Surgeon
Plastic Surgery
University Hospital Lausanne
Lausanne, Vaud, Switzerland

Iris A. Seitz, MD, PhD
Director of Research and International
Collaboration
University Plastic Surgery
Rosalind Franklin University;
Clinical Instructor of Surgery
Chicago Medical School
Chicago, IL, USA

Jesse C. Selber, MD, MPH, FACS
Associate Professor, Director of Clinical
Research
Department of Plastic Surgery
MD Anderson Cancer Center
Houston, TX, USA

Chandan K. Sen, PhD
Professor and Director
Center for Regenerative Medicine and Cell-
Based Therapies
The Ohio State University Wexner Medical
Center
Columbus, OH, USA

Wesley N. Sivak, MD, PhD
Resident in Plastic Surgery
Department of Plastic Surgery
University of Pittsburgh
Pittsburgh, PA, USA

M. Lucy Sudekum
Research Assistant
Thayer School of Engineering at Dartmouth
College
Hanover, NH, USA

**G. Ian Taylor, AO, MBBS, MD, MD(Hon
Bordeaux), FRACS, FRCS(Eng), FRCS(Hon
Edinburgh), FRCSI(Hon), FRSC(Hon
Canada), FACS(Hon)**
Professor
Department of Plastic Surgery
Royal Melbourne Hospital;
Professor
Department of Anatomy
University of Melbourne
Melbourne, Victoria, Australia

Chad M. Teven, MD
Resident
Section of Plastic and Reconstructive Surgery
University of Chicago
Chicago, IL, USA

Ruth Tevlin, MB BAO BCh, MRCSI, MD
Resident in Surgery
Department of Plastic and Reconstructive
Surgery
Stanford University School of Medicine
Stanford, CA, USA

E. Dale Collins Vidal, MD, MS
Chief
Section of Plastic Surgery
Dartmouth–Hitchcock Medical Center
Lebanon, NH, USA

Derrick C. Wan, MD
Associate Professor
Division of Plastic Surgery
Department of Surgery
Director of Maxillofacial Surgery
Lucile Packard Children's Hospital
Stanford University School of Medicine
Stanford, CA, USA

Renata V. Weber, MD
Assistant Professor Surgery (Plastics)
Division of Plastic and Reconstructive Surgery
Albert Einstein College of Medicine
Bronx, NY, USA

Fu-Chan Wei, MD
Professor
Department of Plastic Surgery
Chang Gung Memorial Hospital
Taoyuan, Taiwan

Gordon H. Wilkes, BScMed, MD
Clinical Professor of Surgery
Department of Surgery University of Alberta
Institute for Reconstructive Sciences in Medicine
Misericordia Hospital
Edmonton, Alberta, Canada

**Johan F. Wolfaardt, BDS,
MDent(Prosthodontics), PhD**
Professor
Division of Otolaryngology – Head and Neck
Surgery
Department of Surgery
Faculty of Medicine and Dentistry;
Director of Clinics and International Relations
Institute for Reconstructive Sciences in Medicine
University of Alberta
Covenant Health Group
Alberta Health Services
Alberta, Canada

Kiryu K. Yap, MBBS, BMedSc
Junior Surgical Trainee & PhD Candidate
O'Brien Institute
Department of Surgery, University of Melbourne
Department of Plastic and Reconstructive
Surgery, St. Vincent's Hospital
Melbourne, Australia

Andrew Yee
Research Assistant
Division of Plastic and Reconstructive Surgery
Washington University School of Medicine
St. Louis, MO, USA

Elizabeth R. Zielins, MD
Postdoctoral Research Fellow
Surgery
Stanford University School of Medicine
Stanford, CA, USA

VOLUME TWO

Paul N. Afrooz, MD
Resident
Plastic and Reconstructive Surgery
University of Pittsburgh Medical Center
Pittsburgh, PA, USA

Jamil Ahmad, MD, FRCSC
Director of Research and Education
The Plastic Surgery Clinic
Mississauga;
Assistant Professor
Surgery
University of Toronto
Toronto, Ontario, Canada

Lisa E. Airan, MD
Aesthetic Dermatologist NYC
Private Practice;
Associate Clinical Professor Department of
Dermatology
Mount Sinai School of Medicine
New York, NY, USA

Gary J. Alter, MD
Assistant Clinical Professor
Division of Plastic Surgery
University of California
Los Angeles, CA, USA

Al S. Aly, MD
Professor of Plastic Surgery
Aesthetic and Plastic Surgery Institute University
of California Irvine
Orange, CA, USA

Khalid Al-Zahrani, MD, SSC-PLAST
Assistant Professor
Consultant Plastic Surgeon
King Khalid University Hospital
King Saud University
Riyadh, Saudi Arabia

Bryan Armijo, MD
Plastic Surgery Chief Resident
Department of Plastic and Reconstructive
Surgery
Case Western Reserve/University Hospitals
Cleveland, OH, USA

Daniel C. Baker, MD
Professor of Surgery
Institute of Reconstructive Plastic Surgery
New York University Medical Center
Department of Plastic Surgery
New York, NY, USA

Fritz E. Barton Jr., MD
Clinical Professor
Department of Plastic Surgery
UT Southwestern Medical Center
Dallas, TX, USA

Leslie Baumann, MD
CEO
Baumann Cosmetic and Research Institute
Miami, FL, USA

Miles G. Berry, MS, FRCS(Plast)
Consultant Plastic and Aesthetic Surgeon
Institute of Cosmetic and Reconstructive
Surgery
London, UK

Trevor M. Born, MD
Division of Plastic Surgery
Lenox Hill/Manhattan Eye Ear and Throat
Hospital North Shore-LIJ Hospital
New York, NY, USA;
Clinical Lecturer
Division of Plastic Surgery
University of Toronto Western Division
Toronto, Ontario, Canada

Terrence W. Bruner, MD, MBA
Private Practice
Greenville, SC, USA

Andrés F. Cánchica, MD
Chief Resident of Plastic Surgery
Plastic Surgery Service Dr. Osvaldo Saldanha
São Paulo, Brazil

Joseph F. Capella, MD
Chief Post-bariatric Body Contouring
Division of Plastic Surgery
Hackensack University Medical Center
Hackensack, NJ, USA

Robert F. Centeno, MD, MBA
Medical Director
St. Croix Plastic Surgery and MediSpa;
Chief Medical Quality Officer
Governor Juan F. Luis Hospital and Medical
Center
Christiansted, Saint Croix, United States Virgin
Islands

Ernest S. Chiu, MD, FACS
Associate Professor of Plastic Surgery
Department of Plastic Surgery
New York University
New York, NY, USA

Jong Woo Choi, MD, PhD, MMM
Associate Professor
Department of Plastic and Reconstructive
Surgery
Seoul Asan Medical Center
Seoul, South Korea

Steven R. Cohen, MD
Senior Clinical Research Fellow, Clinical
Professor
Plastic Surgery
University of California
San Diego, CA;
Director
Craniofacial Surgery
Rady Children's Hospital, Private Practice,
FACES+ Plastic Surgery, Skin and Laser Center
La Jolla, CA, USA

Sydney R. Coleman, MD
Assistant Clinical Professor
Plastic Surgery
New York University Medical Center
New York;
Assistant Clinical Professor
Plastic Surgery
University of Pittsburgh Medical Center
Pittsburgh, PA, USA

Mark B. Constantian, MD
Private Practice
Surgery (Plastic Surgery)
St. Joseph Hospital
Nashua, NH, USA;
Adjunct Clinical Professor
Surgery (Plastic Surgery)
University of Wisconsin School of Medicine
Madison, WI, USA;
Visiting Professor
Plastic Surgery
University of Virginia Health System
Charlottesville, VA, USA

Rafael A. Couto, MD
Plastic Surgery Resident
Department of Plastic Surgery
Cleveland Clinic
Cleveland, OH, USA

Albert Cram, MD
Professor Emeritus
University of Iowa
Iowa City Plastic Surgery
Coralville, IO, USA

Phillip Dauwe, MD
Department of Plastic Surgery
University of Texas Southwestern Medical
School
Dallas, TX, USA

Dai M. Davies, FRCS
Consultant and Institute Director
Institute of Cosmetic and Reconstructive
Surgery
London, UK

Jose Abel De la Peña Salcedo, MD, FACS
Plastic Surgeon
Director
Instituto de Cirugia Plastica S.C.
Huixquilucan
Estado de Mexico, Mexico

Barry DiBernardo, MD, FACS
Clinical Associate Professor, Plastic Surgery
Rutgers, New Jersey Medical School
Director New Jersey Plastic Surgery
Montclair, NJ, USA

Felmont F. Eaves III, MD, FACS
Professor of Surgery, Emory University
Medical Director, Emory Aesthetic Center
Medical Director, EAC Ambulatory Surgery
Center
Atlanta, GA, USA

Marco Ellis, MD
Director of Craniofacial Surgery
Northwestern Specialists in Plastic Surgery;
Adjunct Assistant Professor
University of Illinois Chicago Medical Center
Chicago, IL, USA

Dino Elyassnia, MD
Associate Plastic Surgeon
Marten Clinic of Plastic Surgery
San Francisco, CA, USA

Julius Few Jr., MD
Director
The Few Institute for Aesthetic Plastic Surgery;
Clinical Professor
Plastic Surgery
University of Chicago Pritzker School of
Medicine
Chicago, IL, USA

Osvaldo Ribeiro Saldanha Filho, MD
Professor of Plastic Surgery
Plastic Surgery Service Dr. Osvaldo Saldanha
São Paulo, Brazil

Jack Fisher, MD
Associate Clinical Professor
Plastic Surgery
Vanderbilt University
Nashville, TN, USA

Nicholas A. Flugstad, MD
Flugstad Plastic Surgery
Bellevue, WA, USA

**James D. Frame, MBBS, FRCS, FRCSEd,
FRCS(Plast)**
Professor of Aesthetic Plastic Surgery
Anglia Ruskin University
Chelmsford, UK

Jazmina M. Gonzalez, MD
Bitar Cosmetic Surgery Institute
Fairfax, VA, USA

Richard J. Greco, MD
CEO
The Georgia Institute For Plastic Surgery
Savannah, GA, USA

Ronald P. Gruber, MD
Adjunct Associate Clinical Professor
Division of Plastic and Reconstructive Surgery
Stanford University
Stanford, CA
Clinical Association Professor
Division of Plastic and Reconstructive Surgery
University of California San Francisco
San Francisco, CA, USA

Bahman Guyuron, MD, FCVS
Editor in Chief, Aesthetic Plastic Surgery Journal
Emeritus Professor of Plastic Surgery
Case School of Medicine
Cleveland, OH, USA

Joseph P. Hunstad, MD, FACS
Associate Consulting Professor
Division of Plastic Surgery
The University of North Carolina at Chapel Hill;
Private Practice
Huntersville/Charlotte, NC, USA

Clyde H. Ishii, MD, FACS
Assistant Clinical Professor of Surgery
John A. Burns School of Medicine;
Chief, Department of Plastic Surgery
Shriners Hospital
Honolulu Unit
Honolulu, HI, USA

Nicole J. Jarrett, MD
Department of Plastic Surgery
University of Pittsburgh
Pittsburgh, PA, USA

Elizabeth B. Jelks, MD
Private Practice
Jelks Medical
New York, NY, USA

Glenn W. Jelks, MD
Associate Professor
Department of Ophthalmology
Department of Plastic Surgery
New York University School of Medicine
New York, NY, USA

Mark Laurence Jewell, MD
Assistant Clinical Professor Plastic Surgery
Oregon Health Science University
Portland, OR, USA

David M. Kahn, MD
Clinical Associate Professor of Plastic Surgery
Department of Surgery
Stanford University School of Medicine
Stanford, CA, USA

Michael A. C. Kane, BS, MD
Attending Surgeon
Plastic Surgery
Manhattan Eye, Ear, and Throat Hospital
New York, NY, USA

David L. Kaufman, MD, FACS
Private Practice Plastic Surgery
Aesthetic Artistry Surgical and Medical Center
Folsom, CA, USA

Jeffrey Kenkel, MD
Professor and Chairman
Department of Plastic Surgery
UT Southwestern Medical Center
Dallas, TX, USA

Kyung S. Koh, MD, PhD
Professor of Plastic Surgery
Asan Medical Center, University of Ulsan School
of Medicine
Seoul, South Korea

Tracy Leong, MD
Dermatology
Rady Children's Hospital - San Diego;
Sharp Memorial Hospital;
University California San Diego Medical Center
San Diego;
Private Practice, FACES+ Plastic Surgery, Skin
and Laser Center
La Jolla, CA, USA

Steven M. Levine, MD
Assistant Professor of Surgery (Plastic)
Hofstra Medical School, Northwell Health,
New York, NY, USA

Michelle B. Locke, MBChB, MD
Senior Lecturer in Surgery
Department of Surgery
University of Auckland Faculty of Medicine and
Health Sciences;
South Auckland Clinical Campus
Middlemore Hospital
Auckland, New Zealand

Alyssa Lolofie
University of Utah
Salt Lake City, UT, USA

Timothy J. Marten, MD, FACS
Founder and Director
Marten Clinic of Plastic Surgery
San Francisco, CA, USA

Bryan Mendelson, FRCSE, FRACS, FACS
The Centre for Facial Plastic Surgery
Toorak, Victoria, Australia

Constantino G. Mendieta, MD, FACS
Private Practice
Miami, FL, USA

Drew B. Metcalfe, MD
Division of Plastic and Reconstructive Surgery
Emory University
Atlanta, GA, USA

Gabriele C. Miotto, MD
Emory School of Medicine
Atlanta, GA, USA

Foad Nahai, MD
Professor of Surgery
Division of Plastic and Reconstructive Surgery
Department of Surgery
Emory University School of Medicine
Emory Aesthetic Center at Paces
Atlanta, Georgia, USA

Suzan Obagi, MD
Associate Professor of Dermatology
Dermatology
University of Pittsburgh;
Associate Professor of Plastic Surgery
Plastic Surgery
University of Pittsburgh
Pittsburgh, PA, USA

Sabina Aparecida Alvarez de Paiva, MD
Resident of Plastic Surgery
Plastic Surgery Service Dr. Ewaldo Bolivar de
Souza Pinto
São Paulo, Brazil

Galen Perdikis, MD
Assistant Professor of Surgery
Division of Plastic Surgery
Emory University School of Medicine
Atlanta, GA, USA

Jason Posner, MD, FACS
Private Practice
Boca Raton, FL, USA

Dirk F. Richter, MD, PhD
Clinical Professor of Plastic Surgery
University of Bonn
Director and Chief
Dreifaltigkeits-Hospital
Wesseling, Germany

Thomas L. Roberts III, FACS
Plastic Surgery Center of the Carolinas
Spartanburg, SC, USA

Jocelyn Celeste Ledezma Rodriguez, MD
Private Practice
Guadalajara, Jalisco, Mexico

Rod J. Rohrich, MD
Clinical Professor and Founding Chair
Department of Plastic Surgery
Distinguished Teaching Professor
University of Texas Southwestern Medical Center
Founding Partner
Dallas Plastic Surgery Institute
Dallas, TX, USA

E. Victor Ross, MD
Director of Laser and Cosmetic Dermatology
Scripps Clinic
San Diego, CA, USA

J. Peter Rubin, MD, FACS
Chief
Plastic and Reconstructive Surgery
University of Pittsburgh Medical Center;
Associate Professor
Department of Surgery
University of Pittsburgh
Pittsburgh, PA, USA

Ahmad N. Saad, MD
Private Practice
FACES+ Plastic Surgery
Skin and Laser Center
La Jolla, CA, USA

Alesia P. Saboeiro, MD
Attending Physician
Private Practice
New York, NY, USA

Cristianna Bonnetto Saldanha, MD
Plastic Surgery Service Dr. Osvaldo Saldanha
São Paulo, Brazil

Osvaldo Saldanha, MD, PhD
Director of Plastic Surgery Service Dr. Osvaldo
Saldanha;
Professor of Plastic Surgery Department
Universidade Metropolitana de Santos
- UNIMES
São Paulo, Brazil

Renato Saltz, MD, FACS
Saltz Plastic Surgery
President
International Society of Aesthetic Plastic Surgery
Adjunct Professor of Surgery
University of Utah
Past-President, American Society for Aesthetic
Plastic Surgery
Salt Lake City and Park City, UT, USA

Paulo Rodamilans Sanjuan MD
Chief Resident of Plastic Surgery
Plastic Surgery Service Dr. Ewaldo Boliar de
Souza Pinto
São Paulo, Brazil

Nina Schwaiger, MD
Senior Specialist in Plastic and Aesthetic
Surgery
Department of Plastic Surgery
Dreifaltigkeits-Hospital Wesseling
Wesseling, Germany

Douglas S. Steinbrech, MD, FACS
Gotham Plastic Surgery
New York, NY, USA

Phillip J. Stephan, MD
Clinical Faculty
Plastic Surgery
UT Southwestern Medical School;
Plastic Surgeon
Texoma Plastic Surgery
Wichita Falls, TX, USA

David Gonzalez Sosa, MD
Plastic and Reconstructive Surgery
Hospital Quirónsalud Torrevieja
Alicante, Spain

James M. Stuzin, MD
Associate Professor of Surgery
(Plastic) Voluntary
University of Miami Leonard M. Miller School of
Medicine
Miami, FL, USA

Daniel Suissa, MD, MSc
Clinical Instructor
Section of Plastic and Reconstructive Surgery
Yale University
New Haven, CT, USA

Charles H. Thorne, MD
Associate Professor of Plastic Surgery
Department of Plastic Surgery
NYU School of Medicine
New York, NY, USA

Ali Totonchi, MD
Assistant Professor
Plastic Surgery
Case Western Reserve University;
Medical Director Craniofacial Deformity Clinic
Plastic Surgery
MetroHealth Medical center
Cleveland, OH, USA

Jonathan W. Toy, MD, FRCSC
Program Director, Plastic Surgery Residency
Program Assistant Clinical Professor
University of Alberta
Edmonton, Alberta, Canada

Matthew J. Trovato, MD
Dallas Plastic Surgery Institute
Dallas, TX, USA

Simeon H. Wall Jr., MD, FACS
Director
The Wall Center for Plastic Surgery;
Assistant Clinical Professor
Plastic Surgery
LSU Health Sciences Center at Shreveport
Shreveport, LA, USA

Joshua T. Waltzman, MD, MBA
Private Practice
Waltzman Plastic and Reconstructive Surgery
Long Beach, CA, USA

Richard J. Warren, MD, FRCSC
Clinical Professor
Division of Plastic Surgery
University of British Columbia
Vancouver, British Columbia, Canada

Edmund Weisberg, MS, MBE
University of Pennsylvania
Philadelphia, PA, USA

Scott Woehrle, MS BS
Physician Assistant
Department of Plastic Surgery
Jospeh Capella Plastic Surgery
Ramsey, NJ, USA

**Chin-Ho Wong, MBBS, MRCS, MMed(Surg),
FAMS(Plast Surg)**
W Aesthetic Plastic Surgery
Mt Elizabeth Novena Specialist Center
Singapore

Alan Yan, MD
Former Fellow
Adult Reconstructive and Aesthetic
Craniomaxillofacial Surgery
Division of Plastic and Reconstructive Surgery
Massachusetts General Hospital
Boston, MA, USA

Michael J. Yaremchuk, MD
Chief of Craniofacial Surgery
Massachusetts General Hospital;
Clinical Professor of Surgery
Harvard Medical School;
Program Director
Harvard Plastic Surgery Residency Program
Boston, MA, USA

James E. Zins, MD
Chairman
Department of Plastic Surgery
Dermatology and Plastic Surgery Institute
Cleveland Clinic
Cleveland, OH, USA

VOLUME THREE

Neta Adler, MD
Senior Surgeon
Department of Plastic and Reconstructive
Surgery
Hadassah University Hospital
Jerusalem, Israel

Ahmed M. Afifi, MD
Assistant Professor of Plastic Surgery
Department of Surgery
University of Wisconsin
Madison, WI, USA;
Associate Professor
Department of Plastic Surgery
Cairo University
Cairo, Egypt

Marta Alvarado, DDS, MS
Department of Orthodontics
Facultad de Odontología
Universidad de San Carlos de Guatemala
Guatemala

Eric Arnaud, MD
Pediatric Neurosurgeon and Co-Director
Unité de Chirurgie Craniofaciale
Hôpital Necker Enfants Malades
Paris, France

Stephen B. Baker, MD, DDS
Associate Professor and Program Director
Co-Director Inova Hospital for Children
Craniofacial Clinic
Department of Plastic Surgery
Georgetown University Hospital
Georgetown, WA, USA

Scott P. Bartlett, MD
Professor of Surgery
Surgery
University of Pennsylvania;
Chief Division of Plastic Surgery
Surgery
Children's Hospital of Philadelphia
Philadelphia, PA, USA

Bruce S. Bauer, MD
Chief
Division of Plastic Surgery
NorthShore University HealthSystem
Highland Park;
Clinical Professor of Surgery
Department of Surgery
University of Chicago Pritzker School of
Medicine
Chicago, IL, USA

Adriane L. Baylis, PhD
Speech Scientist
Section of Plastic and Reconstructive Surgery
Nationwide Children's Hospital
Columbus, OH, USA

Mike Bentz, MD, FAAP, FACS
Interim Chairman
Department of Surgery
University of Wisconsin;
Chairman Division of Plastic Surgery
Department of Surgery
University of Wisconsin
Madison, WI, USA

Craig Birgfeld, MD, FACS
Associate Professor, Pediatric Plastic and
Craniofacial Surgery
Seattle Children's Hospital
Seattle, WA, USA

William R. Boysen, MD
Resident Physician, Urology
University of Chicago Medicine
Chicago, IL, USA

James P. Bradley, MD
Professor and Chief
Section of Plastic and Reconstructive Surgery
Temple University
Philadelphia, PA, USA

Edward P. Buchanan, MD
Division of Plastic Surgery
Baylor College of Medicine
Houston, TX, USA

Michael R. Bykowski, MD, MS
Plastic Surgery Resident
Plastic Surgery
University of Pittsburgh Medical Center
Pittsburgh, PA, USA

Edward J. Caterson, MD, PhD
Director of Craniofacial Surgery
Division of Plastic Surgery
Brigham and Women's Hospital
Boston, MA, USA

Rodney K. Chan, MD
Chief Plastic and Reconstructive Surgery
Clinical Division and Burn Center
United States Army Institute of Surgical
Research
Joint Base San Antonio, TX, USA

Edward I. Chang, MD
Assistant Professor
Department of Plastic Surgery
The University of Texas M. D. Anderson Cancer
Center
Houston, TX, USA

Constance M. Chen, MD, MPH
Director of Microsurgery
Plastic and Reconstructive Surgery
New York Eye and Ear Infirmary of Mt Sinai;
Clinical Assistant Professor
Plastic and Reconstructive Surgery
Weil Medical College of Cornell University;
Clinical Assistant Professor
Plastic and Reconstructive Surgery
Tulane University School of Medicine
New York, NY, USA

Yu-Ray Chen, MD
Professor of Surgery
Plastic and Reconstructive Surgery
Chang Gung Memorial Hospital
Taoyuan City, Taiwan

Philip Kuo-Ting Chen, MD
Professor
Craniofacial Center
Chang Gung Memorial Hospital
Taoyuan City, Taiwan

Ming-Huei Cheng, MD, MBA
Professor
Division of Reconstructive Microsurgery
Department of Plastic and Reconstructive
Surgery
Chang Gung Memorial Hospital
Taoyuan City, Taiwan

Gerson R. Chinchilla, DDS MS
Director
Department of Orthodontics
Facultad de Odontología
Universidad de San Carlos de Guatemala
Guatemala

Peter G. Cordeiro, MD
Chief
Plastic and Reconstructive Surgery
Memorial Sloan Kettering Cancer Center;
Professor of Surgery
Surgery
Weil Medical College of Cornell University
New York, NY, USA

Alberto Córdova-Aguilar, MD, MPH
Attending Plastic Surgeon
Surgery
Faculty of Medicine Ricardo Palma University
Lima, Peru

Edward H. Davidson, MA(Cantab), MBBS
Resident Plastic Surgeon
Department of Plastic Surgery
University of Pittsburgh
Pittsburgh, PA, USA

Sara R. Dickie, MD
Clinician Educator
Surgery
University of Chicago Hospital Pritzker School of Medicine;
Attending Surgeon
Section of Plastic and Reconstructive Surgery
NorthShore University HealthSystem
Northbrook, IL, USA

Risal S. Djohan, MD
Microsurgery Fellowship Program Director
Plastic Surgery
Cleveland Clinic;
Surgery ASC Quality Improvement Officer
Plastic Surgery
Cleveland Clinic
Cleveland, OH, USA

Amir H. Dorafshar, MBChB, FACS, FAAP
Associate Professor
Plastic and Reconstructive Surgery
Johns Hopkins Medical Institute;
Assistant Professor
Plastic Surgery
R Adams Cowley Shock Trauma Center
Baltimore, MD, USA

Jeffrey A. Fearon, MD
Director
The Craniofacial Center
Dallas, TX, USA

Alexander L. Figueroa, DMD
Craniofacial Orthodontist
Rush Craniofacial Center
Rush University Medical Center
Chicago, IL, USA

Alvaro A. Figueroa, DDS, MS
Co-Director
Rush Craniofacial Center
Rush University Medical Center
Chicago, IL, USA

David M. Fisher, MB, BCh, FRCSC, FACS
Medical Director Cleft Lip and Palate Program
Plastic Surgery
Hospital for Sick Children;
Associate Professor
Surgery
University of Toronto
Toronto, Ontario, Canada

Roberto L. Flores, MD
Associate Professor of Plastic Surgery
Director of Cleft Lip and Palate
Hansjörg Wyss Department of Plastic Surgery
NYU Langone Medical Center
New York, NY, USA

Andrew Foreman, B. Physio, BMBS(Hons), PhD, FRACS
Consultant Surgeon, Department of Otolaryngology - Head and Neck Surgery
University of Adelaide,
Royal Adelaide Hospital,
Adelaide, SA, Australia

Patrick A. Gerety, MD
Assistant Professor of Surgery
Division of Plastic and Reconstructive Surgery
Indiana University and Riley Hospital for Children
Philadelphia, PA, USA

Jesse A. Goldstein, MD
Chief Resident
Department of Plastic Surgery
Georgetown University Hospital
Washington, DC, USA

Arun K. Gosain, MD
Chief
Division of Plastic Surgery
Ann and Robert H. Lurie Children's Hospital of Chicago
Chicago, IL, USA

Lawrence J. Gottlieb, MD
Professor of Surgery
Department of Surgery
Section of Plastic and Reconstructive Surgery
University of Chicago
Chicago, IL, USA

Arin K. Greene, MD, MMSc
Department of Plastic and Oral Surgery
Boston Children's Hospital;
Associate Professor of Surgery
Harvard Medical School
Boston, MA, USA

Patrick J. Gullane, MD, FRCS
Wharton Chair in Head and Neck Surgery
Professor of Surgery, Department of Otolaryngology - Head and Neck Surgery
University of Toronto
Toronto, Ontario, Canada

Mohan S. Gundeti, MB, MCh, FEBU, FRCS(Urol), FEAPU
Associate Professor of Urology in Surgery and Pediatrics, Director Pediatric Urology, Director Centre for Pediatric Robotics and Minimal Invasive Surgery
University of Chicago and Pritzker Medical School Comer Children's Hospital
Chicago, IL, USA

Eyal Gur, MD
Professor of Surgery, Chief
Department of Plastic and Reconstructive Surgery
The Tel Aviv Sourasky Medical Center
Tel Aviv, Israel

Bahman Guyuron, MD, FCVS
Editor in Chief, Aesthetic Plastic Surgery Journal;
Emeritus Professor of Plastic Surgery
Case School of Medicine
Cleveland, OH, USA

Matthew M. Hanasono, MD
Associate Professor
Department of Plastic Surgery
The University of Texas MD Anderson Cancer Center
Houston, TX, USA

Toshinobu Harada, PhD
Professor in Engineering
Department of Systems Engineering
Faculty of Systems Engineering
Wakayama University
Wakayama, Japan

Jill A. Helms, DDS, PhD
Professor
Surgery
Stanford University
Stanford, CA, USA

David L. Hirsch, MD, DDS
Director of Oral Oncology and Reconstruction
Lenox Hill Hospital/Northwell Health
New York, NY, USA

Jung-Ju Huang, MD
Associate Professor
Division of Microsurgery
Plastic and Reconstructive Surgery
Chang Gung Memorial Hospital
Taoyuan, Taiwan

William Y. Hoffman, MD
Professor and Chief
Division of Plastic and Reconstructive Surgery
UCSF
San Francisco, CA, USA

Larry H. Hollier Jr., MD
Division of Plastic Surgery
Baylor College of Medicine
Houston, TX, USA

Richard A. Hopper, MD, MS
Chief
Division of Craniofacial Plastic Surgery
Seattle Children's Hospital;
Surgical Director
Craniofacial Center
Seattle Children's Hospital;
Associate Professor
Department of Surgery
University of Washington
Seattle, WA, USA

Gazi Hussain, MBBS, FRACS
Clinical Senior Lecturer
Macquarie University
Sydney, Australia

Oksana Jackson, MD
Assistant Professor
Plastic Surgery
Perelman School of Medicine at the University of Pennsylvania;
Assistant Professor
Plastic Surgery
The Children's Hospital of Philadelphia
Philadelphia, PA, USA

Syril James, MD
Clinic Marcel Sembat
Boulogne-Billancourt
Paris, France

Leila Jazayeri, MD
Microsurgery Fellow
Plastic and Reconstructive Surgery
Memorial Sloan Kettering Cancer Center
New York, NY, USA

Sahil Kapur, MD
Assistant Professor
Department of Plastic Surgery
University of Texas - MD Anderson Cancer
Center
Houston, TX, USA

Henry K. Kawamoto Jr., MD, DDS
Clinical Professor
Surgery Division of Plastic Surgery
UCLA
Los Angeles, CA, USA

David Y. Khechoyan, MD
Division of Plastic Surgery
Baylor College of Medicine
Houston, TX, USA

Richard E. Kirschner, MD
Section Chief
Plastic and Reconstructive Surgery
Nationwide Children's Hospital;
Senior Vice Chair
Plastic Surgery
The Ohio State University Medical College
Columbus, OH, USA

John C. Koshy, MD
Division of Plastic Surgery
Baylor College of Medicine
Houston, TX, USA

Michael C. Large, MD
Urologic Oncologist
Urology of Indiana
Greenwood, IN, USA

Edward I. Lee, MD
Division of Plastic Surgery
Baylor College of Medicine
Houston, TX, USA

Jamie P. Levine, MD
Chief of Microsurgery
Associate Professor
Plastic Surgery
NYU Langone Medical Center
New York, NY, USA

Jingtao Li, DDS, PhD
Consultant Surgeon
Oral and Maxillofacial Surgery
West China Hospital of Stomatology
Chengdu, Sichuan, People's Republic of China

Lawrence Lin, MD
Division of Plastic Surgery
Baylor College of Medicine
Houston, TX, USA

Joseph E. Losee, MD
Ross H. Musgrave Professor of Pediatric Plastic
Surgery
Department of Plastic Surgery
University of Pittsburgh Medical Center;
Chief, Division of Pediatric Plastic Surgery
Children's Hospital of Pittsburgh
Pittsburgh, PA, USA

David W. Low, MD
Professor of Surgery
Division of Plastic Surgery
Perelman School of Medicine at the University
of Pennsylvania;
Clinical Associate
Department of Surgery
Children's Hospital of Philadelphia
Philadelphia, PA, USA

Ralph T. Manktelow, MD, FRCSC
Professor of Surgery,
The University of Toronto,
Toronto, Ontario, Canada

Paul N. Manson, MD
Distinguished Service Professor
Plastic Surgery
Johns Hopkins University
Baltimore, MD, USA

David W. Mathes, MD
Professor and Chief of the Division of Plastic
and Reconstructive Surgery
Surgery Division of Plastic and Reconstructive
Surgery
University of Colorado
Aurora, CO, USA

Frederick J. Menick, MD
Private Practitioner
Tucson, AZ, USA

Fernando Molina, MD
Director
Craniofacial Anomalies Foundation A.C.
Mexico City;
Professor of Plastic Reconstructive and
Aesthetic Surgery
Medical School
Universidad La Salle
Mexico City, Distrito Federal, Mexico

Laura A. Monson, MD
Division of Plastic Surgery
Baylor College of Medicine
Houston, TX, USA

Reid V. Mueller, MD
Associate Professor
Plastic Surgery
Oregon Health and Science University
Portland, OR, USA

John B. Mulliken, MD
Professor
Department of Plastic and Oral Surgery
Boston Children's Hospital
Harvard Medical School
Boston, MA, USA

Gerhard S. Mundinger, MD
Assistant Professor
Craniofacial, Plastic, and Reconstructive Surgery
Louisiana State University Health Sciences
Center
Children's Hospital of New Orleans
New Orleans, LA, USA

Blake D. Murphy, BSc, PhD, MD
Craniofacial Fellow
Plastic Surgery
Nicklaus Children's Hospital
Miami, FL, USA

**Peter C. Neligan, MB, FRCS(I), FRCSC,
FACS**
Professor of Surgery
Department of Surgery, Division of Plastic
Surgery
University of Washington
Seattle, WA, USA

M. Samuel Noordhoff, MD, FACS
Emeritus Professor in Surgery
Chang Gung University
Taoyuan City, Taiwan

Giovanna Paternoster, MD
Unité de chirurgie crânio-faciale du departement
de neurochirurgie
Hôpital Necker Enfants Malades
Paris, France

Jason Pomerantz, MD
Assistant Professor
Surgery
University of California San Francisco;
Surgical Director
Craniofacial Center
University of California San Francisco
San Francisco, CA, USA

Julian J. Pribaz, MD
Professor of Surgery
University of South Florida, Morsani College of
Medicine
Tampa General Hospital
Tampa, FL, USA

Chad A. Purnell, MD
Division of Plastic Surgery
Lurie Children's Hospital of Northwestern
Feinberg School of Medicine
Chicago, IL, USA

Russell R. Reid, MD, PhD
Associate Professor
Surgery/Section of Plastic and Reconstructive
Surgery
University of Chicago Medicine
Chicago, IL, USA

Eduardo D. Rodriguez, MD, DDS
Helen L. Kimmel Professor of Reconstructive
Plastic Surgery
Chair, Hansjörg Wyss Department of Plastic
Surgery
NYU School of Medicine
NYU Langone Medical Center
New York, NY, USA

Craig Rowin, MD
Craniofacial Fellow
Plastic Surgery
Nicklaus Children's Hospital
Miami, FL, USA

Ruston J. Sanchez, MD
Plastic and Reconstructive Surgery Resident
University of Wisconsin
Madison, WI, USA

Lindsay A. Schuster, DMD, MS
Director Cleft-Craniofacial Orthodontics
Pediatric Plastic Surgery
Children's Hospital of Pittsburgh of UMPC;
Clinical Assistant Professor of Plastic Surgery
Department of Plastic Surgery
University of Pittsburgh School of Medicine
Pittsburgh, PA, USA

Jeremiah Un Chang See, MD
Plastic Surgeon
Department of Plastic and Reconstructive
Surgery
Penang General Hospital
Georgetown, Penang, Malaysia

Pradip R. Shetye, DDS, BDS, MDS
Assistant Professor (Orthodontics)
Hansjörg Wyss Department of Plastic Surgery
NYU Langone Medical Center
New York, NY, USA

Roman Skoracki, MD
Plastic Surgery
The Ohio State University
Columbus, OH, USA

Mark B. Slidell, MD, MPH
Assistant Professor of Surgery
Department of Surgery
Section of Pediatric Surgery
University of Chicago Medicine Biological
Sciences
Chicago, IL, USA

Michael Sosin, MD
Research Fellow
Department of Plastic Surgery Institute of
Reconstructive Plastic Surgery
NYU Langone Medical Center
New York, NY, USA;
Research Fellow
Division of Plastic Reconstructive and
Maxillofacial Surgery
R Adams Cowley Shock Trauma Center
University of Maryland Medical Center
Baltimore, MD, USA;
Resident
Department of Surgery
Medstar Georgetown University Hospital
Washington, DC, USA

**Youssef Tahiri, MD, MSc, FRCSC, FAAP,
FACS**
Associate Professor
Pediatric Plastic & Craniofacial Surgery
Cedars Sinai Medical Center
Los Angeles, CA, USA

Peter J. Taub, MD
Professor
Surgery Pediatrics Dentistry and Medical
Education
Surgery Division of Plastic and Reconstructive
Surgery
Icahn School of Medicine at Mount Sinai
New York, NY, USA

Jesse A. Taylor, MD
Mary Downs Endowed Chair of Pediatric
Craniofacial Treatment and Research;
Director, Penn Craniofacial Fellowship;
Co-Director, CHOP Cleft Team
Plastic, Reconstructive, and Craniofacial Surgery
The University of Pennsylvania and
Children's Hospital of Philadelphia
Philadelphia, PA, USA

Kathryn S. Torok, MD
Assistant Professor
Pediatric Rheumatology
University of Pittsburgh
Pittsburgh, PA, USA

Ali Totonchi, MD
Assistant Professor
Plastic Surgery
Case Western Reserve University;
Medical Director Craniofacial Deformity Clinic
Plastic Surgery
MetroHealth Medical Center
Cleveland, OH, USA

Kris Wilson, MD
Division of Plastic Surgery
Baylor College of Medicine
Houston, TX, USA

S. Anthony Wolfe, MD
Plastic Surgery
Miami Children's Hospital
Miami, FL, USA

Akira Yamada, MD, PhD
Professor of Plastic Surgery
World Craniofacial Foundation
Dallas, TX, USA;
Clinical Assistant Professor
Plastic Surgery
Case Western Reserve University
Cleveland, OH, USA

Peirong Yu, MD
Professor
Plastic Surgery
M. D. Anderson Cancer Center;
Adjunct Professor
Plastic Surgery
Baylor College of Medicine
Houston, TX, USA

**Ronald M. Zuker, MD, FRCSC, FACS,
FRCSEd(Hon)**
Professor of Surgery
Department of Surgery
University of Toronto;
Staff Plastic and Reconstructive Surgeon
Department of Surgery
SickKids Hospital
Toronto, Ontario, Canada

VOLUME FOUR

Christopher E. Attinger, MD
Professor, Interim Chairman
Department of Plastic Surgery
Center for Wound Healing
Medstar Georgetown University Hospital
Washington, DC, USA

Lorenzo Borghese, MD
Plastic Surgeon
Chief of International Missions
Ospedale Pediatrico Bambino Gesù
Rome, Italy

Charles E. Butler, MD, FACS
Professor and Chairman
Department of Plastic Surgery
Charles B. Barker Endowed Chair in Surgery
The University of Texas M. D. Anderson Cancer
Center
Houston, TX, USA

David W. Chang, MD
Professor of Surgery
University of Chicago
Chicago, IL, USA

Karel Claes, MD
Department of Plastic and Reconstructive
Surgery
Ghent University Hospital
Ghent, Belgium

Mark W. Clemens II, MD, FACS
Associate Professor
Plastic Surgery
MD Anderson Cancer Center,
Houston, TX, USA

Shannon M. Colohan, MD, MSc
Assistant Professor of Surgery
University of Washington
Seattle, WA, USA

Peter G. Cordeiro, MD
Chief
Plastic and Reconstructive Surgery
Memorial Sloan Kettering Cancer Center
New York, NY, USA

Salvatore D'Arpa, MD, PhD
Department of Plastic and Reconstructive
Surgery
Ghent University Hospital
Ghent, Belgium

Michael V. DeFazio, MD
Department Plastic Surgery
MedStar Georgetown University Hospital
Washington, DC, USA

A. Lee Dellon, MD, PhD
Professor of Plastic Surgery
Professor of Neurosurgery
Johns Hopkins University
Baltimore, MD, USA

Sara R. Dickie, MD
Clinical Associate of Surgery
University of Chicago Hospitals
Pritzker School of Medicine
Chicago, IL, USA

Ivica Ducic, MD, PhD
Clinical Professor of Surgery
GWU Washington Nerve Institute
McLean, VA, USA

Gregory A. Dumanian, MD
Stuteville Professor of Surgery
Division of Plastic Surgery
Northwestern Feinberg School of Medicine
Chicago, IL, USA

John M. Felder III, MD
Fellow in Hand Surgery
Plastic Surgery
Washington University in Saint Louis
St. Louis, MO, USA

Goetz A. Giessler, MD, PhD
Professor Director
Plastic-Reconstructive, Aesthetic and Hand
Surgery
Gesundheit Nordhessen
Kassel, Germany

Kevin D. Han, MD
Department of Plastic Surgery
MedStar Georgetown University Hospital
Washington, DC, USA

Piet Hoebeke
Department of Urology
Ghent University Hospital
Ghent, Belgium

Joon Pio Hong, MD, PhD, MMM
Professor of Plastic Surgery
Asan Medical Center, University of Ulsan
Seoul, South Korea

Michael A. Howard, MD
Clinical Assistant Professor of Surgery
Plastic Surgery
NorthShore University HealthSystem/University
of Chicago
Chicago, IL, USA

Jeffrey E. Janis, MD, FACS
Professor of Plastic Surgery, Neurosurgery,
Neurology, and Surgery;
Executive Vice Chairman, Department of Plastic
Surgery;
Chief of Plastic Surgery, University Hospitals
Ohio State University Wexner Medical Center
Columbus, OH, USA

Leila Jazayeri, MD
Microsurgery Fellow
Plastic and Reconstructive Surgery
Memorial Sloan Kettering Cancer Center
New York, NY, USA

Grant M. Kleiber, MD
Assistant Professor of Surgery
Division of Plastic and Reconstructive Surgery
Washington University School of Medicine
St. Louis, MO, USA

Stephen J. Kovach III, MD
Assistant Professor
Division of Plastic Surgery
University of Pennsylvania
Philadelphia, PA, USA

Robert Kwon, MD
Southwest Hand and Microsurgery
3108 Midway Road, Suite 103
Plano, TX, USA

**Raphael C. Lee, MS, MD, ScD, FACS,
FAIMBE**
Paul and Allene Russell Professor
Plastic Surgery, Dermatology, Anatomy and
Organismal Biology, Molecular Medicine
University of Chicago
Chicago, IL, USA

L. Scott Levin, MD, FACS
Chairman of Orthopedic Surgery
Department of Orthopaedic Surgery
University of Pennsylvania School of Medicine
Philadelphia, PA, USA

Otway Louie, MD
Associate Professor
Surgery
University of Washington Medical Center
Seattle, WA, USA

Nicolas Lumen, MD, PhD
Head of Clinic
Urology
Ghent University Hospital
Ghent, Belgium

Alessandro Masellis, MD
Plastic Surgeon
Euro-Mediterranean Council for Burns and Fire
Disasters
Palermo, Italy

Michele Masellis, MD
Former Chief of Department of Plastic and
Reconstructive Surgery and Burn Therapy
Department of Plastic and Reconstructive
Surgery and Burn Therapy - ARNAS Ospedale
Civico e Benfratelli
Palermo, Italy

Stephen M. Milner, MB BS, BDS
Professor of Plastic Surgery
Surgery
Johns Hopkins School of Medicine
Baltimore, MD, USA

Arash Momeni, MD
Fellow, Reconstructive Microsurgery
Division of Plastic Surgery
University of Pennsylvania Health System
Philadelphia, PA, USA

Stan Monstrey, MD, PhD
Department of Plastic and Reconstructive
Surgery
Ghent University Hospital
Ghent, Belgium

**Venkateshwaran N, MBBS, MS, DNB, MCh,
MRCS(Intercollegiate)**
Consultant Plastic Surgeon
Jupiter Hospital
Thane, India

Rajiv P. Parikh, MD, MPHS
Resident Physician
Department of Surgery, Division of Plastic and
Reconstructive Surgery
Washington University School of Medicine
St. Louis, MO, USA

Mônica Sarto Piccolo, MD, MSc, PhD
Director
Pronto Socorro para Queimaduras
Goiânia, Goiás, Brazil

Nelson Sarto Piccolo, MD
Chief
Division of Plastic Surgery
Pronto Socorro para Queimaduras
Goiânia, Goiás, Brazil

Maria Thereza Sarto Piccolo, MD, PhD
Scientific Director
Pronto Socorro para Queimaduras
Goiânia, Goiás, Brazil

Vinita Puri, MS, MCh
Professor and Head
Department of Plastic, Reconstructive Surgery
and Burns
Seth G S Medical College and KEM Hospital
Mumbai, Maharashtra, India

Andrea L. Pusic, MD, MHS, FACS
Associate Professor
Plastic and Reconstructive Surgery
Memorial Sloan Kettering Cancer Center
New York, NY, USA

Vinay Rawlani, MD
Division of Plastic Surgery
Northwestern Feinberg School of Medicine
Chicago, IL, USA

Juan L. Rendon, MD, PhD
Clinical Instructor Housestaff
Department of Plastic Surgery
The Ohio State University Wexner Medical
Center
Columbus, OH, USA

Michelle C. Roughton, MD
Assistant Professor
Division of Plastic and Reconstructive Surgery
University of North Carolina at Chapel Hill
Chapel Hill, NC, USA

Hakim K. Said, MD, FACS
Associate Professor
Division of Plastic surgery
University of Washington
Seattle, WA, USA

Michel Saint-Cyr, MD, FRSC(C)
Professor
Plastic Surgery
Mayo Clinic
Rochester, MN, USA

Michael Sauerbier, MD, PhD
Professor, Chair
Department for Plastic, Hand, and
Reconstructive Surgery
Academic Hospital Goethe University Frankfurt
am Main
Frankfurt am Main, Germany

Loren S. Schechter, MD
Associate Professor and Chief
Division of Plastic Surgery
Chicago Medical School
Morton Grove, IL, USA

David H. Song, MD, MBA, FACS
Regional Chief, MedStar Health
Plastic and Reconstructive Surgery
Professor and Chairman
Department of Plastic Surgery
Georgetown University School of Medicine
Washington, DC, USA

Yoo Joon Sur, MD, PhD
Associate Professor
Department of Orthopedic Surgery
The Catholic University of Korea, College of
Medicine
Seoul, Korea

Chad M. Teven, MD
Resident
Section of Plastic and Reconstructive Surgery
University of Chicago
Chicago, IL, USA

VOLUME FIVE

Jamil Ahmad, MD, FRCSC
Director of Research and Education
The Plastic Surgery Clinic
Mississauga, Ontario, Canada;
Assistant Professor of Surgery
University of Toronto
Toronto, Ontario, Canada

Robert J. Allen Sr., MD
Clinical Professor of Plastic Surgery
Department of Plastic Surgery
New York University Medical Center
Charleston, NC, USA

Ryan E. Austin, MD, FRCSC
Plastic Surgeon
The Plastic Surgery Clinic
Mississauga, ON, Canada

Brett Beber, BA, MD, FRCSC
Plastic and Reconstructive Surgeon
Lecturer, Department of Surgery
University of Toronto
Toronto, Ontario, Canada

Philip N. Blondeel, MD
Professor of Plastic Surgery
Department of Plastic Surgery
University Hospital Ghent
Ghent, Belgium

Benjamin J. Brown, MD
Gulf Coast Plastic Surgery
Pensacola, FL, USA

Mitchell H. Brown, MD, MEd, FRCSC
Plastic and Reconstructive Surgeon
Associate Professor, Department of Surgery
University of Toronto
Toronto, Ontario, Canada

M. Bradley Calobrace, MD, FACS
Plastic Surgeon
Calobrace and Mizuguchi Plastic Surgery Center
Departments of Surgery, Divisions of Plastic
Surgery
Clinical Faculty, University of Louisville and
University of Kentucky
Louisville, KY, USA

Grant W. Carlson, MD
Wadley R. Glenn Professor of Surgery
Emory University
Atlanta, GA, USA

Bernard W. Chang, MD
Chief of Plastic and Reconstructive Surgery
Mercy Medical Center
Baltimore, MD, USA

Mark W. Clemens II, MD, FACS
Assistant Professor Plastic Surgery
M. D. Anderson Cancer Center
Houston, TX, USA

Robert Cohen MD, FACS
Medical Director
Plastic Surgery
Scottsdale Center for Plastic Surgery
Paradise Valley, AZ and;
Santa Monica, CA, USA

Amy S. Colwell, MD
Associate Professor
Harvard Medical School
Massachusetts General Hospital
Boston, MA, USA

Edward H. Davidson, MA(Cantab), MB, BS
Resident Plastic Surgeon
Department of Plastic Surgery
University of Pittsburgh Medical Center
Pittsburgh, PA, USA

Emmanuel Delay, MD, PhD
Unité de Chirurgie Plastique et Reconstructrice
Centre Léon Bérard
Lyon, France

Francesco M. Egro, MB ChB, MSc, MRCS
Department of Plastic Surgery
University of Pittsburgh Medical Center
Pittsburgh, PA, USA

Neil A. Fine, MD
President
Northwestern Specialists in Plastic Surgery;
Associate Professor (Clinical) Surgery/Plastics
Northwestern University Fienberg School of
Medicine
Chicago, IL, USA

Jaime Flores, MD
Plastic and Reconstructive Microvascular
Surgeon
Miami, FL, USA

Joshua Fosnot, MD
Assistant Professor of Surgery
Division of Plastic Surgery
The Perelman School of Medicine
University of Pennsylvania Health System
Philadelphia, PA, USA

Allen Gabriel, MD
Clinical Associate Professor
Department of Plastic Surgery
Loma Linda University Medical Center
Loma Linda, CA, USA

Michael S. Gart, MD
Resident Physician
Division of Plastic Surgery
Northwestern University Feinberg School of
Medicine
Chicago, IL, USA

Matthew D. Goodwin, MD
Plastic Surgeon
Plastic Reconstructive and Cosmetic Surgery
Boca Raton Regional Hospital
Boca Raton, FL, USA

Samia Guerid, MD
Cabinet
50 rue de la République
Lyon, France

Moustapha Hamdi, MD, PhD
Professor of Plastic and Reconstructive Surgery
Brussels University Hospital
Vrij Universitaire Brussels
Brussels, Belgium

Alexandra M. Hart, MD
Emory Division of Plastic and Reconstructive
Surgery
Emory University School of Medicine
Atlanta, GA, USA

Emily C. Hartmann, MD, MS
Aesthetic Surgery Fellow
Plastic and Reconstructive Surgery
University of Southern California
Los Angeles, CA, USA

Nima Khavanin, MD
Resident Physician
Department of Plastic and Reconstructive
Surgery
Johns Hopkins Hospital
Baltimore, MD, USA

John Y. S. Kim, MD
Professor and Clinical Director
Department of Surgery
Division of Plastic Surgery
Northwestern University Feinberg School of
Medicine
Chicago, IL, USA

Steven Kronowitz, MD
Owner, Kronowitz Plastics
PLLC;
University of Texas, M. D. Anderson Medical
Center
Houston, TX, USA

John V. Larson, MD
Resident Physician
Division of Plastic and Reconstructive Surgery
Keck School of Medicine of USC
University of Southern California
Los Angeles, CA, USA

Z-Hye Lee, MD
Resident
Department of Plastic Surgery
New York University Medical Center
New York, NY, USA

Frank Lista, MD, FRCSC
Medical Director
The Plastic Surgery Clinic
Mississauga, Ontario, Canada;
Assistant Professor Surgery
University of Toronto
Toronto, Ontario, Canada

Albert Losken, MD, FACS
Professor of plastic surgery and Program
Director
Emory Division of Plastic and Reconstructive
Surgery
Emory University School of Medicine
Atlanta, GA, USA

**Charles M. Malata, BSc(HB), MB ChB,
LRCP, MRCS, FRCS(Glasg), FRCS(Plast)**
Professor of Academic Plastic Surgery
Postgraduate Medical Institute
Faculty of Health Sciences
Anglia Ruskin University
Cambridge and Chelmsford, UK;
Consultant Plastic and Reconstructive Surgeon
Department of Plastic and Reconstructive
Surgery
Cambridge Breast Unit at Addenbrooke's
Hospital
Cambridge University Hospitals NHS
Foundation Trust
Cambridge, UK

Jaume Masià, MD, PhD
Chief and Professor of Plastic Surgery
Sant Pau University Hospital
Barcelona, Spain

G. Patrick Maxwell, MD, FACS
Clinical Professor of Surgery
Department of Plastic Surgery
Loma Linda University Medical Center
Loma Linda, CA, USA

James L. Mayo, MD
Microsurgery Fellow
Plastic Surgery
New York University
New York, NY, USA

Roberto N. Miranda, MD
Professor
Department of Hematopathology
Division of Pathology and Laboratory Medicine
MD Anderson Cancer Center
Houston, TX, USA

**Colin M. Morrison, MSc (Hons) FRCSI
(Plast)**
Consultant Plastic Surgeon
St. Vincent's University Hospital
Dublin, Ireland

Maurice Y. Nahabedian, MD, FACS
Professor and Chief
Section of Plastic Surgery
MedStar Washington Hospital Center
Washington DC, USA;
Vice Chairman
Department of Plastic Surgery
MedStar Georgetown University Hospital
Washington DC, USA

James D. Namnoum, MD
Clinical Professor of Plastic Surgery
Atlanta Plastic Surgery
Emory University School of Medicine
Atlanta, GA, USA

Maria E. Nelson, MD
Assistant Professor of Clinical Surgery
Department of Surgery, Division of Upper GI/
General Surgery, Section of Surgical Oncology
Keck School of Medicine
University of Southern California
Los Angeles, CA, USA

Julie Park, MD
Associate Professor of Surgery
Section of Plastic Surgery
University of Chicago
Chicago, IL, USA

Ketan M. Patel, MD
Assistant Professor of Surgery
Division of Plastic and Reconstructive Surgery
Keck Medical Center of USC
University of Southern California
Los Angeles, CA, USA

**Nakul Gamanlal Patel, BSc(Hons),
MBBS(Lond), FRCS(Plast)**
Senior Microsurgery Fellow
St. Andrew's Centre for Plastic Surgery
Broomfield Hospital
Chelmsford, UK

Gemma Pons, MD, PhD
Head
Microsurgery Unit
Plastic Surgery
Hospital de Sant Pau
Barcelona, Spain

Julian J. Pribaz, MD
Professor of Surgery
Brigham and Women's Hospital
Harvard Medical School
Boston, MA, USA

**Venkat V. Ramakrishnan, MS, FRCS,
FRACS(Plast Surg)**
Consultant Plastic Surgeon
St. Andrew's Centre for Plastic Surgery
Broomfield Hospital
Chelmsford, UK

Elena Rodríguez-Bauzà, MD
Plastic Surgery Department
Hospital Santa Creu i Sant Pau
Barcelona, Spain

Michael R. Schwartz, MD
Board Certified Plastic Surgeon
Private Practice
Westlake Village, CA, USA

Stephen F. Sener, MD
Professor of Surgery, Clinical Scholar
Chief of Breast, Endocrine, and Soft Tissue
Surgery
Department of Surgery, Keck School of
Medicine of USC
Chief of Surgery and Associate Medical Director
Perioperative Services
LAC+USC (LA County) Hospital
Los Angeles, CA, USA

Joseph M. Serletti, MD, FACS
The Henry Royster–William Maul Measey
Professor of Surgery and Chief
Division of Plastic Surgery
University of Pennsylvania Health System
Philadelphia, PA, USA

Deana S. Shenaq, MD
Chief Resident
Department of Surgery - Plastic Surgery
The University of Chicago Hospitals
Chicago, IL, USA

Kenneth C. Shestak, MD
Professor, Department of Plastic Surgery
University of Pittsburgh Medical Center
Pittsburgh, PA, USA

Ron B. Somogyi, MD MSc FRCSC
Plastic and Reconstructive Surgeon
Assistant Professor, Department of Surgery
University of Toronto
Toronto, ON, Canada

David H. Song, MD, MBA, FACS
Regional Chief, MedStar Health
Plastic and Reconstructive Surgery
Professor and Chairman
Department of Plastic Surgery
Georgetown University School of Medicine
Washington, DC, USA

The late Scott L. Spear†, MD
Formerly Professor of Plastic Surgery
Division of Plastic Surgery
Georgetown University
Washington, MD, USA

Michelle A. Spring, MD, FACS
Program Director
Glacier View Plastic Surgery
Kalispell Regional Medical Center
Kalispell, MT, USA

W. Grant Stevens, MD, FACS
Clinical Professor of Surgery
Marina Plastic Surgery Associates;
Keck School of Medicine of USC
Los Angeles, CA, USA

Elizabeth Stirling Craig, MD
Plastic Surgeon and Assistant Professor
Department of Plastic Surgery
University of Texas
MD Anderson Cancer Center
Houston, TX, USA

Simon G. Talbot, MD
Assistant Professor of Surgery
Brigham and Women's Hospital
Harvard Medical School
Boston, MA, USA

Jana Van Thielen, MD
Plastic Surgery Department
Brussels University Hospital
Vrij Universitaire Brussel (VUB)
Brussels, Belgium

Henry Wilson, MD, FACS
Attending Plastic Surgeon
Private Practice
Plastic Surgery Associates
Lynchburg, VA, USA

Kai Yuen Wong, MA, MB BChir, MRCS, FHEA, FRSPH
Specialist Registrar in Plastic Surgery
Department of Plastic and Reconstructive
Surgery
Cambridge University Hospitals NHS
Foundation Trust
Cambridge, UK

VOLUME SIX

Hee Chang Ahn, MD, PhD
Professor
Department of Plastic and Reconstructive
Surgery
Hanyang University Hospital School of Medicine
Seoul, South Korea

Nidal F. Al Deek, MD
Surgeon
Plastic and Reconstructive Surgery
Chang Gung Memorial Hospital
Taipei, Taiwan

Kodi K. Azari, MD, FACS
Reconstructive Transplantation Section Chief
Professor
Department of Orthopedic Surgery
UCLA Medical Center
Santa Monica, CA, USA

Carla Baldrighi, MD
Staff Surgeon
Pediatric Surgery Meyer Children's Hospital
Pediatric Hand and Reconstructive Microsurgery
Unit
Azienda Ospedaliera Universitaria Careggi
Florence, Italy

Gregory H. Borschel, MD, FAAP, FACS
Assistant Professor
University of Toronto Division of Plastic and
Reconstructive Surgery;
Assistant Professor
Institute of Biomaterials and Biomedical
Engineering;
Associate Scientist
The SickKids Research Institute
The Hospital for Sick Children
Toronto, Ontario, Canada

Kirsty Usher Boyd, MD, FRCSC
Assistant Professor
Division of Plastic Surgery, University of Ottawa
Ottawa, Ontario, Canada

Gerald Brandacher, MD
Scientific Director
Department of Plastic and Reconstructive
Surgery
Johns Hopkins University School of Medicine
Baltimore, MD, USA

Lesley Butler, MPH
Clinical Research Coordinator
Charles E. Seay, Jr. Hand Center
Texas Scottish Rite Hospital for Children
Dallas, TX, USA

Ryan P. Calfee, MD
Associate Professor
Department of Orthopedic Surgery
Washington University School of Medicine
St. Louis, MO, USA

Brian T. Carlsen, MD
Associate Professor
Departments of Plastic Surgery and Orthopedic
Surgery
Mayo Clinic
Rochester, MN, USA

David W. Chang, MD
Professor
Division of Plastic and Reconstructive Surgery
The University of Chicago Medicine
Chicago, IL, USA

James Chang, MD
Johnson & Johnson Distinguished Professor
and Chief
Division of Plastic and Reconstructive Surgery
Stanford University Medical Center
Stanford, CA, USA

Robert A. Chase, MD
Holman Professor of Surgery – Emeritus
Stanford University Medical Center
Stanford, CA, USA

Alphonsus K. S. Chong, MBBS, MRCS, MMed(Orth), FAMS (Hand Surg)
Senior Consultant
Department of Hand and Reconstructive
Microsurgery
National University Health System
Singapore;
Assistant Professor
Department of Orthopedic Surgery
Yong Loo Lin School of Medicine
National University of Singapore
Singapore

David Chwei-Chin Chuang, MD
Senior Consultant, Ex-President, Professor
Department of Plastic Surgery
Chang Gung University Hospital
Tao-Yuan, Taiwan

Kevin C. Chung, MD, MS
Chief of Hand Surgery
Michigan Medicine
Charles B G De Nancrede Professor, Assistant
Dean for Faculty Affairs
University of Michigan Medical School
Ann Arbor, Michigan, USA

Christopher Cox, MD
Attending Surgeon
Kaiser Permanente
Walnut Creek, CA, USA

Catherine Curtin, MD
Associate Professor
Department of Surgery Division of Plastic
Surgery
Stanford University
Stanford, CA, USA

Lars B. Dahlin, MD, PhD
Professor and Consultant
Department of Clinical Sciences, Malmö – Hand
Surgery
University of Lund
Malmö, Sweden

Kenneth W. Donohue, MD
Hand Surgery Fellow
Division of Plastic Surgery
Department of Orthopedic Surgery
Baylor College of Medicine
Houston, TX, USA

Gregory A. Dumanian, MD, FACS
Stuteville Professor of Surgery
Division of Plastic Surgery
Northwestern Feinberg School of Medicine
Chicago, IL, USA

William W. Dzwierzynski, MD
Professor and Program Director
Department of Plastic Surgery
Medical College of Wisconsin
Milwaukee, WI, USA

Simon Farnebo, MD, PhD
Associate Professor and Consultant Hand
Surgeon
Department of Plastic Surgery, Hand Surgery
and Burns
Institution of Clinical and Experimental
Medicine, University of Linköping
Linköping, Sweden

Ida K. Fox, MD
Assistant Professor of Plastic Surgery
Department of Surgery
Division of Plastic and Reconstructive Surgery
Washington University School of Medicine
St. Louis, MO, USA

Paige M. Fox, MD, PhD
Assistant Professor
Department of Surgery, Division of Plastic and
Reconstructive Surgery
Stanford University Medical Center
Stanford, CA, USA

Jeffrey B. Friedrich, MD
Professor of Surgery and Orthopedics
Department of Surgery, Division of Plastic
Surgery
University of Washington
Seattle, WA, USA

Steven C. Haase, MD, FACS
Associate Professor
Department of Surgery, Section of Plastic
Surgery
University of Michigan Health
Ann Arbor, MI, USA

Elisabet Hagert, MD, PhD
Associate Professor
Department of Clinical Science and Education
Karolinska Institute;
Chief Hand Surgeon
Hand Foot Surgery Center
Stockholm, Sweden

Warren C. Hammert, MD
Professor of Orthopedic and Plastic Surgery
Chief, Division of Hand Surgery
Department of Orthopedics and Rehabilitation
University of Rochester
Rochester, NY, USA

Isaac Harvey, MD
Clinical Fellow
Department of Pediatric Plastic and
Reconstructive Surgery
Hospital for SickKids
Toronto, Ontario, Canada

Vincent R. Hentz, MD
Emeritus Professor of Surgery and Orthopedic
Surgery (by courtesy)
Stanford University
Stanford, CA, USA

Jonay Hill, MD
Clinical Assistant Professor
Anesthesiology, Perioperative and Pain Medicine
Stanford University School of Medicine
Stanford, CA, USA

Steven E. R. Hovius, MD, PhD
Former Head, Department of Plastic,
Reconstructive and Hand Surgery
Erasmus MC
University Medical Center
Rotterdam, the Netherlands;
Xpert Clinic, Hand and Wrist Center
The Netherlands

Jerry I. Huang, MD
Associate Professor
Department of Orthopedics and Sports
Medicine
University of Washington;
Program Director
University of Washington Hand Fellowship
University of Washington
Seattle, WA, USA

Marco Innocenti, MD
Associate Professor of Plastic Surgery,
University of Florence;
Director, Reconstructive Microsurgery
Department of Oncology
Careggi University Hospital
Florence, Italy

Neil F. Jones, MD, FRCS
Professor and Chief of Hand Surgery
University of California Medical Center;
Professor of Orthopedic Surgery;
Professor of Plastic and Reconstructive Surgery
University of California Irvine
Irvine, CA, USA

Ryosuke Kakinoki, MD, PhD
Professor of Hand Surgery and Microsurgery,
Reconstructive, and Orthopedic Surgery
Department of Orthopedic Surgery
Faculty of Medicine
Kindai University
Osakasayama, Osaka, Japan

Jason R. Kang, MD
Chief Resident
Department of Orthopedic Surgery
Stanford Hospital & Clinics
Redwood City, CA, USA

Joseph S. Khouri, MD
Resident
Division of Plastic Surgery, Department of
Surgery
University of Rochester
Rochester, NY, USA

Todd Kuiken, MD, PhD
Professor
Departments of PM&R, BME, and Surgery
Northwestern University;
Director, Neural Engineering Center for Artificial
Limbs
Rehabilitation Institute of Chicago
Chicago, IL, USA

Donald Lalonde, BSC, MD, MSc, FRCSC
Professor of Surgery
Division of Plastic and Reconstructive Surgery
Saint John Campus of Dalhousie University
Saint John, New Brunswick, Canada

W. P. Andrew Lee, MD
The Milton T. Edgerton MD, Professor and
Chairman
Department of Plastic and Reconstructive
Surgery
Johns Hopkins University School of Medicine
Baltimore, MD, USA

Anais Legrand, MD
Postdoctoral Research Fellow
Plastic and Reconstructive Surgery
Stanford University Medical Center
Stanford, CA, USA

Terry Light, MD
Professor
Department of Orthopedic Surgery
Loyola University Medical Center
Maywood, IL, USA

Jin Xi Lim, MBBS, MRCS
Senior Resident
Department of Hand and Reconstructive
Microsurgery
National University Health System
Singapore

Joseph Lopez, MD, MBA
Resident, Plastic and Reconstructive Surgery
Department of Plastic and Reconstructive
Surgery
Johns Hopkins University School of Medicine
Baltimore, MD, USA

Susan E. Mackinnon, MD
Sydney M. Shoenberg, Jr. and Robert H.
Shoenberg Professor
Department of Surgery, Division of Plastic and
Reconstructive Surgery
Washington University School of Medicine
St. Louis, MO, USA

Brian Mailey, MD
Assistant Professor of Surgery
Institute for Plastic Surgery
Southern Illinois University
Springfield, IL, USA

Steven J. McCabe, MD, MSc, FRCS(C)
Director of Hand and Upper Extremity Program
University of Toronto
Toronto Western Hospital
Toronto, Ontario, Canada

Kai Megerle, MD, PhD
Assistant Professor
Clinic for Plastic Surgery and Hand Surgery
Technical University of Munich
Munich, Germany

Amy M. Moore, MD
Assistant Professor of Surgery
Division of Plastic and Reconstructive Surgery
Department of Surgery
Washington University School of Medicine
St. Louis, MO, USA

Steven L. Moran, MD
Professor and Chair of Plastic Surgery
Division of Plastic Surgery, Division of Hand and
Microsurgery;
Professor of Orthopedics
Rochester, MN, USA

Rebecca L. Neiduski, PhD, OTR/L, CHT
Dean of the School of Health Sciences
Professor of Health Sciences
Elon University
Elon, NC, USA

David T. Netscher, MD
Program Director, Hand Surgery Fellowship;
Clinical Professor, Division of Plastic Surgery
and Department of Orthopedic Surgery
Baylor College of Medicine;
Adjunct Professor of Clinical Surgery (Plastic
Surgery)
Weill Medical College
Cornell University
Houston, TX, USA

Michael W. Neumeister, MD
Professor and Chairman
Division of Plastic Surgery
Springfield Illinois University School of Medicine
Springfield, IL, USA

Shelley Noland, MD
Assistant Professor
Division of Plastic Surgery
Mayo Clinic Arizona
Phoenix, AZ, USA

Christine B. Novak, PT, PhD
Associate Professor
Department of Surgery, Division of Plastic and
Reconstructive Surgery
University of Toronto
Toronto, Ontario, Canada

Scott Oates, MD
Deputy Department Chair;
Professor
Department of Plastic Surgery, Division of
Surgery
The University of Texas MD Anderson Cancer
Center
Houston, TX, USA

Kerby Oberg, MD, PhD
Associate Professor
Department of Pathology and Human Anatomy
Loma Linda University School of Medicine
Loma Linda, CA, USA

Scott Oishi, MD
Director, Charles E. Seay, Jr. Hand Center
Texas Scottish Rite Hospital for Children;
Professor, Department of Plastic Surgery and
Department of Orthopedic Surgery
University of Texas Southwestern Medical Center
Dallas, TX, USA

William C. Pederson, MD, FACS
President and Fellowship Director
The Hand Center of San Antonio;
Adjunct Professor of Surgery
The University of Texas Health Science Center at
San Antonio
San Antonio, TX, USA

Dang T. Pham, MD
General Surgery Resident
Department of Surgery
Houston Methodist Hospital
Houston, TX, USA

Karl-Josef Prommersberger, MD, PhD
Chair, Professor of Orthopedic Surgery
Clinic for Hand Surgery
Bad Neustadt/Saale, Germany

Carina Reinholdt, MD, PhD
Senior Consultant in Hand Surgery
Center for Advanced Reconstruction of
Extremities
Sahlgrenska University Hospital/ Mölndal
Mölndal, Sweden;
Assistant Professor
Department of Orthopedics
Institute for Clinical Sciences
Sahlgrenska Academy
Goteborg, Sweden

Justin M. Sacks, MD, MBA, FACS
Director, Oncological Reconstruction;
Assistant Professor
Department of Plastic and Reconstructive
Surgery
Johns Hopkins School of Medicine
Baltimore, MD, USA

Douglas M. Sammer, MD
Associate Professor of Plastic and Orthopedic
Surgery
Chief of Plastic Surgery at Parkland Memorial
Hospital
Program Director Hand Surgery Fellowship
University of Texas Southwestern Medical Center
Dallas, TX, USA

Subhro K. Sen, MD
Clinical Associate Professor
Plastic and Reconstructive Surgery
Robert A. Chase Hand and Upper Limb Center
Stanford University School of Medicine
Stanford, CA, USA

**Pundrique R. Sharma, MBBS, PhD and
FRCS (Plast)**
Consultant Plastic Surgeon
Department for Plastic and Reconstructive
Surgery
Alder Hey Children's Hospital
Liverpool, UK

Randolph Sherman, MD, FACS
Vice Chair
Department of Surgery
Cedars-Sinai Medical Center
Los Angeles, CA, USA

Jaimie T. Shores, MD
Clinical Director, Hand/Arm Transplant Program
Department of Plastic and Reconstructive
Surgery
Johns Hopkins University School of Medicine
Baltimore, MD, USA

Vanila M. Singh, MD, MACM
Clinical Associate Professor
Anesthesiology, Perioperative and Pain Medicine
Stanford University School of Medicine
Stanford, CA, USA

Jason M. Souza, MD, LCDR, MC, USN
Staff Plastic Surgeon, United States Navy
Walter Reed National Military Medical Center
Bethesda, MD, USA

Amir Taghinia, MD, MPH
Attending Surgeon
Department of Plastic and Oral Surgery
Boston Children's Hospital;
Assistant Professor of Surgery
Harvard Medical School
Boston, MA, USA

David M. K. Tan, MBBS
Senior Consultant
Department of Hand and Reconstructive
Microsurgery
National University Health System
Singapore;
Assistant Professor
Department of Orthopedic Surgery
Yong Loo Lin School of Medicine
National University Singapore
Singapore

Jin Bo Tang, MD
Professor and Chair
Department of Hand Surgery;
Chair, The Hand Surgery Research Center
Affiliated Hospital of Nantong University
Nantong, The People's Republic of China

Johan Thorfinn, MD, PhD
Senior Consultant of Plastic Surgery, Burn Unit;
Co-Director
Department of Plastic Surgery, Hand Surgery
and Burns
Linköping University Hospital
Linköping, Sweden

Michael Tonkin, MBBS, MD, FRACS(Orth), FRCS(Ed Orth)
Professor of Hand Surgery
Department of Hand Surgery and Peripheral
Nerve Surgery
Royal North Shore Hospital
The Children's Hospital at Westmead
University of Sydney Medical School
Sydney, New South Wales, Australia

Joseph Upton III, MD
Staff Surgeon
Department of Plastic and Oral Surgery
Boston Children's Hospital;
Professor of Surgery
Harvard Medical School
Boston, MA, USA

Francisco Valero-Cuevas, PhD
Director
Brain-Body Dynamics Laboratory;
Professor of Biomedical Engineering;
Professor of Biokinesiology and Physical
Therapy;
(By courtesy) Professor of Computer Science
and Aerospace and Mechanical Engineering
The University of Southern California
Los Angeles, CA, USA

Christianne A. van Nieuwenhoven, MD, PhD
Plastic Surgeon/Hand Surgeon
Plastic and Reconstructive Surgery
Erasmus Medical Centre
Rotterdam, the Netherlands

Nicholas B. Vedder, MD
Professor of Surgery and Orthopedics
Chief of Plastic Surgery Vice Chair
Department of Surgery
University of Washington
Seattle, WA, USA

Andrew J. Watt, MD
Attending Hand and Microvascular Surgeon;
Associate Program Director, Buncke Clinic Hand
and Microsurgery Fellowship;
Adjunct Clinical Faculty, Stanford University
Division of Plastic and Reconstructive Surgery
The Buncke Clinic
San Francisco, CA, USA

Fu-Chan Wei, MD
Professor
Department of Plastic Surgery
Chang Gung Memorial Hospital
Taoyuan, Taiwan

Julie Colantoni Woodside, MD
Orthopedic Surgeon
OrthoCarolina
Gastonia, NC, USA

Jeffrey Yao, MD
Associate Professor
Department of Orthopedic Surgery
Stanford Hospital & Clinics
Redwood City, CA, USA

Acknowledgments

My wife, Gabrielle Kane, has always been my rock. She not only encourages me in my work but gives constructive criticism bolstered by her medical expertise as well as by her knowledge and training in education. I can never repay her. The editorial team at Elsevier have made this series possible. Belinda Kuhn leads the group of Alexandra Mortimer, Louise Cook, and the newest addition to the team, Sam Crowe. The Elsevier production team has also been vital in moving this project along. The volume editors, Geoff Gurtner, Peter Rubin, Ed Rodriguez, Joe Losee, David Song, Mo Nahabedian, Jim Chang, and Dan Liu have shaped and refined this edition, making vital changes to keep the series relevant and up-to-date. My colleagues in the University of Washington, headed by Nick Vedder, have provided continued encouragement and support. Finally, and most importantly, the residents and fellows who pass through our program keep us on our toes and ensure that we give them the best possible solutions to their questions.

Peter C. Neligan, MB, FRCS(I), FRCSC, FACS

I'd like to thank all the authors for their commitment to producing this volume, my colleagues and residents at the University of Chicago Medical Center, MedStar Health and Georgetown University School of Medicine who work tirelessly to advance Plastic Surgery; my parents who first inspired me to seek knowledge; and most importantly my wife Janie and my daughters Olivia, Ava, and Ella without whom this and all work loses meaning and significance for me.

David H. Song, MD, MBA, FACS

Dedicated to future plastic surgeons. Take up the torch and lead us forward!

1

Comprehensive lower extremity anatomy

Grant M. Kleiber and Rajiv P. Parikh

SYNOPSIS

- Reconstructive surgery of the lower extremity is dependent on a comprehensive understanding of structural and functional anatomy in order to accurately analyze defects and develop tailored solutions that preserve and restore normal form and function.

- The reconstructive surgeon may be called upon to treat specific tissue defects of the lower extremity, or to harvest tissue for transfer from the many potential donor sites in the lower extremity.

- This chapter aims to provide a comprehensive review of the 3D anatomy of the lower extremity in order to facilitate operative and clinical decision-making by the reconstructive surgeon.

- A detailed description is given of each region of the lower extremity with respect to skeletal support, musculofascial anatomy, vascular supply, lymphatic drainage, neuroanatomy, and skin and soft-tissue elements.

- A broad overview of the available soft-tissue donor sites from each region, donor sites for bone grafts, anatomic basis of common lower extremity flaps, and common points of nerve injury and entrapment are included to provide a clinically relevant discussion of the anatomy of the lower extremity as a framework for common challenges in reconstructive surgery.

Embryology

The first recognizable sign of lower limb growth in the human embryo occurs during the third week of life. The initial limb development begins along the ventrolateral surface. Slow outgrowth of the apical epidermal ridge continues into the fifth week when a small, flattened foot plate develops. The foot plate begins development straight with no dorsiflexion and the plantar surface pointed toward the head. Skeletogenesis occurs in the tibial/fibular region while the foot plate rotates externally. By the sixth week, digital rays appear and external notching occurs. From the sixth to the eighth week chondrification progresses throughout the future bony structures and the lower limb elongates.

The transition from the embryonic to the fetal period occurs during the eighth week. At this point, the phalanges, metatarsals, tarsals, malleoli, tibia, fibula, and femur are all present. The first signs of detectable ossification begin in the foot, specifically in the distal phalanges and metatarsal shaft. The intervening proximal and middle phalanges follow. Tarsal bones begin ossification in the fifth month, first with the talus and the cuboid. Ossification of the remaining regions of the lower extremity continues throughout gestation.

The lower extremity vascular anatomy of the embryo differs from the adult primarily by the development and transient presence of the sciatic artery.[1] This artery arises from the umbilical artery and is separate from the femoral artery as it courses inferiorly along the posterior surface of the thigh, knee, and leg, and is a major contributor to lower extremity vascular supply in early fetal development. The femoral artery passes along the anterior side of the thigh and branches into the primitive posterior tibial, anterior tibial, and peroneal arteries. As the fetus grows, the femoral artery increases in size and the sciatic artery becomes attenuated. In normal development the sciatic artery involutes during the eighth week of gestation and its remnants contribute to the formation of the inferior gluteal, deep femoral, popliteal, and peroneal vessels (Fig. 1.1). However, in 0.01–0.05% of the population a sciatic artery persists throughout fetal development and into adulthood.[2] A persistent sciatic artery can lead to aneurysm formation, thrombosis, and embolization. Although it is a rare anomaly, failure to recognize a persistent sciatic artery can lead to incorrect assumptions of vascular anatomy.

The gluteal region

Gluteal skeletal structure

The pelvis consists of the paired hip bones and the midline sacrum, articulating together at the two sacroiliac joints. The hip bones are formed by the fusion of the ilium, pubis, and ischium. These three bony regions of the pelvis coalesce to

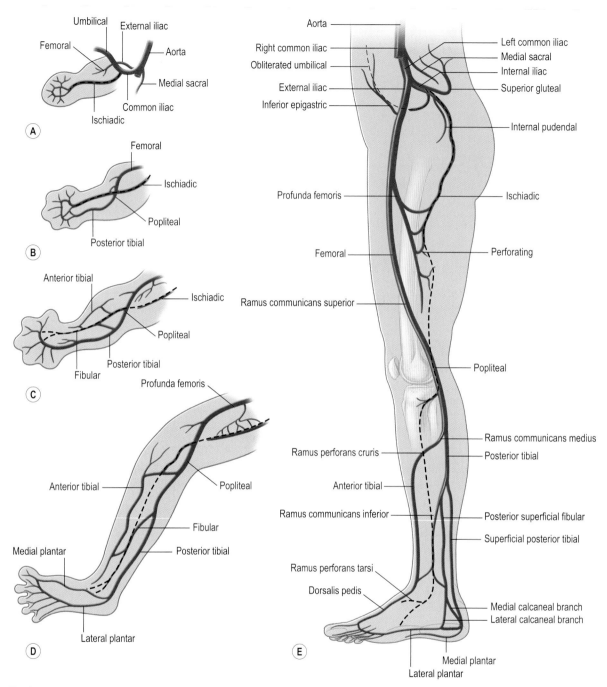

Fig. 1.1 Vascular development of the lower extremity.

form the acetabulum. The large thick bony prominences of the pelvis serve as attachments for the muscles of the hip and thigh (Fig. 1.2). These prominences also become clinically relevant in contributing to the formation of pressure ulcers, most commonly over the ischial tuberosity, sacral prominence, and greater trochanter. Dense ligaments reinforce the pelvis and distribute the numerous opposing forces acting on it. The sacrospinous ligament runs from the sacrum to the ischial spine, bounding the greater sciatic foramen. The sacrotuberous ligament attaches the sacrum to the ischial tuberosity and encloses the lesser sciatic foramen. Running from the anterior superior iliac spine (ASIS) to the pubic tubercle is the inguinal ligament. The actions of the multiple flexors, extensors, and

internal and external rotators on the hip joint serve to stabilize and position the torso during the complex process of ambulation.

Clinical correlation – iliac crest bone graft

The iliac crest serves as a versatile source of autogenous bone graft for reconstructing a variety of defects. Bone grafts can be cortical, cancellous, or corticocancellous in composition. Cortical bone is structurally stable with osteoconductive properties and ideally suited for structural defects requiring immediate mechanical stability. Cancellous bone is osteoinductive, osteogenic, and osteoconductive, undergoes rapid

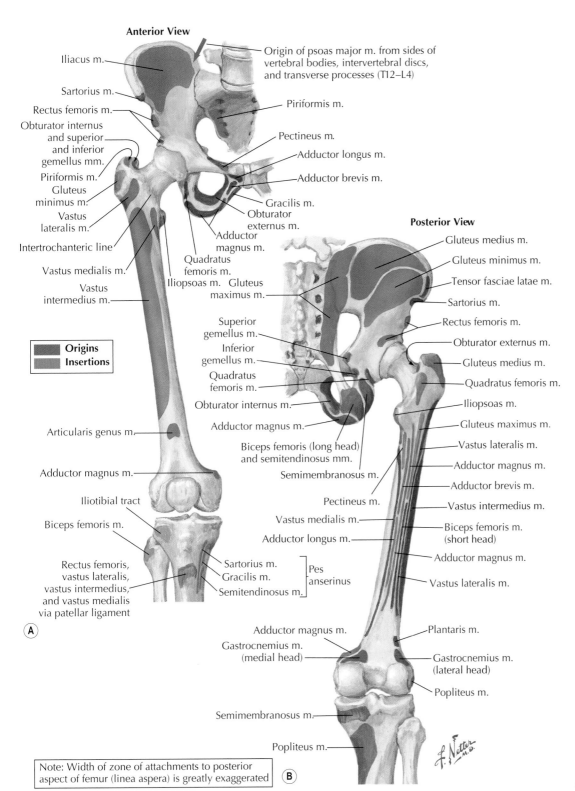

Anterior View

Iliacus m.

Origin of psoas major m. from sides of vertebral bodies, intervertebral discs, and transverse processes (T12–L4)

Sartorius m.

Rectus femoris m.

Obturator internus and superior and inferior gemellus mm.

Piriformis m.

Piriformis m.

Pectineus m.

Gluteus minimus m.

Adductor longus m.

Vastus lateralis m.

Adductor brevis m.

Intertrochanteric line

Gracilis m.

Obturator externus m.

Vastus medialis m.

Adductor magnus m.

Vastus intermedius m.

Quadratus femoris m.

Iliopsoas m. Gluteus maximus m.

Superior gemellus m.

Inferior gemellus m.

Gluteus medius m.

Posterior View

Gluteus medius m.

Gluteus minimus m.

Tensor fasciae latae m.

Sartorius m.

Rectus femoris m.

Obturator externus m.

Gluteus medius m.

Quadratus femoris m.

Quadratus femoris m.

Obturator internus m.

Iliopsoas m.

Gluteus maximus m.

Adductor magnus m.

Vastus lateralis m.

Biceps femoris (long head) and semitendinosus mm.

Adductor magnus m.

Semimembranosus m.

Adductor brevis m.

Pectineus m.

Vastus intermedius m.

Vastus medialis m.

Biceps femoris m. (short head)

Adductor longus m.

Adductor magnus m.

Vastus lateralis m.

Origins
Insertions

Articularis genus m.

Adductor magnus m.

Iliotibial tract

Biceps femoris m.

Rectus femoris, vastus lateralis, vastus intermedius, and vastus medialis via patellar ligament

Sartorius m.
Gracilis m.
Semitendinosus m.

Pes anserinus

Ⓐ

Adductor magnus m.

Gastrocnemius m. (medial head)

Plantaris m.

Gastrocnemius m. (lateral head)

Popliteus m.

Semimembranosus m.

Popliteus m.

Note: Width of zone of attachments to posterior aspect of femur (linea aspera) is greatly exaggerated

Ⓑ

Fig. 1.2 Bony attachments of buttock and thigh muscles. *(From: Netter; www.netterimages .com. © Elsevier Inc. All rights reserved.)*

remodeling and vascularization and is ideally suited for non-unions and bony fusion. Cancellous bone can be obtained between the inner and outer table of the ilium. The anterior and posterior iliac crest are common donor sites for cancellous and corticocancellous bone grafts, with 13 cm³ and 30 cm³ average graft volumes available from the anterior and posterior crest, respectively[3] (Fig. 1.3). Anteriorly, bone graft is most commonly harvested from the iliac tubercle, 3–4 cm posterior and parallel to the ASIS to maximize available bone and minimize risk to the lateral femoral cutaneous nerve. The iliac crest lies deep to a musculofascial layer from the external oblique and the iliacus muscle. The ilioinguinal nerve runs along the medial surface of the iliacus muscle and is at risk during harvest from the anterior crest. The anterior iliac crest

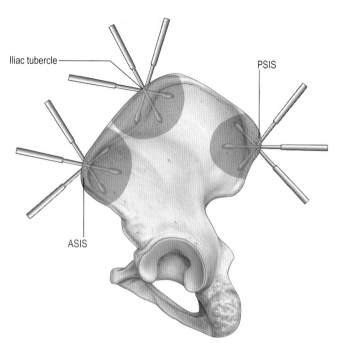

Fig. 1.3 Harvest sites for iliac crest bone graft. ASIS, anterior superior iliac spine; PSIS, posterior superior iliac spine. *(From: Ebraheim NA, Elgafy H, Xu R. Bone-graft harvesting from iliac and fibular donor sites: techniques and complications.* J Am Acad Orthop Surg. *2001;9(3):210–218.)*

provides twice the volume of packed cancellous bone compared to the distal radius or olecranon. Alternatively, tricortical bone grafts can be harvested from the inner and outer table of the anterior ilium, and corticocancellous bone grafts can be harvested to include either the inner or outer table. Posteriorly, the bone is thickest and best harvested in the area superior to a line connecting the posterior superior iliac spine (PSIS) and the apex of the sacroiliac joint. Harvesting from an area approximately 4 cm distal to the PSIS prevents violation of the sacroiliac joint.[4] Unicortical and corticocancellous bone grafts can be obtained from the outer table of the posterior ilium and additional cancellous bone harvested from the inner table of the ilium. The iliac crest can also provide vascularized bone for a variety of composite soft-tissue and bone defects. Corticocancellous, vascularized bone can be obtained from the outer cortex of the ilium on the lateral half of the iliac crest, supplied by the ascending branch of the lateral femoral circumflex system.[5] The inner cortex of the ilium, supplied through nutrient branches off the deep circumflex iliac artery, is another common source of vascularized iliac bone.

Gluteal fascial anatomy

The fascial system of the gluteal region and the lower extremity contains various permutations of a nearly continuous superficial fascial and a deep fascial layer. The superficial system is located in the subcutaneous fat. The deep fascial layer is thicker and frequently can be seen as a dual-layered fibrous band. It usually lies directly over the underlying limb musculature and its proper fascia. The superficial fascia of the gluteal region is contiguous with that over the lower back and continues inferiorly into the proximal thigh. The deep fascia covering the gluteal muscles varies in thickness. Over the maximus it is thin, but over the anterior two-thirds of the

medius it thickens and forms the gluteal aponeurosis. This is attached to the lateral border of the iliac crest superiorly, and splits anteriorly to enclose the tensor fasciae latae and posteriorly to enclose the gluteus maximus.

Muscles of the buttocks

The gluteus maximus is the largest muscle in the body and lies most superficially in the gluteal region, originating from the posterior gluteal line of the ilium and the dorsal portion of the sacrum (Fig. 1.4). The superficial fibers coalesce into a thick tendinous expansion that contributes to the iliotibial band of the fascia lata, while the deep fibers insert on the gluteal tuberosity of the femur. The gluteus maximus acts as a hip extensor when the hip is in a flexed position. In a standing position, the gluteus maximus dorsally rotates the pelvis and torso, maintaining stability. The vascular supply is primarily derived from the inferior gluteal vessels, which supply the inferior two-thirds of the muscle. The superior gluteal vessels supply the superior portion, and the first perforator branch of the profunda femoris contributes to the vascular supply of the muscle laterally. For ease of description, the Mathes–Nahai classification system is used when discussing muscle vascularity (Table 1.1).[6] The gluteus maximus has a type III vascular supply, with two dominant pedicles from the superior and inferior gluteal arteries. Innervation to the gluteus maximus is provided by the inferior gluteal nerve. Underneath the gluteus maximus lie three bursae: the trochanteric, gluteofemoral, and ischiofemoral, which allow frictionless movement over its underlying structures.

The gluteus medius, situated immediately deep to the gluteus maximus, arises from the outer surface of the iliac wing and inserts on the greater trochanter of the femur. It is innervated by the superior gluteal nerve and functions to abduct the hip and medially rotate the femur. Blood supply to this muscle is from the deep branch of the superior gluteal artery (SGA) and from the trochanteric connection.

The gluteus minimus lies deep to the gluteus medius and arises from the outer surface of the ilium. Its fibers join the aponeurosis of the gluteus medius to insert on the greater trochanter, and the two muscles function together to abduct the hip. The gluteus minimus is innervated by the superior gluteal nerve and receives blood supply from the SGA and trochanteric connection. Several small muscles arise from the medial pelvis and insert on the greater trochanter of the femur, functioning collectively to rotate the hip externally.

Table 1.1 Mathes–Nahai classification system for muscle vascular supply	
Muscle vascular supply type	**Description**
I	Single vascular pedicle
II	Dominant vascular pedicle and one or more minor pedicles
III	Two dominant pedicles
IV	Segmental vascular pedicles
V	Single dominant vascular pedicle and secondary segmental pedicles

Superficial dissection

Deeper dissection

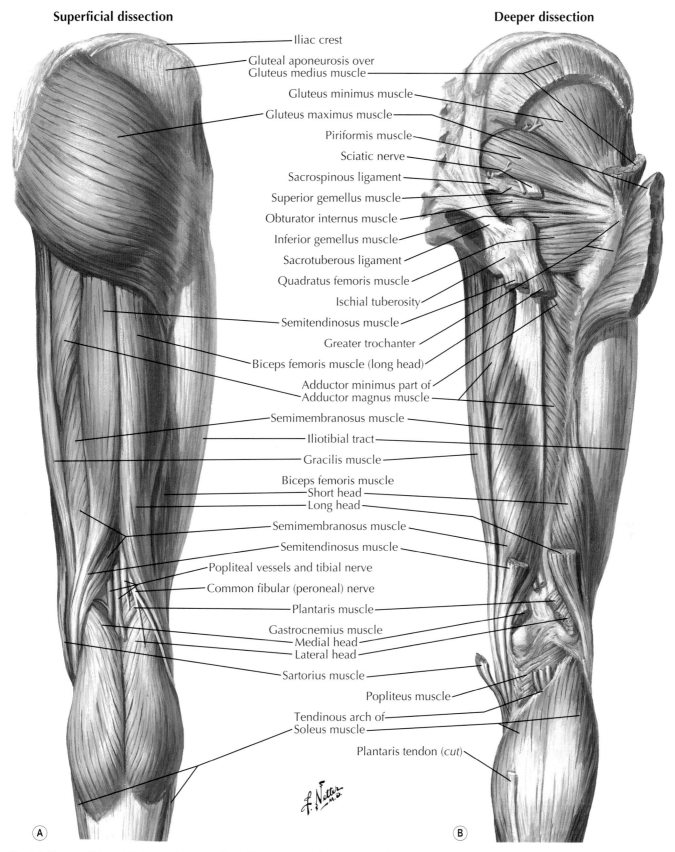

Iliac crest

Gluteal aponeurosis over
Gluteus medius muscle

Gluteus minimus muscle

Gluteus maximus muscle

Piriformis muscle

Sciatic nerve

Sacrospinous ligament

Superior gemellus muscle

Obturator internus muscle

Inferior gemellus muscle

Sacrotuberous ligament

Quadratus femoris muscle

Ischial tuberosity

Semitendinosus muscle

Greater trochanter

Biceps femoris muscle (long head)

Adductor minimus part of
Adductor magnus muscle

Semimembranosus muscle

Iliotibial tract

Gracilis muscle

Biceps femoris muscle
Short head
Long head

Semimembranosus muscle

Semitendinosus muscle

Popliteal vessels and tibial nerve

Common fibular (peroneal) nerve

Plantaris muscle

Gastrocnemius muscle
Medial head
Lateral head

Sartorius muscle

Popliteus muscle

Tendinous arch of
Soleus muscle

Plantaris tendon (*cut*)

Ⓐ

Ⓑ

Fig. 1.4 Muscles of hip and thigh: posterior views. *(From: Netter; www.netterimages.com. © Elsevier Inc. All rights reserved.)*

These muscles include piriformis, superior and inferior gemellus, quadratus femoris, obturator internus, and obturator externus.

Gluteal vasculature

The SGA is the last branch of the posterior trunk of the internal iliac artery. It exits the pelvis through the greater sciatic foramen superior to the piriformis, dividing into two branches (Fig. 1.5). The deep branch runs deep to the gluteus medius, dividing into superior and inferior branches. The superior branch travels laterally to the anterior superior iliac spine and connects with the ascending branch of the lateral circumflex femoral and the deep circumflex iliac. The inferior branch supplies the gluteus medius and minimus, and later joins with the lateral circumflex femoral. The superficial branch of the SGA pierces the gluteus maximus, connecting intramuscularly with branches of the inferior gluteal artery (IGA), and sending musculocutaneous perforators to the overlying skin. The IGA branches from the anterior trunk of the internal iliac and exits the pelvis through the greater sciatic foramen below the piriformis. It runs deep to the gluteus maximus, supplying it and its overlying skin with musculocutaneous perforators. The descending branch of the IGA continues down the posterior thigh, between the semitendinosus and the biceps femoris, running with the posterior cutaneous nerve and connecting with the perforating branches to supply the skin.[7]

Clinical correlation – SGAP and IGAP flaps

Perforating branches from the SGA and IGA can be used to perfuse free and pedicled flaps to reconstruct a variety of soft-tissue defects. There is considerable variability in size, location, and branching pattern of perforators in the gluteal region. Generally, the superior gluteal region is perfused by perforators from the SGA and the inferior gluteal region is perfused by perforators from the IGA. SGA perforators can be reliably found medial and adjacent to a line drawn from the PSIS to the greater trochanter and range in number from 5 to 11. The mean size of SGA perforators is 0.6 mm; however, there is always a perforator greater than 0.8 mm in diameter and, on average, at least 4 perforators per side greater than 0.8 mm.[8] Perforator lengths for pedicle use vary from 4 cm to 10 cm and are dependent on the extent of dissection to the source vessel. The thickness and size of subcutaneous tissue that can be reliably perfused by SGA perforators follows the perforasome theory.[9] Flaps harvested on the superficial fascial plane can be "ultra-thin", with thickness ranging from 5 mm to 11 mm and an average flap size of 125 cm.[2,10] IGA perforators range in number from 4 to 12 perforators each side, with a mean diameter of 0.4–0.6 mm, and perforator lengths vary from 4 cm to 14 cm.[8,11] Perforators from the IGA can perfuse an average of 175 cm[2] of subcutaneous tissue, with thickness ranging from 1 cm to 6 cm depending on indication and patient body habitus.[11]

Gluteal innervation

The posterior cutaneous nerve of the thigh exits the pelvis with the inferior gluteal vessels (Fig. 1.5). Several branches will curl around the inferior border of the gluteus maximus and run superiorly to innervate the overlying skin of the buttocks, while the posterior cutaneous nerve continues to descend down the posterior thigh deep to the fascia lata, sending segmental cutaneous branches to the skin of the posterior thigh. The gluteal muscles are innervated by the superior and inferior gluteal nerves. The superior gluteal nerve runs with the SGA and divides into superior and inferior branches, which course respectively with the superior and inferior branches of the deep SGA, supplying the gluteus medius and minimus. The inferior branch runs laterally to also innervate the tensor fascia latae. The inferior gluteal nerve runs with the IGA, exiting the pelvis below the piriformis and entering the gluteus maximus.

The thigh

The thigh region is generally defined as the cylindrical proximal portion of the lower extremity that extends from the infragluteal crease and the inguinal ligament distally to the tibiofemoral joint. The thigh aids in trunk support and positioning of the knee in space, serving a critical role in ambulation. The muscles of the thigh are some of the largest in the body and often have redundant or overlapping function. Similarly, the corresponding fasciocutaneous coverage in the thigh is relatively redundant. Thorough knowledge of thigh anatomy is key for taking advantage of these redundancies and utilizing the thigh as a generous source of donor tissue for local, regional, and distant reconstructive surgical options.

Thigh skeletal structure

The femur is the longest bone in the body and the predominant bone in the thigh region. The femoral head articulates with the pelvic acetabulum to form the only true ball-and-socket joint in the body, allowing for stability under load as well as smooth multiplanar movement. Two bony prominences emanate from the femoral neck at about 90° from each other – the greater and lesser trochanters. These femoral prominences primarily serve as insertion sites for hip actors (Fig. 1.2). The action of multiple flexors, extensors, and internal and external rotators on the hip joint serves to stabilize and position the torso during the complex process of ambulation.

The vascular supply of the femoral bone arises from multiple sources. The femoral head and neck are encircled by an arterial anastomosis between the medial and lateral circumflex arteries with lesser contribution by the superior and inferior gluteal vessels. The femoral shaft has multiple nutrient foramina supplied by branches from the second perforating artery from the profunda femoris. These foramina usually run along the linea aspera on the posterior surface of the femur in the middle one-third of the femoral shaft. Periosteal vascularity along the femur receives vascular input from either the perforating branches of the profunda or directly from the profunda femoris. The distal metaphyseal region of the femur also has multiple vascular foramina that are derived from the genicular arterial system.

Clinical correlation – medial femoral condyle flap

The arterial anatomy of the distal femur, specifically the medial femoral condyle (MFC) and supracondylar region, has clinical significance as it is the anatomical basis for the MFC

Deep dissection

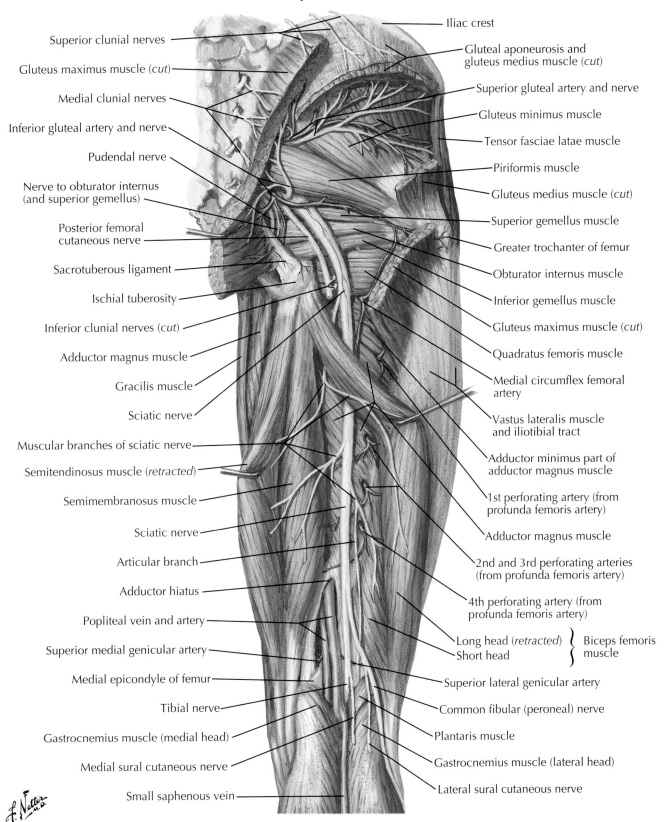

Superior clunial nerves

Gluteus maximus muscle (*cut*)

Medial clunial nerves

Inferior gluteal artery and nerve

Pudendal nerve

Nerve to obturator internus
(and superior gemellus)

Posterior femoral
cutaneous nerve

Sacrotuberous ligament

Ischial tuberosity

Inferior clunial nerves (*cut*)

Adductor magnus muscle

Gracilis muscle

Sciatic nerve

Muscular branches of sciatic nerve

Semitendinosus muscle (*retracted*)

Semimembranosus muscle

Sciatic nerve

Articular branch

Adductor hiatus

Popliteal vein and artery

Superior medial genicular artery

Medial epicondyle of femur

Tibial nerve

Gastrocnemius muscle (medial head)

Medial sural cutaneous nerve

Small saphenous vein

Iliac crest

Gluteal aponeurosis and
gluteus medius muscle (*cut*)

Superior gluteal artery and nerve

Gluteus minimus muscle

Tensor fasciae latae muscle

Piriformis muscle

Gluteus medius muscle (*cut*)

Superior gemellus muscle

Greater trochanter of femur

Obturator internus muscle

Inferior gemellus muscle

Gluteus maximus muscle (*cut*)

Quadratus femoris muscle

Medial circumflex femoral
artery

Vastus lateralis muscle
and iliotibial tract

Adductor minimus part of
adductor magnus muscle

1st perforating artery (from
profunda femoris artery)

Adductor magnus muscle

2nd and 3rd perforating arteries
(from profunda femoris artery)

4th perforating artery (from
profunda femoris artery)

Long head (*retracted*)
Short head } Biceps femoris muscle

Superior lateral genicular artery

Common fibular (peroneal) nerve

Plantaris muscle

Gastrocnemius muscle (lateral head)

Lateral sural cutaneous nerve

Fig. 1.5 Arteries and nerves of thigh: deep dissection (posterior view). *(From: Netter; www.netterimages.com.* © *Elsevier Inc. All rights reserved.)*

perforators to the MFC. Paired venae comitantes provide venous drainage for the MFC flap, often converging to form the short descending genicular vein.

Thigh fascial composition

The thigh has a superficial and deep fascial system. The superficial fascia lies within the subcutaneous fat of the thigh encircling the entire structure. Superficial vessels and nerves pass along and pierce this fascia as they travel to the skin. The thickness of the fascia varies throughout the thigh but thickens proximally in the inguinal region. At the inguinal ligament the superficial fascia fuses with the deep thigh fascia.

The deep fascia is a tough, well-vascularized fibrous tissue that lies beneath the superficial fascia and the subcutaneous fat. This fibrous structure encircles and constrains the thigh musculature in a near-complete sheath. There is varying terminology used to describe the deep fascia of the thigh, and this is often a source of confusion. The deep fascia of the thigh is also called investing fascia or the fascia lata. For simplicity and consistency, it will be referred to as the deep fascia in this text. The deep fascia of the thigh attaches posteriorly to the sacrum and coccyx, anteriorly to the inguinal ligament, and laterally to the iliac crest. At the inguinal ligament, where the superficial fascia joins the deep fascia, there is an opening in both fascial layers called the fossa ovalis. The great saphenous vein, superficial branches of the femoral artery, and lymphatics pass through this opening between the deep and the superficial layers of the thigh (Fig. 1.7). This opening is covered by a membranous layer of the superficial fascia called the cribriform fascia. A thickening of the fibrous tissues is present on the lateral aspect of the deep fascia and is termed the iliotibial band or tract (Fig. 1.8). The iliotibial band is proximally attached to the tensor fascia latae muscle, and together this myofascial unit aids in maintaining knee extension.

Septa pass from the deep fascial sheath to the bones underneath, confining the functional muscle groups within osteofascial compartments. In addition to separating musculature, fascial planes also provide pathways for vessel perforators to travel from deeper vasculature to the overlying skin. There are three functional compartments of the thigh: anterior, posterior, and medial. The anterior compartment contains the knee extensor muscles; the posterior compartment comprises knee flexors; and the medial compartment retains the hip adductors (Fig. 1.9). The medial and lateral intermuscular septa travel from the fascia lata to attach to the femur on the linea aspera along its posterior aspect. These septa then divide the anterior compartment from the posterior compartments and partition the thigh musculature according to knee function. Only the anterior and posterior compartments have definite fascial boundaries. The medial (adductor) compartment is not a true anatomical compartment as it has no defined intermuscular septa separating it. The muscles of the adductor compartment – gracilis, pectineus, adductor longus, adductor brevis, and adductor magnus – form a functional compartment in the proximal aspect of the thigh.

Thigh musculature

The three compartments of the thigh are a well-organized way to approach the thigh musculature (Table 1.2). There are 17

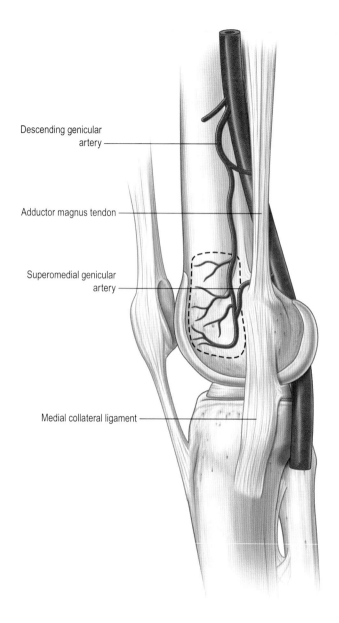

Fig. 1.6 The medial femoral periosteal bone flap. *(From: Netter; www.netterimages.com. © Elsevier Inc. All rights reserved.)*

vascularized corticoperiosteal flap (Fig. 1.6). This flap can be harvested as a corticoperiosteal free or pedicled flap with or without cancellous bone and provides an excellent option for transfer of vascularized bone in the treatment of recalcitrant fracture nonunions.[12] The vascular supply to the MFC is derived from the descending genicular artery (DGA) and/or the superior medial genicular artery. The DGA, the longer and larger of the two vessels, is a medial branch off the superficial femoral artery and originates just proximal to the adductor hiatus, approximately 14 cm proximal to the knee joint. The DGA is the dominant vessel to the MFC 90% of the time, has a mean pedicle length of 8 cm, and has a proximal diameter of at least 1.5 mm, suitable for microsurgical anastomosis.[13,14] The superior medial genicular artery, a branch off the popliteal artery, has a smaller vessel diameter of 0.8 mm and pedicle length of 5 cm, and therefore is less utilized when harvesting a flap.[13] The osteoarticular branch of the DGA provides periosteal perfusion, and there are numerous intraosseous

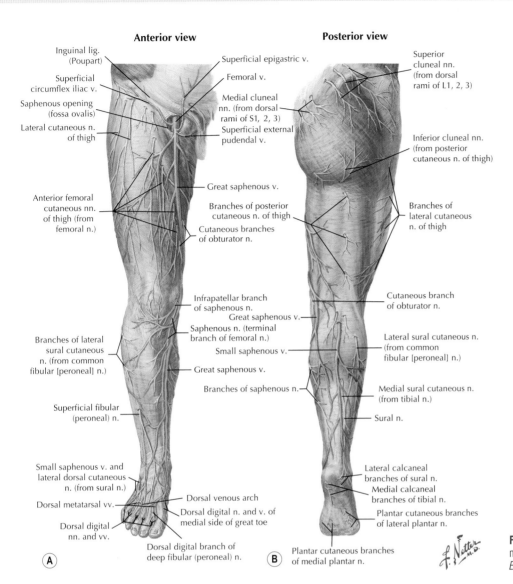

Anterior view

Inguinal lig. (Poupart)
Superficial circumflex iliac v.
Saphenous opening (fossa ovalis)
Lateral cutaneous n. of thigh
Anterior femoral cutaneous nn. of thigh (from femoral n.)
Branches of lateral sural cutaneous n. (from common fibular [peroneal] n.)
Superficial fibular (peroneal) n.
Small saphenous v. and lateral dorsal cutaneous n. (from sural n.)
Dorsal metatarsal vv.
Dorsal digital nn. and vv.

Superficial epigastric v.
Femoral v.
Medial cluneal nn. (from dorsal rami of S1, 2, 3)
Superficial external pudendal v.
Great saphenous v.
Branches of posterior cutaneous n. of thigh
Cutaneous branches of obturator n.
Infrapatellar branch of saphenous n.
Great saphenous v.
Saphenous n. (terminal branch of femoral n.)
Small saphenous v.
Great saphenous v.
Branches of saphenous n.
Dorsal venous arch
Dorsal digital n. and v. of medial side of great toe
Dorsal digital branch of deep fibular (peroneal) n.

(A)

Posterior view

Superior cluneal nn. (from dorsal rami of L1, 2, 3)
Inferior cluneal nn. (from posterior cutaneous n. of thigh)
Branches of lateral cutaneous n. of thigh
Cutaneous branch of obturator n.
Lateral sural cutaneous n. (from common fibular [peroneal] n.)
Medial sural cutaneous n. (from tibial n.)
Sural n.
Lateral calcaneal branches of sural n.
Medial calcaneal branches of tibial n.
Plantar cutaneous branches of lateral plantar n.
Plantar cutaneous branches of medial plantar n.

(B)

Fig. 1.7 Surface anatomy: superficial veins and nerves. *(From: Netter; www.netterimages.com. © Elsevier Inc. All rights reserved.)*

muscles that course through the region of the thigh. The anterior thigh compartment contains the sartorius, articularis genu, and quadriceps femoris comprising the rectus femoris, vastus lateralis, intermedius, and medialis. These muscles are the primary knee extensors. All of the anterior compartment muscles share a single articular function, with the exception of the sartorius and the rectus femoris, which cross both the hip joint and the knee joint. The sartorius muscle is the most superficial muscle of the thigh. It obliquely crosses the anterior thigh from superolateral to medial inferior. The proximal end of the sartorius makes up one of the three limbs of the femoral triangle: the medial border of the sartorius makes up the lateral side, the medial border of the adductor longus makes up the medial side, and the inguinal ligament makes up the superior limb (Fig. 1.10). The femoral triangle denotes the region where the femoral artery, nerve, and vein are transiently uncovered superficially by muscle in the proximal thigh. Here, all three structures radiate multiple branches in multiple directions to supply the vasculature and innervation to the groin region, lower abdomen, and proximal thigh. As the femoral artery, vein, and nerve descend distally in the thigh, they dive under the adductor longus and then proceed to the adductor canal. At the distal end of the sartorius, the

muscle inserts on the proximal, medial surface of the tibia. The sartorius inserts in this region above the gracilis, which then inserts above the semitendinosus (Fig. 1.11). This three-muscle insertion point forms the pes anserinus. The superficial location of the sartorius muscle and its proximity to the femoral triangle make it an ideal flap for muscle transposition coverage over proximal thigh wounds with vessel or prosthetic graft exposure. The vascular anatomy of the sartorius muscle is traditionally described as a type IV, segmental pattern. Six to eight muscular branches enter the sartorius along the length of the muscle from different source vessels. The proximal third is supplied by branches from the superficial circumflex iliac and the lateral circumflex femoral arteries. The middle third receives multiple branches from the superficial femoral artery. The distal third of the muscle is supplied by muscular branches of the descending genicular and superomedial genicular arteries (Fig. 1.12).[15] A recent anatomic study has challenged this purely segmental classification, demonstrating two dominant vascular pedicles.[16] This renewed anatomic understanding of the sartorius muscle suggests that it may be based on a single pedicle, and therefore have a larger arc of rotation for wound coverage.

Text continued on p. 16

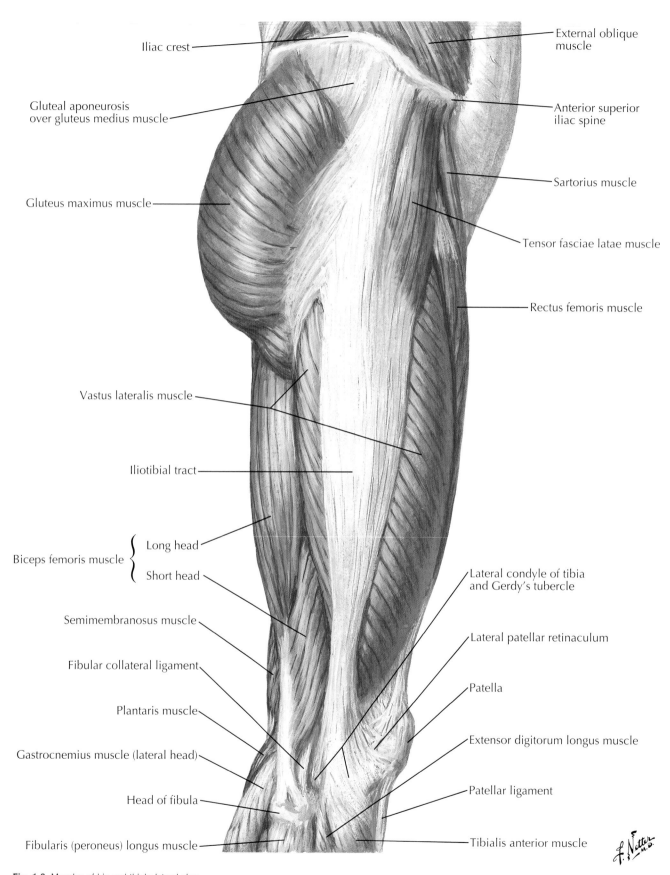

Iliac crest

External oblique muscle

Gluteal aponeurosis over gluteus medius muscle

Anterior superior iliac spine

Sartorius muscle

Gluteus maximus muscle

Tensor fasciae latae muscle

Rectus femoris muscle

Vastus lateralis muscle

Iliotibial tract

Biceps femoris muscle { Long head Short head

Lateral condyle of tibia and Gerdy's tubercle

Lateral patellar retinaculum

Semimembranosus muscle

Fibular collateral ligament

Patella

Plantaris muscle

Extensor digitorum longus muscle

Gastrocnemius muscle (lateral head)

Head of fibula

Patellar ligament

Fibularis (peroneus) longus muscle

Tibialis anterior muscle

Fig. 1.8 Muscles of hip and thigh: lateral view.

Thigh: Serial Cross-Sections

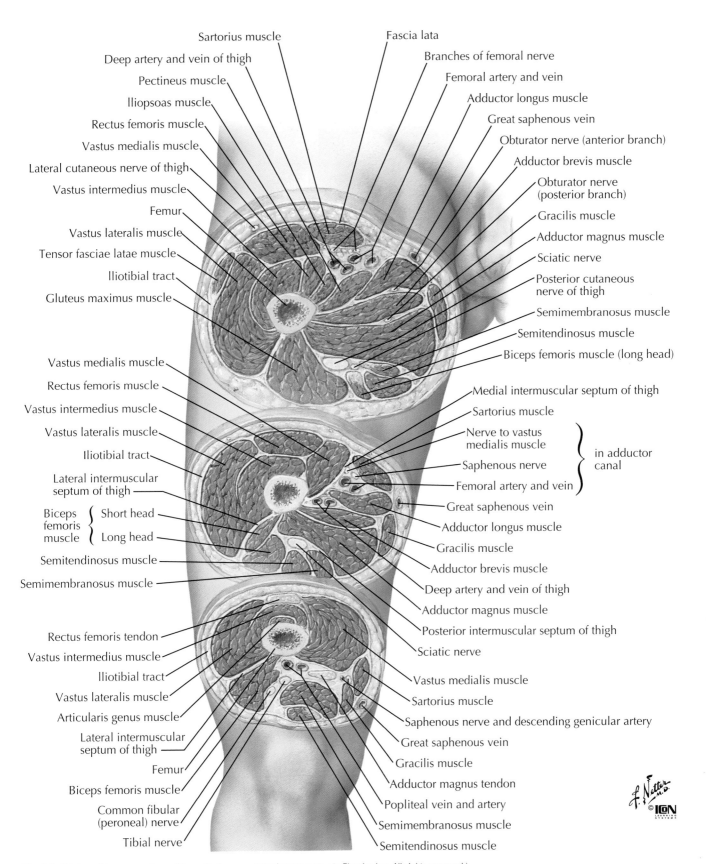

Sartorius muscle
Deep artery and vein of thigh
Pectineus muscle
Iliopsoas muscle
Rectus femoris muscle
Vastus medialis muscle
Lateral cutaneous nerve of thigh
Vastus intermedius muscle
Femur
Vastus lateralis muscle
Tensor fasciae latae muscle
Iliotibial tract
Gluteus maximus muscle

Fascia lata
Branches of femoral nerve
Femoral artery and vein
Adductor longus muscle
Great saphenous vein
Obturator nerve (anterior branch)
Adductor brevis muscle
Obturator nerve (posterior branch)
Gracilis muscle
Adductor magnus muscle
Sciatic nerve
Posterior cutaneous nerve of thigh
Semimembranosus muscle
Semitendinosus muscle
Biceps femoris muscle (long head)

Vastus medialis muscle
Rectus femoris muscle
Vastus intermedius muscle
Vastus lateralis muscle
Iliotibial tract
Lateral intermuscular septum of thigh
Biceps femoris muscle { Short head / Long head }
Semitendinosus muscle
Semimembranosus muscle

Medial intermuscular septum of thigh
Sartorius muscle
Nerve to vastus medialis muscle
Saphenous nerve
Femoral artery and vein
} in adductor canal
Great saphenous vein
Adductor longus muscle
Gracilis muscle
Adductor brevis muscle
Deep artery and vein of thigh
Adductor magnus muscle
Posterior intermuscular septum of thigh
Sciatic nerve

Rectus femoris tendon
Vastus intermedius muscle
Iliotibial tract
Vastus lateralis muscle
Articularis genus muscle
Lateral intermuscular septum of thigh
Femur
Biceps femoris muscle
Common fibular (peroneal) nerve
Tibial nerve

Vastus medialis muscle
Sartorius muscle
Saphenous nerve and descending genicular artery
Great saphenous vein
Gracilis muscle
Adductor magnus tendon
Popliteal vein and artery
Semimembranosus muscle
Semitendinosus muscle

Fig. 1.9 Thigh: serial cross-sections. *(From: Netter; www.netterimages.com.* © Elsevier Inc. All rights reserved.)

Table 1.2 Thigh musculature

		Muscle	Origin	Insertion	Function	Blood supply	Flap blood supply type	Innervation
Hip-related	1	Iliacus	Pelvis – iliac fossa	Lesser trochanter of femur – inferior edge	Hip flexion and internal rotation	–	–	Femoral nerve – intra-abdominal
	2	Psaos major	Thoracic and lumbar spine (T12–L5)	Lesser trochanter of femur – middle region	Hip flexion and internal rotation	–	–	Lumbar spinal nerves
Anterior compartment	3	Sartorius	ASIS	Medial, proximal tibia (pes anserinus)	Flexes, abducts, and externally rotates thigh at hip; flexes, internally rotates leg at knee	Multiple branches for the superficial femoral artery	Segmental (type IV)	Femoral nerve (anterior division)
	4	Rectus femoris	ASIS and ilium	Quadriceps tendon–patella tendon–tibial tuberosity	Hip flexion and knee extension	Descending branch of LCFA (dominant); ascending branch of LCFA (minor), muscular branch of superficial femoral artery (minor)	One dominant and minor pedicles (type II)	Femoral nerve (posterior division)
	5	Vastus lateralis	Shaft of femur – upper intertrochanteric line, base of greater trochanter, lateral linea aspera, lateral supracondylar ridge, and lateral intermuscular septum	Quadriceps tendon–patella tendon–tibial tuberosity (lateral aspect)	Knee extension	Descending branch of LCFA (dominant); transverse branch of LCFA (minor), posterior branches of profunda femoris (minor), branch of superior genicular artery (minor)	One dominant and minor pedicles (type II)	Femoral nerve (posterior division)
	6	Vastus medialis	Shaft of femur – lower intertrochanteric line, spiral line, medial linea aspera and medial intermuscular septum	Quadriceps tendon–patella tendon–tibial tuberosity	Knee extension, patellar stabilization	Branch of superficial femoral artery (dominant); distal branches of the superficial femoral artery (minor), branches of descending genicular artery (minor)	One dominant and minor pedicles (type II)	Femoral nerve (posterior division)

#	Muscle	Origin	Insertion	Action	Blood supply	Pedicles	Nerve supply
7	**Vastus intermedialis**	Shaft of femur – anterior, inferior one-third	Quadriceps tendon–patella tendon–tibial tuberosity	Knee extension	Lateral direct branch from the profunda femoris (dominant); medial direct branch from the profunda femoris (minor)	One dominant and minor pedicles (type II)	Femoral nerve (posterior division)
8	**Articularis genu**	Femur – anterior, distal surface of shaft	Apex of suprapatellar bursa	Retracts bursa as knee extends	Direct branch of profunda femoris	–	Femoral nerve (posterior division)
Posterior compartment							
9	**Biceps femoris**	Long head: ischial tuberosity – posterior surface Short head: linea aspera – middle third and lateral supracondylar ridge of femur	Lateral condyle of tibia & head of fibula	Long head: extends knee Both heads: flexes and laterally rotates knee	Long head: first perforating branch of profunda femoris (dominant); inferior gluteal artery branch (minor), second perforating branch of profunda (minor); short head: second or third perforating branch of profunda (dominant); superior lateral genicular artery (minor)	One dominant and minor pedicles (type II)	Long head: tibial nerve Short head: common peroneal nerve
10	**Semitendinosus**	Ischial tuberosity – medial surface	Medial, proximal tibia (pes anserinus) – below gracilis insertion	Extends hip, flexes, and medially rotates the knee	First perforating branch of profunda femoris (dominant); inferior gluteal artery branch (minor), second or third perforating branch of profunda (minor), superficial femoral artery branch (minor)	One dominant and minor pedicles (type II)	Tibial nerve
11	**Semimembranosus**	Ischial tuberosity – lateral surface	Medial condyle	Extends hip, flexes, and medially rotates the knee	First perforating branch of profunda femoris (dominant); muscular branch of inferior gluteal artery (minor), descending branch of MCFA, inferior medial genicular artery	One dominant and minor pedicles (type II)	Tibial nerve
Adductor compartment							
12	**Adductor magnus**	Pubic bone – ischiopubic ramus	Femoral shaft, inferior – lower gluteal line and linea aspera	Hip adduction, internal hip rotation	Branches from the obturator, profunda femoris, and superficial femoral arteries	–	Obturator nerve (posterior division)

Continued

Table 1.2 Thigh musculature—cont'd

	Muscle	Origin	Insertion	Function	Blood supply	Flap blood supply type	Innervation
13	**Adductor longus**	Pubic bone – pubic tubercle	Femur – inferior aspect of linea aspera	Hip adduction, internal hip rotation	Branch from profunda femoris (artery to the adductors); branches from MCFA, distal branch from the superficial femoral artery	–	Obturator nerve (anterior division)
14	**Adductor brevis**	Pubic bone – superior and inferior ramus	Femur – superior aspect of linea aspera	Hip adduction	Variable – branch of profunda femoris versus branch from MCFA; obturator artery	–	Obturator nerve (anterior division)
15	**Gracilis**	Pubic bone – ischiopubic ramus	Medial, proximal tibia (pes anserinus), below the sartorius	Hip adduction, knee flexion, and internal rotation	Ascending branch of MCFA (dominant); 1–2 branches from the superficial femoral artery	One dominant and minor pedicles (type II)	Obturator nerve (anterior division)
16	**Pectineus**	Pubic bone	Proximal femur – below the lesser trochanter	Hip adduction, knee flexion, and internal rotation	Branches from the MCFA, common femoral, and obturator arteries	–	Femoral nerve (anterior division)
Extracompartmental							
17	**Tensor fascia latae**	Iliac crest	Iliotibial tract-lateral tibia condyle (anterior surface)	Maintains knee extension (assists gluteus maximus) and hip abduction	Ascending branch of the LCFA	One dominant artery (type I)	Superior gluteal nerve

ASIS, anterior superior iliac spine; LCFA, lateral circumflex femoral artery; MCFA, medial circumflex femoral artery.

Superficial dissections

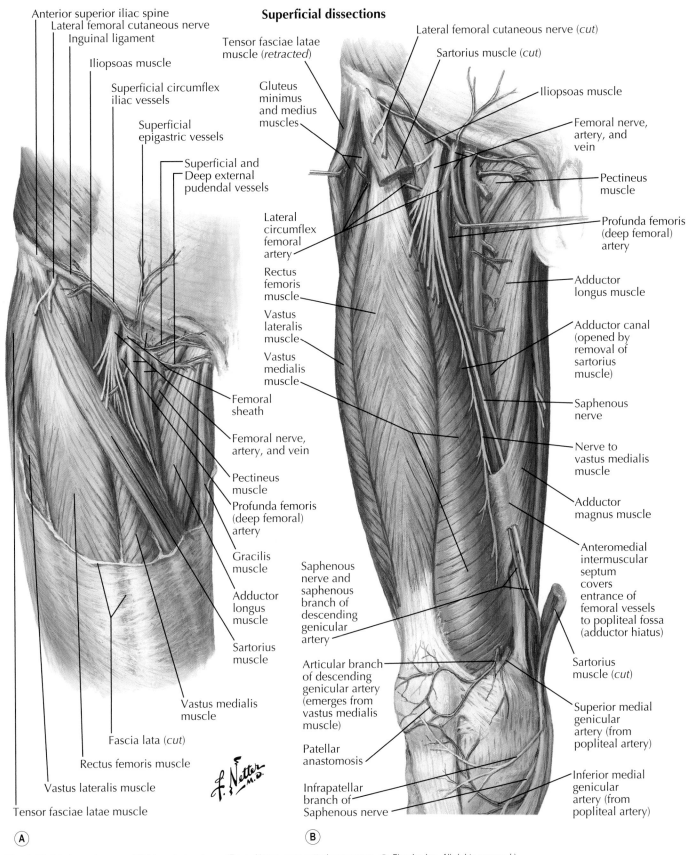

Anterior superior iliac spine
Lateral femoral cutaneous nerve
Inguinal ligament
Iliopsoas muscle
Superficial circumflex iliac vessels
Superficial epigastric vessels
Superficial and Deep external pudendal vessels
Lateral circumflex femoral artery
Rectus femoris muscle
Vastus lateralis muscle
Vastus medialis muscle
Femoral sheath
Femoral nerve, artery, and vein
Pectineus muscle
Profunda femoris (deep femoral) artery
Gracilis muscle
Adductor longus muscle
Sartorius muscle
Vastus medialis muscle
Fascia lata (cut)
Rectus femoris muscle
Vastus lateralis muscle
Tensor fasciae latae muscle

Tensor fasciae latae muscle (retracted)
Gluteus minimus and medius muscles
Saphenous nerve and saphenous branch of descending genicular artery
Articular branch of descending genicular artery (emerges from vastus medialis muscle)
Patellar anastomosis
Infrapatellar branch of Saphenous nerve

Lateral femoral cutaneous nerve (cut)
Sartorius muscle (cut)
Iliopsoas muscle
Femoral nerve, artery, and vein
Pectineus muscle
Profunda femoris (deep femoral) artery
Adductor longus muscle
Adductor canal (opened by removal of sartorius muscle)
Saphenous nerve
Nerve to vastus medialis muscle
Adductor magnus muscle
Anteromedial intermuscular septum covers entrance of femoral vessels to popliteal fossa (adductor hiatus)
Sartorius muscle (cut)
Superior medial genicular artery (from popliteal artery)
Inferior medial genicular artery (from popliteal artery)

A

B

Fig. 1.10 Arteries and nerves of thigh: anterior views. (*From: Netter; www.netterimages.com. © Elsevier Inc. All rights reserved.*)

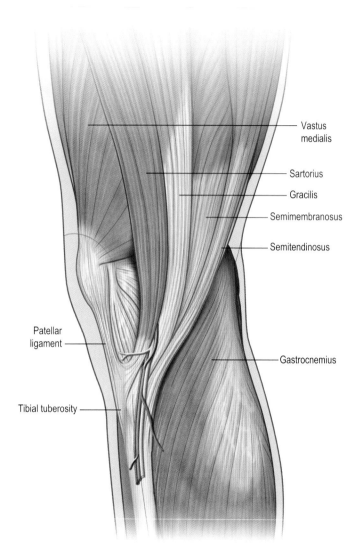

Fig. 1.11 Pes anserinus.

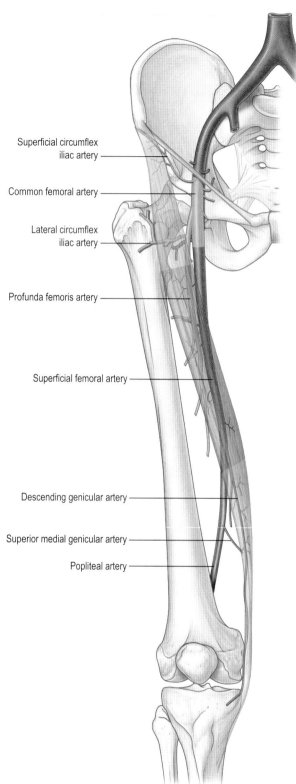

Fig. 1.12 Segmental blood supply to the Sartorius muscle. *(From: Buckland A, Pan WR, Dhar S, et al. Neurovascular anatomy of sartorius muscle flaps: implications for local transposition and facial reanimation.* Plast Reconstr Surg. *2009:123;44–54.)*

The quadriceps muscles act as a unit through the patella and the patellar tendon to extend the lower leg at the knee. Knee extension is critical in ambulation and upright posture maintenance. The redundancy in function of these four muscles ensures this ability, and removal of one of the quadriceps muscles can usually be tolerated with appropriate centralization techniques of the remaining musculature and physical therapy. This recovery potential is a primary factor in the ability to use the type II rectus femoris muscle for regional and distant reconstructions. The dominant pedicle from the descending branch of the lateral circumflex artery allows for wide transposition of the rectus femoris muscle or musculocutaneous flap with minimal impact on knee function.[17]

The posterior compartment musculature comprises the knee flexion muscles, colloquially known as the hamstrings (Table 1.2). The biceps has two heads, each with a slightly different origin and action. All three of these muscles span the posterior knee, with the tendons of the semitendinosus and semimembranosus traveling medially and forming one border of the popliteal fossa and the biceps femoris tendon traveling laterally and forming the other border (Fig. 1.13).

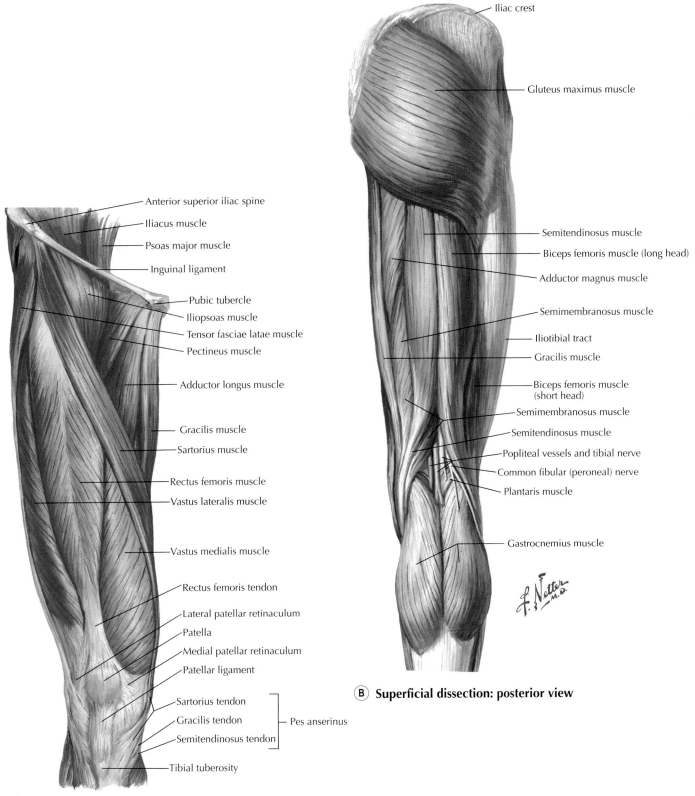

(A) **Superficial dissection: anterior view**

(B) **Superficial dissection: posterior view**

Fig. 1.13 Muscles of the thigh. *(From: Netter; www.netterimages.com. © Elsevier Inc. All rights reserved.)*

Muscles of Hip and Thigh

Anterior view: deep dissection

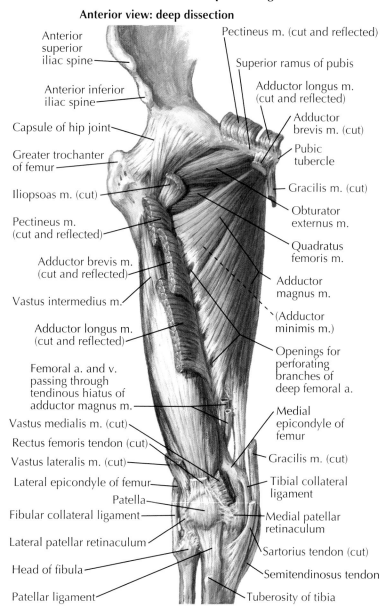

Anterior superior iliac spine

Anterior inferior iliac spine

Capsule of hip joint

Greater trochanter of femur

Iliopsoas m. (cut)

Pectineus m. (cut and reflected)

Adductor brevis m. (cut and reflected)

Vastus intermedius m.

Adductor longus m. (cut and reflected)

Femoral a. and v. passing through tendinous hiatus of adductor magnus m.

Vastus medialis m. (cut)

Rectus femoris tendon (cut)

Vastus lateralis m. (cut)

Lateral epicondyle of femur

Patella

Fibular collateral ligament

Lateral patellar retinaculum

Head of fibula

Patellar ligament

Pectineus m. (cut and reflected)

Superior ramus of pubis

Adductor longus m. (cut and reflected)

Adductor brevis m. (cut)

Pubic tubercle

Gracilis m. (cut)

Obturator externus m.

Quadratus femoris m.

Adductor magnus m.

(Adductor minimis m.)

Openings for perforating branches of deep femoral a.

Medial epicondyle of femur

Gracilis m. (cut)

Tibial collateral ligament

Medial patellar retinaculum

Sartorius tendon (cut)

Semitendinosus tendon

Tuberosity of tibia

Fig. 1.14 Muscles of the thigh, deep dissection: anterior view. *(From: Netter; www.netterimages.com. © Elsevier Inc. All rights reserved.)*

The adductor compartment contains the adductor magnus, brevis, and longus, as well as the gracilis and pectineus muscles (Fig. 1.14). All five muscles cross the hip joint, but only the gracilis crosses the knee. The gracilis is also the most superficial muscle of the adductor compartment. It begins from its origin on the pubic bone as a flat, broad muscle that tapers down into a narrow tendon that inserts into the pes anserinus. The gracilis is often harvested for wound coverage and can be transferred as a pedicled flap for local coverage or a free flap for distant reconstruction. It can also be harvested with its nerve supply for functional upper extremity reconstruction or facial reanimation. The gracilis has a type II vascular supply, perfused from a dominant medial circumflex femoral artery pedicle, with three to six muscular branches entering the muscle on the deep surface adjacent to a branch of the obturator nerve and each branch proceeding distally in

an independent, longitudinal manner, allowing for muscle subdivision when necessary.[18,19] As opposed to the gracilis, the remainder of the adductor muscles do not lend themselves easily for flap transposition due to their position and muscular structure.

The tensor fascia latae is not classically designated in the previously described compartments but is included in the discussion of the thigh because of its intimate relation to thigh musculature and utility in reconstructive surgery. The tensor fascia latae lies on the proximal lateral aspect of the thigh originating from the iliac crest. As it descends distally it is enveloped by the two layers of the iliotibial band (Figs. 1.8 & 1.10). The tensor fascia latae muscle usually ends in the proximal third of the thigh but can extend down to the lateral femoral condyle. Its blood supply is from the ascending or transverse branch of the lateral circumflex femoral arterial system. This allows the muscle and fascia to be included with other flaps based off the same system, if such a composite reconstruction is required.

Thigh vasculature

The primary blood supply to the lower extremity is the femoral artery (Fig. 1.15). It courses with the femoral vein

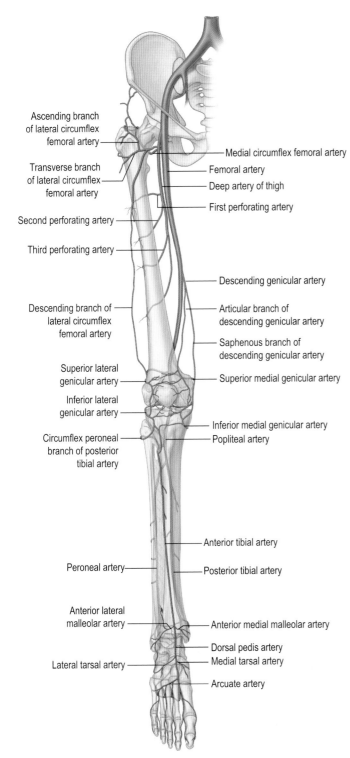

Ascending branch
of lateral circumflex
femoral artery

Transverse branch
of lateral circumflex
femoral artery

Second perforating artery

Third perforating artery

Descending branch of
lateral circumflex
femoral artery

Superior lateral
genicular artery

Inferior lateral
genicular artery

Circumflex peroneal
branch of posterior
tibial artery

Peroneal artery

Anterior lateral
malleolar artery

Lateral tarsal artery

Medial circumflex femoral artery

Femoral artery

Deep artery of thigh

First perforating artery

Descending genicular artery

Articular branch of
descending genicular artery

Saphenous branch of
descending genicular artery

Superior medial genicular artery

Inferior medial genicular artery

Popliteal artery

Anterior tibial artery

Posterior tibial artery

Anterior medial malleolar artery

Dorsal pedis artery

Medial tarsal artery

Arcuate artery

Fig. 1.15 Femoral and profunda arteries.

through the femoral sheath, a short canal composed of the continuation of the transversalis fascia anteriorly and the iliac fascia posteriorly. These fascial layers fuse with the vascular adventitia approximately 4 cm inferior to the inguinal ligament. The femoral artery crosses beneath the sartorius muscle and enters Hunter's canal, a fibromuscular canal bounded laterally by the vastus medialis, inferiorly by the adductor longus and magnus, and anteromedially by the sartorius. The femoral artery exits Hunter's canal through the adductor hiatus, entering the popliteal fossa, at which point it is referred to as the popliteal artery.

In the proximal thigh, the femoral artery bifurcates 4 cm inferior to the inguinal ligament into the profunda femoris (also called the deep femoral artery) and the superficial femoral artery (SFA). Although there is some debate over the terminology of the femoral artery's origin and distal progression, it is usually described as follows: the external iliac artery becomes the femoral artery after it crosses the inguinal ligament, and the femoral artery then branches into the profunda femoris and the SFA. The profunda femoris usually branches from the posterolateral aspect of the femoral artery, then passes deep to the adductor longus muscle, between the insertions of the lateral and the medial intermuscular septa, and runs posterior to the linea aspera of the femur (Figs. 1.9 & 1.16).

Profunda femoris

In the thigh, the profunda femoris is the predominant blood supply source. There are some important contributions to thigh musculature by the SFA (the adductors, sartorius, and the vastus medialis), but the main vascular distribution for the three thigh compartments arises from the profunda femoris. The majority of the pedicles to thigh musculature arise in the proximal two-thirds of the thigh from the six major branches of the profunda femoris: the lateral and medial circumflex arteries and four perforating arteries (Fig. 1.16).

Lateral circumflex femoral arterial system

The lateral circumflex femoral arterial system is particularly relevant to the reconstructive surgeon due to the popularity of flap options that can be harvested on it. Classically, the lateral circumflex femoral artery (LCFA) is described as the second major branch off the profunda femoris, splitting into the ascending, transverse, and descending branches (Fig. 1.16). The ascending branch travels along the intertrochanteric line, supplying the greater trochanter, tensor fascia latae, anterior iliac crest, and skin overlying the hip, before connecting with the superior gluteal and deep circumflex iliac vessels. The transverse branch passes through the vastus lateralis and curls posteriorly around the femur, joining with the medial circumflex artery. The descending branch usually travels in the intermuscular septum between the vastus intermedius and the overlying rectus femoris. From these branches, cutaneous perforators either travel through the musculature (musculocutaneous perforators) or between the musculature along the intervening fibrous septa (septocutaneous perforators).

There is great variability in the LCFA system, and the classical description of the location of the vessels and their courses does not always hold. In 20% of cases, the take-off of the LCFA

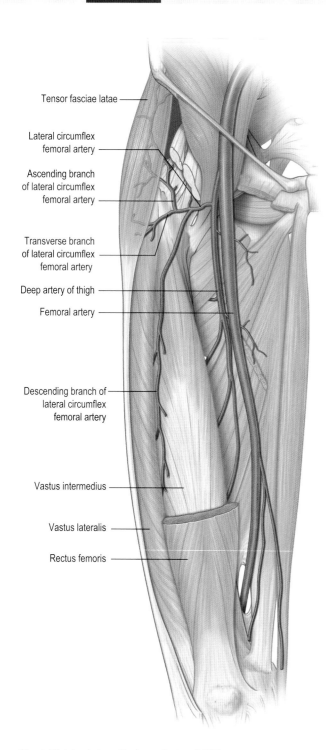

Tensor fasciae latae

Lateral circumflex
femoral artery

Ascending branch
of lateral circumflex
femoral artery

Transverse branch
of lateral circumflex
femoral artery

Deep artery of thigh

Femoral artery

Descending branch of
lateral circumflex
femoral artery

Vastus intermedius

Vastus lateralis

Rectus femoris

Fig. 1.16 Lateral circumflex femoral artery (LCFA).

construction of chimeric flaps with multiple tissue types, including anterolateral thigh skin, fascia lata, vastus lateralis, rectus femoris, tensor fascia latae, and lateral iliac crest (Fig. 1.17).

Clinical correlation – anterolateral thigh flap

The anterolateral thigh (ALT) flap, based on the LCFA system, is one of the most popular soft-tissue flaps for microvascular tissue transfer in reconstructive surgery. There is considerable variability in the arterial anatomy of the ALT flap. Most commonly, perforators from the descending branch of the LCFA supply the ALT flap. However, in up to 44% of cases, there is an oblique branch, arising most commonly from the descending branch of the LCFA or, less frequently, from the transverse branch of the LCFA, which provides the dominant perforator supply to the ALT flap.[20,21] When an oblique branch is present, in over 90% of cases it will supply an additional codominant pedicle to the rectus femoris muscle.[22] The implication of this is that an ALT flap can be reliably harvested on either pedicle without compromising perfusion to the rectus femoris. The superior-most cutaneous perforator is reliably located approximately 17 cm inferior to the ASIS along a line from the ASIS to the lateral patella.[23] The majority of cutaneous perforators will be found within a 3 cm radius around the midpoint of this line.[24,25] Septocutaneous perforators to the ALT flap, which allow for more efficient dissection than musculocutaneous perforators, can be expected to be present in nearly 20% of cases and are more common in the proximal thigh. A major benefit of the ALT flap is the potential for a long vascular pedicle. With a proximal harvest, the pedicle ranges from 4 to 8 cm; however, when harvested distally, the pedicle can reach 20 cm in length.[20]

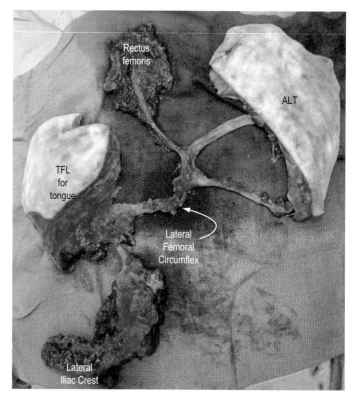

Fig. 1.17 Lateral circumflex femoral artery (LCFA) system. ALT, anterolateral thigh; TFL, tensor fasciae latae. *(Courtesy of Lawrence Gottlieb.)*

is from a different source vessel than the profunda femoris. It can arise from the common femoral artery itself, present as a split artery traveling from the femoral artery and the profunda femoris separately, from a common origin for the profunda femoris and the medial circumflex femoral artery (MCFA), from the MCFA, or even from the external iliac artery.[20] In spite of this multiplicity of anatomic variations, the LCFA system provides a robust interconnected blood supply to skin, muscle, fascia, and bone. This can be exploited for a plethora of flap compositions in a variety of orientations. The numerous independent branches of the LCFA system allow for

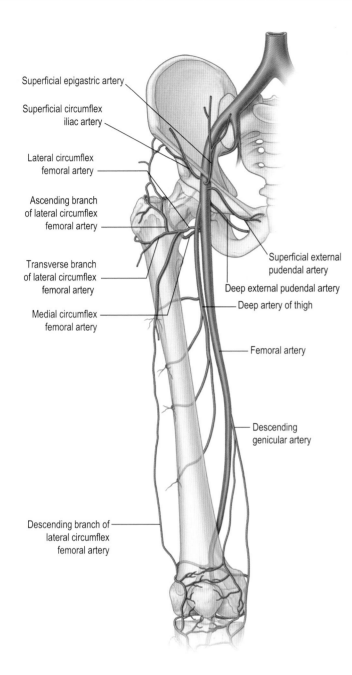

Superficial epigastric artery

Superficial circumflex
iliac artery

Lateral circumflex
femoral artery

Ascending branch
of lateral circumflex
femoral artery

Transverse branch
of lateral circumflex
femoral artery

Medial circumflex
femoral artery

Superficial external
pudendal artery

Deep external pudendal artery

Deep artery of thigh

Femoral artery

Descending
genicular artery

Descending branch of
lateral circumflex
femoral artery

Fig. 1.18 Profunda femoris perforating branches.

Medial circumflex femoral arterial system

The MCFA emerges from the medial and posterior aspect of the profunda, winds around the medial side of the femur, passes between the pectineus and the psoas major, and then between the obturator externus and the adductor brevis to supply the adductor compartment (Fig. 1.18). As the artery passes between the quadratus femoris and the adductor magnus, it splits into descending and transverse branches. The transverse branch passes posteriorly to the femur and joins the transverse branch of the LCFA and the IGA, known as the cruciate connection. The descending branch of the MCFA branches into several muscular branches to supply the gracilis muscle. The MCFA system mirrors the LCFA system as a nexus of branches that supply multiple different muscles

and cutaneous regions. Branches of the MCFA are typically smaller than those of the LCFA. However, patients with small or absent LCFA perforators tend to have larger branches from the MCFA, suggesting a reciprocal dominance of blood supply.[26]

Profunda femoris perforating branches

There are typically four perforating branches of the profunda femoris that arise distal to the circumflex arteries. Their name is derived from the course of the vessels traveling posteriorly near the linea aspera of the femur. These vessels perforate the tendon of the adductor magnus under small tendinous arches to supply the posterior thigh. The first perforating branch emerges from the profunda femoris above the adductor brevis, the second from in front of the adductor, and the third immediately below it. The distal aspect of the profunda becomes the fourth perforator (Fig. 1.18). The first perforating branch supplies the adductor brevis, adductor magnus, biceps femoris, and gluteus maximus. The second perforating branch is larger than the first and divides into an ascending and descending branch. These branches supply the posterior compartment muscles and the endosteal blood supply to the femoral bone. The third and fourth perforating branches also supply the posterior femoral muscles and join with branches of the MCFA and the popliteal artery.

Innervation of the thigh

Motor innervation

The nerve supply of the compartments in the thigh follows a "one compartment, one nerve" pattern. The femoral nerve supplies the anterior compartment, the obturator nerve supplies the medial compartment, and the sciatic nerve supplies the musculature of the posterior compartment. Innervation to the thigh is derived originally from the lumbosacral plexus. The femoral nerve, arising from the L2–L4 nerve roots, passes beneath the inguinal ligament and splits into anterior and posterior divisions around the lateral femoral circumflex artery (Fig. 1.19). The anterior division supplies motor innervation to the sartorius and gives off the intermediate and medial cutaneous nerves of the thigh. The posterior division of the femoral nerve provides motor innervation to the quadriceps and sensory fibers to the knee joint, and also gives rise to the saphenous nerve. The obturator nerve, also arising from the L2–L4 spinal roots, enters the thigh through the obturator foramen and splits into anterior and posterior branches. The anterior branch of the obturator nerve provides motor innervation to the adductor longus brevis and gracilis and sensory innervation to the hip joint, and communicates with the saphenous nerve to innervate the medial leg. The posterior branch of the obturator nerve innervates the adductor magnus and supplies sensory innervation to a portion of the knee joint capsule. The sciatic nerve is the largest nerve in the body, arising from the L4–S3 nerve roots and entering the thigh through the sciatic foramen inferior to the piriformis (Fig. 1.20). It divides into its two major components, the tibial and the common peroneal nerve, at a variable point within the thigh. The tibial nerve supplies all hamstring muscles with the exception of the short head of the biceps femoris, which is innervated by the common peroneal nerve.

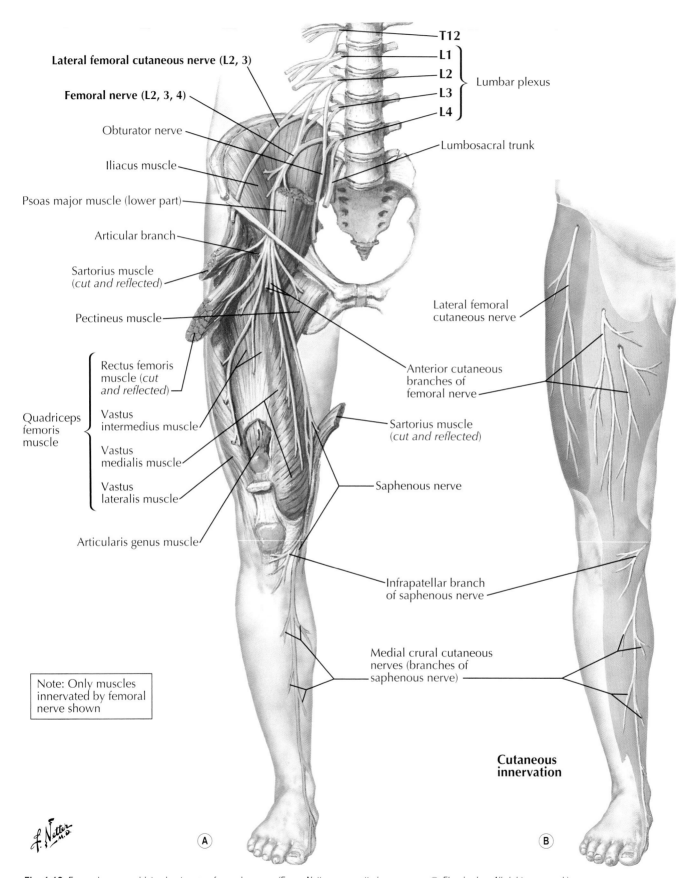

Lateral femoral cutaneous nerve (L2, 3)

Femoral nerve (L2, 3, 4)

Obturator nerve

Iliacus muscle

Psoas major muscle (lower part)

Articular branch

Sartorius muscle
(*cut and reflected*)

Pectineus muscle

Rectus femoris
muscle (*cut
and reflected*)

Quadriceps
femoris
muscle

Vastus
intermedius muscle

Vastus
medialis muscle

Vastus
lateralis muscle

Articularis genus muscle

Note: Only muscles
innervated by femoral
nerve shown

T12

L1
L2
L3
L4

Lumbar plexus

Lumbosacral trunk

Lateral femoral
cutaneous nerve

Anterior cutaneous
branches of
femoral nerve

Sartorius muscle
(*cut and reflected*)

Saphenous nerve

Infrapatellar branch
of saphenous nerve

Medial crural cutaneous
nerves (branches of
saphenous nerve)

Cutaneous
innervation

Ⓐ

Ⓑ

Fig. 1.19 Femoral nerve and lateral cutaneous femoral nerves. (*From: Netter; www.netterimages.com.* © *Elsevier Inc. All rights reserved.*)

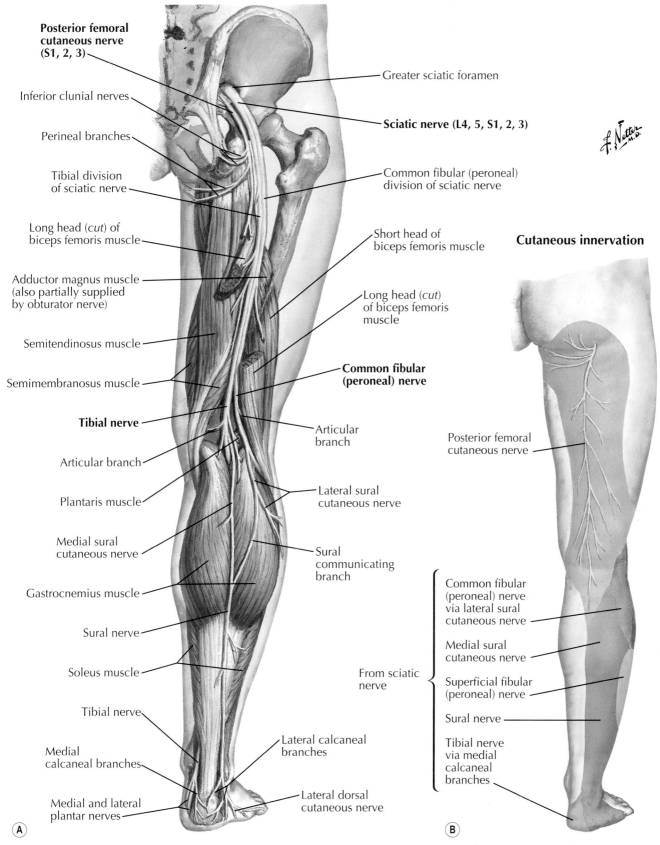

Posterior femoral cutaneous nerve (S1, 2, 3)

Inferior clunial nerves

Perineal branches

Tibial division of sciatic nerve

Long head (*cut*) of biceps femoris muscle

Adductor magnus muscle (also partially supplied by obturator nerve)

Semitendinosus muscle

Semimembranosus muscle

Tibial nerve

Articular branch

Plantaris muscle

Medial sural cutaneous nerve

Gastrocnemius muscle

Sural nerve

Soleus muscle

Tibial nerve

Medial calcaneal branches

Medial and lateral plantar nerves

Greater sciatic foramen

Sciatic nerve (L4, 5, S1, 2, 3)

Common fibular (peroneal) division of sciatic nerve

Short head of biceps femoris muscle

Long head (*cut*) of biceps femoris muscle

Common fibular (peroneal) nerve

Articular branch

Lateral sural cutaneous nerve

Sural communicating branch

Lateral calcaneal branches

Lateral dorsal cutaneous nerve

Cutaneous innervation

Posterior femoral cutaneous nerve

From sciatic nerve

Common fibular (peroneal) nerve via lateral sural cutaneous nerve

Medial sural cutaneous nerve

Superficial fibular (peroneal) nerve

Sural nerve

Tibial nerve via medial calcaneal branches

(A)

(B)

Fig. 1.20 Sciatic nerve (L4, L5; S1, S2, S3) and posterior femoral cutaneous nerve (S1, S2, S3). *(From: Netter; www.netterimages.com. © Elsevier Inc. All rights reserved.)*

Cutaneous innervation

The cutaneous innervation of the thigh is shared by two pure cutaneous nerves directly branching from the lumbosacral plexus (lateral and posterior femoral cutaneous nerves) and cutaneous branches from two mixed nerves (femoral and obturator) (Figs. 1.19–1.21).

The lateral femoral cutaneous nerve arises from the dorsal branches of the second and third lumbar rami. It travels from intra-abdominal and behind the descending colon to exit to the thigh underneath or through the inguinal ligament. The nerve may become entrapped or compressed at this point in a condition known as meralgia paresthetica. The lateral femoral cutaneous nerve divides into an anterior and posterior branch. The anterior branch pierces the fascia lata and becomes superficial ≈10 cm below the ASIS. The posterior branch pierces the fascia lata more superiorly than the anterior branch. The posterior branch supplies the cutaneous region around the greater trochanter and midthigh. The anterior branch supplies the anterolateral skin of the thigh down to the knee.

The posterior femoral cutaneous nerve arises from the first and second sacral rami. It leaves the pelvis via the greater sciatic foramen and descends distally under the gluteus maximus with the inferior gluteal vessels. It travels down the thigh superficial to the long head of the biceps femoris but still under the fascia lata. It pierces the deep fascia behind the knee, and its terminal branches continue down to the midcalf. The posterior femoral cutaneous nerve supplies the majority of the posterior thigh skin via branches that pierce the fascia lata to travel superficially. The skin over the popliteal fossa is also supplied by the posterior femoral cutaneous nerve.

The femoral nerve course has been described previously. Its anterior division supplies the medial superior and inferior thigh skin by way of the intermediate cutaneous and medial cutaneous nerve of the thigh. The obturator nerve arises from the second to the fourth lumbar rami. It exits the pelvis, initially descending within the psoas major then finally through the obturator foramen, anterosuperior to the obturator vessels. It branches into an anterior and posterior division. The branches off the anterior division give cutaneous innervation to the inferomedial thigh (Fig. 1.21).

The leg

As the lower extremity extends distally, the anatomic structures narrow significantly and the tissues become more compact. The amount of redundant soft tissue present in the thigh is not available in the leg, and there is less redundancy of similar functioning muscles. These issues make the leg more of a target for tissue reconstruction, rather than a source of donor tissue.

Knee skeletal structure

The knee is the largest synovial joint in the body. It comprises the two largest long bones of the body (femur and tibia) and the largest sesamoid bone (patella). The tendons of the vastus lateralis, vastus medialis, vastus intermedialis, and rectus femoris all come to a confluence at the superior surface of the patella and then insert on the smooth proximal region of the tibial tuberosity as the patellar tendon (Fig. 1.22). The

tibial tuberosity is a small, raised triangular area where the anterior condylar surfaces merge. The primary functional role of the patella is to assist in knee extension, amplifying the extensor force by 30%.[27]

The knee comprises two joints, the patellofemoral and the tibiofemoral joint. The patellofemoral joint assists in producing leg flexion and extension at the tibiofemoral joint. The tibiofemoral joint is a bicompartmental synovial joint whose stability and range of motion are governed by a complex interplay between the bony anatomy and its soft-tissue constraints. The femoral condyles, their articular surfaces on the tibia, and the intercondylar regions are all uniquely and asymmetrically shaped. This gives the knee lateral translocation and rotational movement beyond any hinge joint. The medial collateral ligament, lateral collateral ligament, posterior cruciate, anterior cruciate, popliteofibular, transverse, coronary, and tibiofibular ligaments all work in cooperation with the muscular attachments to provide knee joint stability. The medial and lateral menisci are semilunar cartilaginous structures connected to the surrounding peripheral ligaments that deepen the articulation surface between the tibia and the femoral condyles.

Leg skeletal structure

The shafts of both the tibia and the fibula form triangular cross-sectional shapes. The apex of the tibia is oriented anteriorly with a smooth curvilinear medial surface and a shelf-like lateral surface that brackets the lateral compartment musculature. The triangular apex of the fibula is oriented laterally and 90° to that of the tibia. The interosseous membrane crosses the leg in the anterior one-third area and is attached between the interosseous crests of the tibia and the fibula (Fig. 1.23). The vascular supply to the tibia and fibula is provided from multiple sources. The tibia receives major endosteal vascularity through the proximal nutrient foramen that lies near the soleal line, a bony ridge on the posterior superior aspect of the tibia that serves as the origin of the soleus, flexor digitorum longus, and tibialis posterior muscles (Fig. 1.23).[28] The endosteal blood supply to the tibia enters this area after branching off the posterior tibial artery as it exits the popliteal fossa. This branch may also stem from the popliteal bifurcation of the anterior tibial artery and the tibioperoneal trunk. The periosteal supply to the tibial shaft arises from multiple segmental branches directly from the anterior tibial artery and from perforating branches from the surrounding musculature. The distal tibia is supplied by branches from the connection around the ankle between the peroneal and posterior tibial vessels.

The fibular shaft receives its endosteal blood supply from a branch of the peroneal artery that enters the bone through a nutrient foramen in the middle one-third of the shaft. The nutritive branch enters the fibula on the posteromedial surface, posterior to the interosseous membrane.[29] The fibula also receives a periosteal blood supply from multiple branches from the peroneal artery. The fibular head receives a separate blood supply. The anterior tibial artery gives off recurrent branches and both the inferior lateral genicular arteries may supply the fibular head and neck. The distal metaphyseal region of the fibula is supplied by the ankle connection between the peroneal and the posterior tibial vessels similar to the distal tibia.

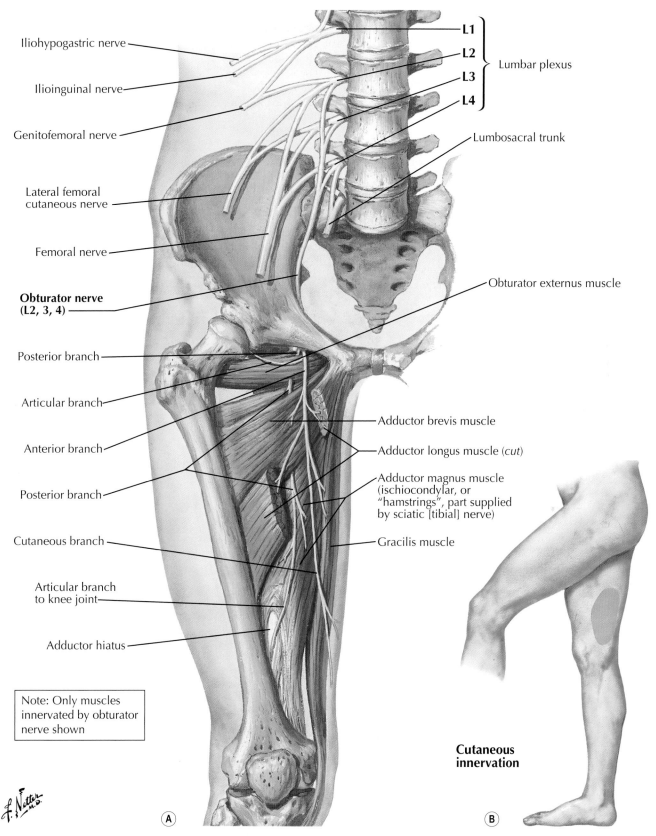

Iliohypogastric nerve

Ilioinguinal nerve

Genitofemoral nerve

Lateral femoral cutaneous nerve

Femoral nerve

Obturator nerve (L2, 3, 4)

Posterior branch

Articular branch

Anterior branch

Posterior branch

Cutaneous branch

Articular branch to knee joint

Adductor hiatus

L1
L2
L3
L4

Lumbar plexus

Lumbosacral trunk

Obturator externus muscle

Adductor brevis muscle

Adductor longus muscle (cut)

Adductor magnus muscle (ischiocondylar, or "hamstrings", part supplied by sciatic [tibial] nerve)

Gracilis muscle

Note: Only muscles innervated by obturator nerve shown

Cutaneous innervation

Ⓐ

Ⓑ

Fig. 1.21 Obturator nerve. *(From: Netter; www.netterimages.com. © Elsevier Inc. All rights reserved.)*

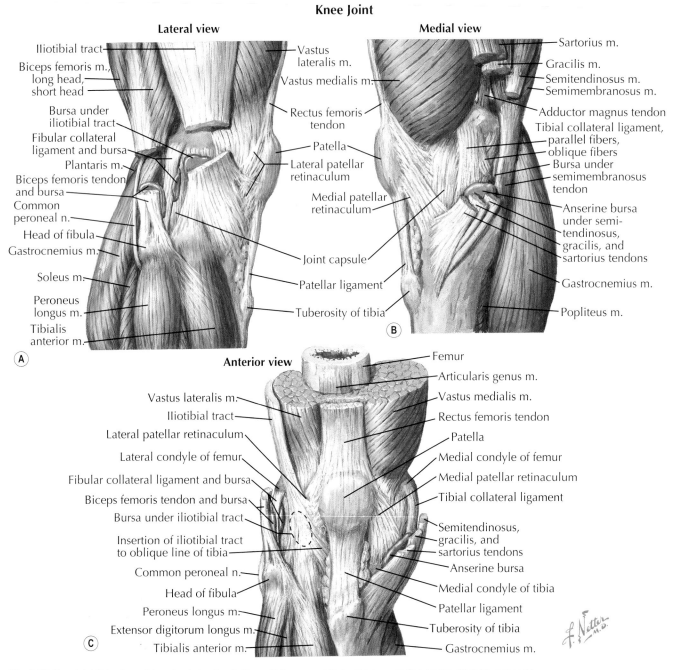

Fig. 1.22 Knee joint (lateral, medial, and anterior views). *(From: Netter; www.netterimages.com. © Elsevier Inc. All rights reserved.)*

Clinical correlation – fibula osteocutaneous flap

The fibula flap, initially described as an osseous free flap and later modified to include a cutaneous paddle, is a workhorse flap in microvascular reconstruction of bony defects. The proximal 6 cm of the fibula should be maintained to protect the peroneal nerve and the attachments of the peroneus muscles, and the distal 6 cm should be preserved to maintain ankle stability. To reliably harvest this as an osteocutaneous flap, incorporation of peroneal artery perforators is essential. Peroneal artery perforators to the skin can be identified using common anatomic landmarks: the proximal fibular head is the proximal landmark, and the lateral malleolus is the distal landmark, creating the fibula axis. The highest concentration of septocutaneous perforators is found at the 60% mark from

the fibular head to the lateral malleolus.[30] Therefore to reliably capture these perforators, the cutaneous paddle should be designed over the third quarter of the fibula, or centered between 20 and 25 cm from the fibula head in adult patients.[31]

Leg fascial composition

The fascial structure of the leg is in continuation with the fascial system of the thigh. The superficial fascia of the leg lies within the subcutaneous tissue. It is often present in two or more layers of areolar tissue, but the layers can also be densely adherent and appear as one. In the leg, the greater and lesser saphenous veins and the sural and saphenous nerve travel along the superficial fascia (Fig. 1.24).

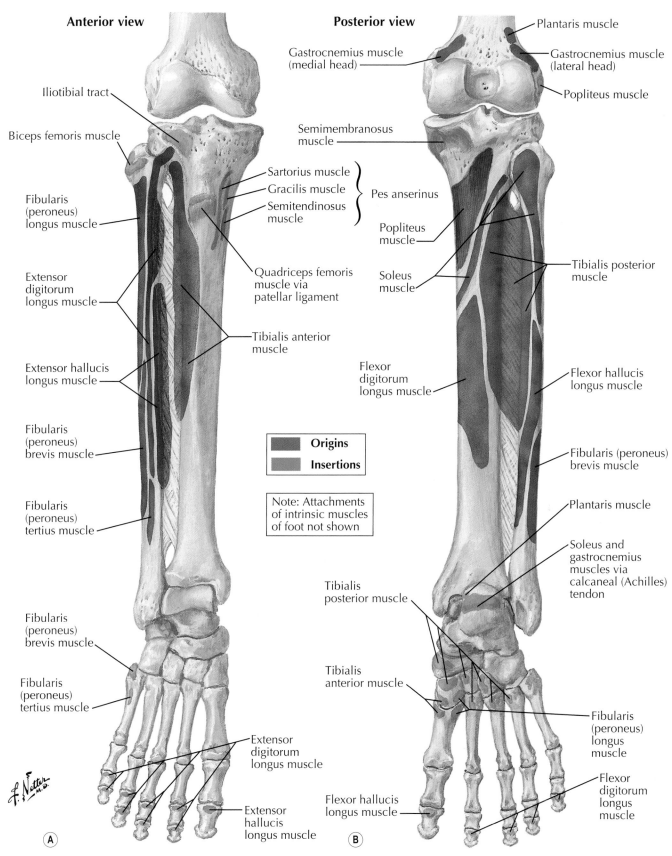

Anterior view

Iliotibial tract

Biceps femoris muscle

Fibularis (peroneus) longus muscle

Extensor digitorum longus muscle

Extensor hallucis longus muscle

Fibularis (peroneus) brevis muscle

Fibularis (peroneus) tertius muscle

Fibularis (peroneus) brevis muscle

Fibularis (peroneus) tertius muscle

Extensor digitorum longus muscle

Extensor hallucis longus muscle

Posterior view

Gastrocnemius muscle (medial head)

Semimembranosus muscle

Sartorius muscle
Gracilis muscle
Semitendinosus muscle

Pes anserinus

Quadriceps femoris muscle via patellar ligament

Tibialis anterior muscle

Popliteus muscle

Soleus muscle

Flexor digitorum longus muscle

Plantaris muscle

Gastrocnemius muscle (lateral head)

Popliteus muscle

Tibialis posterior muscle

Flexor hallucis longus muscle

Fibularis (peroneus) brevis muscle

Plantaris muscle

Soleus and gastrocnemius muscles via calcaneal (Achilles) tendon

Tibialis posterior muscle

Tibialis anterior muscle

Fibularis (peroneus) longus muscle

Flexor hallucis longus muscle

Flexor digitorum longus muscle

Origins
Insertions

Note: Attachments of intrinsic muscles of foot not shown

Ⓐ **Ⓑ**

Fig. 1.23 Bony attachments of muscles of leg. *(From: Netter; www.netterimages.com. © Elsevier Inc. All rights reserved.)*

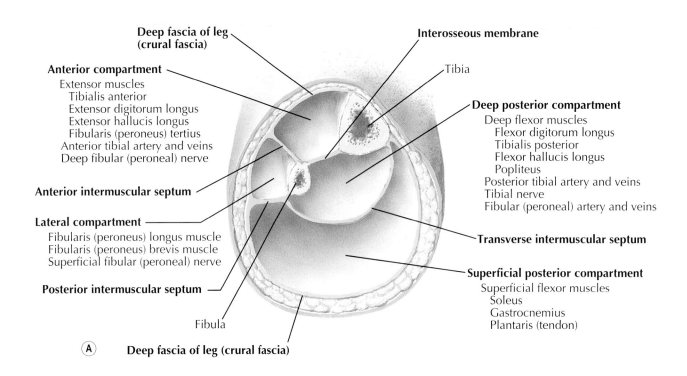

Deep fascia of leg
(crural fascia)

Interosseous membrane

Tibia

Anterior compartment
Extensor muscles
Tibialis anterior
Extensor digitorum longus
Extensor hallucis longus
Fibularis (peroneus) tertius
Anterior tibial artery and veins
Deep fibular (peroneal) nerve

Deep posterior compartment
Deep flexor muscles
Flexor digitorum longus
Tibialis posterior
Flexor hallucis longus
Popliteus
Posterior tibial artery and veins
Tibial nerve
Fibular (peroneal) artery and veins

Anterior intermuscular septum

Lateral compartment
Fibularis (peroneus) longus muscle
Fibularis (peroneus) brevis muscle
Superficial fibular (peroneal) nerve

Transverse intermuscular septum

Superficial posterior compartment
Superficial flexor muscles
Soleus
Gastrocnemius
Plantaris (tendon)

Posterior intermuscular septum

Fibula

(A) **Deep fascia of leg (crural fascia)**

Cross-section just above middle of leg

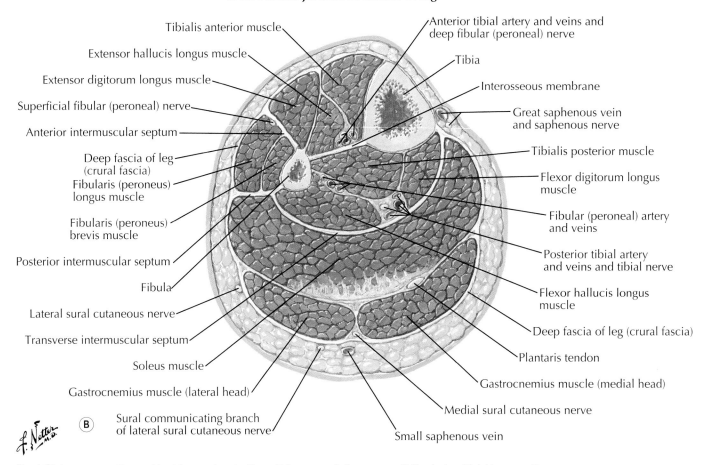

Tibialis anterior muscle

Anterior tibial artery and veins and
deep fibular (peroneal) nerve

Extensor hallucis longus muscle

Tibia

Extensor digitorum longus muscle

Interosseous membrane

Superficial fibular (peroneal) nerve

Great saphenous vein
and saphenous nerve

Anterior intermuscular septum

Tibialis posterior muscle

Deep fascia of leg
(crural fascia)
Fibularis (peroneus)
longus muscle

Flexor digitorum longus
muscle

Fibularis (peroneus)
brevis muscle

Fibular (peroneal) artery
and veins

Posterior intermuscular septum

Posterior tibial artery
and veins and tibial nerve

Fibula

Flexor hallucis longus
muscle

Lateral sural cutaneous nerve

Transverse intermuscular septum

Deep fascia of leg (crural fascia)

Soleus muscle

Plantaris tendon

Gastrocnemius muscle (lateral head)

Gastrocnemius muscle (medial head)

Sural communicating branch
of lateral sural cutaneous nerve

Medial sural cutaneous nerve

Small saphenous vein

(B)

Fig. 1.24 Leg: cross-sections and fascial compartments. *(From: Netter; www.netterimages.com.* © *Elsevier Inc. All rights reserved.)*

The deep fascia of the leg (also called the investing fascia or fascia cruris) constrains the leg musculature. The deep fascia is actually a continuation of the deep fascia of the thigh and receives fascial expansions from the tendons of the knee extensors and flexors. The deep fascia varies in thickness in different regions and is closely attached to the tissue structures beneath it.

The interosseous membrane of the leg is a band of dense fibrous fibers oriented obliquely that extends between the interosseous crests of the tibia and the fibula (Fig. 1.24). It separates the anterior and posterior compartments of the leg. The muscles that lie directly on the membrane (tibialis anterior, extensor hallucis longus; tibialis posterior, flexor hallucis longus) use the membrane as a muscular origin. At the superior aspect of the interosseous membrane is an oval aperture that allows for passage of the anterior tibial vessels traveling from the popliteal bifurcation in the popliteal fossa to the anterior leg. At the inferior edge of the interosseous membrane there is another opening that allows for the passage of perforating branches from the distal peroneal artery.

Lower leg compartments

Intermuscular septa radiate from the tibia and fibula to the investing deep fascia and divide the leg musculature into compartments (Fig. 1.24). These compartments organize the musculature into groups of similar function. These intermuscular septa divide the leg into anterior, lateral, and posterior compartments. The boundaries of the anterior muscle compartment are the tibial surface medially, the interosseous membrane as the floor, the deep fascia as the roof, and the intermuscular septum, which divides the anterior compartment from the lateral compartment, as the lateral wall. The lateral compartment boundaries are as follows: the floor is the anterior surface of the fibula, the roof is the investing fascia of the leg, and the other wall is the intermuscular septum dividing the lateral from the posterior compartment. The posterior compartment is the largest of the three major compartments and lies posterior to the interosseous membrane. The transverse intermuscular septum creates a division line from the lateral deep fascia wall to the medial deep fascia wall, separating the posterior compartment into the deep and superficial layers. The superficial layer is the only compartment that does not have a bony component. The medial surface of the tibia is bare, with no muscular peripheral coverage, and therefore there is no medial compartment.

Clinical correlation – compartment syndrome

The functional advantage of osteofascial compartment organization can turn problematic when the compartment volume is pathologically expanded against its fascial constraints. Trauma, infection, and intravenous extravasation of liquids can increase compartmental volume through edema, inflammation, and/or direct volume addition.[32] As the volume of a compartment increases, so does the intracompartmental pressure due to the rigid nature of the fascial boundaries. As intracompartmental pressure rises above capillary and arterial filling pressure, perfusion and vascular inflow decreases, leading to tissue ischemia. Because the investing fascia of the leg is thickest on the anterior surface, the anterior compartment is the least expansile of the four major compartments of the leg. The posterior aspect of the investing fascia of the leg is more pliable; therefore, the superficial posterior compartment is much more expansile and slightly less at risk for compartment syndrome.

Leg musculature

Anterior compartment

The composition of the compartments of the leg follows a congruent order, with the muscular components of each compartment sharing similar functions. The anterior compartment comprises four muscles (tibialis anterior, extensor digitorum longus, extensor hallucis longus, and peroneus tertius), one major artery (anterior tibial), and one major mixed nerve (deep peroneal) (Figs. 1.25 & 1.26). These muscles are responsible for dorsiflexion of the ankle, foot, and toes. The tibialis anterior is the most superficial muscle in the compartment, overlying the anterior tibial vessels and the deep peroneal nerve in the proximal leg. Its tendon passes through the medial compartments of the superior and inferior extensor retinacula to insert on the medial cuneiform and first metatarsal base. Its specific mechanism of action is foot dorsiflexion and inversion. The tibialis receives its blood supply from the anterior tibial artery, usually in branches organized in two columns. These columns give off 8–12 branches that segmentally supply the muscle. The extensor digitorum longus lies lateral to the tibialis anterior in the anterior compartment, travels distally in the lateral aspect of the ankle and transitions to tendon around the same point as the tibialis anterior. It divides into four slips that proceed to the second through fifth toes. The extensor digitorum longus extends the toes, dorsiflexes synergistically with the tibialis anterior and extensor hallucis, as well as everts the foot. It has a segmental blood supply from the anterior tibial artery similar to that of the tibialis anterior. The extensor hallucis longus shares the origin of the extensor digitorum longus but inserts on the base of the distal phalanx of the first toe. Its mechanism of action is dorsiflexion of the first toe and foot. Like all muscles in the anterior compartment, its blood supply is segmental from the anterior tibial artery. This segmental vascularity limits the mobility and arc of rotation of anterior-compartment muscle flaps. The peroneus tertius is a muscle unique to the human species. Along with the popliteus, it is the shortest muscle in the leg. Its mechanism of action is to work in collaboration with the other muscles of the anterior compartment to dorsiflex and evert the foot. All the muscles of the anterior compartment are innervated by the deep peroneal nerve.

Lateral compartment

The lateral compartment comprises only two muscles – the peroneus longus and brevis, which originate from, and are anatomically related to, the fibula (Figs. 1.23 & 1.25). The peroneus longus is the more superficial of the two and has a more superior origin on the fibula than the brevis (Table 1.3). Both muscles transition to tendons at the ankle, course in a groove behind the lateral malleolus, and ultimately travel on the plantar surface of the foot to their insertions. The peroneus brevis inserts on the plantar surface of the base of the fifth metatarsal. The peroneus longus crosses the foot traveling beneath the midsole musculature to insert on the plantar surface of the base of the first metatarsal. Both muscles work

Text continued on p. 34

Muscles of Leg (Superficial Dissection): Anterior View

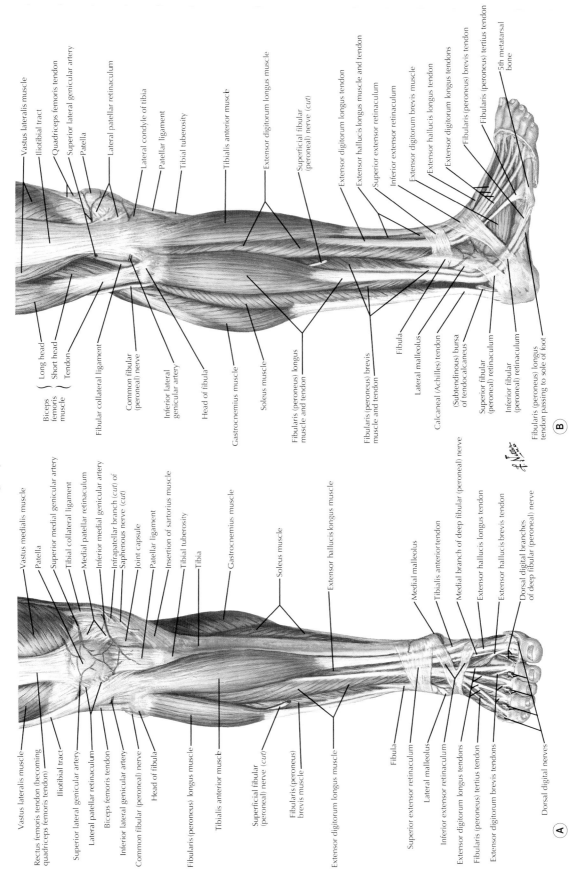

Vastus lateralis muscle
Iliotibial tract
Quadriceps femoris tendon
Superior lateral genicular artery
Patella
Lateral patellar retinaculum
Lateral condyle of tibia
Patellar ligament
Tibial tuberosity
Tibialis anterior muscle
Extensor digitorum longus muscle
Superficial fibular (peroneal) nerve (cut)
Extensor digitorum longus tendon
Extensor hallucis longus muscle and tendon
Superior extensor retinaculum
Inferior extensor retinaculum
Extensor digitorum brevis muscle
Extensor hallucis longus tendon
Extensor digitorum longus tendons
Fibularis (peroneus) brevis tendon
Fibularis (peroneus) tertius tendon
5th metatarsal bone

Biceps femoris muscle:
  Long head
  Short head
  Tendon
Fibular collateral ligament
Common fibular (peroneal) nerve
Inferior lateral genicular artery
Head of fibula
Gastrocnemius muscle
Soleus muscle
Fibularis (peroneus) longus muscle and tendon
Fibularis (peroneus) brevis muscle and tendon
Fibula
Lateral malleolus
Calcaneal (Achilles) tendon
(Subtendinous) bursa of tendocalcaneus
Superior fibular (peroneal) retinaculum
Inferior fibular (peroneal) retinaculum
Fibularis (peroneus) longus tendon passing to sole of foot

B

Vastus lateralis muscle
Rectus femoris tendon (becoming quadriceps femoris tendon)
Iliotibial tract
Superior lateral genicular artery
Lateral patellar retinaculum
Biceps femoris tendon
Inferior lateral genicular artery
Common fibular (peroneal) nerve
Head of fibula
Fibularis (peroneus) longus muscle
Tibialis anterior muscle
Superficial fibular (peroneal) nerve (cut)
Fibularis (peroneus) brevis muscle
Extensor digitorum longus muscle

Vastus medialis muscle
Patella
Superior medial genicular artery
Tibial collateral ligament
Medial patellar retinaculum
Inferior medial genicular artery
Infrapatellar branch (cut) of saphenous nerve (cut)
Joint capsule
Patellar ligament
Insertion of sartorius muscle
Tibial tuberosity
Tibia
Gastrocnemius muscle
Soleus muscle
Extensor hallucis longus muscle
Medial malleolus
Tibialis anterior tendon
Medial branch of deep fibular (peroneal) nerve
Extensor hallucis longus tendon
Extensor hallucis brevis tendon
Dorsal digital branches of deep fibular (peroneal) nerve

Fibula
Superior extensor retinaculum
Lateral malleolus
Inferior extensor retinaculum
Extensor digitorum longus tendons
Fibularis (peroneus) tertius tendon
Extensor digitorum brevis tendons
Dorsal digital nerves

A

Fig. 1.25 Muscles of leg (superficial dissection): anterior view. *(From: Netter, www.netterimages.com.*

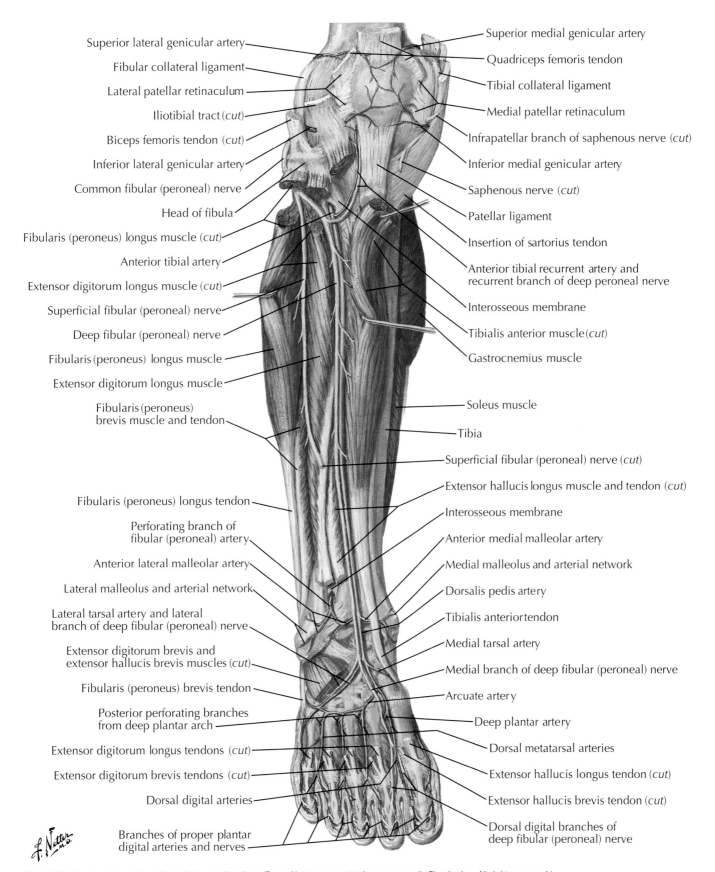

Superior lateral genicular artery

Fibular collateral ligament

Lateral patellar retinaculum

Iliotibial tract *(cut)*

Biceps femoris tendon *(cut)*

Inferior lateral genicular artery

Common fibular (peroneal) nerve

Head of fibula

Fibularis (peroneus) longus muscle *(cut)*

Anterior tibial artery

Extensor digitorum longus muscle *(cut)*

Superficial fibular (peroneal) nerve

Deep fibular (peroneal) nerve

Fibularis (peroneus) longus muscle

Extensor digitorum longus muscle

Fibularis (peroneus) brevis muscle and tendon

Fibularis (peroneus) longus tendon

Perforating branch of fibular (peroneal) artery

Anterior lateral malleolar artery

Lateral malleolus and arterial network

Lateral tarsal artery and lateral branch of deep fibular (peroneal) nerve

Extensor digitorum brevis and extensor hallucis brevis muscles *(cut)*

Fibularis (peroneus) brevis tendon

Posterior perforating branches from deep plantar arch

Extensor digitorum longus tendons *(cut)*

Extensor digitorum brevis tendons *(cut)*

Dorsal digital arteries

Branches of proper plantar digital arteries and nerves

Superior medial genicular artery

Quadriceps femoris tendon

Tibial collateral ligament

Medial patellar retinaculum

Infrapatellar branch of saphenous nerve *(cut)*

Inferior medial genicular artery

Saphenous nerve *(cut)*

Patellar ligament

Insertion of sartorius tendon

Anterior tibial recurrent artery and recurrent branch of deep peroneal nerve

Interosseous membrane

Tibialis anterior muscle *(cut)*

Gastrocnemius muscle

Soleus muscle

Tibia

Superficial fibular (peroneal) nerve *(cut)*

Extensor hallucis longus muscle and tendon *(cut)*

Interosseous membrane

Anterior medial malleolar artery

Medial malleolus and arterial network

Dorsalis pedis artery

Tibialis anterior tendon

Medial tarsal artery

Medial branch of deep fibular (peroneal) nerve

Arcuate artery

Deep plantar artery

Dorsal metatarsal arteries

Extensor hallucis longus tendon *(cut)*

Extensor hallucis brevis tendon *(cut)*

Dorsal digital branches of deep fibular (peroneal) nerve

Fig. 1.26 Muscles of leg (deep dissection): anterior view. *(From: Netter; www.netterimages.com.* © *Elsevier Inc. All rights reserved.)*

Table 1.3 Leg musculature

	Muscle	Origin	Insertion	Function	Muscle	Blood supply	Flap blood supply type	Innervation
Anterior compartment	1 Tibialis anterior	Shaft of tibia and interosseous membrane	Medial cuneiform and base of first metatarsal	Foot dorsiflexion and inversion	Tibialis anterior	Anterior tibial	Segmental (IV)	Deep peroneal nerve
	2 Extensor digitorum longus	Shaft of fibula and interosseous membrane	Extensor expansion of lateral four toes	Foot and II–V toe dorsiflexion and foot eversion	Extensor digitorum longus	Anterior tibial	Segmental (IV)	Deep peroneal nerve
	3 Extensor hallucis longus	Shaft of fibula and interosseous membrane	Base of distal phalanx of big toe	First-toe dorsiflexion	Extensor hallucis longus	Anterior tibial	Segmental (IV)	Deep peroneal nerve
	4 Peroneus tertius	Shaft of fibula and interosseous membrane	Base of fifth metatarsal bone	Dorsiflexes (extends) foot; everts foot at subtalar and transverse tarsal joints	Peroneus tertius	Anterior tibial	Segmental (IV)	Deep peroneal nerve
Lateral compartment	5 Peroneus longus	Shaft of fibula	Base of first metatarsal and medial cuneiform	Plantarflexes foot; everts foot at subtalar and transverse tarsal joints; supports lateral longitudinal and transverse arches of foot	Peroneus longus	Peroneal	Dominant pedicle and minor pedicle(s) (II)	Superficial peroneal nerve
	6 Peroneus brevis	Shaft of fibula	Base of fifth metatarsal bone	Plantarflexes foot; everts foot at subtalar and transverse tarsal joints; supports lateral longitudinal arch	Peroneus brevis	Peroneal	Dominant pedicle and minor pedicle(s) (II)	Superficial peroneal nerve

Compartment		Muscle	Origin	Insertion	Action	Muscle	Blood supply	Vascular pattern	Nerve
Superficial posterior compartment	7	Medial gastrocnemius	Medial femoral condyle	Calcaneum via Achilles tendon	Plantarflexes foot; flexes leg	Medial gastrocnemius	Posterior tibial	One vascular pedicle (I)	Tibial nerve
	8	Lateral gastrocnemius	Lateral femoral condyle	Calcaneum via Achilles tendon	Plantarflexes foot; flexes leg	Lateral gastrocnemius	Posterior tibial	One vascular pedicle (I)	Tibial nerve
	9	Plantaris	Lateral supracondylar ridge of femur	Calcaneum	Plantarflexes foot; flexes leg	Plantaris	Posterior tibial	Segmental (IV)	Tibial nerve
	10	Soleus	Shafts of tibia and fibula	Calcaneum via Achilles tendon	Foot plantarflexion	Soleus	Posterior tibial	Dominant pedicles and minor pedicle (II)	Tibial nerve
Deep posterior compartment	11	Popliteus	Lateral condyle of femur	Shaft of medial tibia	Flexes leg; unlocks full extension of knee by laterally rotating femur on tibia	Popliteus	Medial and lateral genicular arteries	Segmental (IV)	Tibial nerve
	12	Flexor digitorum longus	Shaft of tibia	Distal phalanges of lateral four toes	Flexes distal phalanges of lateral four toes; plantarflexes foot; supports medial and lateral longitudinal arches of foot	Flexor digitorum longus	Posterior tibial branches	Segmental (IV)	Tibial nerve
	13	Flexor hallucis longus	Shaft of fibula	Base of distal phalanx of big toe	Flexes distal phalanx of big toe; plantarflexes foot; supports medial longitudinal arch	Flexor hallucis longus	Peroneal branches	Segmental (IV)	Tibial nerve
	14	Tibialis posterior	Shafts of tibia and fibula and interosseous membrane	Tuberosity of navicular bone and the medial cuneiform	Plantarflexes foot; inverts foot at subtalar and transverse tarsal joints; supports medial longitudinal arch of foot	Tibialis posterior	Posterior tibial and peroneal	Segmental (IV)	Tibial nerve

together to evert and plantarflex the foot. The blood supply for both muscles is the same, type II, with the major pedicle branching from the peroneal artery in the proximal one-third and a distal minor branch coming off the anterior tibial artery in the distal two-thirds of the muscles. There is no major vessel within the lateral compartment, so both pedicles must traverse the intermuscular septa to reach their target muscles. Both muscles are innervated by the superficial branch of the peroneal nerve.

Posterior compartment – superficial layer

The posterior compartment is the largest compartment of the leg and is divided into deep and superficial layers by the deep transverse fascia. The superficial group contains four muscles – medial and lateral gastrocnemius, soleus, and plantaris (Fig. 1.24). The gastrocnemius and plantaris muscles originate on the femur and insert on the calcaneus (Table 1.3). Therefore these muscles cause activity on both the knee (flexion) and ankle joints (plantar flexion). The medial head of the gastrocnemius is larger and longer than the lateral head. The proximal aspect of the gastrocnemius defines the inferior border of the popliteal fossa (the superior border is marked by the terminus of the biceps femoris, semitendinosus, and semimembranosus). The lateral head overlies the biceps femoris, and the medial head overlies the semimembranosus. The muscle mass of the gastrocnemius extends to midcalf and transitions to its tendinous component more proximally than the soleus muscle. Of note, in 10–30% of individuals, a sesamoid bone can be present in the proximal tendon of the lateral head of the gastrocnemius. Located behind the femoral condyle, this sesamoid body is called the fabella and can be either fibrocartilaginous or bony. Radiographically, the fabella can mistakenly be identified as a foreign body or an osteophyte.[33]

Each head of the gastrocnemius is supplied by a sural branch off the popliteal artery. The medial sural artery always arises more proximally from the popliteal artery than the lateral, usually at the level of the tibiofemoral joint line. Each sural artery enters the deep surface of the gastrocnemius at about the midpoint of the popliteal fossa, paired with a motor branch from the tibial nerve. These muscles follow a single major pedicle vascular supply pattern (type I), but also have some small connecting vessels between the muscle heads. The plantaris muscle is a small, expendable muscle that lies between the gastrocnemius muscles and the soleus. It is absent in approximately 10% of the population, and its tendon, often used as a source for tendon grafting, is located medial and anterior to the Achilles tendon.[34] The soleus is a broad, flat muscle that works synergistically with the other muscles of the compartment to plantarflex the foot. In the proximal calf, the gastrocnemius overlies the soleus. However, the muscle belly of the soleus continues much more distally than the gastrocnemius until its musculotendinous transition into the Achilles. The tendons of the gastrocnemius, soleus, and plantaris coalesce to create the broad, thick Achilles tendon that inserts into the posterior calcaneus. The soleus has a type II blood supply with three major dominant pedicles feeding it from the popliteal, peroneal, and posterior tibial arteries. Proximally, near the soleal origin, the popliteal artery sends two branches to the soleus; just below the tibioperoneal bifurcation, the peroneal artery contributes two branches; and the posterior tibial artery delivers two major pedicle branches

in the proximal one-third of the soleus. Additionally, there are minor pedicles that flow as segmental branches from the posterior tibial artery in the distal one-third of the leg. Because of the multiple different vascular supplies, basing an entire soleus muscle flap off one or two closely related pedicles usually results in some ischemia of the muscle area most distant from the arterial inflow. Of note, the muscles of the superficial posterior compartment create a "muscle pump" effect which helps facilitate venous return. There is an intramuscular venous plexus within the soleus that is important for adequate lower extremity venous return, especially when an upright position is maintained. Consequently, most distal deep venous thromboses are seen in either the soleus or gastrocnemius.

Posterior compartment – deep layer

The deep posterior compartment comprises four muscles – popliteus, flexor digitorum longus, flexor hallucis longus, and tibialis posterior (Table 1.3). These muscles function to flex the toes and plantarflex the ankle. All muscles in this compartment are innervated by the tibial nerve (Fig. 1.27). The popliteus is a flat muscle that travels obliquely across the popliteal fossa from its origin on the posterior aspect of the lateral femoral condyle to the posterior aspect of the proximal tibial shaft. The popliteus is characterized as the muscle that "unlocks" the knee joint from full extension. It rotates the tibia medially on the femur to allow the beginning of knee flexion. The flexor digitorum longus descends down the leg, and its tendon courses posterior to the medial malleolus and across the sole of the foot to insert to the plantar surfaces of the base of the distal phalanges. The flexor hallucis longus travels from the fibular origin down to the ankle with most of the muscle belly uniquely still present at the calcaneal level. It crosses the sole of the foot under the flexor digitorum longus to insert into the base of the plantar surface of the first-toe distal phalanx. Slips of tendons connect the flexor digitorum longus and the flexor hallucis longus. This allows coordinated flexion between the great toe and the other toes to maintain balance. The blood supply for the flexor digitorum longus comes from multiple segmental branches of the posterior tibial artery. The flexor hallucis longus, originating from the fibula, is supplied by the peroneal artery via multiple segmental branches. The tibialis posterior is the deepest muscle of the posterior compartment. As the tibialis posterior progresses to the musculotendinous junction, it courses behind the medial malleolus with the flexor digitorum longus and crosses the plantar surface of the foot beneath the flexor retinaculum, inserting onto the navicular and the medial cuneiform. It receives a segmental blood supply from multiple branches of the posterior tibial artery (Fig. 1.28).

Leg vasculature

The lower leg is entirely supplied by branches from the popliteal artery (Fig. 1.29). The popliteal artery is an extension of the femoral artery after it exits the adductor canal and crosses the popliteal fossa. Prior to entering the fossa, it gives off multiple genicular branches that form a rich vascular plexus that wraps anteriorly around the knee. The superior genicular arteries connect with descending branches from the LCFA and superficial femoral artery (Fig. 1.18). As the popliteal artery

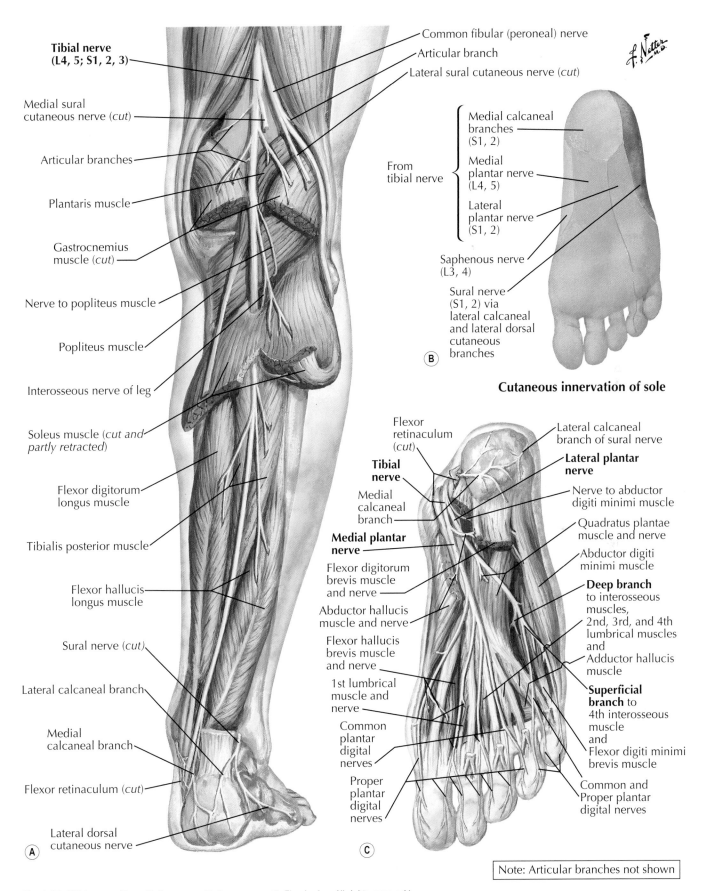

Common fibular (peroneal) nerve

Articular branch

Lateral sural cutaneous nerve (cut)

Tibial nerve (L4, 5; S1, 2, 3)

Medial sural cutaneous nerve (cut)

Articular branches

Plantaris muscle

Gastrocnemius muscle (cut)

Nerve to popliteus muscle

Popliteus muscle

Interosseous nerve of leg

Soleus muscle (cut and partly retracted)

Flexor digitorum longus muscle

Tibialis posterior muscle

Flexor hallucis longus muscle

Sural nerve (cut)

Lateral calcaneal branch

Medial calcaneal branch

Flexor retinaculum (cut)

Lateral dorsal cutaneous nerve

(A)

From tibial nerve
{
Medial calcaneal branches (S1, 2)

Medial plantar nerve (L4, 5)

Lateral plantar nerve (S1, 2)
}

Saphenous nerve (L3, 4)

Sural nerve (S1, 2) via lateral calcaneal and lateral dorsal cutaneous branches

(B)

Cutaneous innervation of sole

Flexor retinaculum (cut)

Tibial nerve

Medial calcaneal branch

Medial plantar nerve

Flexor digitorum brevis muscle and nerve

Abductor hallucis muscle and nerve

Flexor hallucis brevis muscle and nerve

1st lumbrical muscle and nerve

Common plantar digital nerves

Proper plantar digital nerves

Lateral calcaneal branch of sural nerve

Lateral plantar nerve

Nerve to abductor digiti minimi muscle

Quadratus plantae muscle and nerve

Abductor digiti minimi muscle

Deep branch to interosseous muscles, 2nd, 3rd, and 4th lumbrical muscles and Adductor hallucis muscle

Superficial branch to 4th interosseous muscle and Flexor digiti minimi brevis muscle

Common and Proper plantar digital nerves

(C)

Note: Articular branches not shown

Fig. 1.27 Tibial nerve. (From: Netter; www.netterimages.com. © Elsevier Inc. All rights reserved.)

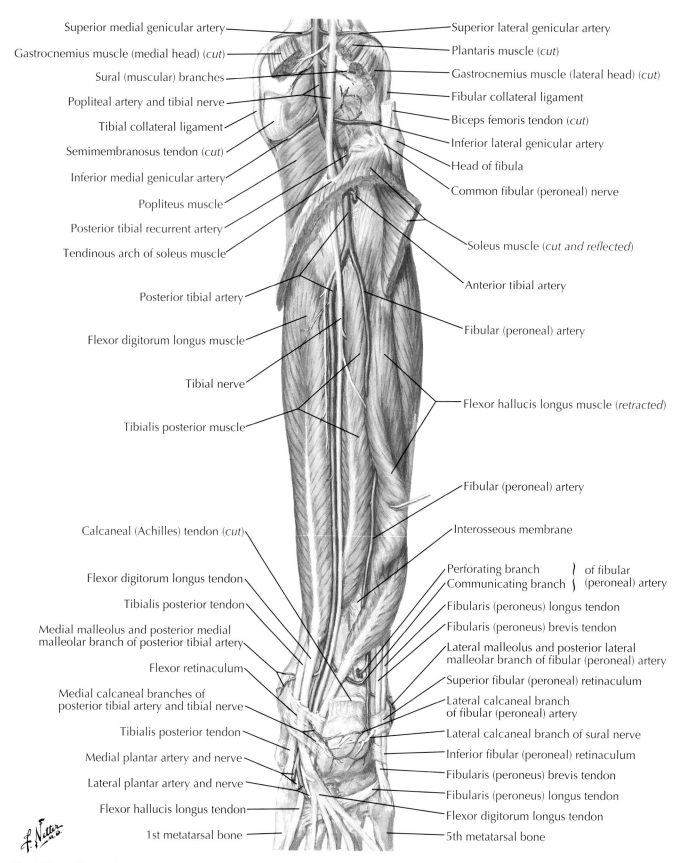

Superior medial genicular artery

Gastrocnemius muscle (medial head) (cut)

Sural (muscular) branches

Popliteal artery and tibial nerve

Tibial collateral ligament

Semimembranosus tendon (cut)

Inferior medial genicular artery

Popliteus muscle

Posterior tibial recurrent artery

Tendinous arch of soleus muscle

Posterior tibial artery

Flexor digitorum longus muscle

Tibial nerve

Tibialis posterior muscle

Calcaneal (Achilles) tendon (cut)

Flexor digitorum longus tendon

Tibialis posterior tendon

Medial malleolus and posterior medial
malleolar branch of posterior tibial artery

Flexor retinaculum

Medial calcaneal branches of
posterior tibial artery and tibial nerve

Tibialis posterior tendon

Medial plantar artery and nerve

Lateral plantar artery and nerve

Flexor hallucis longus tendon

1st metatarsal bone

Superior lateral genicular artery

Plantaris muscle (cut)

Gastrocnemius muscle (lateral head) (cut)

Fibular collateral ligament

Biceps femoris tendon (cut)

Inferior lateral genicular artery

Head of fibula

Common fibular (peroneal) nerve

Soleus muscle (cut and reflected)

Anterior tibial artery

Fibular (peroneal) artery

Flexor hallucis longus muscle (retracted)

Fibular (peroneal) artery

Interosseous membrane

Perforating branch } of fibular
Communicating branch } (peroneal) artery

Fibularis (peroneus) longus tendon

Fibularis (peroneus) brevis tendon

Lateral malleolus and posterior lateral
malleolar branch of fibular (peroneal) artery

Superior fibular (peroneal) retinaculum

Lateral calcaneal branch
of fibular (peroneal) artery

Lateral calcaneal branch of sural nerve

Inferior fibular (peroneal) retinaculum

Fibularis (peroneus) brevis tendon

Fibularis (peroneus) longus tendon

Flexor digitorum longus tendon

5th metatarsal bone

Fig. 1.28 Muscles, arteries, and nerves of the leg: deep dissection (posterior view). *(From: Netter; www.netterimages.com. © Elsevier Inc. All rights reserved.)*

exits the popliteal fossa, at the distal edge of the popliteus, it produces its first terminal branch, the anterior tibial artery.

The anterior tibial artery passes between the heads of the tibialis posterior and penetrates through the oval aperture in the superior aspect of the interosseous membrane. It then enters the anterior compartment and descends along the anterior surface of the interosseous membrane until it reaches the ankle. At the ankle, the anterior tibial artery is positioned midway between the lateral and the medial malleoli on the anterior surface of the ankle and enters the foot as the dorsalis pedis artery.

After the anterior tibial artery branches from the popliteal artery, there is usually a short segment of vessel known as the tibioperoneal trunk, which divides into the peroneal and posterior tibial vessels (Fig. 1.30). Both arteries remain in the deep layer of the posterior compartment with the peroneal artery traveling deeper and laterally, closely related to the fibula. The posterior tibial artery descends down the leg, initially slightly more superficially than the peroneal artery, and then courses deeper to just under the deep transverse fascia. As it progresses distally, it becomes more superficially located until it is only covered by skin and subcutaneous fat as it traverses the ankle posterior to the medial malleolus. The tibial nerve runs with the posterior tibial artery in the calf. Approximately five fasciocutaneous perforators emerge between the flexor digitorum longus and the soleus to pass through the deep fascia to the skin (Fig. 1.31). As the posterior tibial artery rounds the medial malleolus, it divides into its terminal branches – the medial and lateral plantar arteries.

Leg nerve anatomy

Leg innervation is derived from the tibial and peroneal branches of the sciatic nerve. The sciatic nerve bifurcates into the tibial and common peroneal nerves in the popliteal fossa. The tibial nerve continues down the deep posterior compartment running alongside the posterior tibial artery (Fig. 1.28). It innervates all the musculature of both the deep and the superficial posterior compartments. The tibial nerve accompanies the posterior tibial artery to the ankle, and they course together behind the medial malleolus under the flexor retinaculum. As the tibial nerve leaves the ankle and enters the plantar surface of the foot, it bifurcates into the medial and lateral plantar nerves.

In the popliteal fossa, the common peroneal nerve branches off laterally from the sciatic nerve and then passes from the posterior to the lateral aspect of the leg. It curves laterally around the fibular neck, passing beneath the posterior crural intermuscular septum that acts as an anatomic compression point. The peroneal nerve continues deep to the peroneus longus, the extensor digitorum longus, and the tibialis anterior. The nerve divides into superficial and deep peroneal nerves beneath the peroneus longus (Fig. 1.32). The superficial peroneal nerve travels distally down the leg between the peroneus and the extensor digitorum longus. In the proximal two-thirds of the leg, it gives off its motor innervation to the muscles of the lateral compartment. As the superficial peroneal nerve continues to the lateral compartment, it pierces the fascia between the distal and the middle thirds. Here it bifurcates into medial and lateral branches that provide innervation to the skin of the lower leg and foot.

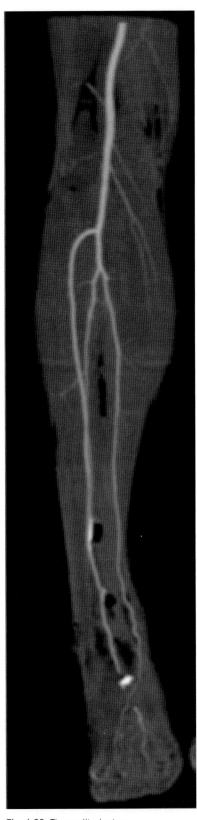

Fig. 1.29 The popliteal artery.

The deep peroneal nerve begins its course splitting from the common peroneal nerve between the fibula and the proximal part of the peroneus longus. It crosses medially from the lateral leg compartment to the deep aspect of the anterior compartment. There, it travels down the leg in front of the interosseous membrane, behind the extensor digitorum longus. It descends to the ankle alongside the anterior tibial artery and sends terminal branches into the foot joints and first webspace.

Lower leg motor innervation

The motor innervation of the leg muscles follows a "one compartment, one nerve" principle. The muscles of the anterior compartment are innervated by the deep peroneal nerve; the muscles of the lateral compartment are innervated by the superficial peroneal nerve; and, the muscles of the posterior compartment (both superficial and deep layers) are innervated by the tibial nerve.

Lower leg cutaneous innervation

Cutaneous innervation of the leg is shared by branches of the major mixed nerves of the lower extremity (femoral and sciatic nerves) and the posterior cutaneous nerve of the thigh (Figs. 1.19 & 1.20). The nerves that innervate the skin surfaces of the knee and leg are saphenous, posterior femoral cutaneous, common peroneal, superficial peroneal, and sural nerves.

The saphenous nerve branches from the femoral nerve in the middle one-third of the thigh. It travels within the adductor canal, passing medially and underneath the sartorius, and then heads superficially between the sartorius and the gracilis. Here, the saphenous nerve pierces the fascia and enters the subcutaneous space. As it descends inferiorly, it gives off an infrapatellar branch that innervates the medial knee and medial crural branches that supply the entire medial leg.

The posterior femoral cutaneous nerve, described in detail earlier in the chapter, sends off multiple branches to the posterior thigh and continues distally to innervate the posterior knee where it also forms communicating branches with the sural nerve.

The course of the common peroneal nerve in the proximal leg has previously been discussed. As it curves lateral to the fibula neck the common peroneal nerve gives off cutaneous branches that innervate the lateral knee skin. Beneath the peroneus longus muscle, the common peroneal nerve divides into superficial and deep peroneal nerves (Fig. 1.32).

The superficial peroneal nerve is responsible for the cutaneous nerve supply for the middle one-third area of the anterolateral leg (Fig. 1.32). The superficial peroneal nerve cutaneous innervation continues distally to the anterior ankle. Both the superficial and the deep peroneal branches exit the ankle into the foot to give dorsal cutaneous innervation. In the dorsal foot, the deep peroneal nerve courses below the superior extensor retinaculum, whereas the superficial peroneal nerve passes above the retinaculum in the subcutaneous space. The majority of the dorsal foot is innervated by the peroneal nerve, and only the first webspace is innervated by the deep peroneal nerve. The cutaneous innervation of the lateral side of the dorsum of the foot is also provided by the sural nerve via the lateral dorsal cutaneous branch.

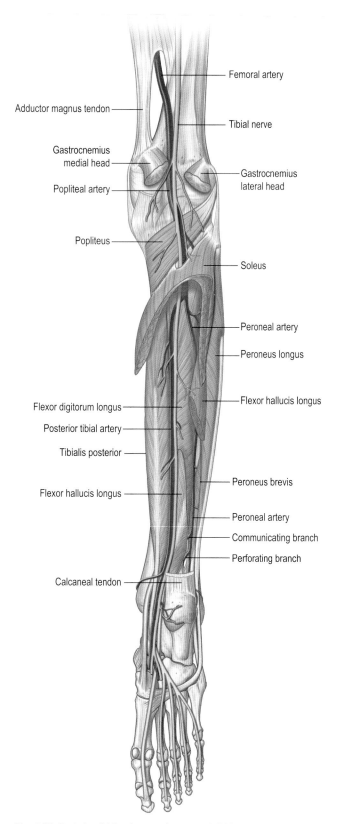

Adductor magnus tendon

Gastrocnemius medial head

Popliteal artery

Popliteus

Flexor digitorum longus

Posterior tibial artery

Tibialis posterior

Flexor hallucis longus

Calcaneal tendon

Femoral artery

Tibial nerve

Gastrocnemius lateral head

Soleus

Peroneal artery

Peroneus longus

Flexor hallucis longus

Peroneus brevis

Peroneal artery

Communicating branch

Perforating branch

Fig. 1.30 Posterior tibial and peroneal artery and tibial nerve.

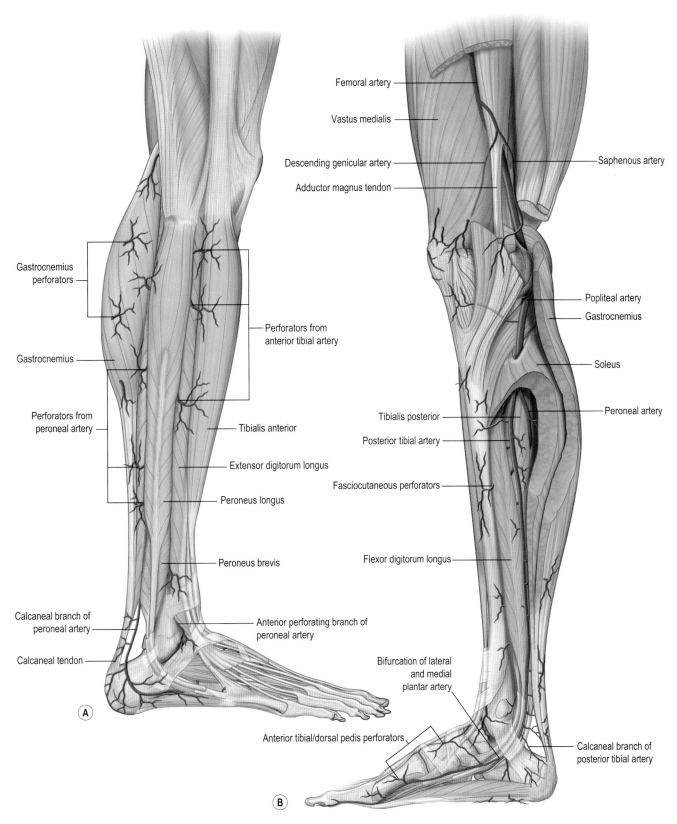

Femoral artery

Vastus medialis

Descending genicular artery

Adductor magnus tendon

Saphenous artery

Gastrocnemius perforators

Perforators from anterior tibial artery

Gastrocnemius

Popliteal artery

Gastrocnemius

Soleus

Perforators from peroneal artery

Peroneal artery

Tibialis posterior

Posterior tibial artery

Tibialis anterior

Extensor digitorum longus

Fasciocutaneous perforators

Peroneus longus

Peroneus brevis

Flexor digitorum longus

Calcaneal branch of peroneal artery

Anterior perforating branch of peroneal artery

Calcaneal tendon

Bifurcation of lateral and medial plantar artery

A

Anterior tibial/dorsal pedis perforators

Calcaneal branch of posterior tibial artery

B

Fig. 1.31 Leg vasculature.

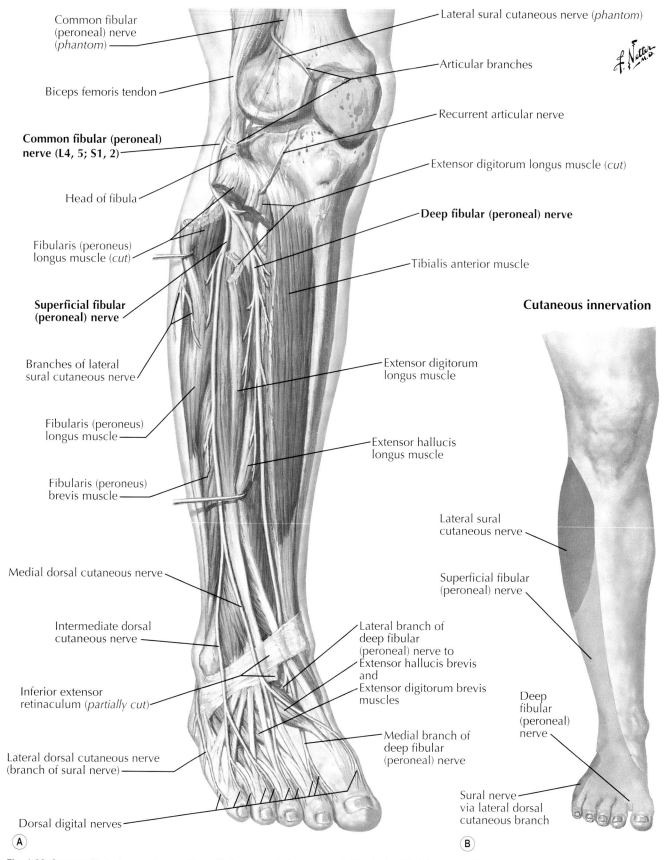

Common fibular (peroneal) nerve (*phantom*)

Biceps femoris tendon

Common fibular (peroneal) nerve (L4, 5; S1, 2)

Head of fibula

Fibularis (peroneus) longus muscle (*cut*)

Superficial fibular (peroneal) nerve

Branches of lateral sural cutaneous nerve

Fibularis (peroneus) longus muscle

Fibularis (peroneus) brevis muscle

Medial dorsal cutaneous nerve

Intermediate dorsal cutaneous nerve

Inferior extensor retinaculum (*partially cut*)

Lateral dorsal cutaneous nerve (branch of sural nerve)

Dorsal digital nerves

Lateral sural cutaneous nerve (*phantom*)

Articular branches

Recurrent articular nerve

Extensor digitorum longus muscle (*cut*)

Deep fibular (peroneal) nerve

Tibialis anterior muscle

Extensor digitorum longus muscle

Extensor hallucis longus muscle

Lateral branch of deep fibular (peroneal) nerve to Extensor hallucis brevis and Extensor digitorum brevis muscles

Medial branch of deep fibular (peroneal) nerve

Cutaneous innervation

Lateral sural cutaneous nerve

Superficial fibular (peroneal) nerve

Deep fibular (peroneal) nerve

Sural nerve via lateral dorsal cutaneous branch

A

B

Fig. 1.32 Common fibular (peroneal) nerve. *(From: Netter; www.netterimages.com. © Elsevier Inc. All rights reserved.)*

The sural nerve system is an intercommunicating complex of nerve branches that travel between the common peroneal and the tibial nerves. There is a medial sural branch from the tibial nerve that supplies the medial posterior portion of the leg and a lateral sural nerve from the common peroneal nerve that supplies the lateral posterior portion of the leg. The true sural nerve is composed of several different possible intercommunicating cutaneous branches of the leg. The branches coalesce in the proximal leg and form the sural nerve. The sural nerve pierces the deep fascia of the leg at the inferior edge of the gastrocnemius head median raphe. It travels down the leg in the subcutaneous space with the lesser saphenous vein. It innervates the distal one-third of the posterolateral leg.

The sural nerve is of specific clinical importance as it is commonly harvested for use as a nerve graft. The distal sural nerve is located approximately 1 cm posterior to the lateral malleolus and has an intimate relationship with the short saphenous vein.[35] This superficial location, the relatively small number of branches present, and the tolerable anesthetic defect in the lateral lower leg and foot left after harvest make the use of the sural nerve graft very appealing for nerve reconstruction.

The ankle and foot

The ankle and foot region has significant functional responsibility for ambulation and upright positioning. It is an area of frequent concern in reconstructive surgery, as there is only thin soft-tissue coverage over highly complex and compact osteoligamentous structures. Adequate ambulation and balance rely on a proper interplay between proprioception and sensation, musculotendinous performance, and bony alignment. Proficient reconstruction of the ankle and foot requires a focus on maintaining these essential anatomic interactions.

Ankle and foot skeletal structure

There are 28 major bones in the human foot. The bony arrangement produces an intricate system, reinforced by the surrounding ligament system that supports the entire weight of the body. The ankle is the region of transition from the leg to the foot and orientation of bones and muscles from vertical to horizontal.

Ankle

The ankle comprises two joints: (1) the ankle joint – the articulation between the distal surfaces of the fibula (lateral malleolus) and tibia (medial malleolus) to the superior aspect of the talus; and (2) the subtalar joint – the articulation of the inferior aspect of the talus to the superior aspect of the calcaneus and four bones (lateral malleolus, medial malleolus, talus, and calcaneus). Strong ligaments support this structure throughout its multiplanar movement. The anterior and posterior inferior tibiofibular ligaments, the interosseous ligament, and the interosseous membrane act synergistically to stabilize the joint. The ankle joint is a hinged synovial joint with plantarflexion and dorsiflexion movements, but the addition of the subtalar joint allows the ankle to have comprehensive range of motion, including rotational and inversion–eversion movements.

Foot

The tarsal bones are arranged in a proximal and distal row, analogous to the carpal bones in the wrist. The talus and calcaneus make up the proximal row in the foot, while the medial, intermediate, and lateral cuneiforms and the cuboid comprise the distal row. The navicular bone is interspersed between the talus and the cuneiform. The bones of the toes are very similar to the hand with the second through fifth toes consisting of metatarsal, proximal, middle, and distal phalanges. The first toe – similar to the thumb – does not contain a middle phalanx (Fig. 1.33).

Ankle and foot fascial composition

The retinacula of the ankle are important structural elements for maintaining normal function of the foot. They restrain the tendons crossing the ankle, preventing bowstringing and subluxation. Additionally, they keep the tendons closely adapted to the bony structure of the ankle for maximum stability. Three retinacula separate the musculotendinous units crossing the ankle into groups: the extensor retinacula on the dorsum of the foot, the flexor retinaculum on the medial ankle, and the peroneal retinaculum on the lateral ankle.

Extensor retinacula

Two retinacular bands restrain the dorsal tendons of the foot and ankle – the superior and inferior extensor retinacula. This retinacular system contains the tibialis anterior, extensor hallucis longus, extensor digitorum longus, and peroneus tertius (Table 1.4). The superior extensor retinaculum attaches to the distal tibia and fibula just superior to the malleoli. The inferior extensor retinaculum is a Y-shaped band inserting laterally on the superior calcaneus and medially on the medial malleolus and the plantar aponeurosis (Fig. 1.34).

Table 1.4 Retinacular contents at the ankle
Extensor retinaculum
Anterior tibial vessels Deep peroneal nerve Tibialis anterior Extensor hallucis longus Extensor digitorum longus Peroneus tertius
Flexor retinaculum
Tibialis posterior Flexor digitorum longus Posterior tibial vessels Tibial nerve Flexor hallucis longus
Peroneal retinaculum
Peroneus longus tendon Peroneus brevis tendon

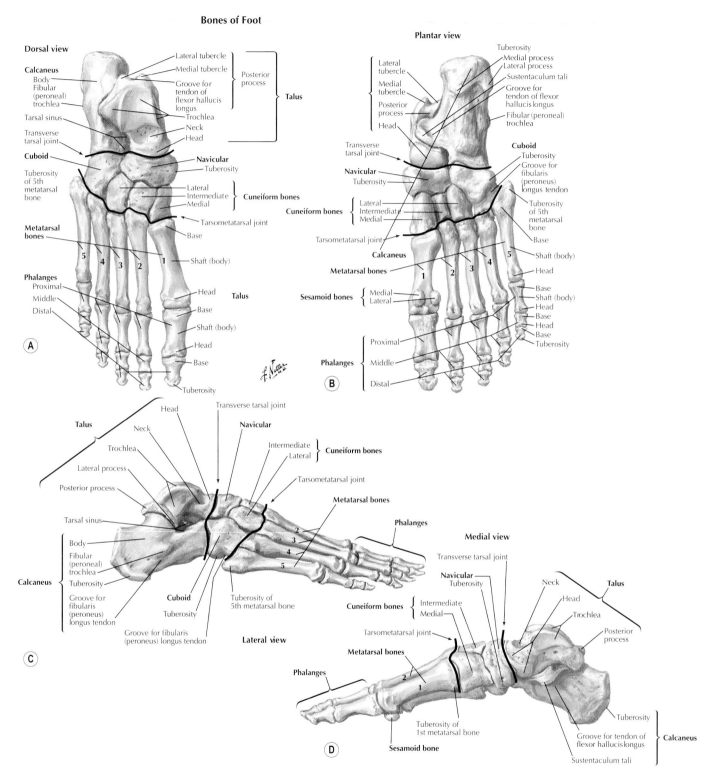

Fig. 1.33 Bones of the foot. *(From: Netter; www.netterimages.com.* © *Elsevier Inc. All rights reserved.)*

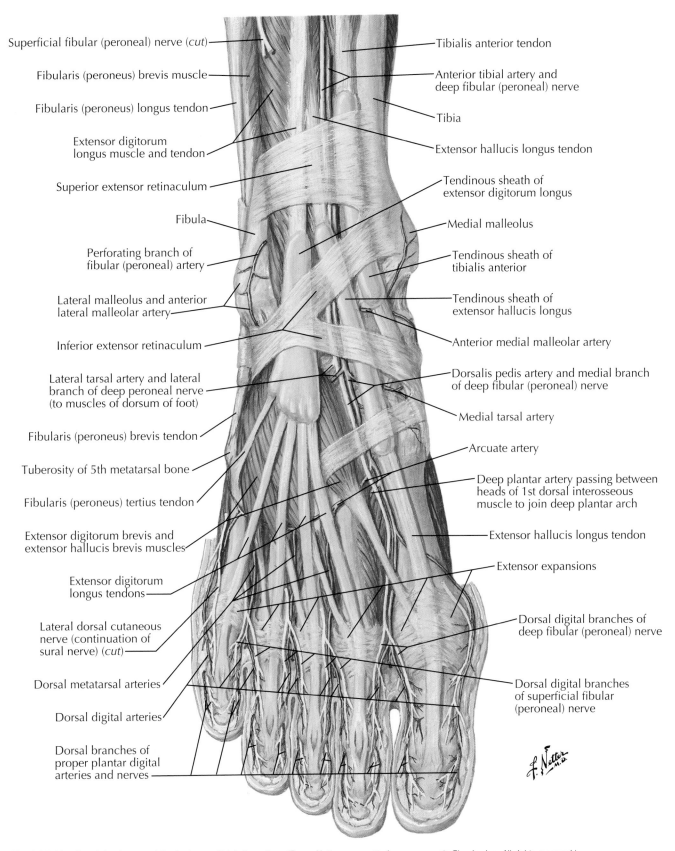

Superficial fibular (peroneal) nerve (*cut*)

Fibularis (peroneus) brevis muscle

Fibularis (peroneus) longus tendon

Extensor digitorum longus muscle and tendon

Superior extensor retinaculum

Fibula

Perforating branch of fibular (peroneal) artery

Lateral malleolus and anterior lateral malleolar artery

Inferior extensor retinaculum

Lateral tarsal artery and lateral branch of deep peroneal nerve (to muscles of dorsum of foot)

Fibularis (peroneus) brevis tendon

Tuberosity of 5th metatarsal bone

Fibularis (peroneus) tertius tendon

Extensor digitorum brevis and extensor hallucis brevis muscles

Extensor digitorum longus tendons

Lateral dorsal cutaneous nerve (continuation of sural nerve) (*cut*)

Dorsal metatarsal arteries

Dorsal digital arteries

Dorsal branches of proper plantar digital arteries and nerves

Tibialis anterior tendon

Anterior tibial artery and deep fibular (peroneal) nerve

Tibia

Extensor hallucis longus tendon

Tendinous sheath of extensor digitorum longus

Medial malleolus

Tendinous sheath of tibialis anterior

Tendinous sheath of extensor hallucis longus

Anterior medial malleolar artery

Dorsalis pedis artery and medial branch of deep fibular (peroneal) nerve

Medial tarsal artery

Arcuate artery

Deep plantar artery passing between heads of 1st dorsal interosseous muscle to join deep plantar arch

Extensor hallucis longus tendon

Extensor expansions

Dorsal digital branches of deep fibular (peroneal) nerve

Dorsal digital branches of superficial fibular (peroneal) nerve

Fig. 1.34 Muscles of the dorsum of the foot: superficial dissection. *(From: Netter; www.netterimages.com.*

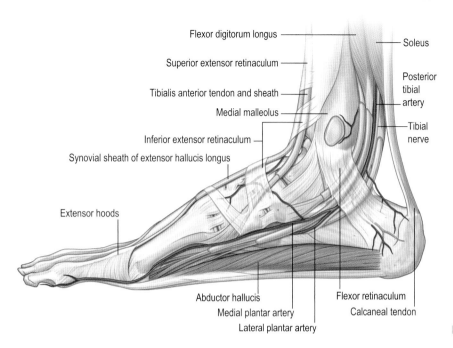

Flexor digitorum longus
Soleus
Superior extensor retinaculum
Posterior tibial artery
Tibialis anterior tendon and sheath
Medial malleolus
Tibial nerve
Inferior extensor retinaculum
Synovial sheath of extensor hallucis longus
Extensor hoods
Abductor hallucis
Flexor retinaculum
Medial plantar artery
Calcaneal tendon
Lateral plantar artery

Fig. 1.35 Fascial components of foot.

Flexor retinaculum

The flexor retinaculum (also called the laciniate ligament) is a medial ankle-located fascial band that restricts bowstringing of the plantar-flexing tendons traveling from the leg to the foot behind the medial malleolus (Fig. 1.35). The retinaculum is attached to the medial malleolus and fans out to the calcaneus and plantar aponeurosis. The flexor retinaculum retains the tendons of the flexor digitorum longus, flexor hallucis longus, and the tibialis posterior, the posterior tibial vessels, and the tibial nerve (Table 1.4). The tendons are usually located anteriorly and the neurovascular structures posteriorly.

An osteoligamentous passageway is created superficially by the flexor retinaculum and deeply by the talus and calcaneus. This structure is also called the tarsal tunnel and is analogous in many ways to the carpal tunnel of the hand. Both tunnels contain flexor tendons and a mixed motor and sensory nerve that gives supply to intrinsic muscles and the glabrous skin of the distal extremity. There is very little elasticity in the ligament roofs of both tunnels and none in the bony floor. As the tarsal tunnel courses distally, it becomes septated into medial and lateral tarsal tunnels, which contain the medial and lateral plantar neurovascular structures.

Peroneal retinaculum

On the lateral aspect of the ankle, the tendons of the peroneus longus and brevis are held in position by a dual-positioned fascial band – the peroneal retinaculum. The superior peroneal retinaculum extends from the posterior surface of the lateral malleolus to the calcaneus. The inferior peroneal retinaculum retains the tendons by attaching from the inferolateral surface of the calcaneus and inserting on the superior surface of the calcaneus

The peroneal retinaculum retains only two structures: the peroneus longus tendon and the peroneus brevis tendon

(Table 1.4). As the peroneal artery passes distally from the leg to the foot, it exits from the deep region of the ankle to pass superficially to the peroneal retinaculum and provides vascular supply to the calcaneal and lateral malleolar regions of the ankle.

Plantar fascia

The plantar fascia (also called the plantar aponeurosis) is a thick fibrous band that constrains the intrinsic structures of the foot deeper to it and serves as the fixed base for the densely adherent glabrous skin superficial to it. It is analogous to the palmar fascia of the hand in providing a stable base for overlying skin to resist shear forces and to facilitate ambulation. In the multilayered sole of the foot, the plantar fascia is the first defined structure beneath the subcutaneous fat. Proximally, the plantar fascia is attached to the calcaneus and, distally, it divides into five slips that are joined by transverse fibers and then insert to the dermis beyond the metatarsal heads via retinacula cutis skin ligaments (Fig. 1.36). It is joined at a right angle, just distal to the metatarsal heads, by the transverse metatarsal ligament. The plantar fascia is not uniform in its consistency: it is strongest and thickest centrally and thins laterally and distally.

Fascial compartments of the foot

The foot can be divided into several distinct fascial compartments (Table 1.5). These divide the foot musculature into distinct functional units. The plantar compartments include the medial, central, lateral, and interosseous compartments. The central compartment is further subdivided into adductor, deep, and superficial compartments (Fig. 1.37). The interosseous compartment is actually four separate spaces divided by the metatarsals. There are several distinct fascial layers in the dorsum of the foot, but this can effectively be thought of as a single functional compartment.

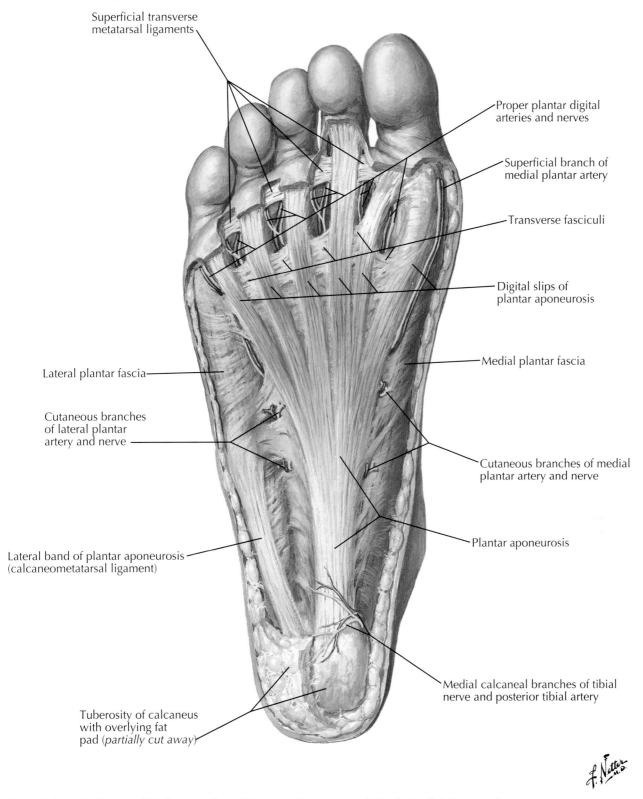

Superficial transverse metatarsal ligaments

Proper plantar digital arteries and nerves

Superficial branch of medial plantar artery

Transverse fasciculi

Digital slips of plantar aponeurosis

Medial plantar fascia

Lateral plantar fascia

Cutaneous branches of lateral plantar artery and nerve

Cutaneous branches of medial plantar artery and nerve

Plantar aponeurosis

Lateral band of plantar aponeurosis (calcaneometatarsal ligament)

Medial calcaneal branches of tibial nerve and posterior tibial artery

Tuberosity of calcaneus with overlying fat pad (*partially cut away*)

Fig. 1.36 Sole of the foot: superficial dissection. *(From: Netter; www.netterimages.com. © Elsevier Inc. All rights reserved.)*

Table 1.5 Fascial compartments of the foot	
Plantar	
Medial compartment	Contains abductor hallucis and flexor hallucis brevis
Central compartment	Contains flexor digitorum brevis, lumbricals, flexor accessorius, and adductor hallucis
Lateral compartment	Contains abductor digiti minimi and flexor digit minimi brevis
Interosseous compartment	Contains the seven interossei
Dorsal compartment	Although several fascial layers in dorsum, effectively there is one dorsal compartment

Similar to the leg, conditions that cause increased intra-compartmental pressure can lead quickly to compartment syndrome of the foot. Release of the surrounding fascial attachments is essential to avoid tissue ischemia and necrosis. Crush injuries, calcaneal fractures, and tarsometatarsal joint dislocations are the most common causes for foot compartment syndrome.

Foot musculature

The foot and ankle are acted upon by both extrinsic and intrinsic musculature. The extrinsic muscles all originate from proximal to the foot and have been described in the leg section. The intrinsic muscles of the foot originate and insert within the foot and act primarily on the toes. Their secondary function is to maintain postural balance through stabilization of the osteocartilaginous architecture of the foot.

The plantar muscles of the foot can be thought of as organized by layers from sole of the foot progressing deep to the bony structures (Table 1.6). The first layer consists of muscles found just beneath the plantar aponeurosis – the flexor digitorum brevis, the abductor hallucis, and the abductor digiti minimi (Fig. 1.38). These muscles extend from calcaneus to toes and create a functional group that assists in maintaining foot concavity. All three have been described as local pedicled muscle flaps, and all have type I vascular supply. The flexor digitorum brevis is supplied by branches of the posterior tibial artery via the medial and lateral plantar arteries on its proximal deep surface. The abductor hallucis is supplied by a dominant pedicle on its deep surface and by a branch of the medial plantar artery in the proximal foot. The abductor digiti minimi muscle receives its dominant pedicle from a lateral branch of the proximal lateral plantar artery.

The first layer for the plantar foot is separated from the second layer by the tendons of the extrinsic muscles of the flexor digitorum longus and the flexor hallucis longus. Also, the medial and lateral plantar artery and nerve course in this intermediary plane (Fig. 1.39). The second layer consists of the quadratus plantae muscle and the lumbrical muscles of the foot. The quadratus plantae is one of the few muscles of the foot that does not have an analogous structure in the hand. It has two heads extending from the medial and lateral border of the calcaneus, inserts into the tendon of the flexor digitorum longus, and aids in plantarflexion of the second to fifth toes. The lumbricals of the foot mirror those of the hand in their unique attribute of both originating and inserting on tendons. These four muscles arise from the medial side of the flexor digitorum longus and insert on the extensor system of the second through fifth phalanges (Fig. 1.39). The foot lumbricals follow the same course as those of the hand and flex

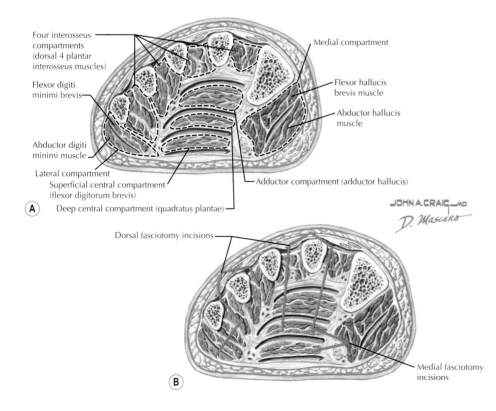

Fig. 1.37 Muscles of the foot and ankle. (From: Netter; www.netterimages.com. © Elsevier Inc. All rights reserved.)

Table 1.6 Muscles of the foot		
Plantar musculature		
First layer	Abductor hallucis Flexor digitorum brevis Abductor digiti minimi	All three extend from calcaneus to toes and create a functional group that assists in maintaining foot concavity
Second layer	Flexor digitorum accessorius Lumbrical muscles	Injury to the motor supply branch for the tibial nerve to the lumbricals can cause clawing of the toes
Third layer	Flexor hallucis brevis Adductor hallucis Flexor digiti minimi brevis	Highly interrelated musculature that contributes in the maintenance of the longitudinal plantar arch
Fourth layer (interosseous compartment)	Dorsal interossei Plantar interossei	The adduction–abduction activity of the interossei is based through the axis of the second toe (dissimilar from the third finger in the hand). Therefore the second toe is the least mobile of the metatarsophalangeal joints. Tendons of the tibialis posterior and the peroneus longus are considered part of the fourth layer
Dorsal musculature	Extensor digitorum brevis	Additional extensor of toes; if it or the extensor digitorum longus are cut, then the toes still extend and do not impede ambulation. Useful muscle flap for small skin defects and as joint interposition to prevent fusion (e.g., calcaneonavicular bar). Major vascular pedicle from dorsalis pedis perforator and minor pedicle from peroneal artery perforator
	Extensor hallucis brevis	Closely associated with the extensor digitorum brevis and sometimes considered as variant slip of the extensor digitorum brevis

the metatarsophalangeal joints and extend the interphalangeal joints.

The third layer consists of the flexor hallucis brevis, the adductor hallucis, and flexor digiti minimi brevis (Fig. 1.39). These form a small, deep intrinsic musculature that contributes in the maintenance of the longitudinal plantar arch and participates in the stabilization of intrinsic foot osteoligamentous intercalation and balance.

The fourth layer is the interosseous compartment that contains both the plantar and the dorsal interossei. The three plantar interosseous muscles adduct the toes. The four dorsal interosseous muscles abduct the toes. The adduction–abduction activity of the interossei is based through the axis of the second toe, making this toe the least mobile at the metatarsophalangeal joints. Tendons of the tibialis posterior and the peroneus longus are considered part of the fourth layer.

The dorsum of the foot contains two muscles – the extensor digitorum brevis and extensor hallucis brevis (Fig. 1.34). These muscles perform accessory toe extension function to the extrinsic toe extensors. The loss of these muscles does not significantly affect toe extension or impede ambulation. The extensor digitorum brevis extends the second through fifth toes while the extensor hallucis brevis extends the great toe. The extensor digitorum brevis receives its blood supply from the lateral tarsal artery, a branch off the dorsalis pedis. The extensor digitorum brevis is a useful muscle flap for small skin defects of the proximal foot and ankle. It can also be used as joint interposition to prevent fusion in nearby tarsal joints (e.g., calcaneonavicular bar).

Foot and ankle vasculature

The foot and ankle receive blood supply from three proximal sources: the dorsalis pedis artery, the terminal branches of the posterior tibial artery, and the terminal branches of the peroneal artery.

Dorsalis pedis artery

The dorsalis pedis is a direct extension from the anterior tibial artery and is the major vascular supply for the dorsum of the foot. It passes from underneath the extensor retinaculum and travels underneath the extensor digitorum brevis, passing between the tendons of the extensor hallucis longus medially and the extensor digitorum longus laterally. As it crosses over the tarsus and continues over the space between the first and the second metatarsal, it gives off a major terminal branch that dives deep between the first intermetatarsal space and joins the lateral plantar artery to complete the plantar arterial arch (Fig. 1.40). This branching is significant because it provides communication between the dorsal foot circulation, primarily supplied by the dorsalis pedis, and the plantar circulation, supplied by the posterior tibial artery (via the lateral and medial plantar arteries). Another major terminal branch from the dorsalis pedis is the first dorsal metatarsal artery that courses distally and supplies the dorsal skin of the first and second toes. In the mid-forefoot the dorsalis pedis (and variably the first dorsal metatarsal artery) gives off septocutaneous branches that supply the dorsal skin of the medial two-thirds of the foot. This area of skin can be harvested with the dorsalis pedis artery as a fasciocutaneous dorsalis pedis flap.

Posterior tibial artery – medial and lateral plantar arteries

The posterior tibial artery runs beneath the flexor retinaculum and splits into the medial and lateral plantar arteries as it enters the sole of the foot in between the first and second

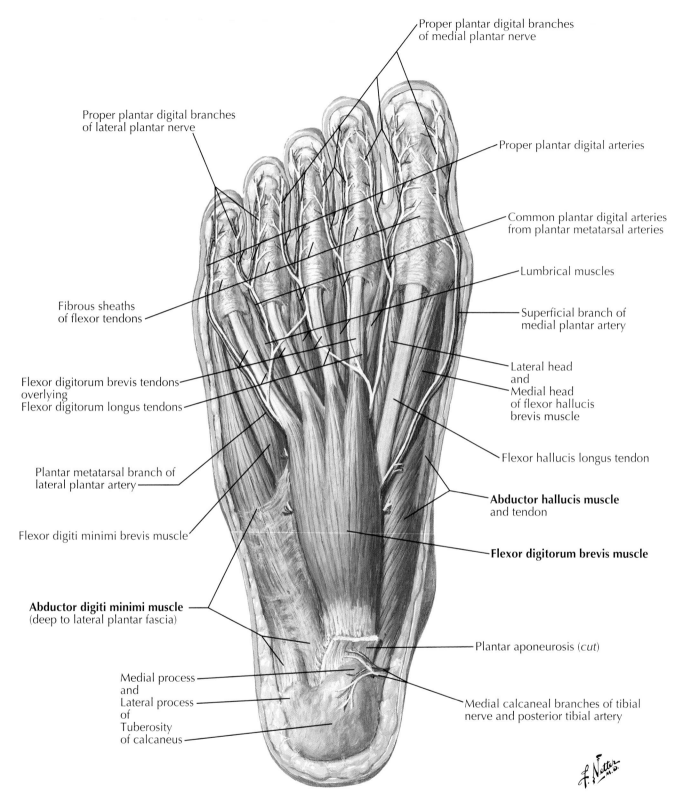

Proper plantar digital branches
of medial plantar nerve

Proper plantar digital branches
of lateral plantar nerve

Proper plantar digital arteries

Common plantar digital arteries
from plantar metatarsal arteries

Lumbrical muscles

Fibrous sheaths
of flexor tendons

Superficial branch of
medial plantar artery

Lateral head
and
Medial head
of flexor hallucis
brevis muscle

Flexor digitorum brevis tendons
overlying
Flexor digitorum longus tendons

Flexor hallucis longus tendon

Abductor hallucis muscle
and tendon

Plantar metatarsal branch of
lateral plantar artery

Flexor digitorum brevis muscle

Flexor digiti minimi brevis muscle

Abductor digiti minimi muscle
(deep to lateral plantar fascia)

Plantar aponeurosis (*cut*)

Medial process
and
Lateral process
of
Tuberosity
of calcaneus

Medial calcaneal branches of tibial
nerve and posterior tibial artery

Fig. 1.38 Muscles of the sole of the foot: first layer. *(From: Netter; www.netterimages.com.* © *Elsevier Inc. All rights reserved.)*

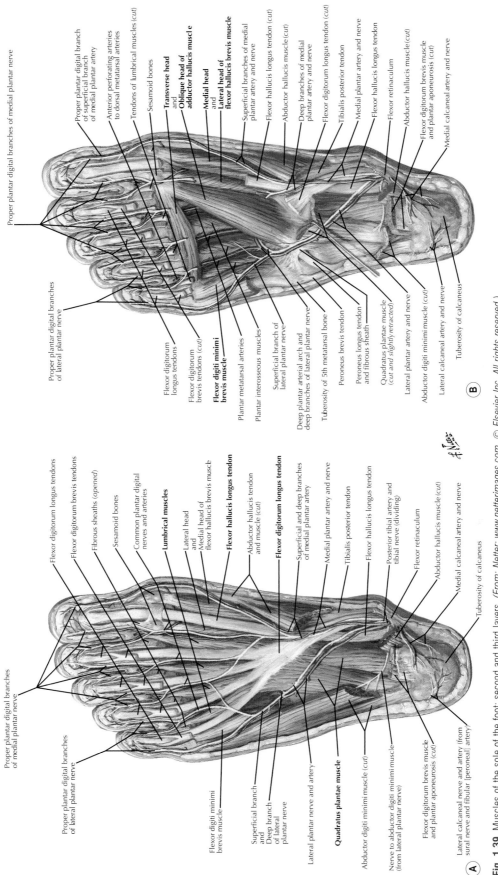

Muscles of the Sole of the Foot: Second Layer

Muscles of the Sole of the Foot: Third Layer

Fig. 1.39 Muscles of the sole of the foot: second and third layers. *(From: Netter; www.netterimages.com. © Elsevier Inc. All rights reserved.)*

Dorsal view

Medial dorsal cutaneous nerve Supplies skin on medial sides and dorsum of foot and adjacent sides of 2nd and 3rd toes

Intermediate dorsal cutaneous nerve Supplies skin on lateral side of dorsum of foot, ankle, and adjacent sides of 3rd, 4th and 5th toes

Deep peroneal nerve Supplies the muscles: tibialis anterior, extensor hallucis longus, extensor digitorum longus, and peroneus tertius of the ankle joint

Superficial peroneal nerve

Anterior tibial artery

Sural nerve Supplies dorsal and calcaneal areas of the skin of the foot

Lateral dorsal cutaneous nerve (branch of the sural nerve)

Lateral tarsal arteries

Tibial nerve

Posterior tibial artery

Dorsal digital arteries

Dorsal metatarsal arteries

Arcuate artery

Medial tarsal arteries

Dorsalis pedis artery

Anterior lateral malleolar arteries

Anterior and posterior medial malleolar arteries

Saphenous nerve Supplies the skin on the medial side of the foot, and often the allucial metatarsophalangeal joint

(A)

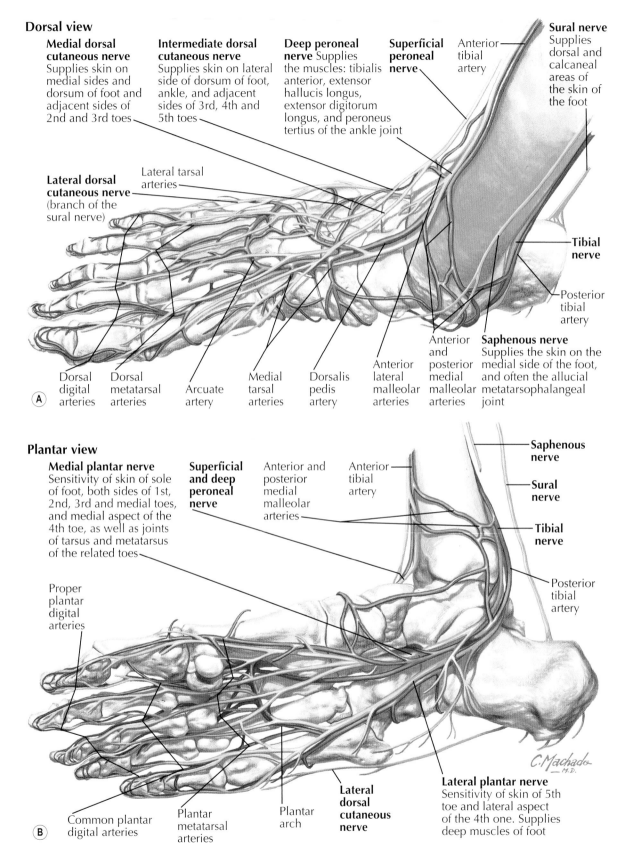

Plantar view

Medial plantar nerve Sensitivity of skin of sole of foot, both sides of 1st, 2nd, 3rd and medial toes, and medial aspect of the 4th toe, as well as joints of tarsus and metatarsus of the related toes

Superficial and deep peroneal nerve

Anterior and posterior medial malleolar arteries

Anterior tibial artery

Saphenous nerve

Sural nerve

Tibial nerve

Posterior tibial artery

Proper plantar digital arteries

C. Machado
_M.D.

Common plantar digital arteries

Plantar metatarsal arteries

Plantar arch

Lateral dorsal cutaneous nerve

Lateral plantar nerve Sensitivity of skin of 5th toe and lateral aspect of the 4th one. Supplies deep muscles of foot

(B)

Fig. 1.40 Anatomy of the foot: nerves. *(From: Netter; www.netterimages.com. © Elsevier Inc. All rights reserved.)*

layers (Fig. 1.39). The bifurcation occurs under the abductor hallucis muscle, and both the lateral and medial plantar arteries arborize to give branches to the toes. The medial plantar artery has a smaller caliber than the lateral plantar artery, runs along the medial side of the foot, and contributes to the plantar digital arteries of the first through third toes. The lateral plantar artery is analogous to the ulnar artery in the hand and similarly is the dominant blood supply for the plantar arterial arch (Fig. 1.40). At the first intermetatarsal space, a perforating branch from the dorsalis pedis traverses the foot to the plantar surface and connects with the plantar arterial arch via the lateral plantar artery. Together, the dorsalis pedis branch and the lateral plantar arch feed the toes through metatarsal branches. These branches join with branches from the medial plantar artery to complete the connecting blood supply to the toes.

Peroneal arterial branches

In the distal leg, the peroneal artery primarily contributes to the ankle blood supply (Fig. 1.41). The terminal branches of the peroneal artery join with the lateral malleolar and calcaneal branches of the posterior tibial artery system at the posterior ankle and heel. The peroneal artery usually terminates at the level of the calcaneus. However, the size and contribution of the peroneal arterial system is inversely proportional to the other arteries of the ankle and foot. Depending on the size and perfusion from the posterior tibial and anterior tibial arterial systems, the peroneal artery system may have an expanded contribution to the foot and ankle vascular supply. A dominant peroneal artery is seen in 7–12% of the population. In up to 5%, the peroneal artery may be the only blood supply to the foot, known as peronea arteria magna.[36,37] These variants stress the importance of preoperative evaluation of the leg vasculature prior to fibula harvest.

Ankle and foot nerve anatomy

Foot cutaneous innervation

The cutaneous innervation of the foot is shared by the superficial peroneal, deep peroneal, saphenous, sural, and tibial terminal branches (medial calcaneal, medial plantar, and lateral plantar) (Fig. 1.40). As discussed above, the dorsum of the foot is innervated mostly by the superficial peroneal nerve. The first webspace is supplied by the deep peroneal nerve and the lateral foot by the sural nerve. The saphenous nerve innervates the proximal anteromedial foot and ankle. The cutaneous sensation of the sole of the foot is primarily innervated by the tibial nerve and its branches – medial calcaneal, medial plantar, and lateral plantar (Fig. 1.27).

Foot motor innervation

The motor supply to the intrinsic muscle of the foot comes from the same nerves as the cutaneous innervation and is organized similarly. The dorsal muscles of the extensor hallucis brevis and the extensor digitorum brevis are innervated by the deep peroneal nerve. All the intrinsic muscles of the plantar surface are innervated by the tibial nerve via the medial and lateral plantar nerves.

The medial and lateral plantar nerves follow the course of the corresponding medial and lateral plantar arteries. The medial plantar nerve follows an innervation pattern similar to the median nerve. The muscles to the great toe (abductor hallucis, flexor digitorum brevis, flexor hallucis brevis, and first lumbrical) and the medial plantar cutaneous region, including the first through to the third toes, are supplied by the medial plantar nerve. The lateral plantar nerve mirrors the ulnar nerve as it innervates the deep muscles (interossei, second through fourth lumbricals, adductor hallucis, flexor digitorum brevis and flexor digitorum accessorius, and abductor digiti minimi) and the lateral side of the plantar skin, including the fourth and fifth toes.

Conclusion

The reconstructive surgeon may be called upon to treat specific tissue defects of the lower extremity, or to harvest tissue for transfer from the many potential donor sites in the lower extremity. Therefore an intricate understanding of the structural and functional anatomy of the lower extremity is essential. This chapter provides the reader with a comprehensive review of the 3D anatomy of the lower extremity. With a thorough anatomical foundation, the reconstructive options discussed in the following chapters will be better appreciated. It is our goal that this chapter serves as a valuable resource for readers, of all experience levels, to facilitate operative planning and clinical decision-making in reconstructive surgery.

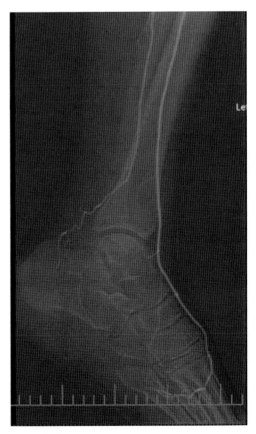

Fig. 1.41 The peroneal artery.

Access the complete reference list online at **http://www.expertconsult.com**

4. Ebraheim NA, Elgafy H, Xu R. Bone-graft harvesting from iliac and fibular donor sites: techniques and complications. *J Am Acad Orthop Surg.* 2001;9(3):210–218.

6. Mathes SJ, Nahai F. Classification of the vascular anatomy of muscles: experimental and clinical correlation. *Plast Reconstr Surg.* 1981;67(2):177–187. *This landmark article, one of the most cited in the reconstructive surgery literature, first proposed a classification system for flaps based on the vascular anatomy of muscles. This classification system is used ubiquitously in reconstructive surgery and knowledge of the vascular pattern of each muscle facilitates the choice and design of flaps throughout the body.*

8. Rozen WM, Ting JW, Grinsell D, Ashton MW. Superior and inferior gluteal artery perforators: in-vivo anatomical study and planning for breast reconstruction. *J Plast Reconstr Aesthet Surg.* 2011;64(2):217–225.

13. Yamamoto H, Jones DB Jr, Moran SL, et al. The arterial anatomy of the medial femoral condyle and its clinical implications. *J Hand Surg [Eur].* 2010;35(7):569–574. *An excellent overview of the arterial anatomy of the medial femoral condyle region, including intraosseous and extraosseous vascular anatomy, is provided in this article. This study demonstrates the reliability and usefulness of the medial femoral condyle as a source for vascularized periosteal and bone grafts.*

15. Buckland A, Pan WR, Dhar S, et al. Neurovascular anatomy of sartorius muscle flaps: implications for local transposition and facial reanimation. *Plast Reconstr Surg.* 2009;123(1):44–54. *This article, from Dr. G. Ian Taylor's lab, describes the neural and vascular anatomy of the sartorius muscle, with particular emphasis on the supply for local, regional and free tissue transfer. It provides exquisite illustrations and objective data, from cadaveric dissections, regarding the neurovascular anatomy of the sartorius muscle and is an essential article for any reconstructive surgeon operating in the lower extremity.*

16. Mojallal A, Wong C, Shipkov C, et al. Redefining the vascular anatomy and clinical applications of the sartorius muscle and myocutaneous flap. *Plast Reconstr Surg.* 2011;127(5):1946–1957.

20. Lakhiani C, Lee MR, Saint-Cyr M. Vascular anatomy of the anterolateral thigh flap: a systematic review. *Plast Reconstr Surg.* 2012;130(6):1254–1268.

21. Wong CH, Wei FC, Fu B, et al. Alternative vascular pedicle of the anterolateral thigh flap: the oblique branch of the lateral circumflex femoral artery. *Plast Reconstr Surg.* 2009;123(2):571–577. *This article, derived from the extensive experience at Chang Gung Memorial Hospital with anterolateral thigh flap harvest and transfer, further clarifies the vascular anatomy of the anterolateral thigh region and proposes the existence, in a proportion of patients, of an oblique branch of the lateral circumflex femoral artery. The reliability of harvesting an anterolateral thigh flap using the oblique branch as the vascular pedicle and the clinical implications of the presence of this oblique branch are detailed in this study.*

30. Iorio ML, Cheerharan M, Olding M. A systematic review and pooled analysis of peroneal artery perforators for fibula osteocutaneous and perforator flaps. *Plast Reconstr Surg.* 2012;130(3):600–607. *This article represents a significant contribution to the literature by conclusively demonstrating the optimal design for fibular osteocutaneous and perforator flaps based on the distribution of the peroneal artery perforators. This systematic review and pooled analysis comprehensively analyzes the existing literature, including clinical and cadaveric reports, to provide the most up-to-date data to guide reconstructive surgeons in the design and harvest of osteocutaneous and perforator flaps along the lateral lower leg.*

36. Rosson GD, Singh NK. Devascularizing complications of free fibula harvest: peronea arteria magna. *J Reconstr Microsurg.* 2005;21(8):533–538.

Management of lower extremity trauma

Yoo Joon Sur, Shannon M. Colohan, and Michel Saint-Cyr

Access video and video lecture content for this chapter online at expertconsult.com

SYNOPSIS

- Lower extremity trauma is common and often associated with other injuries.
- An Advanced Trauma Life Support (ATLS) approach is required in order to evaluate properly a patient with lower extremity injuries.
- Initial management includes fracture reduction to reduce bleeding, and appropriate radiologic investigations.
- External fixation is useful in the temporization of complex fractures until definitive fixation can be achieved.
- Evidence-based practice with regard to antibiotics, anticoagulation, and timing of reconstruction is recommended.
- A multidisciplinary approach is required in the acute and rehabilitative phases of a patient with lower extremity trauma.

 Access the Historical Perspective section online at
http://www.expertconsult.com

Introduction

Major injuries are a significant cause of death and disability worldwide. Injuries are among the leading causes of death in the USA, with unintentional injuries as the fourth leading cause of death in all ages.[1] During the years 1999–2013 unintentional injuries were the leading cause of death for those aged 1–44 years, and the third leading cause of death in those aged 45–54 years.[2] In the most recent National Vital Statistics Report (2010), motor vehicle collisions (MVCs) were responsible for 18.6% of injury-related deaths.[3] The World Health Organization ranked MVCs as the ninth leading cause of disability-adjusted life years and predicted an increase in ranking to seventh by 2030.[4] According to the National Trauma Bank's Annual Report (2014),[5] the greatest number of incidents occur between the ages of 25 and 34 years, with a case-fatality

rate of 3.76. The highest case-fatality rate occurred in those >85 years of age (8.69). Males have a higher case fatality rate beyond age 15.

The majority of our trauma systems were designed following experience gained in military combats. These have been further modified and improved with the development of standardized trauma protocols, such as those published by ATLS, and the establishment of scoring systems such as the Glasgow Coma Scale (GCS), Injury Severity Scale (ISS), and Trauma and Injury Severity Score (TRISS). Furthermore, scoring systems specific to lower extremity trauma have been developed and include the Mangled Extremity Severity Score (MESS), Limb Salvage Index (LSI), Predictive Salvage Index (PSI), the Hanover Fracture Scale-97 (HFS-97), and the Nerve Injury, Ischemia, Soft-tissue Injury, Skeletal Injury, Shock, and Age of patient score (NISSSA).

The management of a patient with lower extremity trauma involves a multidisciplinary approach. Following the initial provision of emergent trauma care and evaluation by general, vascular, and orthopedic surgery colleagues, the plastic surgeon is often involved in the management of extremity coverage and reconstruction of both salvaged and amputated limbs. This is often done in conjunction with orthopedics, thus emphasizing Levin's concept of the "orthoplastic approach".[6] The current literature is constantly evolving to reflect changes in practice regarding the criteria for limb salvage, timing of reconstruction, and appropriate supportive and adjunctive patient care.

Basic science and disease process

The body's response to trauma is a complex orchestration of inflammatory and immune responses. There is interplay between those mediators produced at the site of injury (e.g., cytokines, growth factors, nitric oxide, and platelet-activating factors) and the activation of local and systemic polymorphonuclear neutrophils, lymphocytes, and macrophages.[16] The changes in hemodynamics and immune and metabolic responses following trauma are largely due to the effects of cytokines. Cytokines act through specific cellular receptors and activate intracellular signaling pathways that regulate gene transcription.

The amplitude of the inflammatory response is often related to the severity of the injury. In addition to the initial response to the trauma, a secondary response, or secondary hit phenomenon, occurs with further interventions, including surgical management of fractures and reconstruction.[17-19] There has been increasing focus on methods of avoiding or decreasing the effect of this second hit.

Those patients who succumb to their injury in the third peak of the trimodal distribution (days to weeks postinjury) may be victims of a hyperactive inflammatory response that leads to systemic inflammatory response syndrome, acute respiratory distress syndrome, and, ultimately, multiple-organ failure syndrome.[20]

Diagnosis and patient presentation

Lower extremity trauma is often seen in the setting of poly-trauma, emphasizing the need to follow protocols during the assessment and management of these patients. Vigilance to rule out other injuries is important, as complex lower-extremity injuries can be a significant form of distracting injury. Death due to trauma is often described as having a trimodal distribution.[20] Immediate death is attributed to central nervous system etiologies, including severe brain injury and high spinal cord injury, or major vessel/cardiac injury. Salvage of these patients is rare, emphasizing the need for prevention of such injuries. The second peak occurs within minutes to hours, and deaths are comprised of subdural/epidural hematomas, hemopneumothorax, intra-abdominal major-organ lacerations, pelvic fracture, and hemorrhage from multiple combined injuries. Finally, the third peak occurs within days to weeks and is due to sepsis or multiple-organ failure, pulmonary embolism, and unrecoverable head injury.

The assessment of the patient with lower extremity trauma starts with triage, to insure that the patient is treated in the appropriate facility capable of managing the injuries. The ultimate goal is to provide timely care (in the "golden hour") to minimize secondary injury. In patients presenting with lower extremity injuries, associated life-threatening injuries may be present in 10–17%.[21] It is therefore paramount to use a protocol-based assessment of the patient such as the ATLS algorithm. Beginning with the primary survey, the airway is maintained or secured while providing cervical spine control, followed by assessment of breathing. Once this is complete, a circulatory exam is carried out, ensuring proper end-organ perfusion and peripheral circulation, as well as control of bleeding. The appropriate monitors are placed, two large-bore intravenous lines are inserted for fluid resuscitation, and a Foley catheter is inserted once a proper rectal/genitourinary screening exam is complete. Any areas of obvious hemorrhage are compressed, and splints or pelvic binders are placed to stabilize orthopedic injuries. Following this, a screening neurological exam is performed to assess the patient's level of consciousness (Table 2.1), cranial nerve function, lateralizing signs, and peripheral nerve function including documentation of motor/sensory levels. If it can be safely done, the neurological exam is especially important to perform prior to

Table 2.1 Glasgow coma scale		
Eye opening	Spontaneously	4
	To speech	3
	To pain	2
	None	1
Verbal response	Oriented	5
	Confused	4
	Inappropriate	3
	Incomprehensible	2
	None	1
	None – intubated	1T
Motor response	Obeys commands	6
	Localizes to pain	5
	Withdraws from pain	4
	Flexion to pain (decorticate)	3
	Extension to pain (decerebrate)	2
	None	1
Maximum score		15
Minimum score		3 (3T if intubated)

analgesia, sedating medications, or intubation. Finally, head-to-toe examination of the patient is done in a manner that exposes the patient while preventing hypothermia. Once the primary survey is complete, a secondary survey is carried out, and appropriate radiologic and laboratory investigations are ordered. These may include, but are not limited to, cervical spine, chest, and pelvic X-rays; diagnostic peritoneal lavage, or Focused Assessment with Sonography for Trauma (FAST); computed tomography (CT) scan or angiography; specific extremity X-rays; and laboratory tests including hematologic and chemistry profiles, arterial blood gas, cross-match, and toxicology screen.

Concerning lower extremity injuries, it is not only important to assess the injury itself, but also to be aware of its possible complications, such as significant bleeding or fat embolism from long bone injuries, rhabdomyolysis from crush injury, and acute compartment syndrome. In the initial management of these injuries, splinting helps to control blood loss and reduce pain. During the secondary survey, an appropriate history-taking helps determine the mechanism of injury and anticipated degree of injury. The physical examination of the lower extremity includes examination of the skin, neurological status, circulatory status, and skeletal or ligamentous injury. The degree of soft-tissue damage and contamination is important, as these patients will often require prophylactic broad-spectrum antibiotic coverage and tetanus immunization if not up to date (Table 2.2). Neurological examination

Table 2.2 Tetanus prophylaxis immunization schedule

History of tetanus immunization	Tetanus-prone wound		Non-tetanus-prone wound	
	TD	TIG	TD	TIG
Unknown or <3 doses	Yes	Yes	Yes	No
≥3 doses	No*	No	No†	No

TD, tetanus/diphtheria vaccine; TIG, tetanus immune globulin.
*Yes, if >5 years since last booster. †Yes, if >10 years since last booster.

should include motor/sensory function and deep tendon reflexes. Assessment of posterior tibial nerve function can be particularly important in guiding decisions regarding limb salvage. Any circulatory compromise suggests possible arterial injury. Initial management should include fracture reduction, and, if pulses are still not restored, appropriate angiographic studies should be sought along with consultation of an orthopedic or vascular surgery colleague. Vascular injury should be suspected in cases of active hemorrhage, expanding or pulsatile hematoma, thrill/bruit over wound, absent distal pulses, or distal ischemic manifestations (the five "Ps": pain, pallor, paralysis, paresthesia, and poikilothermy).[22] Ischemic time should be estimated for any amputated or vascular-compromised segments. X-rays should be obtained of all areas of suspected injury, including the joint above and below the injury site.

Several grading systems exist to classify lower extremity trauma. The systems most commonly used are the Gustilo and the Byrd systems, in which tibial fractures are classified based on the size of the wound, amount of soft-tissue injury, degree of bony injury, and presence of vascular injury (Table 2.3).[23,24]

Patient selection

When managing the patient with complex lower extremity trauma, it is important to recognize that futile attempts at limb salvage may be associated with physical, mental, social, and financial implications.[25] Despite advances in microsurgical reconstruction, bony regeneration, and infection control, many patients undergo a number of surgeries only to have eventual amputation. It is important to identify such patients at the outset and provide them with the best option that maximizes function and recovery.

Amputation versus salvage

The establishment of the MESS by Johansen et al. in 1990 was the first effort to produce a set of guidelines that would help a physician to decide between salvage and amputation.[26] This score relied on four criteria: (1) skeletal/soft-tissue injury; (2) limb ischemia; (3) shock; and (4) patient age (Table 2.4). A score of 7 or greater was used as the cutoff point in favor of amputation. Unfortunately, even with this tool there was still

Table 2.3 Classification of lower extremity injury

System	Grade	Details
Gustilo	I	Wound <1 cm Simple fracture, no comminution
	II	Wound >1 cm Minimal soft-tissue damage Moderate comminution/contamination
	III	Extensive soft-tissue damage, comminuted fracture, unstable
	IIIA	Adequate soft-tissue coverage
	IIIB	Extensive soft-tissue loss with periosteal stripping and exposed bone
	IIIC	Arterial injury requiring repair

System	Type	
Byrd	I	Wound <2 cm Low-energy causing spiral or oblique fracture pattern
	II	Wound >2 cm, contusion of skin/muscle Moderate-energy force causing comminuted or displaced fracture
	III	Extensive skin loss and devitalized muscle High-energy force causing significantly displaced fracture with severe comminution, segmental fracture, or bone defect
	IV	Degloving or associated vascular injury requiring repair Extensive energy forces with type III fracture pattern

Table 2.4 Mangled extremity severity score (MESS) criteria	
Variable	**Points**
A Skeletal/soft-tissue injury	
Low-energy (stab, simple fracture, civilian gunshot wound)	1
Medium-energy (open/multiple fractures, dislocation)	2
High-energy (close-range shotgun, military gunshot wound, crush)	3
Very-high-energy (above + gross contamination)	4
B Limb ischemia*	
Pulse reduced or absent; perfusion normal	1
Pulseless, paresthesias, diminished capillary refill	2
Cool, paralyzed, insensate, numb	3
C Shock	
Systolic blood pressure always >90 mmHg	1
Transient hypotension	2
Persistent hypotension	3
D Age	
<30 years	1
30–50 years	2
>50 years	3
Maximum score possible	16
Threshold score for amputation	7

*Score doubled for ischemia time >6 h.

is important to guard against delay in amputation for limbs that are not salvageable. Discrimination was moderately good in assessing salvage versus amputation of the limb. Overall, the analysis did not validate the clinical utility of any of the lower extremity injury severity scores, and advised for their cautious application when making decisions regarding limb salvage. Additionally, these scores are not predictive of functional recovery in patients who undergo successful limb reconstruction, as shown by Ly et al.[29]

Unfortunately, despite a number of studies, there are still no definite criteria for amputation. Several proposed criteria have since been refuted following proper outcome studies. For example, it is a widely held belief that tibial nerve injury or absence of plantar foot sensation is an indication for amputation. However, a study by Bosse et al.,[30] examining functional outcomes of patients with severe lower extremity injuries, found that more than half of the patients who initially presented with an insensate foot that underwent salvage regained sensation by 2 years. The authors concluded that initial plantar sensation was not prognostic of long-term plantar sensation status or functional outcome, and that this should therefore not be a criterion in limb salvage algorithms.

Risk factors that may contribute to or predict the need for amputation include:[22]

- Gustilo grade IIIC tibial injuries
- Sciatic or tibial nerve injury
- Prolonged ischemia (>4–6 h)/muscle necrosis
- Crush or destructive soft-tissue injury
- Significant wound contamination
- Multiple/severely comminuted fractures; segmental bone loss
- Old age or severe comorbidity
- Apparent futility of revascularization or failed revascularization.

In addition to these risk factors, several prognostic factors for limb salvage have been identified.[22] These include mechanism of injury, anatomy of injury (e.g., popliteal artery injury has worst prognosis), presence of associated injuries, age and physiologic health of the patient, and clinical presentation (e.g., shock and obvious limb ischemia). The environmental circumstances may also play a role in determining salvage, with higher amputation rates in combat zones, austere environments, and multicasualty events.

Treatment and surgical techniques

Timing of treatment

There is no debate that a patient with complex trauma should undergo thorough irrigation of open fractures and debridement of devitalized tissue. This is considered to be of paramount importance for the prevention of infection. It is commonly taught that the standard of care is to take patients to the operating room within 6 h of injury.[31,32] However, this timeframe is not supported by evidence and was recently addressed in a subgroup analysis of the LEAP study.[33] Among those patients who developed major infections, significant factors included bone loss >2 cm and Gustilo grade IIIC fractures. Factors such as degree of nerve/muscle damage, size of skin defect, injury severity score, and surgeon's

debate over definitive criteria for amputation, and this led to the recent multicenter study entitled the Lower Extremity Assessment Project (LEAP), carried out at eight level I trauma centers in the USA.[27] This study looked prospectively at patients with traumatic amputations below the distal femur, Gustilo grade III (A–C) open tibia fractures, devascular injuries below the distal femur, major soft-tissue injuries below the distal femur excluding the foot, open pilon fractures (grade III), open ankle fractures (grade IIIB), and severe open hindfoot and midfoot injuries with degloving and nerve injury. The goal of the study was to define the characteristics of the individuals sustaining lower extremity trauma. A total of 601 patients were enrolled, and the patient demographics were primarily male (77%), Caucasian (72%), and young (71% between 20 and 45 years old). The results demonstrated that the patients who sustained a high degree of extremity trauma had several disadvantages prior to their injury (social, economic, and personality), and that quality of life and functional outcome data seemed more related to these than to the injury.

A subset of the LEAP studies assessed several available clinical decision-making scores relating to injury severity,[28] which included MESS, LSI, PSI, NISSSA, and HFS-97. When applying these scores to the open tibial fracture group, MESS, PSI, and LSI demonstrated high specificity (91%, 87%, and 97%, respectively) but low sensitivity (46%, each). Specificity is important to insure that a minimal number of salvageable limbs are incorrectly assigned to amputation, and sensitivity assessment of the degree of contamination were non-predictive of infection. Regarding their treatment, patients who were managed with intramedullary (IM) nail had a lower incidence of infection compared with those who were externally fixated or treated with plate/screw fixation. There was no significant difference in terms of mean time to debridement between patients who developed infection and those who did not. Time from initial debridement to eventual soft-tissue coverage was also not a risk factor for infection. Multivariate regression showed that delayed admission of patients to a primary trauma center (>2 h postinjury) or delayed transfer from an outside institution to primary trauma center resulted in higher rates of infection. It is unclear whether delay in admission to a trauma center was in fact a surrogate marker indicative of a higher degree of injury.

With regard to the timing of reconstruction of lower extremity trauma, most believe that early reconstruction leads to better outcome. This follows the study by Godina[34] in which the timing of microsurgical reconstruction was analyzed with respect to flap failure, infection, bone-healing time, length of hospital stay, and number of operative procedures. This study stratified patients into three groups of repair: (1) within 72 h; (2) between 72 h and 3 months; and (3) beyond 3 months postinjury. The study concluded that reconstruction within 72 h showed the best outcomes for all analyzed factors. Those reconstructed between 72 h and 3 months postinjury had the highest flap failure rates and highest rates of infection. Those reconstructed beyond 3 months had the longest time to bone healing and the greatest number of operations (Table 2.5). Criticisms of Godina's study include the fact that the initial 100 patients in the series were treated in a delayed fashion with average operative times of 6–8 h, whereas those subsequently treated in an immediate fashion (when microsurgical experience was improved) had shorter operative times.[35] Patients were also not randomized to their treatment regimens, had variable reconstruction (i.e., different flap choices), and upper/lower extremity reconstruction outcomes were pooled. There have been several subsequent studies on this topic – and the results have varied from indifference to favoritism of immediate reconstruction.[23,35–39] Again, the majority of these have been retrospective reviews, where patients were not randomized to treatment, with non-standardized reconstructive options.

It is important to recognize that immediate reconstruction is not the answer for all patients under all circumstances. The surgeon has to be highly skilled to perform single-stage debridement and immediate reconstruction. The patient must also not have other life-threatening injuries or multiple comorbidities.[40] In some cases, serial debridement, vacuum-assisted closure, and delayed reconstruction may be preferred.

Fracture management

The initial orthopedic management of an open lower extremity fracture has traditionally involved external fixation, in an effort to avoid implantation of metal in a contaminated field. Recently, more orthopedic surgeons perform internal fixation using IM nail or minimally invasive plate osteosynthesis (MIPO) technique.[40] The safety of an unreamed IM nail is thought to be equivalent to external fixation with respect to union, delayed union, deep infection, and chronic osteomyelitis.[41] Use of external fixators may be associated with pin tract infection, and may interfere with access for microvascular reconstruction.

Vascular injury

True vascular injury in the setting of lower extremity trauma is rare. Most definitive signs of vascular compromise can be attributed to soft-tissue and bone bleeding, traction of intact arteries with pulse loss (i.e., due to displaced fractures), or compartment syndrome. However, it is prudent to rule out vascular injury, and therefore liberal use of imaging should be carried out in the presence of hard signs. Traditionally, the arteriogram was the gold standard in the diagnosis of vascular injuries. Although it is accurate in diagnosing vascular injury, it has several disadvantages, including cost, duration of procedure, potential delay to repair, and need for a specialized team to perform it.[42] There is also an associated risk of morbidity in the form of contrast allergy and percutaneous vascular access-related complications. The advent of CT angiography (CTA) has helped provide rapid diagnosis of vascular injury with lower morbidity. It also enables multiple parts of the body to be assessed. CT angiographic signs of arterial injury include active extravasation of contrast material, pseudoaneurysm formation, abrupt narrowing of an artery, loss of opacification of an arterial segment, and arteriovenous fistula formation.[42] Studies comparing CTA and conventional angiography have demonstrated a high sensitivity and specificity of CTA for arterial injury that was confirmed with conventional angiography. There is also a significant cost saving – in one institution savings exceeded $13 000 per patient when performing CTA alone.[43]

There is no doubt that "time is muscle", and prompt repair of any vascular injury should be carried out. Permanent ischemic injury may occur anywhere from 2 to 12 h postinjury according to the literature. This wide range may be due to variation in injury mechanism, presence of collateral flow, and level of injury.[44] The decision to perform a definitive vascular repair in the setting of lower extremity trauma depends on the clinical circumstances. There are some situations in which the patient is best served with temporary intraluminal shunting following distal thrombectomy and heparinization. These include unstable fractures, gross contamination of the wound

Table 2.5 Godina's results on the timing of microsurgical repair			
	Early (<72 h)	Delayed (72 h–3 months)	Late (>3 months)
Number of patients	134	167	231
Free flap failures	0.75%	12%	22%
Postoperative infection	1.5%	17.5%	6%
Bone healing time (average)	6.8 months	12.3 months	29 months
Time in hospital (average)	27 days	130 days	256 days
Number of surgeries (average)	1.3	4.1	7.8

bed, soft-tissue deficits that would lead to an exposed reconstruction/repair, unstable patient, unavailable resources/ surgical expertise in vascular repair, and coincident life-threatening injury.[22]

In combined injuries involving bone and vascular disruption, the operative sequence of repair has been debated. In one systematic review,[45] survival of the extremity was directly related to ischemic time, with a steep increase in incidence beyond 3–4 h of ischemic time. Those favoring immediate vascular repair believe that the reversal of ischemia is most important, whereas those favoring skeletal fixation prior to vascular repair argue that stabilization of the bony fragments first will avoid disruption of a vascular repair during bony manipulation. There have been several reports of fracture fixation following vascular repair, with no disruption of the repair.[46–48] A meta-analysis comparing the outcomes of surgical sequence in 14 published studies did not demonstrate a clear difference among groups regarding incidence of subsequent amputation.[49]

Reconstructive options

In patients with lower extremity trauma, it is important to consider all options for reconstruction and choose one that is most reliable or will provide the best functional outcome. The reconstructive ladder is often considered but, in major lower extremity trauma where soft-tissue damage is extensive and the zone of injury is wide, local options are often eliminated, emphasizing the need for free flap coverage. When choosing a reconstructive option, consideration is given to the size and location of the defect, functional needs (i.e., innervated flap), zone of injury, anticipated location of vascular anastomosis for free flap reconstruction, and, accordingly, length of vascular pedicle required for vascular anastomosis. Consideration should also be given to the need for future operative interventions (e.g., tendon or bone reconstruction). Regardless of flap options chosen for reconstruction, adequate debridement of all non-viable tissue is imperative. High-energy trauma can result in significant soft-tissue destruction with a need for extensive debridement of non-viable tissue (Fig. 2.1).

The following is a brief overview of flap options that will be described in more detail in subsequent chapters on lower-extremity reconstruction.

Local flaps

There are a variety of local flap options available in lower extremity reconstruction. Based on anatomic and angiographic studies, local flaps may be safely performed when based on known perforators. Local flaps are advantageous as they offer a viable reconstructive option with shorter operative times and less complexity;[50] they also provide tissue that is similar in composition to the area of the defect. Patients should be screened for comorbidities that would compromise vascular supply of the lower extremity, and have an appropriate vascular examination. A number of local flap options are discussed in the following sections.

Perforator flaps

The lower extremity is an anatomic region where perforators available as a flap pedicle are plentiful (Figs. 2.2 & 2.3). They have been mapped out in extensive detail through cadaveric

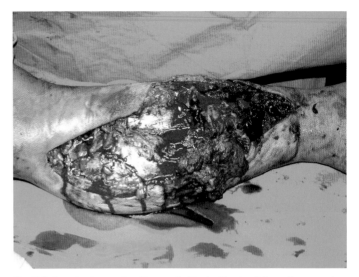

Fig. 2.1 Complex lower extremity wound with significant soft-tissue trauma and devitalization. This wound will require extensive debridement of non-viable skin, muscle, and bone prior to flap coverage in order to prevent infection.

injection studies and angiographic investigations. In the gluteal region, most of perforators are musculocutaneous and arise from the superior and inferior gluteal arteries, with minor contributions from the iliolumbar and internal pudendal arteries. They are the basis for commonly used gluteal perforator flaps including the superior and inferior gluteal artery perforator flaps.

In the hip and thigh region, there are a combination of musculocutaneous and septocutaneous perforators from six source arteries originating from the common femoral artery.[51] The anteromedial thigh (AMT) is supplied by perforators of the lateral circumflex femoral artery (LCFA) and superficial

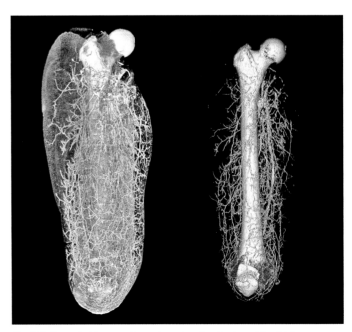

Fig. 2.2 Computed tomography angiography of perforators of the thigh demonstrating a rich density of available cutaneous perforators for flap design and harvest.

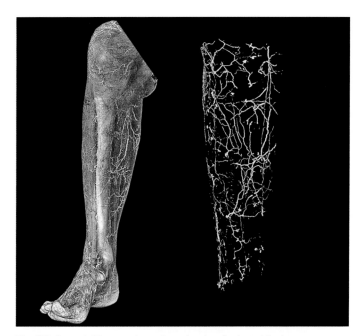

Fig. 2.3 Computed tomography angiography of perforators of the leg, demonstrating a rich density of available cutaneous perforators for flap design and harvest.

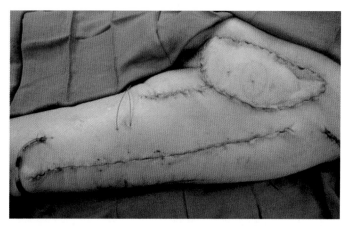

Fig. 2.5 Pedicled anterolateral thigh flap tunneled and inset with primary closure of the donor site.

femoral artery. The anterolateral thigh (ALT) is primarily supplied by the three terminal branches (ascending, transverse, and descending branches) of the LCFA. Perforators of these branches supply the tensor fasciae latae perforator flap and the ALT flap (Figs. 2.4 & 2.5). Just superior to these areas is the superficial circumflex iliac artery, which provides perforators to the free superficial circumflex iliac artery perforator flap and contributes to the groin flap. Perforators from the medial circumflex femoral, profunda femoris, and popliteal arteries supply the posteromedial thigh. The posterolateral thigh is supplied by the profunda femoris and inferior gluteal arteries. Inferiorly, the medial and lateral superior genicular arteries supply the region around the knee and are sources of local perforator flaps in knee reconstruction (Figs. 2.6 & 2.7).

Surrounding the knee are musculocutaneous perforators from the superficial femoral artery, as well as several septocutaneous perforators from the descending genicular, medial/lateral superior and inferior genicular, anterior tibial recurrent, and popliteal arteries[51] (Figs. 2.8–2.10). The saphenous artery is a superficial branch of the descending genicular artery, arising medially with the saphenous nerve and vein, and is the basis of the descending genicular artery perforator flap, which may incorporate the nerve to create an innervated flap. Posteriorly, the sural arteries (medial/lateral) arise from the popliteal trunk and may be sources of local perforator flaps, including the more reliable medial sural artery perforator flap.

Within the leg, perforators arise from the posterior tibial, anterior tibial, and peroneal arteries. The posterior tibial artery perforator flap incorporates perforators emerging from the intermuscular septum between the soleus and the flexor digitorum longus. The anterior tibial artery perforator flap is based on perforators that occur in two rows – one between the tibia and the tibialis anterior muscle, and the other from the anterior crural septum between the extensor digitorum longus and peroneus longus. The peroneal artery perforator flap is nourished by perforators that emerge from the posterior crural septum between the peroneus longus and the soleus (Figs. 2.11–2.15).

In the foot, the terminal branches of the anterior tibial, posterior tibial, and peroneal arteries are sources of perforator flaps. These include the lateral calcaneal artery perforator flap and medial plantar artery perforator-based flaps (medialis pedis flap, instep flap, and abductor hallucis muscle flap) (Fig. 2.16).

Muscle-based flaps

In the thigh, a number of local muscles may be used to reconstruct defects. These include the gracilis flap, which is based on the ascending branch of the medial circumflex femoral artery. As a local flap, this is commonly used to reconstruct the groin, perineum, and ischium. The sartorius flap, which is based on the superficial femoral artery (type IV vascular supply), may be used to cover groin defects and exposed femoral vessels, and is rarely used as a distally based flap to cover small knee defects. The anterior thigh musculature may provide coverage of the inferior abdomen, groin, perineum,

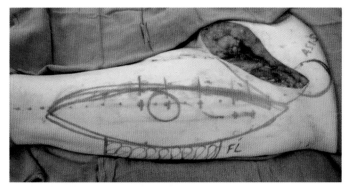

Fig. 2.4 A 66-year-old female with a recurrent squamous cell carcinoma on the left groin following wide excision. Ample laxity was found in the anterior thigh region.

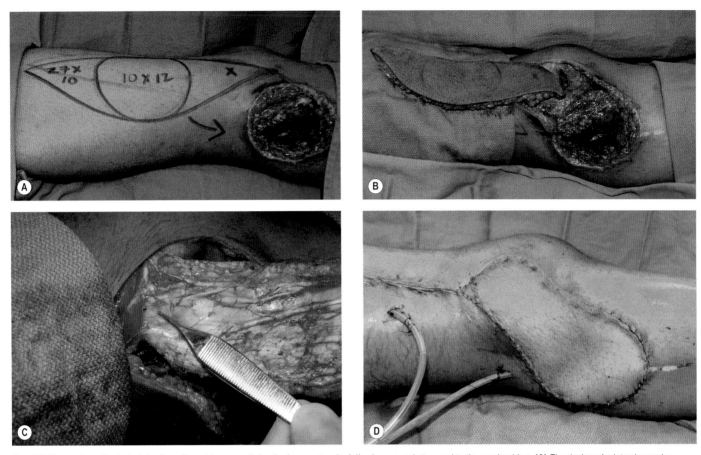

Fig. 2.6 Exposed popliteal arterial vein graft used to revascularize the lower extremity following a gunshot wound to the proximal leg. **(A)** The design of a lateral superior genicular artery pedicle perforator flap with the long axis of the flap designed parallel to the long axis of the thigh. **(B)** The pedicle perforator flap harvested based on a single lateral superior genicular artery perforator. **(C)** The perforator following subfascial harvest of the flap. **(D)** Flap inset with no tension and primary closure of the donor site.

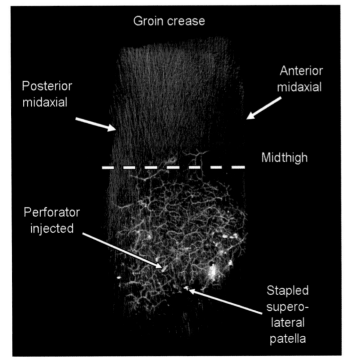

Fig. 2.7 Computed tomography angiography following lead oxide injection of a single lateral superior genicular artery perforator. Perfusion is seen to extend proximally up to the midthigh region and to the anterior and posterior midaxial lines bilaterally.

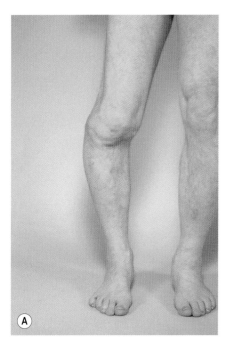
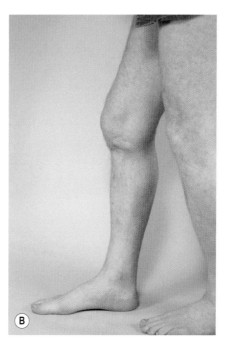
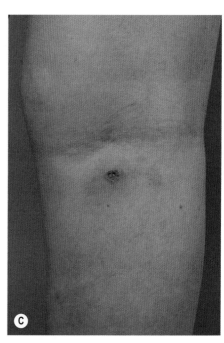

Fig. 2.8 A 64-year-old male with post-traumatic deformity and subsequent arthritis of right knee. Soft-tissue augmentation of medial side of the knee is needed for total knee replacement arthroplasty.

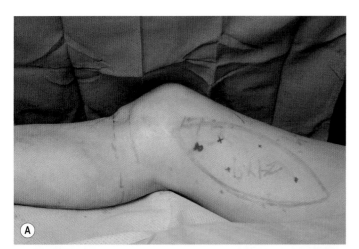
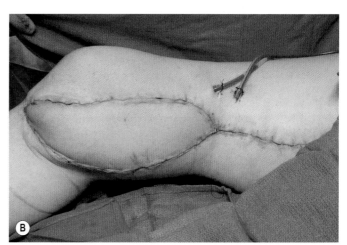
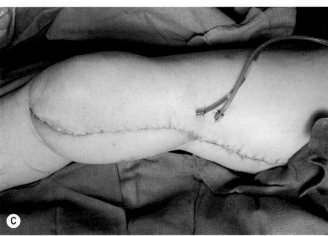

Fig. 2.9 Pedicled superficial femoral artery perforator flap was performed to augment medial side of the knee.

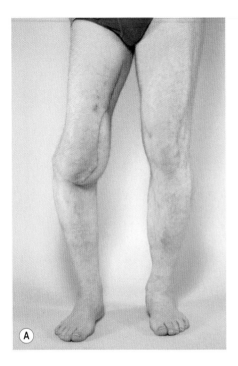
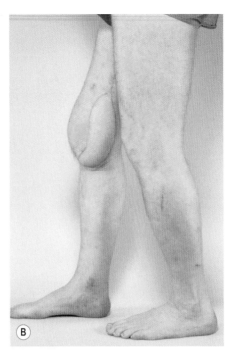

Fig. 2.10 Three months postoperatively with well-perfused flap and sufficient soft tissue on medial side of the knee.

and ischium, and includes the rectus femoris (based on profunda femoris artery), vastus lateralis (descending branch of LCFA), and vastus medialis (superficial femoral artery) flaps. Laterally, the tensor fasciae latae flap (ascending branch of LCFA) may be used for similar applications, and may additionally reach the trochanteric region and sacrum for pressure sore reconstruction. Posteriorly, the biceps femoris flap (profunda femoris) is used primarily for pressure sore reconstruction.

In the lower leg, the most commonly used muscle flaps include the gastrocnemius and soleus flaps. The gastrocnemius has medial and lateral heads, based on the medial and lateral sural arteries, respectively. The medial head is most commonly used as it is longer and has better reach. This is

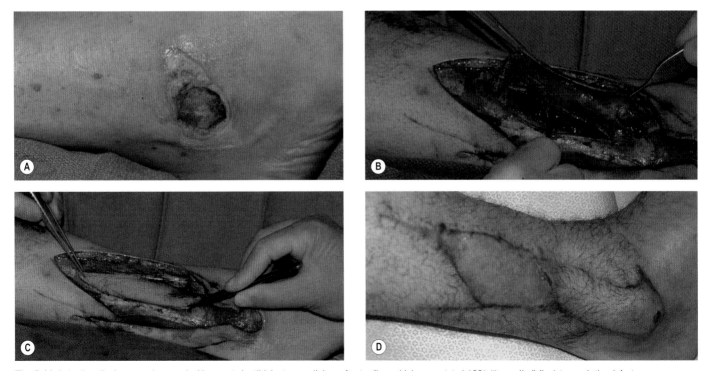

Fig. 2.11 Lateral malleolus wound covered with an anterior tibial artery pedicle perforator flap, which was rotated 180° ("propeller" flap) to reach the defect.

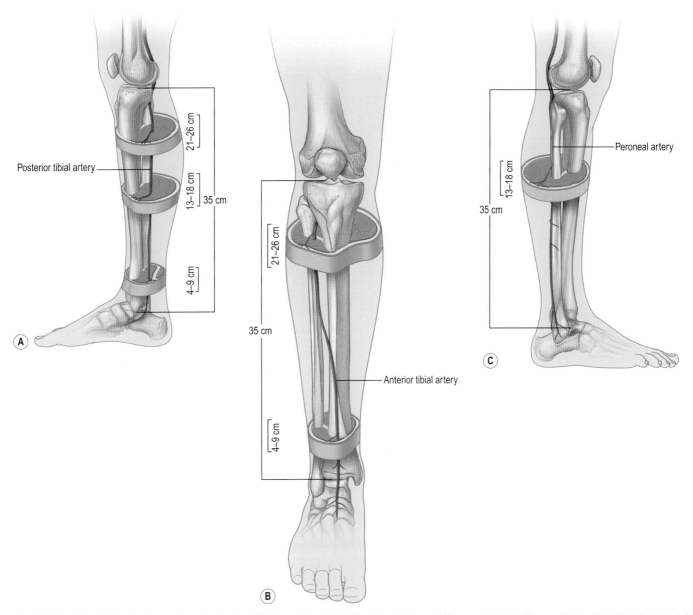

Fig. 2.12 Location of all major clusters of perforators from **(A)** the posterior tibial, **(B)** anterior tibial, and **(C)** peroneal arteries. These perforator cluster locations can help in the design and planning of local pedicle perforator flaps in the lower extremity.

used primarily in knee and upper-third leg coverage (Figs. 2.17 & 2.18). The soleus flap is based on perforators from the popliteal, posterior tibial, and peroneal arteries. Distally, segmental perforators from the posterior tibial artery allow for a reverse soleus flap. A number of other smaller muscle-based flaps have been described (extensor hallucis longus, flexor hallucis longus, extensor digitorum longus, flexor digitorum longus, and peroneus brevis/longus flaps), but these flaps provide minimal bulk, and often suboptimal, coverage in larger defects.

The foot is a source of several small local muscular flaps, including the abductor digiti minimi, abductor hallucis, and flexor digitorum brevis flaps.

Fascial-based flaps (Video 2.1 ○)

In the thigh, the ALT flap has become a workhorse flap and is used primarily as a free flap. This flap is based on the descending branch of the LCFA, which arises from the profunda femoris artery. This flap is described as having three cutaneous perforators – A, B, and C – that lie along a line marked from the anterior superior iliac spine to the supero-lateral corner of the patella.[52] These perforators may have a septocutaneous course between the vastus lateralis and the rectus femoris, or a musculocutaneous course through the vastus lateralis. Dissection can be performed suprafascially or subfascially. An extended ALT flap has been described that

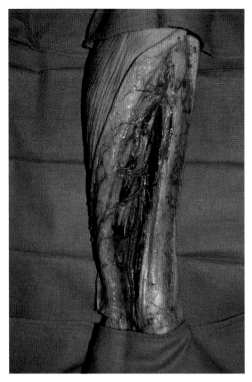

Fig. 2.13 Cadaver dissection of the leg with arterial red latex injection and venous blue latex injection of the posterior tibial artery (PTA) and vein respectively. Perforators of the PTA are shown with their associated venae comitantes. Perforators from the PTA are among the largest in the lower extremity and can form the basis for various local pedicle perforator flaps for anterior tibial and lateral coverage in the distal third of the leg.

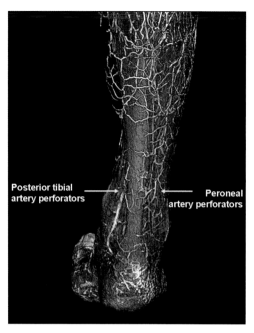

Fig. 2.14 Computed tomography angiography of posterior tibial artery and peroneal artery perforators of the leg demonstrating a rich density of available cutaneous perforators for local flap design and harvest.

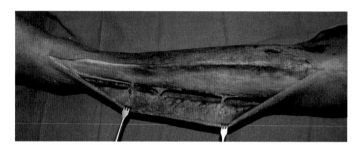

Fig. 2.15 Cadaver dissection showing peroneal artery perforators.

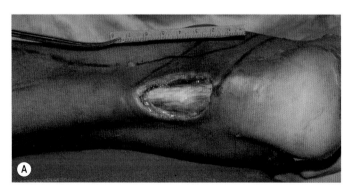

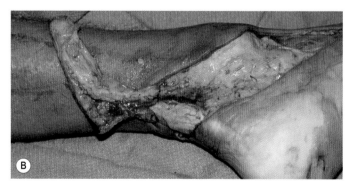

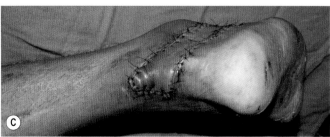

Fig. 2.16 **(A)** A 4 cm defect with exposure of the Achilles tendon following wound debridement. **(B)** Harvest of a calcaneal artery flap for Achilles tendon coverage. **(C)** Achilles coverage and flap inset following transfer.

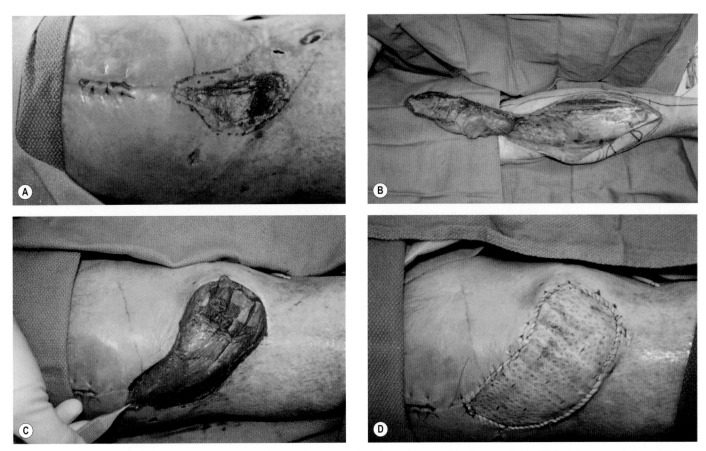

Fig. 2.17 (A) Exposed left patellar tendon with soft-tissue defect in a 56-year-old male patient with an underlying knee prosthesis. **(B)** Posterior approach via a midline incision for harvest of a medial gastrocnemius muscle flap. The posterior and anterior surface of the muscle fascia can be scored to achieve greater length and the muscle origin can also be detached for the same purpose. **(C)** Wound was debrided and defect covered with a tunneled pedicle medial gastrocnemius muscle flap. Tunnel must be adequately released so that no pressure is exerted on the muscle and its pedicle. **(D)** Final flap inset and coverage with a split-thickness skin graft.

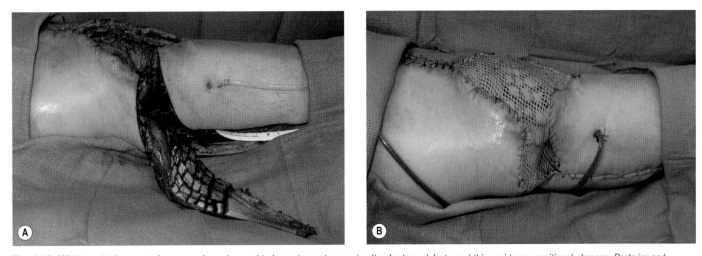

Fig. 2.18 (A) Alternatively, an anterior approach can be used to harvest a gastrocnemius flap for knee defects, and this avoids any positional changes. Posterior and anterior muscle fascia scoring are also performed in order to maximize muscle length. The tendinous portion of the muscle can also be used to anchor the flap and provide additional well-vascularized tissue. **(B)** Final flap inset and split-thickness skin grafting with complete wound coverage.

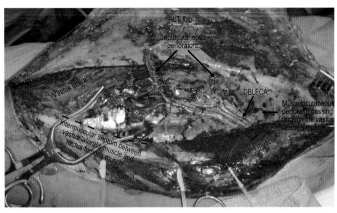

Fig. 2.19 Anterolateral thigh (ALT) flap harvest showing perforators originating from the descending branch of the lateral circumflex femoral artery (DBLCFA). The DBLCFA is seen coursing between the vastus lateralis laterally and the rectus femoris medially. Once the rectus femoris muscle has been dissected and retracted medially, all perforators from the DBLCFA become easily visible. The most direct and least intramuscular perforator is then selected for flap harvest.

incorporates distal linking vessels between LCFA, common femoral, and superficial femoral arteries[53] (Figs. 2.19–2.22). Additionally, the reverse ALT flap has also been described as a distally based pedicled flap in lower extremity reconstruction.[54] Consideration may be given to supercharging this flap through anastomosis of the proximal LCFA to leg donor vessels (e.g., anterior tibial artery) if vascularity is questionable.[55]

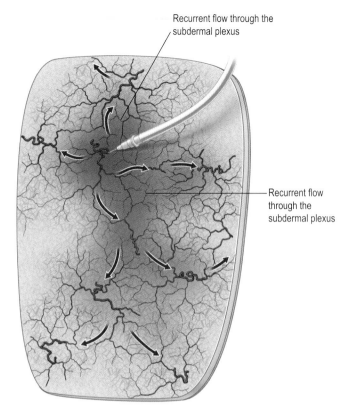

Fig. 2.21 A large (extended) anterolateral thigh flap can be harvested based on a single perforator. High arterial filling pressures from the selected perforator allow interperforator flow and increased flap vascular territory.

Multidirectional interperforator flow

⟶ = direction of interperforator flow
⚬ = perforator

Fig. 2.20 Interperforator flow allows communication with multiple adjacent perforators via direct and indirect linking vessels.

In the leg, the sural artery flap and reverse sural artery flap provide coverage of the knee and calcaneal region, respectively. The sural artery flap is based on a direct cutaneous branch of the sural artery and lesser saphenous vein. The reverse sural artery flap is primarily based on septocutaneous perforators from the peroneal artery and includes the lesser saphenous vein and median cutaneous sural nerve[56] (Fig. 2.23). Venous congestion and partial flap ischemia are possible complications of the reverse sural artery flap and can be overcome by a two-stage delay procedure or venous supercharging[57,58] (Fig. 2.24).

Free tissue transfer – muscle

Larger defects of the lower extremity that require obliteration of dead space often warrant the use of a muscle-based free flap in combination with split-thickness skin graft. Commonly used muscles include the latissimus dorsi (thoracodorsal artery) (Figs. 2.25–2.27), rectus abdominis (deep inferior epigastric artery) (Fig. 2.28), serratus anterior (lateral thoracic artery or branch to serratus anterior from thoracodorsal artery), and gracilis (ascending branch of medial circumflex femoral artery) (Figs. 2.29 & 2.30). For small to moderate defects, muscle-sparing versions of the latissimus dorsi and rectus abdominis flaps can be excellent options without sacrificing donor site function.

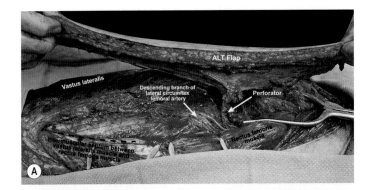

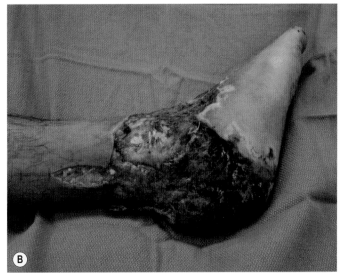

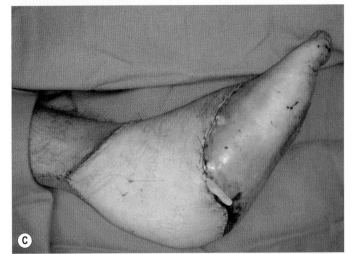

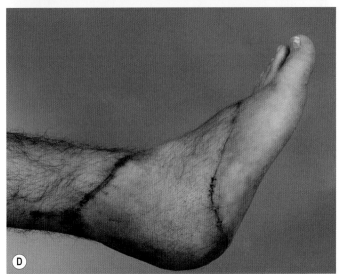

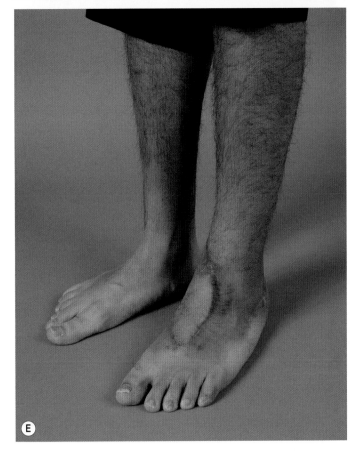

Fig. 2.22 Large degloving injury of the left lower extremity with exposure of the medial malleolus, Achilles tendon, calcaneus, and extensor tendons. Following radical debridement, resurfacing was done with an extended anterolateral thigh (ALT) flap. The ALT flap was later liposuctioned for improved contour, and the patient was able to wear his normal footwear and ambulate at his preinjury level.

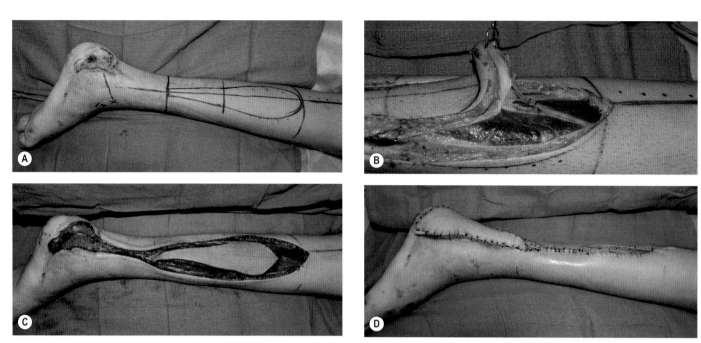

Fig. 2.23 (A) Left lower extremity defect with exposed Achilles tendon and calcaneus. Sural artery flap designed along a vertical axis centered from the midpoint between the lateral malleolus and the Achilles tendon and the midpoint of the popliteal fossa. Maximal peroneal perforator density can be found within 8 cm of the lower transverse line. This location represents the proximal extent of the sural artery flap. The sural artery flap can be safely extended to three-quarters of the leg proximally. A delay procedure can be considered in patients with advanced age and medical comorbidities (e.g., diabetes) in order to maximize arterial perfusion and venous outflow. **(B)** Subfascial elevation of the sural artery flap from proximal to distal with early identification of the sural nerve and artery, which are incorporated into the flap. Note that this flap is principally based on peroneal perforators and can alternatively be harvested without sacrifice of the sural nerve. **(C)** Sural artery flap *in situ* following elevation and recipient site debridement. **(D)** Final flap inset without tension. Donor site is closed primarily and the addition of a split-thickness skin graft as needed. Liberal use of skin grafting should be done proximal to the flap base in order to minimize undue pressure on the perforators.

Free tissue transfer – fasciocutaneous ▶

One of the most versatile and popular fasciocutaneous free flaps used in lower extremity reconstruction is the ALT flap. This can be converted into a sensate flap by incorporating the lateral femoral cutaneous nerve, which is useful in distal third of a leg and foot reconstruction where sensation is important. This flap is described above. The ALT flap can also be harvested as a thinner adipofascial flap that allows primary donor site closure. This is very useful in patients who have an unsuitable ALT donor site due to excessive thickness (Figs. 2.31 & 2.32).

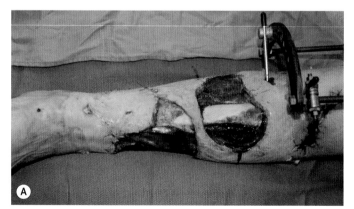

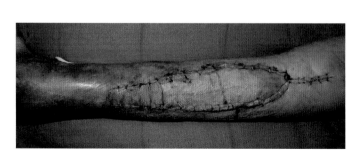

Fig. 2.24 Two weeks postsurgical delay procedure of a sural artery flap in a diabetic 84-year-old patient. This delay procedure allows for a clear demarcation of flap viability. Note the proximal ischemic portion of the flap was discarded prior to definitive flap transfer.

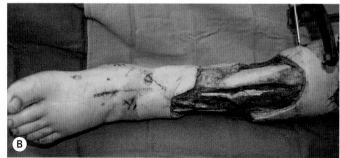

Fig. 2.25 (A) Complex left lower extremity defect with a comminuted fracture of the proximal tibia. **(B)** Defect following radical debridement and conversion of multiple wound units to a simpler single wound unit.

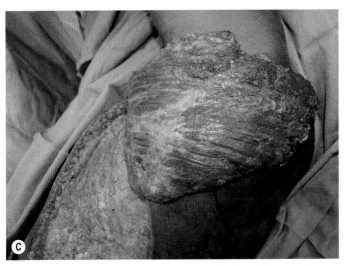

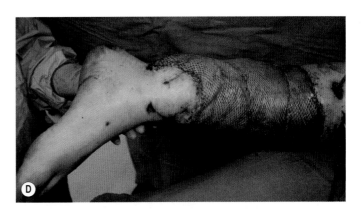

Fig. 2.25, cont'd **(C)** Free latissimus dorsi muscle flap harvested to provide coverage of a large surface area. This muscle flap also allows important deep space obliteration in cases involving comminuted fractures with complex 3D wound defects. **(D)** Circumferential coverage of the lower extremity wound with a latissimus dorsi flap and split-thickness skin graft. Anastomosis was performed to the posterior tibial artery and vein distal to the zone of injury. Vessels distal to the zone of injury have the advantage of being more superficial, which facilitates vessel access and microsurgery.

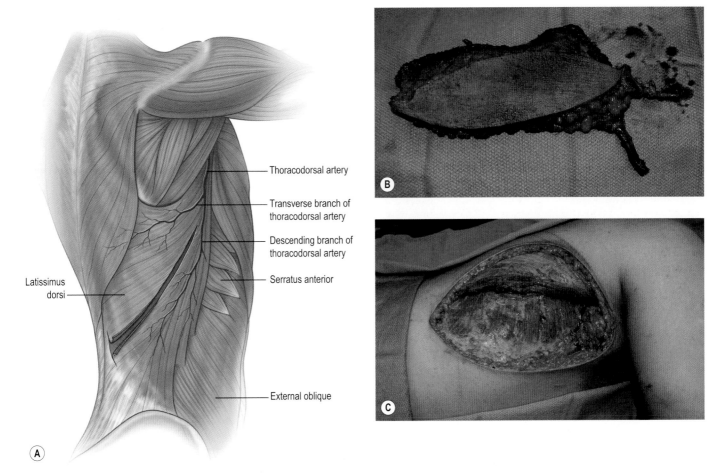

Fig. 2.26 **(A)** Alternatively, for smaller defects of the lower extremity, a free muscle-sparing latissimus dorsi flap can be used. This flap retains all of the advantages of its full latissimus dorsi counterpart without sacrificing donor muscle function. The muscle-sparing latissimus dorsi flap can be based on either the descending or transverse branch of the thoracodorsal artery and vein. **(B)** Muscle-sparing latissimus dorsi myocutaneous flap for lower extremity reconstruction. **(C)** Donor site following free muscle-sparing latissimus dorsi flap harvest. Note preservation of the anterior axillary line and the majority of the latissimus dorsi muscle.

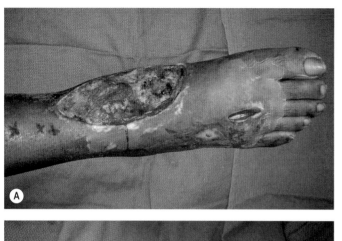

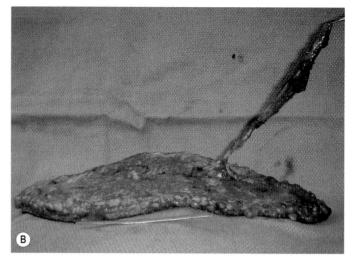

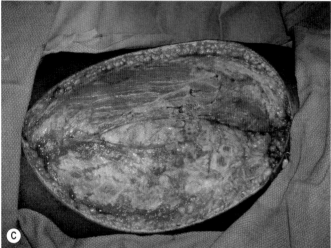

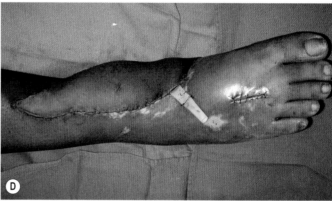

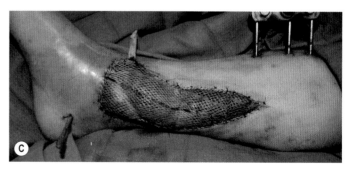

Fig. 2.27 (A) Right ankle wound with exposed medial malleolus and soft-tissue defect in a 45-year-old patient. **(B)** Thin thoracodorsal artery perforator flap harvested for resurfacing a medial ankle defect. **(C)** Thoracodorsal artery perforator flap donor site with preservation of entire latissimus dorsi muscle. Flap was based on a direct cutaneous branch, which followed the anterior border of the latissimus dorsi muscle. **(D)** Thoracodorsal artery perforator flap (8 × 20 cm) used to resurface the medial right ankle and malleolus.

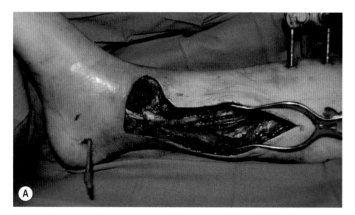

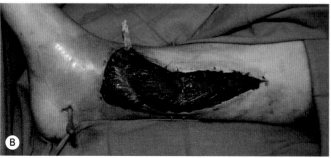

Fig. 2.28 (A) Right medial ankle defect with exposed medial malleolus and tendons. Radical debridement was performed, and posterior tibial artery and vein were prepared as recipient vessels. Posterior tibial vessels are our recipient vessels of choice for medial and anteromedial defects. They provide large, dependable vessels that are usually well protected deep from the zone of injury. **(B)** Coverage of the medial ankle defect with a free muscle-sparing rectus flap. **(C)** Final inset and coverage with a split-thickness skin graft. Note that the external fixator can be temporarily dismantled for better vascular access and easier microsurgery.

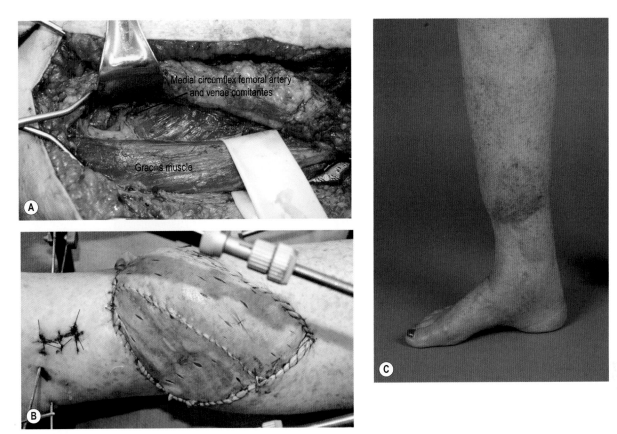

Fig. 2.29 **(A)** Dissection of a free gracilis flap with exposure of the medial circumflex femoral artery and venae comitantes. **(B)** Gracilis free flap inset with sheet split-thickness skin graft. **(C)** Final postoperative result after 1 year with low-profile contouring of the free gracilis flap. Note that this patient underwent minor debulking of the gracilis muscle at 6 months postoperatively. A dermatome was used for muscle debulking and also for split-thickness skin graft removal. The skin graft was recycled back on to the gracilis flap immediately following muscle shaving in order to avoid another skin graft donor site.

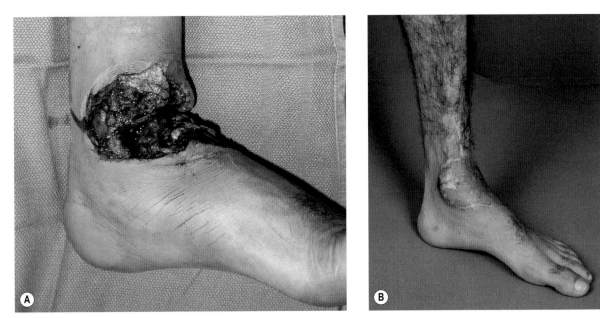

Fig. 2.30 **(A)** Exposed extensor tendons, left talus, distal tibia, and fibula, with significant dead space. This open joint creates a complex 3D defect, which can be effectively obliterated with an expendable free gracilis flap. **(B)** Postoperative result after 6 months with good contouring of the anterior ankle and minimal bulk. Denervated muscle atrophies significantly over time and contours well to its recipient site.

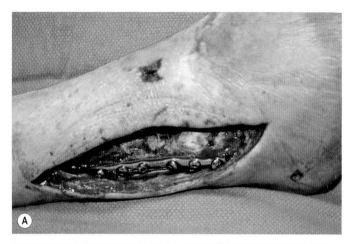

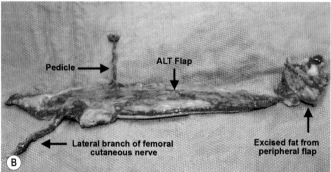

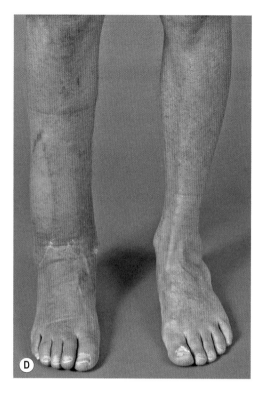

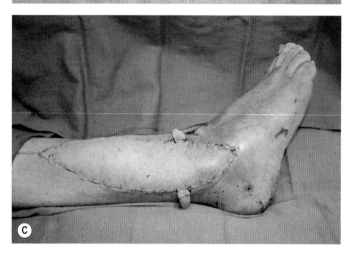

Fig. 2.31 (A–C) Right lateral ankle soft-tissue defect and exposed hardware resurfaced with a thinned and neurotized anterolateral thigh flap based on a lateral branch of the femoral cutaneous nerve. The periphery of the flap can also be thinned for better inset and less bulk. We do not recommend aggressive primary thinning of the anterolateral thigh flap and prefer to do this secondarily if necessary. **(D)** Postoperative results 6 months later with stable right-leg wound coverage and healed donor site. ALT, anteromedial thigh.

Other fasciocutaneous free flaps used in lower extremity reconstruction include the radial forearm flap and the AMT flap. The radial forearm flap is based on the radial artery, which runs proximally between the brachioradialis and pronator teres. It can be made sensate through the incorporation of the lateral or medial antebrachial cutaneous nerves. The AMT flap is supplied by a septocutaneous branch of the LCFA, commonly arising between the medial border of the rectus femoris and the sartorius[59] (Fig. 2.33). It provides a large skin paddle, with a well-hidden donor site. Additionally, it can be designed as a vascular flow-through flap for combined soft-tissue/vascular reconstruction.

Skeletal reconstruction

Options for bony reconstruction of the lower extremity include autogenous cancellous bone graft, vascularized bone graft, and distraction osteogenesis. Autogenous cancellous bone grafts are typically used to fill small defects in bone (Fig. 2.34). While it is possible to bridge larger gaps (8–10 cm) with autogenous cancellous bone graft, it is not favorable. In this situation, vascularized bone graft or distraction osteogenesis is preferred. The most commonly used donor of vascularized bone graft is the fibula based on segmental and nutrient vessels of the peroneal artery. Alternative options

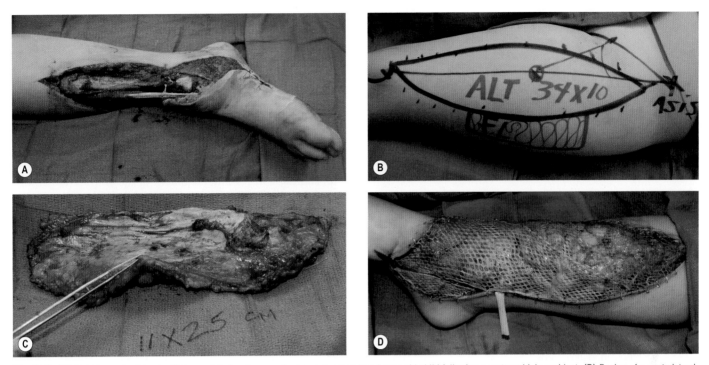

Fig. 2.32 (A) Right leg anterolateral soft-tissue defect and exposed extensor tendons in a 9-year-old child following a motor vehicle accident. **(B)** Design of a contralateral extended anterolateral thigh (ALT) flap. **(C)** The ALT flap was converted into an adipofascial ALT flap in order to minimize bulk and maximize flap size while allowing primary donor site closure. A 25×11 cm adipofascial ALT flap was used for reconstruction and permitted entire wound coverage. **(D)** Adipofascial anterolateral thigh flap inset and coverage with a split-thickness skin graft. The posterior tibial artery and vein were used as reliable recipient vessels.

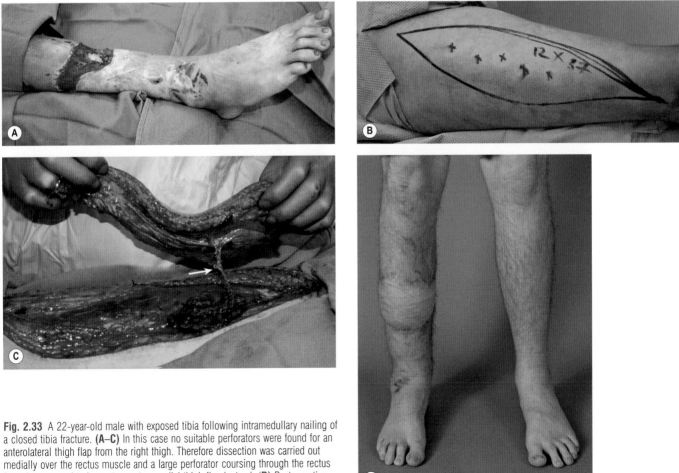

Fig. 2.33 A 22-year-old male with exposed tibia following intramedullary nailing of a closed tibia fracture. **(A–C)** In this case no suitable perforators were found for an anterolateral thigh flap from the right thigh. Therefore dissection was carried out medially over the rectus muscle and a large perforator coursing through the rectus femoris was used to harvest an anteromedial thigh flap instead. **(D)** Postoperative results 6 months later with stable right-leg wound coverage and healed donor site.

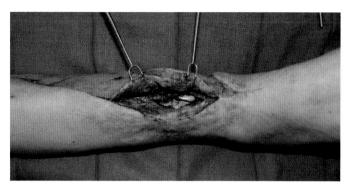

Fig. 2.34 Elevation of previous free muscle-sparing rectus muscle to medial distal third of right leg in order to remove methyl methacrylate and place definitive bone graft. Healed muscle flaps can be easily re-elevated during secondary procedures such as bone grafting or hardware removal.

include the vascularized iliac crest graft (deep circumflex iliac artery) and the vascularized scapular graft (circumflex scapular artery). Grafted vascularized bone will hypertrophy over time, but it takes months to a few years. For defects over 10 cm, distraction osteogenesis is considered. This involves the division of cortical bone with preservation of the continuity of cancellous bone and bloody supply at metaphysis (corticotomy). Half pins are applied to both segments of the bone, and an external fixator is applied. Distraction starts about 10–14 days later with a rate of 1 mm per day. The whole process can take more than 1 year. It can be very arduous and accompany complications such as pin site infection, pain, and nonunion.

Negative-pressure wound therapy in lower extremity defects

As advances in wound care have evolved over the past decade, there is increasing reliance on their use in the management of complex soft-tissue wounds. In particular, the use of commercially available Negative Pressure Wound Therapy (NPWT) devices is becoming more commonplace. It is thought that NPWT provides edema control and facilitation of wound closure via the application of soft-tissue macrostrain forces, stimulation of fibroblast proliferation, and tissue granulation via macrostrain at a cellular level, suppression of destructive wound proteases, facilitation of bacterial clearance from the wound, and prevention of cross-contamination in a hospital environment.[60] DeFranzo et al.[61] used a NPWT system in 75 patients with exposed tendon, bone, or hardware, excluding those with frank osteomyelitis. All wounds underwent surgical debridement until viable tissues were present in the wound base, prior to the application of the NPWT device. The authors found that granulation tissue was often present by the second dressing change, with a reduction in wound edema and bacterial count. All patients achieved stable wound coverage via delayed primary closure, skin graft, or local flap, with no need for free tissue reconstruction. In their assessment of trends in lower extremity reconstruction, Parrett et al.[50] found that there was a trend down the reconstructive ladder, with a decreasing incidence of free flap reconstruction and more frequent use of NPWT devices. They stated that at their center the NPWT system was used in 50% of open fractures and

most Gustilo grade III tibial fractures, with closure being achieved through delayed primary, secondary, and skin graft methods. This is not only cost-effective but also makes it possible to avoid flap surgery related complications. Additionally, NPWT systems can be used in fasciotomy wounds and incisional edema management.[62]

Amputation

In the situation where amputation is indicated, or the trauma has resulted in a complete/near-complete amputation, it is important to consider management of the amputation stump from a prosthetic standpoint. Preservation of length and creation of stable soft-tissue coverage are of paramount importance. If at all possible, maintaining a below-knee amputation length is important, as this is better tolerated and has much less energy demand for mobilization. In cases where there is inadequate soft-tissue coverage of a below-knee amputation bony stump, it is possible to use free flaps to maintain length. These can include musculocutaneous and fasciocutaneous options, similar to those discussed above. One can also consider the use of "spare parts" surgery, whereby portions of the amputated extremity (if intact/appropriate) can be used to reconstruct the remaining defect. Finally, if there is muscle coverage of the bony stump but no skin coverage, the use of skin grafts is appropriate to provide soft-tissue coverage.

Treatment of associated complications

Rhabdomyolysis

The concept of acute renal failure associated with crush injuries was first documented by Bywaters and Beal in 1941. It was their observation that patients who had been buried for several hours (during the Blitzkrieg attacks in London) presented with swelling and anesthesia of their limbs, with progression to pallor, coldness, sweating, and unstable vital signs (shock). Eventually arterial pulses diminished and urine output dropped, coincident with an increase in albumin and dark brown casts within it. Patients subsequently developed hyperkalemia and renal failure, leading to an accelerated death.

The pathophysiology of rhabdomyolysis involves muscle injury and resultant myocyte damage, which results in sodium and calcium influx into the cytoplasm and potassium efflux into the extracellular fluid.[63] As a result of this myocyte damage, a large quantity of breakdown products are released into the blood stream, and some of them, such as myoglobin, induce renal failure. The diagnosis of rhabdomyolysis is supported by a positive urine dipstick for hemoglobin, in addition to laboratory confirmation of myoglobin and quantitative assessment. The severity of acute renal failure that ensues can be predicted by the presence of a urine myoglobin concentration >20 mg/L.[64] Renal failure associated with rhabdomyolysis has three main mechanisms: (1) tubular obstruction; (2) tubular damage by oxidant injury; and (3) vasoconstriction.[63]

In the treatment of rhabdomyolysis, the most important component is early volume replacement to prevent the development of renal failure. Alkalinization of the urine using sodium bicarbonate (to a target pH 7.0) may be beneficial for washout of myoglobin and the prevention of lipid peroxidation and renal vasoconstriction. The use of mannitol is more controversial and may not be better than volume expansion alone.[65]

Fat embolism

Fat embolism is a rare entity, but occurs most commonly as a result of long bone fractures and polytrauma. It may be related to excessive pseudomotion of unstable fracture or internal fixation with IM nail. It is most common in young males aged 10–40 years and is rare in children and the elderly. This may be related to the low fat content of bone marrow in children and the minimal trauma fractures that tend to occur in the elderly.[66]

Two theories regarding the pathophysiologic mechanism of fat embolism syndrome (FES) exist – the mechanical hypothesis and the biochemical hypothesis. The mechanical hypothesis postulates that an increase in IM pressure forces marrow particles, fat, or bone fragments into the circulation via the open venous sinusoids. This leads to obstruction of peripheral and lung microcirculation. This results in ventilation–perfusion mismatch, low partial pressure of oxygen, and low oxygen saturation. Cerebral and renal embolization may contribute to the symptoms. The biochemical hypothesis postulates that physiochemical alteration occurs when fat globules are acted upon by lipoprotein lipase, resulting in the release of free fatty acids. This results in the release of toxic intermediates that can cause direct injury to pneumocytes and lung endothelial cells.[67]

FES is characterized by progressive respiratory insufficiency, deteriorating mental status, and petechial rash (major diagnostic criteria). Minor diagnostic criteria include pyrexia, tachycardia, retinal changes, jaundice, oliguria/anuria, thrombocytopenia, high erythrocyte sedimentation rate, and fat macroglobulinemia. According to Gurd and Wilson, the diagnosis of FES involves two major criteria, or one major plus four minor criteria plus fat microglobulinemia.[68] Typically, FES occurs within 24–72 h after injury and is largely a clinical diagnosis. Laboratory investigations may include an arterial blood gas to diagnose hypoxemia and cytologic examination of urine, blood, or sputum looking for fat globules. Chest radiography may be normal in these patients, prompting investigation with chest CT or bronchoalveolar lavage looking for fat-laden macrophages.[69] Because of the lack of specific diagnostic criteria or investigations, the incidence of FES is likely to be underestimated.

Once FES is suspected, the management is largely supportive and usually involves management of the hypoxemia. Prophylactic measures in those considered at risk for FES are most important. These include early stabilization of long bone/pelvic fractures, minimizing IM pressures during reaming, and irrigation of marrow prior to insertion of prostheses. Pharmacologic therapies have been disappointing and, despite initial interest in using steroids, there have not been any level 1 studies supporting their use.

Compartment syndrome

Compartment syndrome is a rare, but potentially devastating, complication of lower extremity trauma. Undiagnosed compartment syndrome can lead to nerve damage and muscle necrosis. Acute compartment syndrome involves a build-up of pressure within a non-elastic muscle compartment that is surrounded by fascia and bone. In the lower extremity there are four compartments: (1) anterior; (2) lateral; (3) superficial posterior; and (4) deep posterior. Compartment syndrome typically results from bleeding or edema within the compartment. Edema can create a barrier to perfusion, which results in hypoxia and acidosis. This is a self-perpetuating cycle, as this leads to further capillary permeability and fluid extravasation, worsening the edematous state.[70] The pathophysiology of compartment syndrome involves increasing interstitial pressure. This leads to increased intraluminal venous pressure in an effort to avoid vascular collapse. As a result, there is a decreased gradient between arterioles and veins, and capillary blood flow thus decreases and results in ischemia. The muscle undergoes ischemic scar formation, and necrosis leads to myoglobinemia.

The classic description of compartment syndrome was provided by Griffiths, in which he described the "four Ps" – pain, paresthesia, paresis, and pain with stretch.[71] This has been further expanded to "six Ps" with the addition of pulselessness and poikilothermia. Compartment syndrome is relatively uncommon, but should be anticipated in situations of high-velocity trauma, in patients on blood thinners, and with lower extremity vascular occlusion or disruption. Pain is the earliest and most sensitive clinical sign. Confirmation of the diagnosis can be achieved by measuring the intracompartmental pressure. The absolute threshold for fasciotomy has been debated, with some favoring pressures greater than 30 mmHg and others looking at the difference between compartment pressure and mean arterial pressure (<30 mmHg below mean arterial pressure significant), or diastolic pressure (<30 mmHg below diastolic pressure significant).[70]

Following diagnosis, the treatment consists of urgent surgical decompression of all four compartments. Multiple approaches have been described, but the most common techniques are release via a single lateral incision or combined anterolateral and posteromedial incisions. The single-incision technique involves an incision in line with the fibula extending from just distal to the head of fibula to 3–4 cm proximal to the lateral malleolus. Longitudinal fasciotomies of the anterior and lateral compartments are performed, followed by subcutaneous dissection posteriorly to access the superficial and deep posterior compartments. In the two-incision technique, an anterolateral incision is placed between the tibial crest and the fibula over the anterior intermuscular septum. Fasciotomies of the anterior and lateral compartments are carried out through this incision. The posteromedial incision is placed 2 cm posterior to the posteromedial edge of the tibia. This allows access to the superficial posterior compartment, and, following division of the soleal bridge, the deep compartment can be accessed.

Postoperative care

Antibiotics

In 2009 the EAST practice management group published updated guidelines for antibiotic use in open fractures.[72] Based on their literature review, they made several recommendations. These include level I recommendations: antibiotics with Gram-positive coverage to start at time of injury, with the addition of Gram-negative coverage in Gustilo grade III injuries. Also, high-dose penicillin should be added in the presence of fecal or possible clostridial contamination. They suggest that aminoglycosides do not offer an advantage over cephalosporin/aminoglycoside regimens, and they may have a detrimental effect on fracture healing. Level II recommendations include discontinuation of antibiotics within 24 h of wound closure (grade I and II fractures) or 72 h postinjury/24 h post soft-tissue coverage in grade III fractures. A single dose of aminoglycoside is appropriate for grade II and III fractures.

Anticoagulation

Death from venous thromboembolism (VTE) is preventable, which is why the use of VTE protocols is on the rise. The prophylaxis of VTE is one of the goals of improved surgical care identified by the Surgical Care Improvement Project.[73] Victims of major trauma have the highest risk of VTE.[74] Proposed risk factors include spinal cord injury, lower extremity fractures, pelvic fractures, surgery, femoral central venous lines, age, immobility, and delay in initiating thromboprophylaxis.[74]

Two of the commonly used anticoagulants include unfractionated heparin (UH) and low-molecular-weight heparin (LMWH). UH acts on antithrombin, catalyzing the reaction between antithrombin and thrombin (factor IIa) as well as factor Xa.[75] This inhibits the procoagulant activity of thrombin. LMWH is a depolymerized form of UH and exerts its action via factor Xa, with less effect on antithrombin. Until now, few studies existed comparing the efficacy and safety of pharmacoprophylaxis using these drugs. One retrospective study comparing protocols of UH and LMWH found that there was no difference in incidence of VTE or bleeding complications between the two drugs and that 5000 U three times a day of UH was much cheaper than 40 mg per day of LMWH.[74]

Blood loss

Hemorrhage in the setting of lower extremity trauma is common, especially with long bone or combined injuries. It may account for as much as 40% of trauma-related mortality and is the second leading cause of death after injury.[76] As many as 30% of patients may require massive transfusion during the initial postinjury period. This is classified as transfusion of 10 or more units of packed red blood cells in the first 24 h following injury.[77,78] Unfortunately, there is no ideal strategy for the management of post-traumatic hemorrhagic shock. The current trend for prevention of hemorrhagic shock is a brief "damage control" surgery, rapid fluid resuscitation, and sufficient administration of blood products. In damage control surgery, there are four phases: (1) recognizing a patient who warrants the "damage control" approach; (2) salvage surgery for control of hemorrhage, contamination, and stabilization of long bone and pelvic fractures; (3) intensive care unit management for restoration of physiologic and immunologic baseline functions; and (4) scheduled reconstructive surgeries for definitive management of the injury once the patient is stable enough.[79]

The threshold for starting blood transfusion is also debated. According to ATLS protocols, blood products should be considered in patients who are non-responders or transient responders to fluid resuscitation, with estimated blood loss >30%. The original Transfusion Requirements In Critical Care (TRICC) trial looking at transfusion protocols provides a rough estimate of when to transfuse, suggesting that a restrictive approach (transfusing when hemoglobin <7 g/dL) may be safe.[80] However, this study population may not be equivalent to a patient involved in lower extremity trauma. It may be more accurate to follow base deficit and serum lactate in the assessment of bleeding and shock. Transfusion strategy also involves multiple components, including red blood cells, fresh frozen plasma, and platelets. The ratio of each varies significantly in the literature and is beyond the scope of this chapter. Additionally, it is important to avoid other factors that may contribute to coagulopathy, such as hypothermia, and all attempts should be made to control any such preventable factors.

Outcomes, prognosis, and complications

Outcomes and prognosis

Functional outcomes

One of the most important criteria of the functional recovery in patients sustaining lower extremity trauma is their return to work. Studies have demonstrated that more than one-quarter of these patients have not returned to work at 1 year postinjury. Butcher et al.[81] investigated functional recovery of patients who did not return to work by 1 year. Using the Sickness Impact Profile (SIP) questionnaire, they determined that return to work occurred in 72% of their patients by 12 months, and 82% had returned to work by 30 months. Among them, 64% of patients had no disability, 17% had mild disability, 12% had moderate disability, and 7% had severe disability. This study did not differentiate between those who underwent limb salvage and those with amputation.

Mackenzie et al.[82] examined functional outcomes in those patients who underwent amputation following trauma-related lower extremity injury. Study participants were part of the original LEAP cohort that had undergone amputation as a result of their injury. Patients were stratified according to level of amputation – above-knee, through-knee, and below-knee. At 24 months, patients with through-knee amputation had the highest SIP scores. There was a modest degree of disability among all patient groups. Overall, patients with through-knee amputation had worse outcomes with lower self-selected walking speed, ability to perform functional transfers, and ability to walk and stair-climb. There were no significant differences in SIP scores between those with below-knee and those with above-knee amputations.

Amputation versus salvage

A systematic review of outcomes and complications in patients undergoing reconstruction and amputation of grade IIIB and IIIC tibial injuries assessed 26 studies in the published literature.[83] It was found that hospital stay was longer in the amputation group (63.7 vs. 56.9 days), but this was statistically insignificant. Of those initially reconstructed, the pooled secondary amputation rate was 5.1% in type IIIB fractures and 28.7% in type IIIC fractures. When regressed against the year of study publication, the secondary amputation rate decreased – likely due to improved operative technique and increasing incidence of successful salvage. The rate of osteomyelitis in limb salvage patients was variable, with a range of 4–56%. Complete flap loss was 5.8% (pooled result; range 0–15%). Overall, this study did not reveal a superior strategy in treating patients with lower limb-threatening injuries, as the outcomes of salvage and amputation groups were similar.

Patient satisfaction

Very few studies have examined the differences between patient's and physician's satisfaction in lower extremity trauma. The LEAP study looked at this issue in 463 patients with unilateral lower extremity injuries. Patients' satisfaction was evaluated at 12 and 24 months postinjury via a structured clinical interview. Surgeons were asked to evaluate their satisfaction with the clinical recovery and cosmetic recovery of the lower extremity at the 24-month mark. The results demonstrated that there was poor agreement between the surgeons' and patients' satisfaction with both overall and cosmetic outcomes.[84] Surgeons and patients differed particularly on the cosmetic outcome, with patients being less satisfied than their surgeons. Patients and surgeons were more likely to disagree regarding overall outcome when the injury severity score was greater than 17, complications that required hospital admission occurred, patients were dissatisfied with their care, or when patients failed to return to work within 1 year. Disagreement regarding cosmetic outcome was greater when patients were female, had sustained a traumatic amputation (patients were more satisfied in this group), had complications requiring hospital admission, or were dissatisfied with their care. On the whole, 66% of patients were satisfied with their overall outcome at 2 years, and 34% were not.[85] No pre-existing patient factors were identified to be predictive of this. The factors that correlated with satisfaction were measures of physical function, psychological distress, clinical recovery, and return to work.

Cost-utility

There have been two large studies looking at cost utility in lower extremity trauma. This is especially important as reconstructive endeavors are considered not only to be technically demanding and time-consuming, but they can be associated with a high risk of complications and rehabilitation time. It is important to justify this from a patient care and economic perspective. In 2007, Mackenzie et al.[86] conducted a multicenter study estimating the healthcare costs for 545 patients with unilateral limb-threatening lower extremity trauma. This was part of the original LEAP study. They found that, when costs associated with re-hospitalization and postacute care were added to the initial cost of hospitalization, the 2-year overall cost was similar between salvage and amputation groups. However, when prosthesis-related costs were added, the amputation group required a much higher cost of treatment, with an initial $10 000 difference in cost and a projected lifetime cost that was three times higher ($509 275 vs. $163 282) than the salvage group. In a study by Chung et al.[87] a cost-utility analysis demonstrated that, independently of ongoing prosthesis-related needs and remaining years of life, amputation is more expensive overall. They estimated that amputation will cost a 40-year-old patient $93 606–$154 636 more than limb salvage. This study suggested that surgeons should select limb salvage more aggressively, in particular for patients where amputation is not clearly indicated.

Complications

Wound complications

The goal of reconstruction is to provide soft-tissue coverage that creates a closed wound, provides vascularized tissue, and prevents secondary complications of the injury including late infection and nonunion. A subset of the LEAP study specifically examined wound complications as stratified by type of reconstruction. It was found that those reconstructed with free flaps were more likely to have multicompartment functional compromise in the leg with more severe soft-tissue injury. Despite this, there was no overall difference in complication rates between patients reconstructed with local rotational flaps and those reconstructed with free tissue transfer. However, when patients were further stratified by underlying osseous injury, regression analysis demonstrated that this was an important predictor of wound complication. In patients with ASIF/OTA type C injury, those with rotational flap reconstruction were 4.3 times more likely to have a wound complication requiring operative intervention than those with free flap reconstruction.[88] Interestingly, there was not an increased rate of wound complications when the patients were stratified by time to reconstruction, suggesting that, in this cohort, time to reconstruction was not an important predictor, as is suggested by Godina.[34]

Osteomyelitis

It has been shown that the tibia is the most common site of infected nonunion and chronic post-traumatic osteomyelitis.[89] This is associated with morbidity and may be limb-threatening. In this regard, it is important to prevent the occurrence of osteomyelitis and treat it early and aggressively. The LEAP study had an incidence of 7.7% for osteomyelitis, with 84% of these patients requiring operative intervention and hospitalization.[90]

It is thought that an aggregation of microbe colonies called "biofilm" is the key in the development and persistence of infection.[91] The most common organism in chronic osteomyelitis is *Staphylococcus aureus*, which may be commonly combined with other pathogens such as *Pseudomonas aeruginosa*. Four anatomic types of osteomyelitis exist: (1) medullary (IM bone surface); (2) superficial (bone surface); (3) localized (full-thickness cortex extending into medullary canal); and (4) diffuse (circumferential bone involvement). Furthermore, the patient can be classified according to physiologic status: good systemic defenses (type A), systemic/local/combined deficiency in wound healing (type B), or severe local/systemic factors (type C). Infection may be clinically silent, emphasizing the need for a high index of suspicion. Diagnosis relies on clinical findings, laboratory tests (erythrocyte sedimentation rate and C-reactive protein), diagnostic imaging (X-ray, magnetic resonance imaging, and technetium-99m bone scan), and, the gold standard, bone culture. The management of osteomyelitis includes debridement and antibiotics, in conjunction with fracture stabilization. It is necessary to remove all operative hardware, debride infected bony sequestra aggressively, and ream out the IM canal if rod fixation was used. It cannot be overemphasized how important it is to perform extensive bony debridement until viable bone with punctate bleeding is achieved. It is possible to use local antibiotic therapy in the form of antibiotic-impregnated beads, placed in the defect site following debridement. Systemic antibiotic therapy should be broad initially and tailored according to culture results. If internal fixation is removed and the fracture is not healed or in a state of nonunion, a temporary external fixator may be placed until the infection is eradicated. The secondary stages of reconstruction involve local or free tissue coverage (usually within 1 week of initial debridement), followed by management of bony defects or ununited fractures. Bone-grafting procedures are carried out once the soft-tissue envelope has healed and infection is under control, typically 6–8 weeks after soft-tissue coverage.

In some situations amputation is inevitable; these include extensive bone defects, poor soft-tissue coverage, neurovascular compromise, anticipated poor function, and multiple comorbidities.[91]

Nonunion

In the LEAP study, nonunion was among the most common complications, with an incidence of 23.7%. Of these, 83% required operative intervention and 72% required inpatient care.[90]

Chronic pain

It has long been suspected that chronic pain has been a complication of traumatic injury, but to date there has been little prospective evidence to document this. The LEAP study addressed chronic pain in a prospective cohort analysis of patients with severe lower extremity trauma.[92] A total of 397 patients were followed for 7 years after discharge, with a follow-up rate of 72%. Data were collected regarding injury and treatment characteristics, socio-demographics, and predictors of pain. Predictors included functional outcomes (ambulation, mobility, body care, and communication), depression and anxiety scores, and pain intensity scores. This study demonstrated a high level of long-term chronic pain, with more than one-quarter of the study population reporting pain that interfered with daily activities and 40% reporting clinically significant pain intensity. The chronic pain levels in the study group were comparable to those of back pain and headache populations at pain clinics. The multivariate analysis did not identify any predictors of pain related to the injury and treatment, suggesting that the onset of chronic pain is independent of injury characteristics and surgical treatment decisions – supporting prior studies by Ashburn and Fine.[93] Protective factors included years of education and increased self-efficiency for return to usual major activities. Risk factors included alcohol use in the month prior to injury; symptoms of anxiety, depression, and sleep irregularities at 3 months postinjury; and, the strongest risk factor, intensity of acute pain at 3 months postinjury. Narcotic use at 3 months appeared to be protective as well, perhaps supporting the central sensitization theory for the development of chronic pain.

Secondary procedures

A variety of secondary procedures may be required following lower extremity reconstruction and limb salvage. These can fall into two broad categories: (1) secondary cosmetic procedures to improve the quality and appearance of the reconstruction (e.g., flap debulking); and (2) secondary functional procedures to finalize the reconstruction (e.g., delayed bone graft).

Secondary cosmetic procedures

One of the most frequent secondary procedures required to improve the appearance of the reconstruction is flap debulking. For fasciocutaneous flap and perforator flaps we prefer to wait a minimum of 3 months, preferably 6 months prior to any debulking procedures. Liposuction is the most common method of debulking. If redundant skin requires excision, we usually perform this 3 months following liposuction in order not to compromise vascularity and limit skin excision to 50% or less of the flap circumference. Combined aggressive liposuction with flap skin excision should be avoided whenever possible in order to prevent complications. Several sessions of debulking may be required in certain flaps in order to provide the lowest profile resurfacing possible, for example, flaps for medial or lateral malleolus reconstruction (Figs. 2.35–2.38).

For muscle flaps or myocutaneous flaps, debulking procedures can also be required but less frequently with free muscle flaps alone. Denervated muscle undergoes significant atrophy over time and provides excellent contouring for lower-extremity reconstruction. The skin paddle from a myocutaneous flap can also be removed as a split-thickness skin graft or thin full-thickness skin graft with a dermatome and then reused to cover the underlying muscle following excision of excess subcutaneous tissue. If required, the muscle can also be debulked, and we prefer to use the dermatome for this to shave the muscle from superficial to deep, making sure to protect the pedicle at all times. For skin-grafted muscle flaps, a dermatome can also be used to remove the skin graft from the flap temporarily. The muscle is then debulked with progressive shaving using a dermatome, and the skin graft is recycled to cover the muscle once debulking is completed. We prefer to use the tourniquet for all debulking procedures, perform meticulous hemostasis, and use a negative-pressure dressing to secure the skin graft following debulking (Figs. 2.29A, 2.39 & 2.40).

Secondary functional procedures

Secondary procedures to restore function of the lower extremity are numerous and include secondary bone graft, hardware removal or replacement, tendon reconstruction, and nerve repair/graft. For any anticipated orthopedic procedure, close collaboration with orthopedic surgery is important in order to re-elevate the flap safely. Muscle and skin flaps can be easily re-elevated, although skin flaps provide the greatest flexibility and ease for re-elevation, which is why we prefer to use them if secondary procedures are anticipated. The tourniquet is also used for secondary procedures and elevation of flaps.

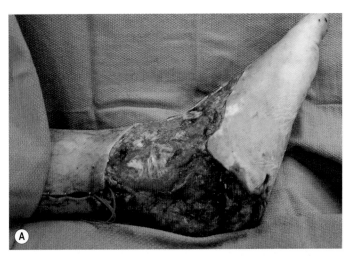
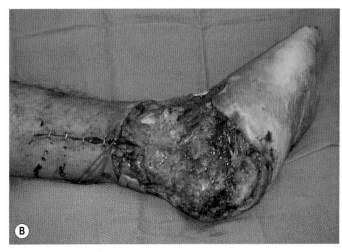

Fig. 2.35 Extensive degloving injury following a motorcycle accident in a 24-year-old man, with exposure of the calcaneus, medial malleolus, and extensor tendons.

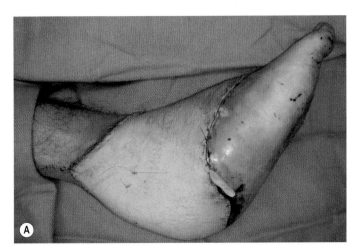
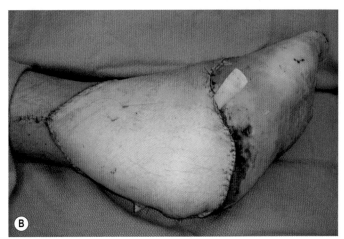

Fig. 2.36 Resurfacing of the lower extremity defect with an extended free anterolateral thigh flap (384 cm^2).

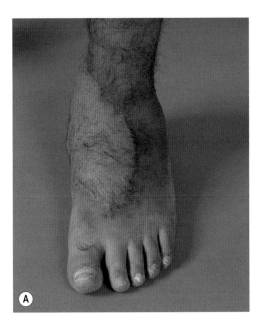
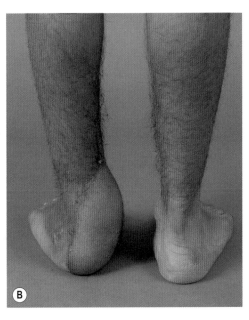

Fig. 2.37 Appearance of the anterolateral thigh flap following liposuction at 6 months following initial surgery. A total of 75 cc of lipoaspirate was removed.

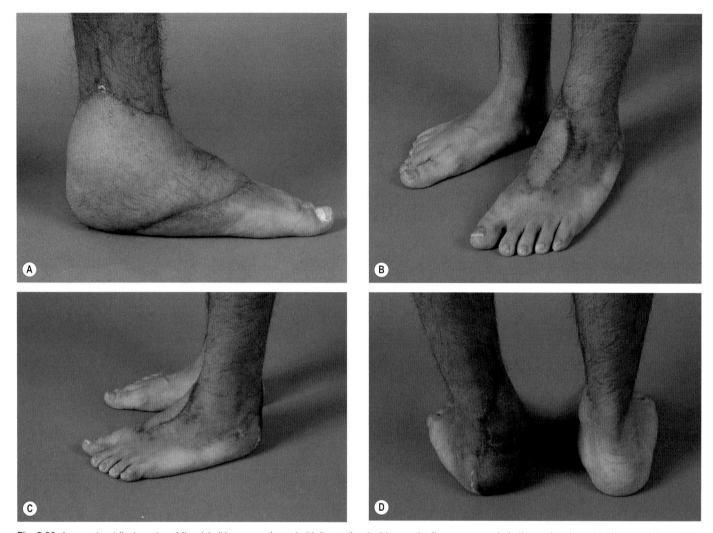

Fig. 2.38 A second and final session of flap debulking was performed with liposuction. In this case the flap was aggressively liposuctioned, even in the area of the pedicle, to minimize bulk. If the peripheral flap incision is kept intact, then aggressive liposuction can be performed while maintaining adequate vascularity.

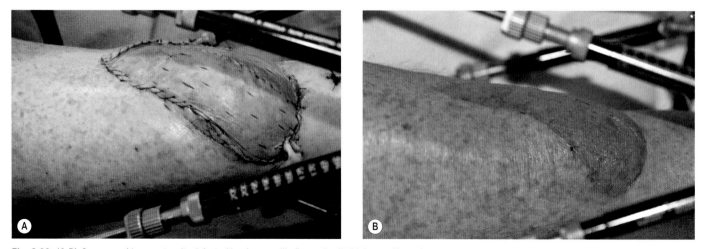

Fig. 2.39 (A,B) Coverage of lower extremity defect with a free gracilis flap and split-thickness skin graft.

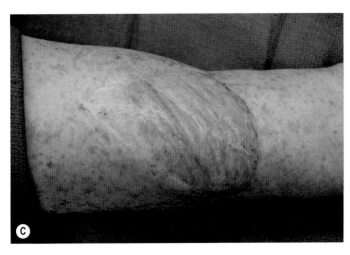

Fig. 2.39, cont'd (C) Appearance of the gracilis muscle flap at 3 months following surgery. Note significant muscle atrophy over time.

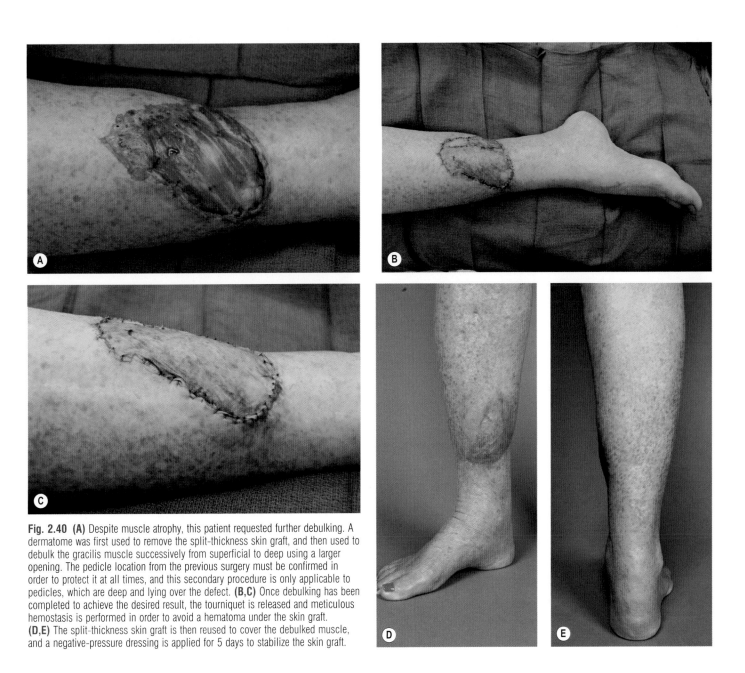

Fig. 2.40 (A) Despite muscle atrophy, this patient requested further debulking. A dermatome was first used to remove the split-thickness skin graft, and then used to debulk the gracilis muscle successively from superficial to deep using a larger opening. The pedicle location from the previous surgery must be confirmed in order to protect it at all times, and this secondary procedure is only applicable to pedicles, which are deep and lying over the defect. **(B,C)** Once debulking has been completed to achieve the desired result, the tourniquet is released and meticulous hemostasis is performed in order to avoid a hematoma under the skin graft. **(D,E)** The split-thickness skin graft is then reused to cover the debulked muscle, and a negative-pressure dressing is applied for 5 days to stabilize the skin graft.

Access the complete reference list online at   **http://www.expertconsult.com**

6. Levin LS. The reconstructive ladder. An orthoplastic approach. *Orthop Clin North Am.* 1993;24(3):393–409.

17. Keel M, Trentz O. Pathophysiology of polytrauma. *Injury.* 2005;36(6):691–709.

22. Management of Complex Extremity Trauma. American College of Surgeons. The Committee on Trauma. [Online] Available from: <http://www.facs.org/quality-programs/trauma/publications>.

24. Gustilo RB, Mendoza RM, Williams DN. Problems in the management of type III (severe) open fractures: a new classification of type III open fractures. *J Trauma.* 1984;24(8):742–746.

27. Higgins TF, Klatt JB, Beals TC. Lower Extremity Assessment Project (LEAP) – the best available evidence on limb-threatening lower extremity trauma. *Orthop Clin North Am.* 2010;41(2):233–239. *An overview of the LEAP protocol and substudy analyses. A total of 601 patients were enrolled and followed for a period of 44 months at 8 centers. The LEAP study attempted to assess the characteristics of the patients sustaining lower extremity injury, environmental characteristics of the injury, physical and mental aspects of the injury, secondary medical issues arising from the injury, and functional status. It was found that social, economic, and personality disadvantages that existed prior to the injury play a large role in the functional and quality-of-life outcomes measured in the study. It was also found that the functional outcomes 2 years postinjury were similar between those undergoing limb salvage and those that underwent amputation.*

29. Ly TV, Travison TG, Castillo RC, et al. Ability of lower-extremity injury severity scores to predict functional outcome after limb salvage. *J Bone Joint Surg Am.* 2008;90(8):1738–1743.

34. Godina M. Early microsurgical reconstruction of complex trauma of the extremities. *Plast Reconstr Surg.* 1986;78(3):285–292. *Landmark paper examining the timing of microsurgical reconstruction in extremity trauma. This study divided patients into 3 groups according to time of reconstruction: <72 h, 72 h–3 months, >3 months. Godina examined the incidence of flap failure, infection, bone-healing time, length of hospital stay, and number of operative procedures. He found that outcomes were the best in the group reconstructed within 72 h. Those reconstructed between 72 h and 3 months had the highest rate of infection, and those reconstructed >3 months postinjury had the longest bone-healing time and required the greatest number of operations.*

40. Ong YS, Levin LS. Lower limb salvage in trauma. *Plast Reconstr Surg.* 2010;125(2):582–588. *An overview of the management of lower extremity trauma, including initial management, decision-making for salvage versus amputation, timing of reconstruction, and choice of flap. This paper also reviews outcomes of reconstruction, including flap failure, late complications, and function.*

50. Parrett BM, Talbot SG, Pribaz JJ, et al. A review of local and regional flaps for distal leg reconstruction. *J Reconstr Microsurg.* 2009;25(7):445–455. *A thorough review of local and regional flap options available in distal leg reconstruction. This paper outlines the preoperative work-up and provides an algorithmic approach to select an appropriate flap for reconstruction. Several flaps are reviewed in detail, including their indications, design, surgical technique, and complications/pitfalls.*

82. MacKenzie EJ, Bosse MJ, Castillo RC, et al. Functional outcomes following trauma-related lower-extremity amputation. *J Bone Joint Surg Am.* 2004;86(8):1636–1645. *A subset of the LEAP study, 161 patients who underwent above-the-ankle amputation following lower extremity trauma were followed prospectively for a total of 24 months. Outcomes included functional measures using the Sickness Inventory Profile (SIP), pain assessments, and degree of independence assessment. The SIP was not different between those amputated above- versus below-the-knee. Physical function was affected by the level of amputation, with walking speeds higher in below-the-knee amputation patients.*

3

Lymphatic reconstruction of the extremities

David W. Chang

Access video content for this chapter online at expertconsult.com

SYNOPSIS

- Direct excision with skin grafting is reserved for the most extreme cases in which function is severely affected.
- Liposuction for reduction of excess adipose deposition requires lifelong postoperative compression garments.
- Reductive procedures alone or as an adjunct are effective in gross reduction of volume; however, they may carry significant morbidity.
- Lymphovenous bypass (LVB) appears to be most effective at the early stages of lymphedema before destruction of lymphatic vessel smooth muscle and development of irreversible tissue fibrosis.
- LVB alone may be more effective in addressing the upper extremity vs. lower extremity lymphedema.
- Vascularized lymph node transfers (VLNT) can be harvested from numerous locations such as the groin, axilla, supraclavicular, and submental regions. They can also be transferred to proximal (groin/axilla) or distal (wrist/ankle) areas of the affected limb.
- Harvest of VLNT should be performed carefully to prevent donor limb lymphedema.
- VLNT may be combined with LVB in patients with moderate to severe lymphedema.

Introduction

Lymphedema is a chronic, debilitating disease affecting up to 250 million people worldwide. It is caused by an accumulation of lymphatic fluid leading to progressive tissue fibrosis, fat hypertrophy, and destruction of lymphatic vessels.[1–3] Lymphedema may be classified as primary due to abnormal development of the lymphatic system or secondary due to acquired damage to the lymphatic system. Globally, the most common cause is filariasis, but in the USA and most developed countries, cancer and its treatments are the most common cause. There is currently no cure for this disease, and we are still searching for the "gold" standard treatment for lymphedema.

Most common and essential treatment for lymphedema is complex decongestive lymphatic therapy including compression garments. These therapies are labor intensive, time consuming, expensive, and often not covered by insurance. They also require strict lifetime compliance, which leads to high rates of non-compliance and patient dissatisfaction. Surgery may be considered when conservative measures fail. Goals of surgical intervention include weight reduction of the affected region, reduced frequency of infections, prevention of disease progression, improvement in limb function and cosmesis, and overall improvement in patient's quality of life.

Evaluation techniques

There are many modalities in place to evaluate lymphedema. The International Society of Lymphology has created a clinical staging system to help document disease progression. In stage I, the limb is swollen, feels heavy, and has pitting edema partially reversible with elevation. In stage II, the limb is swollen, the skin is brawny, and tissue fibrosis has started, leading to non-pitting edema that is not reversible with elevation. In stage III, there is enormous swelling of the involved extremity with fibrosis and hardening of the dermal tissues. Skin papillomas, acanthosis, fat deposits, and warty overgrowths may be present.

Currently, the most definitive tool for evaluation of lymphedema is lymphoscintigraphy, in which a radioactive dye is injected into the affected limb to visualize the lymphatics and quantify the lymphatic flow by calculating a lymphatic transport index. The index ranges from 0 (optimal flow) to 45 (no flow). A transport index below 10 is considered normal. Indocyanine green (ICG) lymphangiography is a newer technology to help us visualize superficial lymphatics and determine the severity of the disease. ICG is a fluorescent dye that is activated when it binds to protein and imaged using near-infrared technology. A staging system has been proposed based on ICG lymphangiography findings.[4] In stage I, there are many patent lymphatic vessels, with minimal, patchy dermal backflow. Stage II shows a moderate number of patent lymphatic vessels, with segmental dermal backflow. Stage III shows few patent lymphatic vessels, with extensive dermal backflow involving the entire extremity. Stage IV shows no patent lymphatic vessels, with severe dermal backflow involving the entire extremity. Knowing the lymphedema disease stage helps guide appropriate surgical intervention. Postoperatively, one of the most common and simple methods to determine improvement is to perform serial circumferential measurements or limb volumes. Other means to measure outcomes include bio-impedance and quality-of-life questionnaires.

Surgical management

Options for surgical treatment of lymphedema can be divided into two categories: excisional and physiologic treatment. Excisional treatment usually involves reductive procedures such as liposuction and excisional debulking with skin grafting (Charles procedure). Physiologic treatment is aimed at restoring or reconstructing the physiologic drainage of the lymph fluid. Several different strategies to achieve this have been proposed, such as buried flaps, direct repair of lymphatics, bypass grafting of lymphatics, lymphaticovenular anastomosis, and vascularized lymph node transfers. The outcomes of such procedures vary. The aim of this chapter is to present the overview of therapies that have been described and tested.

Reductive/excisional techniques

Direct excision (Video 3.4 ○)

In 1912, Charles wrote a book chapter entitled "Elephantiasis Scroti" in which he described a treatment for scrotal lymphedema that he learned while spending time in Calcutta with his mentor McLeod. This procedure involved excision of the lymphedematous scrotal tissue and coverage with thigh advancement flaps. Charles suggested this technique could be applied to treat lymphedema in other areas of the body including the lower extremities, but would require preoperative arrangements for skin graft coverage.[5,6] This idea of treating lower extremity lymphedema with radical excision down to deep fascia and covering with a skin graft was not actually reported until 1940, when Macey from the Mayo Clinic published his experience. What we currently consider the "Charles procedure" was reported in 1947 by Poth from Galveston, who reported utilizing the skin from the excised specimen to cover the exposed limb.[7,8]

Although some have advocated the abandonment of such procedures, there are some cases of severe refractory lymphedema that have been successfully treated with radical excision and skin grafting.[9,10] Undoubtedly, although this can be an effective way of reducing bulk and allowing function of some extremities, there are also significant risks. In addition to contour irregularities, scarring, and poor cosmesis, there are risks of infection, hematoma, blood loss requiring transfusions, and possible loss of skin grafts resulting in more surgery. Alternatively, staged elliptical excision of skin and subcutaneous tissue can also be performed to minimize morbidity or to address specific pockets of tissue. For some patients suffering with severe impairment in use of their limb, recurrent infections, skin ulcerations, chronic pain, and poor quality of life, radical excision may be their only, and possibly best, option for returning to function (Fig. 3.1).

Liposuction

The accumulation of lymphatic fluid in the limb results in increased deposition and hypertrophy of the adipose tissue. Liposuction, in which a fenestrated metallic cannula connected to vacuum suction is used to aspirate subcutaneous fat, was originally developed for body contouring but since then has been used for the treatment of lymphedema. O'Brien *et al.* reported an average of 20–23% reduction using liposuction to treat lymphedema for a mixed cohort of patients.[11] Brorson and Svensson compared the combined use of liposuction and compression therapy to therapy alone in stage II patients and reported 115% reduction in volume compared to 54%. This was maintained at 4 years with average reduction of 106% (66–179%).[12]

One of the theoretical risks of liposuction is further damage to existing lymphatic vessels. Cadaveric and imaging studies have shown that performing liposuction longitudinally to the limb minimizes this damage and that further impairment to already delayed transport of lymphatic fluid does not seem to occur.[13–15] In addition to volumetric reduction, functional improvement was also reported by Qi *et al.* when liposuction was combined with physiologic treatments. The incidence of cellulitis (6.5±4.3 vs. 0.7±0.8 episodes/year) was drastically improved albeit confounded by the mixture of procedures performed.[16]

In general, treatment of lymphedema with circumferential liposuction is considered safe with quick recovery within 48 h.[17] Complications are few and usually limited to minor wound healing problems and paresthesias. The use of tumescence and tourniquets during liposuction can greatly decrease the blood loss and need for transfusions.

While liposuction can aggressively debulk hypertrophied adipose tissue in the lymphedematous limb, the primary disadvantage of liposuction is the lifelong need for continuous (24 h) use of compression garments postoperatively to maintain the new equilibrium.[18] In the Brorson series, patients that discontinued use of compression garments rapidly re-accumulated fluid.[12]

Physiologic treatment

Another approach to surgically treat lymphedema is to create a new path for lymphatic drainage or repair the lymphatic dysfunction. This concept was first described by Kondoleon in 1912 and expounded upon by Sistrunk in 1927 where they sought to establish new pathways between the deep and superficial systems.[19–21] Sistrunk removed skin and soft tissue through an elliptical incision along the medial arm and wide excision of the deep fascia. Thompson expanded this procedure by embedding the de-epithelialized skin flaps from the entire length of the elliptical incision along the neurovascular bundle. The theory was to facilitate spontaneous lymphangiogenesis from the superficial system that can be drained away by the deep system. Although some have reported favorable results with these methods, there have been no objective data that demonstrates lymphangiogenesis via this approach.[22]

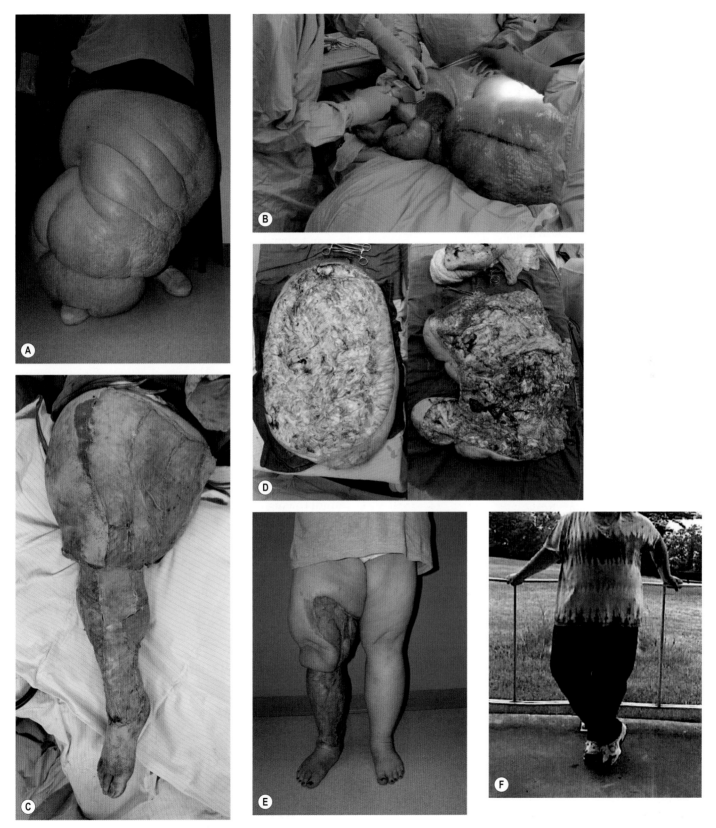

Fig. 3.1 An example of Charles procedure. Skin and subcutaneous lymphedematous tissue is excised to the deep fascia. Skin graft can be harvested from the specimen or contralateral thigh and used to cover the defect. Patient's remark in her letter, "My first hiking/outing in 13 years. My first pair of jeans in 13 years and in 14 years a pair of new balance sneakers." *(From: Cheng MH, Chang DW, Patel K.* Principles and Practice of Lymphedema Surgery. *New York: Elsevier; 2015.)*

Flap interposition

The basis behind flap interposition is to place functioning lymphatic vessels contained within a segment of vascularized tissue into an affected area to siphon or bypass excess lymph fluid. In 1935, Gilles and Fraser were the first to treat lower extremity lymphedema by attaching a flap of skin and subcutaneous tissue from the arm to the leg and keeping the arm by the patient's side.[23,24] In the second stage, the flap was divided and the flap was transferred to the trunk. The theory was to use the flap from the arm to re-establish lymphatic flow and then to eventually bypass the groin region and restore lymphatic flow to the trunk.

Goldsmith et al. reported the use of greater omentum flaps to upper and lower extremity lymphedema.[25] The greater omentum was pedicled off the ipsilateral gastroepiploic vessel and transferred to the extremity via a subcutaneous tunnel. The excess lymph fluid in the extremity was expected to drain into the abdominal lymphatic system through the rich network of lymph vessels in the greater omentum. In the series of 22 patients, 38% of lower extremity and 56% of upper extremity experienced good results. Despite this moderate improvement, the operation did not gain popularity due to the high incidence of complications including bowel obstruction, pulmonary embolus, and hernia.

Since then other authors reported small series using a variety of pedicled, free muscle, and myocutaneous flaps (tensor fascia lata, deltopectoral, latissimus, and serratus) for the treatment of extremity and head and neck lymphedema.[26–29] No prospective or long-term studies have demonstrated the efficacy of these procedures, and they remain anecdotal for the most part.

Lymphatic–lymphatic bypass

Some investigators have attempted to bypass fibrosed lymphatics by using lymphatic or vein grafts to link distal lymphatics to more proximal lymphatic channels. Baumeister and Suida attempted to bridge areas of stenosed lymphatic vessels with autologous lymphatic grafts in the upper and lower extremities.[30] For the upper extremity, healthy lymphatic vessels from the medial thigh are harvested as a composite graft and buried in a subcutaneous tunnel between the supraclavicular shoulder region and the upper arm. The lymphatic vessels at either end are microscopically identified and anastomosed to the recipient lymphatics. To treat unilateral lower extremity lymphedema, the lymphatics of the graft spans across the affected thigh and the contralateral groin region. In 55 patients tested, there was an 80% reduction of volume at 3-year follow-up. The patency of the lymphatic grafts were tested with lymphoscintigraphy and demonstrated new lymphatic drainage patterns and 30% faster clearance of radioisotope than in preoperative images. Ho and colleagues performed similar procedures and noted that the microlymphatic bypass must be carried out before the lymphatics were permanently damaged by back-pressure and recurrent infection.[31] In addition to the drawback of long incisions at donor and recipient sites, the harvest of lymphatics from a functional extremity may predispose that extremity to lymphedema.

Alternatively, vein grafts have been used to perform distal to proximal lymphatic bypasses. Campisi et al. reported a series of 39 patients using lymphatic–venous–lymphatic bypasses in upper and lower extremities when LVB could not be performed.[32] In their procedure, multiple distal lymphatic channels are sutured into the cut distal end of an autologous vein graft that provides a conduit to more proximal lymph vessels inserted into the other end of the vein graft. Patients were followed for as long as 5 years demonstrating improvement in edema and function.

Lymphovenous bypass (LVB) and lymphovenous anastomosis (LVA) (Videos 3.1 and 3.3)

The final destination of lymphatic fluid in the lymph vessels is return to the venous system by way of the thoracic ducts. LVB attempts to return the lymphatic fluid to the venous system earlier along the pathway. A lymphovenous shunt was first described by Jacobson in 1962 in a canine model.[33] This was followed by Yamada who first experimented in dogs before applying the technique in a series of patients with lower extremity lymphedema.[34] In cases involving filariasis, Sedlacek described the use of end-to-side LVB using the saphenous vein.[35] While others also used the saphenous vein, concern over venous hypertension in larger caliber vessels resulted in attempts to bypass to venules. Yamada was the first to describe end-to-end anastomosis between a lymphatic and venule, hence LVA. The use of "supermicrosurgery" to anastomose vessels <0.8 mm in diameter has recently gained popularity around the world.[4,36–38,39]

Results of LVB have been favorable, but outcomes have been difficult to standardize. In 1990 O'Brien et al. reported long-term follow-up on 90 patients, some of whom received LVB-only and others who had LVB with adjunctive reductive procedures.[40] In the cohort that received LVB-only, subjective improvement occurred in 73% of patients and objective improvement was documented in 42% of patients with an average of 44% reduction in volume. At 4-year follow-up, 74% of patients were able to discontinue conservative measures completely and the incidence of cellulitis decreased by 58%. Results with LVA operations have likewise been difficult to generalize with a wide range of results, differing follow-up times, variable postoperative therapy protocols, non-standard volumetric measurements, and no metrics on patient outcomes. Subjective measures of improvement have ranged from 95% to 50% of patients. Variable volumetric improvements have ranged from 75% decrease in 73% of patients to no change in 50% of patients, with average reduction in volume of 55%.[4,36,41–43] In the few studies that included incidence of cellulitis, most demonstrated a significant decrease after LVA/LVB.[36,40,44] Finally, a portion of patients were able to completely discontinue use of compression garments even over long-term follow-up.[36]

In a recent report of the author's experience with 100 patients undergoing LVA (89 upper extremity and 11 lower extremity), symptom improvement was reported in 96% of patients and quantitative improvement was noted by 74%. The overall mean volume differential reduction at 12 months follow-up was 42%. This reduction was significantly larger in patients with earlier stage (stage I or II) vs. later stage (stage III or IV) lymphedema as determined with ICG (61% vs. 17%).[4] LVB alone is best indicated in patients with mild to moderate upper extremity lymphedema where there are still some functioning lymphatic vessels and there is minimal tissue fibrosis.

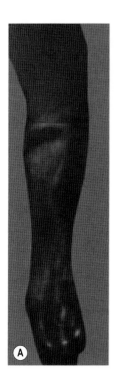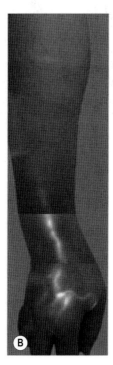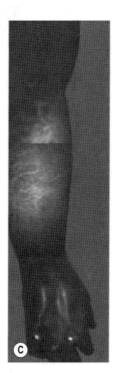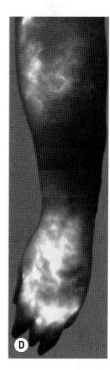

Fig. 3.2 Lymphedema classification based on indocyanine green lymphangiographic findings. **(A)** Stage I: many patent lymphatic vessels, with minimal, patchy dermal backflow. **(B)** Stage II: moderate number of patent lymphatic vessels, with segmental dermal backflow. **(C)** Stage III: few patent lymphatic vessels, with extensive dermal backflow involving the entire arm. **(D)** Stage IV: no patent lymphatic vessels seen with severe dermal backflow involving the entire arm and extending to the dorsum of the hand. *(From: Chang DW, Suami H, Skoracki R. A prospective analysis of 100 consecutive lymphovenous bypass cases for treatment of extremity lymphedema.* Plast Reconstr Surg. *2013;132(5):1305–1314.)*

In a subsequent study, skin tissue changes in patients before and after LVB were analyzed to assess whether these procedures can reverse the pathologic tissue changes associated with lymphedema.[45–47] Biopsy specimens were fixed and analyzed for inflammation, fibrosis, hyperkeratosis, and lymphangiogenesis. Histologic analysis demonstrated a significant decrease in tissue CD4+ cell inflammation in lymphedematous limb (but not normal limb) biopsies ($p < 0.01$). These changes were associated with significantly decreased tissue fibrosis as demonstrated by decreased collagen type I deposition and transforming growth factor-β1 (TGF-β1) expression ($p < 0.01$). In addition, we found a significant decrease in epidermal thickness, decreased numbers of proliferating basal keratinocytes, and decreased numbers of LYVE-1+lymphatic vessels in lymphedematous limbs after LVB. We have shown, for the first time, that microsurgical LVB not only improves symptomatology of lymphedema but also helps to improve pathologic changes in the skin. These findings suggest that some of the pathologic changes of lymphedema are reversible and may be related to lymphatic fluid stasis.

Recent technological advancements with fluorescence lymphangiography have provided surgeons with much better ability to perform real-time identification and evaluation of existing lymphatics.[48,49] Injection of ICG dye into the dermis and evaluation with near-infrared laser angiography immediately displays the severity of the process and location of vessels if present (Fig. 3.2). In early stage disease, it is easy to identify discrete functioning lymphatic channels. In late stage disease significant dermal backflow is present. This improves operative efficiency and allows for limited dissection and morbidity to the patient, as well as quicker recovery. The surgery is then performed using short horizontal incisions at the marked locations along the length of the extremity. Dissection is performed at the superficial subcutaneous plane to locate a venule and lymphatic channel, confirmed with isosulfan blue or ICG lymphangiography, and the LVA is

performed. After completion of the anastomosis, patency can be confirmed with isosulfan blue passing from the lymphatic to the venule, or with ICG lymphangiography.

The following is the author's preferred method for LVA. After the patient is anesthetized, ICG is injected into the dermis of the webspace and superficial lymphatics are evaluated with near-infrared fluorescence (Fig. 3.3). Dissection is performed under the microscope in the superficial subcutaneous plane to locate a good venule and lymph channel. Lymphatics are confirmed with isosulfan blue and ICG. Once a bypass site is determined, the lymphatic is anastomosed to the venule either end-to-side or end-to-end depending on the vessel size match (Fig. 3.4). After the anastomosis is complete, the patency is confirmed with isosulfan blue and ICG (Fig. 3.5). The incision is closed under the microscope as well to ensure no damage to the delicate superficial anastomosis. Postoperatively the patient's limb is wrapped by the lymphedema physical therapist. Wrapping is performed in lieu of compression garments for about 1 month postoperatively to avoid shear injury to the delicate anastomoses.[4]

Most reported series of lymphatic bypass surgery have reported low complications rates, primarily consisting of minor wound healing problems and cellulitis.[4,40,42,50] Most cases of wound healing problems healed spontaneously, and cases of cellulitis were treated with a short course of antibiotics. In general LVA may be best indicated in patients with mild upper extremity lymphedema who still have a moderate amount of functioning lymphatic vessels and minimal irreversible tissue fibrosis.[4]

Vascularized lymph node transfers (VLNT) (Video 3.2 ▶)

Another approach to treating lymphedema is to replenish the missing lymph nodes of the affected extremity by harvesting healthy lymph nodes from one area of the body and

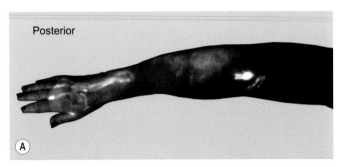
Posterior

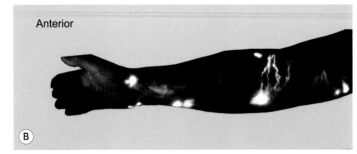
Anterior

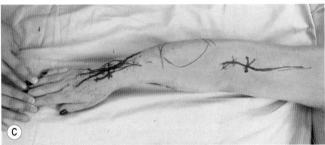

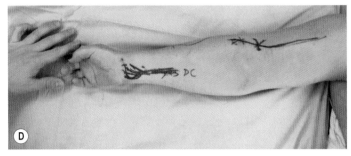

Fig. 3.3 Indocyanine green (ICG) lymphangiography is performed by intradermal injection of ICG into each finger/toe web of the lymphedematous limb. An infrared camera **(A,B)** is used to visualize and mark the visible lymphatic pathways **(C,D)**. *(From: Chang DW, Suami H, Skoracki R. A prospective analysis of 100 consecutive lymphovenous bypass cases for treatment of extremity lymphedema.* Plast Reconstr Surg. *2013;132(5):1305–1314.)*

transplanting them as a free tissue transfer to either the affected basin or a non-anatomic area on the affected limb. It is unclear whether the orthotopically placed lymph nodes act as a sponge to absorb lymphatic fluid and direct it into the vascular network, or if the transferred nodes induce lymphangiogenesis, or perhaps both.[51–53] Although some researchers have experimented in animal models with grafting avascular whole nodes or cut up lymph nodes, their viability is highly variable.[54,55] In general, it has been shown that preserving the

vascular supply during transfer results in greater improvements in the degree of edema and in lymphatic function.[56]

In 1982, Clodius first reported the use of VLNT in humans for treatment of lower extremity lymphedema in two patients. In the first patient, a pedicled groin flap including the inguinal lymph nodes was transferred to the contralateral inguinal region of the affected lower extremity resulting in a stable volume reduction. In the second patient, a free groin flap was transferred to the medial knee to bridge a lymphatic defect caused by trauma. This patient initially experienced limb volume reduction, but his lymphedema recurred within 6 months postoperatively.[20] Since then, many surgeons have worked at perfecting the technique. In 2006, Becker reported favorable long-term outcomes in 24 patients who underwent free transfer of nodes from the groin to either the axilla or elbow of the affected upper extremity, including objective evidence of functioning transplanted lymph nodes with lymphoscintigraphy in 30% of the patients.[57]

The harvest of vascularized lymph nodes has been described using groin, thoracic, submental, supraclavicular nodes, and omentum. The lymph nodes in the groin have been described as being spread over five regions – central (saphenofemoral junction), superomedial, superolateral, inferomedial, and inferolateral.[58] Since nodes that drain the lower limb are located medially and centrally, it is more advisable to harvest the laterally based nodes that drain the suprailiac region. The superior row of nodes is supplied by the superficial circumflex iliac artery, whereas the medial column is supplied by branches off the femoral artery.[59,60] Although controversy exists regarding the safety for harvesting medial nodes, there is agreement in preserving the deeper lymphatics and nodes inferior to the inguinal ligament, and many have advocated using the reverse sentinel node mapping technique to avoid causing secondary donor site lymphedema.

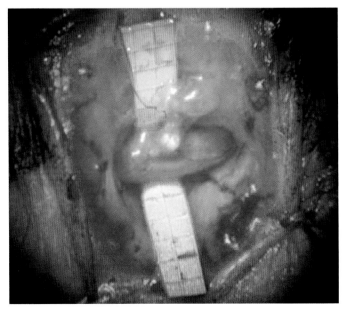

Fig. 3.4 The lymphatic vessel is anastomosed to the venule either end-to-side or end-to-end depending on the vessel size match.

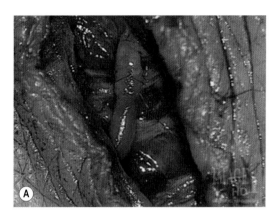

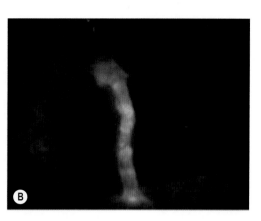

Fig. 3.5 The patency of the bypass is confirmed by observing the isosulfan blue dye pass from the lymphatic through the anastomosis into the venule (A). Alternatively, indocyanine green (ICG) may be also be used if the operating microscope has capability for ICG fluoroscopy (B). *(From: Chang DW, Suami H, Skoracki R. A prospective analysis of 100 consecutive lymphovenous bypass cases for treatment of extremity lymphedema. Plast Reconstr Surg. 2013;132(5):1305–1314.)*

Saaristo combined vascularized lymph node transfer with autologous breast reconstruction and also reported favorable outcomes, with one-third of patients no longer needing compression therapy and evidence of improved lymphatic flow on lymphoscintigraphy in five of six cases.[61] The lateral, superficial groin lymph nodes are harvested for transfer leaving behind the deeper lymph nodes that drain the leg. The desired nodes are usually located deep to Scarpa's fascia within a 3 cm radius of a point 3 cm inferior and perpendicular to a point one-third the distance from the pubic tubercle to the anterior superior iliac spine, clustered at the junction of the superior inferior epigastric and superficial circumflex iliac veins. Reverse lymphatic mapping with technetium and ICG is performed to decrease the risk of causing donor site lymphedema. In combined breast reconstruction cases, this tissue is taken as an extension of the abdominal tissue based on the deep inferior epigastric system used to reconstruct the breast (Fig. 3.6). In these cases, the superficial circumflex iliac vein is anastomosed in the axilla in addition to the arterial and venous anastomosis of the deep inferior epigastric vessels to the internal mammary vessels for the breast reconstruction.[62,63]

Cheng *et al.* described the use of submental lymph nodes based off the submental branch of the facial artery, taking care to avoid injury to the marginal mandibular branch. The author has advocated for the use of supraclavicular nodes based off the transverse cervical artery (Fig. 3.7).[64] Dissection of this flap can be tedious as there is frequent anatomic variation, and care must be taken to avoid injury to the lymphatic ducts. Additionally, while a skin paddle can be included in the flap design, its vascularity is not always reliable.

The other consideration when performing this surgery is where to place the transplanted tissue in the affected limb: anatomic vs. non-anatomic. The theory behind placement in non-anatomic sites is that they work as a "lymphatic pump". Pulsations from the arterial anastomosis act as a pump providing a strong hydrostatic force into the flap and then the low-pressure flap vein acts as suction. Since lymph has lower colloid osmotic pressure than blood, lymphatic fluid is drawn into the capillaries. It is also theorized that a "catchment" effect is at play with non-anatomic placement as well. Distal flap placement allows gravitational drainage of the limb, and as interstitial pressures normalize old lymphatic channels may open allowing improved lymphatic drainage. Proponents of non-anatomic placement also believe it is better to avoid the scarred bed present in anatomic placement. A disadvantage to non-anatomic placement is the presence of a visible, bulky flap on the extremity. It also is commonly difficult to primarily close the recipient site due to compression on the pedicle and skin grafts are often needed. The advantages of anatomic placement are excision of scar tissue, which is likely contributing to the lymphedema and placement of healthy vascularized lymph nodes to promote lymphangiogenesis where lymphatics are known to be deficient. Additionally there is abundant surrounding soft tissue to allow easy closure and the scar is usually well hidden. In the upper extremity, vascularized lymph nodes have been placed in the axilla, elbow, or wrist. In the lower extremity, vascularized lymph nodes have been placed in the ankle, knee, or groin.[63]

In treating upper extremity lymphedema, recipient sites have included the wrist, elbow, and axillary regions. As most upper extremity lymphedema results from prior surgery with or without radiation to the axilla, it is important to perform wide excision of the scar that may be enveloping nerves, muscles, and recipient vessels (e.g. thoracodorsal), to both ensure a healthy bed for lymphangiogenesis and to remove scar that would prevent bridging of lymphatics in the recipient bed. Becker *et al.* reported treating upper extremity

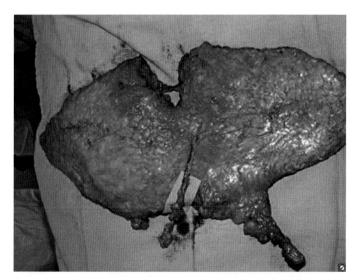

Fig. 3.6 An example of a free deep inferior epigastric perforator flap with lymph node flap based on superficial circumflex iliac artery for simultaneous breast reconstruction and lymph node transfer.

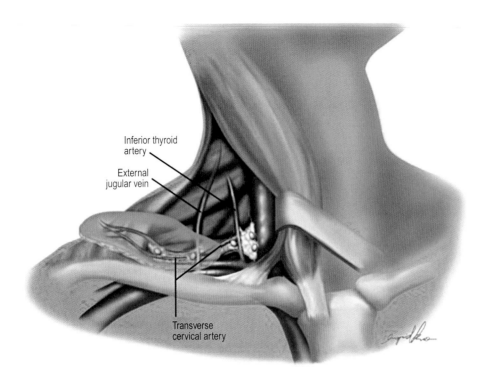

Inferior thyroid artery

External jugular vein

Transverse cervical artery

Fig. 3.7 A supraclavicular lymph node transfer based off the transverse cervical artery. *(From: Cheng MH, Chang DW, Patel K. Principles and Practice of Lymphedema Surgery.* New York: Elsevier; 2015.)

lymphedema by transferring inguinal lymph nodes to the axillary region.[57] The anterior recurrent ulnar artery and basilica vein or the radial artery and its vena comitantes have been used by Cheng and Gharb as recipient vessels at elbow.[59,60] In contrast, the radial artery at the level of the wrist has been used by Lin *et al.*, as recipient vessels for groin nodes based off the superficial circumflex iliac vessels.[65]

For the lower extremity, the ankle and groin are the most common recipient sites. Similar to the axilla, the groin may often require extensive lysis or excision of scars from previous surgery and radiotherapy.[51,64,66] The use of the ankle for recipient site in the lower extremity follows along the logic that the gravitational forces that keep the lymphatic fluid from rising up to the groin are difficult to overcome.[64,66] Instead placement of the vascularized lymph nodes at the level of the ankle would take advantage of these forces to facilitate drainage into the flap at the level of the ankle.

For isolated extremity lymphedema, the author tends to harvest the supraclavicular nodes and place the tissue in the anatomic location. It is important to excise all scar in the recipient site as it hinders lymphatic flow and inhibits lymphangiogenesis. If it is difficult to access or remove scar in the anatomic location, the author's preference is to place the vascularized lymph nodes just distal on the limb to the site of lymphatic obstruction. For example, in a patient who had removal of pelvic lymph nodes via laparotomy, the flap would be placed in the proximal thigh along the femoral artery and saphenous vein. Additionally, if a patient has no definitive site of injury or primary lymphedema with edema localized to the distal limb, the author prefers to place lymph nodes at the medial portion of the leg along the posterior tibial vessels as opposed to the dorsum of the ankle. This results in a less bulky flap and allows better ease in wearing shoes.

A recent meta-analysis looked at five quantitative studies reporting outcomes with vascularized lymph node transfer. One of these studies provided level III evidence, and the remaining were level IV. Subjective improvement was reported by 100% of patients, 91% had a quantitative improvement, and 78% were able to discontinue compression therapy. Complications included infection (8%), lymphorrhea (15%), re-exploration (3%), and need for additional procedures (36%).[19] As mentioned previously, although helpful in summarizing outcomes, these results should be interpreted with scrutiny given the great amount of heterogeneity between the studies. The largest series included in the meta-analysis was

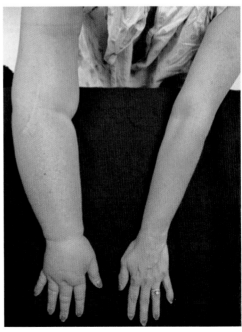

Fig. 3.8 A woman with lymphedema of her right arm for 5 years following right mastectomy and radiation therapy. Her right arm is 81% larger than her left arm.

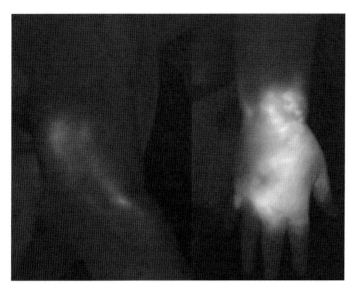

Fig. 3.9 Preoperative indocyanine green lymphangiography shows severe lymphatic dermal backflow in the hand and patent lymphatic vessels at the elbow.

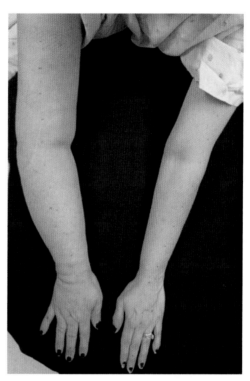

Fig. 3.11 At 12 months, her right arm had 57% reduction in excess volume.

from Becker who reported experience with 24 patients.[21] Since then, that group has reported operating on 1500 patients with an average 3-year follow-up, and they have briefly commented on their outcomes, although they have not published detailed results. They reported 98% of patients have some degree of improvement, with 40% of clinical stage I or II patients experiencing normalization of their affected extremity.[24]

While the literature for vascularized lymph nodes is still in its early stages, results have been favorable with an average volume reduction of 47%.[43,63] The indications for VLNT are still unclear, but some have advocated criteria based on total occlusion on lymphoscintigraphy, international society of lymphedema stage II with repeated episodes of cellulitis, no acute cellulitis, and more than 12-months of follow-up.[59]

VLNT offers an exciting new horizon for physiologic treatment of more advanced stage lymphedema. Furthermore, for patients with moderate to severe lymphedema, combining both VLNT and LVA may optimize the chances for improvement of lymphedema as these two approaches work via different mechanisms. VLNT is done proximally and LVA is done distally to take advantage of both procedures (Figs. 3.8–3.11).

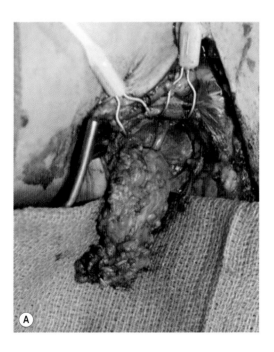

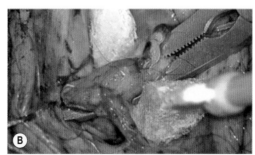

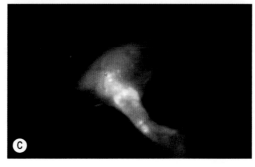

Fig. 3.10 A vascularized lymph node transfer to the axilla and four lymphovenous bypasses were performed on the arm. Lymphazurin and Indocyanine Green (ICGN) demonstrate patency of one of the E–S anastomosis.

Prophylactic surgery

As we have gained more experience with lymphatic surgery, the idea of prophylactic surgery has been proposed. Boccardo *et al.* have proposed a procedure named lymphatic microsurgical preventing healing approach (LYMPHA). This involves anastomosing arm lymphatics to a collateral branch of the axillary vein at the time of nodal dissection to prevent lymphedema. They have reported 4-year outcomes in 74 patients undergoing this procedure, and only 3 patients have developed lymphedema determined by volumetry and lymphoscintigraphy.[26] This 4% risk of lymphedema compares favorably to the 13–65% incidence of lymphedema in women undergoing axillary lymph node dissection. Although these results are intriguing, further study needs to be performed before this can truly be determined to be efficacious or oncologically safe.

Summary

The surgical treatment of lymphedema has been attempted since the early 20th century. This has obviously been a difficult problem to solve for surgeons and an even more difficult problem for the patients who are afflicted. Recent technological advances have enabled surgeons to refine previous techniques and develop new ones. Despite variability in protocols and reported outcomes, LVA and VLNT offer promising solutions for the future. In general, early intervention before the development of lymphatic fibrosis and adipose deposition results in improved final outcomes. Consensus in grading systems, reporting of outcomes, and standardized protocol will help to facilitate the next phase of evolution in the treatment of lymphedema.

⊕ Access the complete reference list online at **http://www.expertconsult.com**

4. Chang DW, Suami H, Skoracki R. A prospective analysis of 100 consecutive lymphovenous bypass cases for treatment of extremity lymphedema. *Plast Reconstr Surg.* 2013;132(5):1305–1314. *In a recent report of the author's experience with 100 patients undergoing LVA, symptom improvement was reported in 96% of patients and quantitative improvement was noted by 74%. The overall mean volume differential reduction at 12 months follow-up was 42%. This reduction was significantly larger in patients with earlier stage (stage I or II) vs. later stage (stage III or IV) lymphedema as determined with indocyanine green (61% vs. 17%). Lymphovenous bypass alone is best indicated in patients with mild to moderate upper extremity lymphedema where there are still some functioning lymphatic vessels and there is minimal tissue fibrosis.*

39. Koshima I, Kawada S, Moriguchi T, Kajiwara Y. Ultrastructural observations of lymphatic vessels in lymphedema in human extremities. *Plast Reconstr Surg.* 1996;97(2):397–405. *Koshima biopsied lymphatic trunks and demonstrated that the proximal-to-distal destruction of the endothelial and smooth muscle cells within the tunica media is a key step for lymphedema progression. Clinical experiences have been consistent with Koshima's findings in that subdermal lymphatic vessels are easily identifiable at the distal arm but much more difficult to identify in the proximal arm.*

42. Chang DW. Lymphaticovenular bypass for lymphedema management in breast cancer patients: a prospective study. *Plast Reconstr Surg.* 2010;126(3):752–758.

47. Ghanta S, Cuzzone D, Torrisi J, et al. Lymphaticovenous bypass decreases pathologic skin changes in upper extremity breast cancer-related lymphedema. *Lymphat Res Biol.* 2015;13(1):46–53. *In this study, it was demonstrated for the first time that microsurgical LVB not only improves symptomatology of lymphedema but also helps to improve pathologic changes in the skin. These findings suggest that some of the pathologic changes of lymphedema are reversible and may be related to lymphatic fluid stasis.*

49. Suami H, Chang DW, Yamada K, Kimata Y. Use of indocyanine green fluorescent lymphography for evaluating dynamic lymphatic status. *Plast Reconstr Surg.* 2011;127(3):74e. *Recent technological advancements with fluorescence lymphangiography have provided surgeons with much better ability to perform real-time identification and evaluation of existing lymphatics.[12] ICG dye into the dermis and evaluation with near-infrared laser angiography immediately displays the severity of the process and location of vessels if present. This improves operative efficiency and allows for limited dissection and morbidity of the patient, as well as quicker recovery.*

57. Becker C, Assouad J, Riquet M, Hidden G. Postmastectomy lymphedema: long-term results following microsurgical lymph node transplantation. *Ann Surg.* 2006;243(3):313–315.

61. Saaristo AM, Niemi TS, Viitanen TP, et al. Microvascular breast reconstruction and lymph node transfer for postmastectomy lymphedema patients. *Ann Surg.* 2012;255(3):468–473. *Saaristo combined vascularized lymph node transfer with autologous breast reconstruction and also reported favorable outcomes, with one-third of patients no longer needing compression therapy and evidence of improved lymphatic flow on lymphoscintigraphy in five of six cases. The lateral, superficial groin lymph nodes are harvested for transfer leaving behind the deeper lymph nodes that drain the leg.*

62. Ngyuen A, Chang EI, Suami H, Chang DW. An algorithmic approach to simultaneous vascularized lymph node transfer with microvascular breast reconstruction. *Ann Surg Oncol.* 2015;22(9):2919–2924.

64. Althubaiti GA, Crosby MA, Chang DW. Vascularized supraclavicular lymph node transfer for lower extremity lymphedema treatment. *Plast Reconstr Surg.* 2013;131(1):133e–135e.

65. Lin CH, Ali R, Chen SC, et al. Vascularized groin lymph node transfer using the wrist as a recipient site for management of postmastectomy upper extremity lymphedema. *Plast Reconstr Surg.* 2009;123(4):1265–1275.

4

Lower extremity sarcoma reconstruction

Goetz A. Giessler and Michael Sauerbier

SYNOPSIS

- Any lesion in the lower extremity with a clinical history of pain, continuous growth, size over 5 cm, or deep subfascial localization is suspicious of a sarcomatous malignancy and should be surgically biopsied according to established surgical rules.

- Still the single statistically proven modality of curing sarcomas and prolonging postsurgical lifespan is surgical excision with wide margins resulting in a postoperative R_0-status. To date, no other neoadjuvant or postoperative treatment modality can replace this approach. If wide margins cannot be achieved, adjuvant therapy is indicated for extremity preservation.

- Plastic surgical lower extremity sarcoma reconstruction is – especially in bone sarcoma reconstruction – the classical field of an interdisciplinary, multimodal approach, and is most commonly together with tumor- and orthopedic surgeons, oncologic radiotherapists, and oncologists.

- Modern oncoplastic reconstructive surgery can provide adequate reconstructive options for almost any defect size and composition, and so radical tumor excision can be combined with over 95% extremity preservation today.

- The plastic reconstructions in sarcoma related limb-sparing surgery (LSS) are often demanding and complex and consist of the full spectrum of plastic surgical options. They should be performed in specialized centers and specifically adapted to the patient and case profile.

 Access the Historical Perspective section online at
http://www.expertconsult.com

Introduction

Soft-tissue and bone sarcomas

Soft-tissue tumors are a highly heterogenous group of about 100 different tumor entities, which are still classified histogenetically according to the main adult tissue component they resemble most. The malignant subgroup among them is called sarcomas, which not only have the potential to grow locally invasive or even demonstrate destructive growth but also have a variable risk of recurrence and metastatic potential. As the term "*sarcoma*" (derived from the Greek word $\sigma\alpha\rho\xi$ "*sarx*"="meat") itself does not necessarily imply fast, expansive growth, or metastasis, a further subclassification system into more aggressive sarcomas (high-grade, poorly differentiated) or less aggressive (low-grade, well differentiated) types does exist. Some lesions like the atypical fibroxanthoma are called "pseudosarcomas", as they demonstrate a benign clinical course but are histologically malignant. However, usually well-differentiated tumors show low-grade characteristics and *vice versa*.

Primary bone sarcomas are even less frequent than soft-tissue sarcomas, and most malignant osseous lesions are metastatic, especially in advanced age. Despite having a low incidence, bone sarcomas have a high significance for both patient and surgeon due to their impact on extremity function and overall mobility. Limb preserving surgery after wide tumor resections frequently poses a real challenge for the reconstructive surgeon.

Sarcomas can occur in every part of the body, as they derive from mesodermic tissue like muscle, nerve, bone cartilage, blood vessels, or fat. The therapeutic mainstay for soft-tissue sarcomas is based on surgical excision, whereas radiotherapy and less so chemotherapy are used as adjunct adjuvant therapeutic modalities. In primary osseous sarcomas neoadjuvant chemotherapy plays a more important role. The complexity of the surgical resection and the subsequent plastic surgical reconstruction differs considerably depending on the localization.

Like any oncologic discipline, sarcoma treatment is a typical field of modern interdisciplinary and multimodal therapy. Lower extremity sarcoma reconstruction is – especially in bone sarcoma reconstruction – also a fascinating field for an effective interaction between the surgical disciplines of orthopedic, oncologic, pediatric, and podiatric surgeons and plastic reconstructive (micro-)surgeons.

Modern plastic reconstructive surgery can provide adequate reconstructive options for almost any defect size and composition, so considerations about defect size should not play a role during tumor excision. Today, over 95% of the extremities can be preserved after radical tumor excision. The plastic reconstructive procedures are often demanding and complex and frequently encompass the full spectrum of plastic surgical options. These procedures may be best performed in specialized centers where regimens individually adapted to patient and case profiles may be optimized.

Sarcomas in the lower extremity

Sarcomas in the lower extremity are more common than in the upper limb (74% vs. 26%) and represent the most common location of sarcomas in the body overall (45%).[1] Currently, they are safely treatable by extremity preservation in most cases, if properly performed according to the rules described in this chapter and in the pertinent current literature. In this context, several studies have now demonstrated that LSS is oncologically not inferior to amputation in the treatment of lower extremity sarcoma.[9] While amputation was still the keystone of previous surgical therapy several decades ago, it usually represents only an important last line therapeutic modality today. The common misconceptions that amputations have a better outcome both in tumor safety and quality of life have both definitely been proven wrong.[2-4]

Sarcomas are rare, and a "soft tissue swelling" is often misinterpreted by both patient and physician because of this fact. This can considerably delay proper diagnosis. Still, tumor manifestations in the extremities are often detected a bit earlier than in the trunk, as the extremities are constantly under personal "visual" control in daily life. This might be even truer for tumors on the upper extremity than on the lower.

Due to the highly functional anatomy of our extremities with vessels, nerves, tendons, bones, and muscles in the close vicinity, even smaller tumors can represent a challenge to both the resecting tumor surgeon as well as the reconstructive plastic surgeon. Preservation of the lower extremity in sarcoma reconstruction differs from alike manifestations in the upper extremity[5] in several key points that have to be considered carefully:

- Stability and weight-bearing capability are usually regarded higher than functional mobility or range of motion in the lower extremity.
- Postoperative appearance is usually less important. In most urban cultures the reconstructed legs with their scars and possible voluminous flaps can easily be hidden in clothing and have a less important role in social interaction than the upper extremity (i.e., handshaking).
- Weight-bearing demands are higher and atherosclerotic vessel damage and orthostatic venous pressure are more profound in the lower extremity. Both may play a major role in free tissue transfer.
- Nerve regeneration is less successful in the lower extremity at any age.
- Wound healing is slower, and the risk for an infectious complication is higher.

Basic science/disease process

Epidemiology soft-tissue sarcomas

Soft-tissue sarcomas are a rare disease entity with an incidence of 1:100000 in adults and 10–15% in children. This accounts for an incidence of about 10600 new cases in 2009 in the USA representing 1–2% of all malignancies (www.seer.cancer.gov). There is no overall significant gender predisposition, and the overall median age at presentation is between 50 and 60 years of age.

With about 45% of all sarcomas occurring in the lower extremity, 15% in the upper extremity, 10% in the head and neck region, 15% in the retroperitoneal space, and the remaining 15% in the abdomen and the chest wall,[6] the musculoskeletal system of the extremities and the abdominal and thoracic walls are the most common predilection sites. Extremity sarcomas are most common in the thigh (50–60%).

While most cases of soft-tissue sarcomas are sporadic, there are some genetic and non-genetic risk factors summarized in Table 4.1. Up to 60% of all soft-tissue sarcomas contain a somatic mutation of p53.[7] A detailed description of the various risk factors is beyond the scope of this chapter, but there are several strong associations to be mentioned: a history of radiation exposure accounts for up to 5.5% of all sarcomas. The risk is dose dependent, and the latency period between radiation and clinical tumor manifestation is around 5 years. Over 80% of radiation-associated sarcomas are high-grade types.[8] Neurofibromatosis type NF-1 is strongly associated with the cumulative lifetime risk of up to 13% for the occurrence of malignant peripheral nerve sheath tumors (MPNST).

Table 4.1 **Predisposing factors for soft-tissue sarcomas**	
Genetic	Neurofibromatosis NF-1 (von Recklinghausen disease)
	Retinoblastoma
	Gardner's syndrome
	Werner's syndrome
	Bloom's syndrome
	Fumarate hydratase leiomyosarcoma syndrome
	Diamond–Blackfan anemia
Mechanical	Li–Fraumeni syndrome
	Postparturition
Chemical	Chronic irritation
	Polyvinylchloride (PVC)
	Hemochromatosis
	Dioxin (TCDD) "Agent Orange"
Radiation	Arsenic
	Traumatic–accidental
Lymphedema	Post-therapeutic
	Parasitic (filariasis)
	Iatrogenic
	Stewart–Treves syndrome
Infectious (viral)	Congenital
	Kaposi sarcoma (HHV-8)
HHV-8, human herpes virus-8; TCDD, 2,3,7,8-tetrachlorodibenzodioxin.	

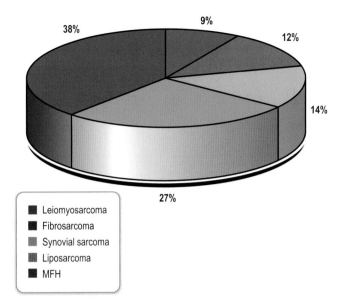

38% | 9% | 12% | 14% | 27%

- Leiomyosarcoma
- Fibrosarcoma
- Synovial sarcoma
- Liposarcoma
- MFH

Fig. 4.1 Distribution of histopathologic types in extremity soft-tissue sarcomas. MFH, malignant fibrous histiocytoma. *(From: Weitz J, Antonescu CR, Brennan MF. Localized extremity soft-tissue sarcoma: improved knowledge with unchanged survival over time. J Clin Oncol. 2003;21:2719–2725.)*

The sarcoma subtype is determined by light- and electron microscopy, immunohistochemistry, and cytogenetic analysis. If it results in a tumor that cannot be designated accordingly, a descriptive evaluation is given for an "unclassified sarcoma". Obtaining reference pathologies for soft- and bone-tissue sarcomas should be standard, as the rate of diagnostic agreement among specialists is below 75%.[9,10] The most common histopathologic subtype distribution in extremities in the largest series in the literature is shown in Fig. 4.1.

Bone sarcomas

About 2600 new primary bone sarcomas occur each year in the USA (www.seer.cancer.gov). The overall median age at diagnosis is 39 years. Many predisposing factors for bone sarcomas are similar to those for soft-tissue sarcomas (like retinoblastoma, Li–Fraumeni syndrome, radiation, and others) (Table 4.1). Paget's disease, bone infarction, and fibrous dysplasia may also represent risk factors for bone sarcomas.

The most common type is the osteogenic sarcoma, which has a predilection for the metaphyses around the knee in about 50% of cases. It is the third most common cancer in the young (www.nhs.uk) with a second peak around age 60. The male to female ratio is almost 2:1 in large studies, and for this specific tumor the median age at diagnosis is 17 years. Only 6.4% present initially with pathologic fractures, whereas the majority are detected in the workup of a painful mass or swollen extremity.[11,12] It commonly arises in the medulla, but as a juxtacortical osteogenic sarcoma it arises from the external surface – most commonly the posterior aspect of the femur.

The spindle cell mesenchymal sarcoma group contains chondrosarcomas, intraosseous malignant fibrous histiocytomas (MFHs), and fibrosarcomas. The tumors of this group only have an incidence of about two-thirds of the incidence of osteogenic sarcomas and primarily occur in an older population. Chondrosarcomas are slow growing and relatively resistant to adjuvant therapy.

Ewing's sarcoma is classically located in the femur diaphysis in teenagers, and only 20% occur in middle-aged adults. If found extradiaphyseal, it is very common in the pelvis. It is the most common primary bone malignancy of the fibula. The Ewing's sarcoma is very radiation sensitive.

Tumor growth and metastasizing

Sarcomas in the extremity may spread locally by continuous expanding growth irrespective of anatomic borders. In many cases it mistakingly seems that the tumor has developed a bordering capsule to surrounding "healthy tissue". However, this capsule is part of the tumor, and soft-tissue satellite-like or intraosseous skip-lesion tumor manifestations are beyond this capsule. This fact represents the main justification for a modern wide-resection concept in sarcoma surgery.

Hematogenic spread is most common in soft-tissue and bone sarcomas. For lower extremity tumors, the primary site for metastasis is the lung. Lymphatic metastases are present in less than 5% of all soft-tissue sarcomas (rhabdomyosarcoma, angiosarcoma, and epitheloid-like sarcoma).[13,14]

Diagnosis/patient presentation/imaging

A detailed history and physical examination is the first initial and very important step to professional tumor surgery. In sarcomatous lesions, the patient often relates the tumor causally to an – often minor – traumatic event, bringing the lesion into clinical attention to the patient. Acute trauma, however, is not a proven predisposing factor for sarcoma development. Because of this, there is often a considerable time lag between this initial recognition and the first presentation of the lesion to a medical professional. Furthermore, the rationale of the lesion is often erratically misinterpreted and then causes a variety of inadequate treatments by both lays and physicians, further delaying proper diagnosis. The average duration of any symptoms before seeing a physician is 6 months in all soft-tissue sarcomas, but possibly shorter in extremity manifestation.[3] So in adults, lesions that (1) have not disappeared after 4 weeks, (2) are located subfascially or in the popliteal or groin flexion creases, (3) continue to grow or are symptomatic (i.e., pain and paresthesias), or (4) are already larger than 5 cm on detection should generally be biopsied as they are highly suspicious for malignancy.

It is not unusual that sarcomas are found by physicians in the context of a workup for a completely different medical problem (i.e., chronic venous insufficiency in the leg). Coincidental findings like articular pain and joint effusions are common especially with osseous sarcomas, whereas clinically manifest neurovascular symptoms are relatively rare at initial presentation. Two-thirds of sarcoma patients present with a painless mass during their first clinical examination, and only one-third have current pain or have had a history of pain in the affected region.

The thorough physical examination is not only focused on the affected extremity but includes the complete body. The pertaining lymph node stations should be examined as well, even though lymphatic spread is uncommon in the majority of all sarcoma types. The general health status should be assessed and optimized by all relevant medical specialties. This is especially important in multimorbid patients with concomitant acute and chronic comorbidities in the context of the planned operative procedures. Terminal illnesses and comorbidities have to be taken into consideration for the extent of both resection and reconstructive surgery.

Clinical assessment and staging of the patient must be completed by adequate imaging diagnostics for evaluating local and generalized tumor manifestations. Any imaging of the tumor region must be performed before any surgical biopsy as the latter may confound the picture to a considerable extent.

Gadolinium contrast-enhanced magnetic resonance imaging (MRI) is currently the diagnostic mainstay to define exact tumor location, its relation to neighboring neurovascular structures and muscular compartments, to determine its homogeneity, integrity, and vascularization, and its presumed main tissue component. MRI is specifically useful for detecting skip lesions. It allows 3D planning of the resection and helps to assess the necessary reconstruction procedures preoperatively.

Modern spiral computerized tomography (CT) scans are indispensable for clarifying the detailed anatomy of osseous sarcomas, determining the extent to which skeletal structures are affected by neighboring soft-tissue tumors, and aiding in operative planning of these sarcomatous entities. Thoracic and abdominal CT-scans are the diagnostics of choice for staging of high-grade sarcomas of the extremities and detect intrapulmonary and abdominal metastases. In recurrent disease, positron emission tomography (PET) CT can augment the information about suspicious lesions in selected cases, though not accepted as a standard instrument for the preoperative workup (see Chapter 7).[16–18]

CT-angiography with 3D-reconstructions is a valuable tool in determining the overall vascular status of the affected leg, the underlying generalized vessel disease, and the vascularity of the tumor, and showing vascular displacements, collateral perfusion systems, vessel invasion, and tumor-related occlusion. They also provide valuable information about the feasibility of microvascular anastomoses and the presence of suitable recipient vessels, especially in elderly patients.

Plain X-ray films demonstrate specific periosteal or cortical signs, osteolysis, and paraosseous calcifications in diaphyseal and metaphyseal bony lesions. Even today, a plain radiograph remains the diagnostic method of choice for primary bone sarcomas (Fig. 4.2). A plain chest radiograph is still considered the standard for clinical staging in low-grade extremity lesions.

Ultrasound with or without contrast media is a cheap, fast, and painless adjunctive diagnostic measure that may be especially helpful in highly vascularized tumors. Ultrasound was often the diagnostic device of coincidental tumor findings but is also used for getting an initial overall picture of the lesion.

A 99m-Tc-pyrophosphate bone scan is essential to bone tumor staging and screening for multicentric disease or metastases.

A special laboratory workup for soft-tissue sarcomas does not exist, whereas elevated alkaline phosphatase and lactate dehydrogenase over 400 U/L are independent predictors of an unfavorable outcome in bone sarcomas.[19]

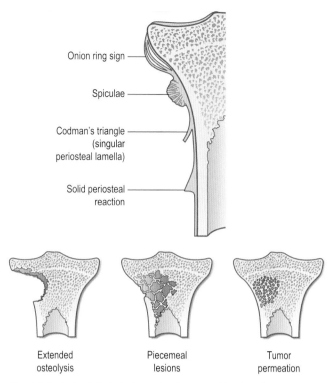

Onion ring sign

Spiculae

Codman's triangle (singular periosteal lamella)

Solid periosteal reaction

Extended osteolysis

Piecemeal lesions

Tumor permeation

Fig. 4.2 Typical radiologic features of malignant and benign primary osseous tumors.

Patient profile/general considerations/ treatment planning

Patient profile

The goals of surgery in sarcoma reconstruction in the lower extremity depend on the individual case profile, which is composed of personal factors and the available reconstructive options. The most important personal factors that need to be taken into consideration are age, size, and weight; concomitant chronic diseases relevant to general health and operability; medications; social status; functional and aesthetic conceptions; previous operations; and tissue quality of the affected extremity.

The pertinent reconstructive options that need to be discussed with the patient are the relevant operative methods according to the applicable steps of the reconstructive ladder, counterweighing their advantages and disadvantages for the actual tumor stage, location, oncologic safety, and potential adjuvant procedures (i.e., irradiation).

General considerations

Above all, the prime goal should be an R_0-resection with tumor-free and adequately wide margins, which provides the best chance of complete surgical cure of the disease. This might create a considerable surgical defect and can imply major surgical reconstructive procedures for the patient. The extent of adequate wide tissue resection is almost never realized by the patient presenting with a palpable mass and has to be explained to him or her in detail.

If surgical cure is not possible, resection of as much tumor mass as possible (tumor debulking) is paramount (R_1/R_2) and usually followed by adjuvant radio- and (less frequently) chemotherapy according to the recommendations of a multidisciplinary tumor board. At this point, the reconstructive goal should aim for a functional lower extremity capable of full weight-bearing that appears as aesthetically pleasing as possible in the given case and circumstances. The surgical therapy should create a status for the patient to be integrated in social life, allowing him or her to wear normal clothing and having a closed skin envelope. In selected cases, creating a stable open chronic wound is the only remaining palliative option; however, it should be free of copious discharge and secretions and avoid any olfactory nuisances. For example, a stable open wound producing minimal drainage that can be treated by daily dressing changes at home may offer a higher quality of life than performing another resection and reconstructive effort that may force the patient to stay in the clinic during his or her last days.

Treatment planning

Each case should be discussed in the multidisciplinary tumor board with all relevant medical disciplines involved in the setup of a treatment plan (tumor surgeon, medical oncologist, orthopedic surgeon, plastic surgeon, internal medicine, psychologist, radiologist, oncologic radiotherapy specialist, prosthetic technician, etc.). For optimal planning and strategy development, all diagnostic procedures, the radiologic imaging, and the definitive histology should already be present (see below).

A thorough and complete discussion of the tumor-board treatment recommendations are explained to and discussed with the patient including all operative options (including amputation) and neoadjuvant or adjuvant chemo- or radiotherapy. It is important for many patients to have an outline of the timeframe for the various surgical or multimodal therapeutic options.

Finally, tumor staging is done according to the current staging systems for soft-tissue sarcomas. The American Joint Committee on Cancer (AJCC) system is designed for extremity sarcomas (Table 4.2), including most but not all histologic subtypes. Dermatofibrosarcoma protuberans (DFSP) and angiosarcoma, among others, are exempt from staging with the AJCC. For primary bone sarcomas like the osteogenic sarcoma, the Musculoskeletal Tumor Society (Table 4.3) staging system is used.

Surgery

To date, no other treatment modality provides better cure for sarcomas than adequate surgery. Oncologic safety is paramount, but preservation of the leg or foot should be achieved to preserve patient integrity, which is usually possible. This avoids the need for prosthesis adaptation and use, and prosthesis-related problems. Several considerations in sarcoma-related defect reconstruction need to be mentioned that differ from sarcoma-related surgery at the upper extremity. The capability for stable weight-bearing is more important than joint mobility in the lower extremity, whereas preservation or restoration of sensitivity is less important on the leg and foot than on the arm or hand. While sensitivity should be

Table 4.2 American Joint Committee on Cancer staging system: predisposing factors for soft-tissue sarcomas

Classification and staging	Characteristic
Primary tumor (T)	
T1	Tumor 5 cm or less in greatest dimension
T1a	Superficial tumor (in relation to investing fascia)
T1b	Deep tumor (visceral and retroperitoneal sarcomas are defined as deep tumors)
T2	Tumor larger than 5 cm in greatest dimension
T2a	Superficial tumor
T2b	Deep tumor
Regional lymph nodes (N)	
N0	No evidence of nodal metastasis
N1	Nodal metastasis present
Distant metastasis (M)	
M0	No distant metastasis
M1	Distant metastasis present
Grade (G)	
G1	Low-grade
G2 and G3	High-grade
Staging	
Stage I	Low-grade tumors, no evidence of regional nodes or distant metastases (T1a, T1b, T2a, T2b)
Stage II	High-grade small tumors (T1a and b) and superficial large tumors (T2a), no evidence of regional nodes or distal metastases
Stage III	High-grade deep tumors larger than 5 cm (T2b), no evidence of regional nodes or distant metastases
Stage IV	Any tumor with regional nodes or distant metastases

(Reproduced from Papagelopoulos PJ, Mavrogenis AF, Mastorakos DP, et al. Current concepts for management of soft-tissue sarcomas of the extremities. *J Surg Orthop Adv.* 2008;17:204–215.)

Table 4.3 Musculoskeletal Tumor Society staging system

Stage	Characteristic
IA	Low-grade, intracompartmental
IB	Low-grade, extracompartmental
IIA	High-grade, intracompartmental
IIB	High-grade, extracompartmental
IIIA	Low- or high-grade, intracompartental with metastases
IIIB	Low- or high-grade, extracompartental with metastases

(Reproduced from Papagelopoulos PJ, Mavrogenis AF, Mastorakos DP, et al. Current concepts for management of soft-tissue sarcomas of the extremities. *J Surg Orthop Adv.* 2008;17:204–215.)

preserved as much as possible, in selective cases, asensitive "stilt-legs" are considered superior to amputations, especially in elderly patients that would have problems adapting to prosthesis handling. Not being able to preserve the main nerves and thereby sensitivity is not an indication for amputation by itself!

Radiotherapy

Radiotherapy is the primary adjunctive treatment method in sarcoma management today. Neoadjuvant radiation in large sarcomas uses external beam irradiation that helps in tumor shrinkage and thickening of the tumor capsule, which facilitates adequate resection and the achievement of negative margins during wide resection and reduces potential surgical tumor seeding. The disadvantages of preoperative irradiation are a higher rate of wound healing complications compared to postoperative radiotherapy and the creation of necrotic tumor material for the pathologist.[2]

Intraoperative radiation comprises a single dose electron radiation and has indications for use in the lower extremity for locations around the groin and foot. It is especially effective when the tumor dose is increased relative to the normal tissue dose. However, its availability is limited even in modern tumor centers.

Postoperative irradiation is done with brachytherapy and electron beam therapy both used in solitary and combination regimens. Brachytherapy is especially useful after resection of local recurrences in a previously irradiated field.

Chemotherapy

To date, any adjuvant or neoadjuvant chemotherapy for sarcomas should only be conducted in clinical studies (EORTC, COSS, EURO-Ewing, etc.). The various protocols are beyond the scope of this chapter and are changing rapidly. The reader is therefore advised to consult the pertinent most recent literature on that matter.

Isolated extremity perfusion or hyperthermia is currently indicated for patients that would otherwise require primary amputation. The precise selection criteria have not been clearly defined yet, and valid comparisons to other approaches are lacking.[2]

Treatment/surgical resection techniques

Histologic confirmation, grading, and subtyping of the presumed malignant sarcomatous tumor on the lower extremity must be achieved before the overall treatment strategy is planned in the tumor board and definitive, usually more extensive, surgery is initiated. However, not all known biopsy techniques are useful for a correct and safe diagnosis of a sarcoma.

Biopsy techniques

Fine-needle or core-needle aspirations

These techniques gain only a very small amount of tissue even in the hands of an experienced clinician. While tissue aspiration with a 23-gauge needle usually harvests only a very small number of cells, the volume of tissue gained from a core-needle biopsy is a bit higher. Still, both methods have the disadvantage of not representing the tumor tissue components correctly, especially in larger tumors, which makes it very difficult for the histopathologist to find the exact diagnosis, perform the necessary number of different studies, and determine the correct grading. However, if combined with CT-scan or ultrasound guided needle placement, core biopsies may achieve a correct diagnosis in up to 90% of cases under optimal circumstances. Fine-needle aspirations only reach 56–72%.[20–22] While single core-biopsies may harvest too little tissue for an extensive pathologic workup with several stainings and immunohistochemical diagnostics, they provide the advantage of gathering tissue from different parts of the tumor to create a comprehensive picture.[22]

Both methods are atraumatic and only very rarely cause dangerous tumor-cell dissipating hematomas. In several institutions, core biopsies are reserved for surgically unresectable tumors (i.e., retroperitoneal lesions) to determine tissue type and guide an eventual neoadjuvant therapy,[3] while others use it as a prime diagnostic tissue sampling method.[22]

In summary, fine needle biopsies do not have a place in sarcoma diagnosis in the lower extremities, and both core biopsy and open surgical biopsy are very operator dependent: if poorly performed, the risk of getting an inadequate diagnostic sample or tumor seeding is high, respectively.[23,24] Bone forming lesions are very difficult to adequately sample percutaneously, and open biopsies are preferable.[25]

Excisional biopsy

Excisional biopsies aim for the removal in toto of all tumor tissue with primary closure of the surrounding tissue and are therefore reserved for lesions less than 3–5 cm in diameter and with epifascial location. As the definitive diagnosis is not known beforehand, no tissue margin of defined thickness is left with this procedure.

Any surgical biopsy on the lower extremity should be performed with a pressurized tourniquet (no exsanguination!) if tumor location permits. The bloodless field not only aids in exact and atraumatic safe dissection but also inhibits possible tumor cell contamination during surgery.

Before incising the skin, it is absolutely necessary that the surgeon already imagines any secondary, definitive tumor resections and has possible muscle and tendon transfers and local flap options in mind. The biopsy incision should interfere as little as possible with these factors. Usually, a longitudinal incision as short as possible for an adequate exposure directly over the tumor is made, providing the shortest reasonable access route to the neoplasm.

The tumor should be excised in a no-touch/no-see technique including any pseudocapsule (if present) without opening it. Any "shelling-out" of the tumor should not be performed as in sarcomas this capsule is part of the tumor and its remaining walls do contain tumor cells.

After the excision, it may be useful to mark the resection bed with titanium or vitallium microclips to make later excision easier, if malignancy was affirmed. Localization sutures are fixed to the tumor, and both instruments and gloves are changed.

Meticulous hemostasis and the placement of a closed suction drainage within the wound to prevent possible tumor seeding through a hematoma are paramount before a multilayered skin closure is done. The skin should be closed with single interrupted stitches or intracutaneous sutures. Mattress sutures or separate drainage perforations leave stitch marks too far away from the incision and, as they all have to be excised in case of malignancy, this would enlarge the amount of tissue to be resected. A sterile circular compressive dressing is placed, and the affected extremity is immobilized – especially in procedures close to joints. Temporary splinting for a few days assists well here.[3]

Incisional biopsy

The surgical resection of a representative part of the sarcoma is the gold standard in diagnosis of extremity tumors for any lesions that are larger than 3–5 cm and of subfascial location. This technique should only be performed by an experienced surgeon, as the gathering of respective tissue specimens and the handling of the tissue is crucial to the success of the procedure. The advantages of getting adequate tissue for a full range of diagnostics greatly outweigh the disadvantages by opening the tumor and introducing the potential for tumor cell seeding in the path of the access route.

Again, the procedure should be performed with a tourniquet, as detailed dissection is possible and intraoperative contamination of surrounding tissue areas during resection of the histologic specimen with potentially tumor-cell containing blood is minimized.

The guidelines for the skin incision are practically the same as for the excisional biopsies with regard to keeping any further operative options in mind. An incision parallel to the axis of the extremity is made. It should be as short as possible for an adequate exposure directly over the tumor providing the shortest reasonable access route to the neoplasm. The incision must not unnecessarily interfere with later procedures needed to cover the defect.

A properly conducted incision biopsy should harvest a relevantly large, at least $2\times1\times1$ cm, tissue block from all areas of the tumor including the capsule. It is a common misconception to want to gain tissue only from the central portion, as this area often contains considerable amounts of necrotic tissue that are not adequate for pathology and makes definitive histologic classification impossible. The tissue block removed should be manipulated as little as possible and should not come into contact with the wound edges of the surgical access route. Any instrument used to hold or manipulate the biopsy specimen must not be used for wound closure or retraction, etc. After removal of the tumor block, localization sutures are tied and both instruments and gloves are changed.

Meticulous hemostasis and the placement of a closed suction drainage within the wound to prevent possible tumor seeding through a hematoma are paramount before a multilayered skin closure is done. The skin should be closed with single interrupted stitches or intracutaneous sutures. Mattress sutures or separate drainage perforations leave stitch marks too far away from the incision and, as they all have to be excised in case of malignancy, this would enlarge the amount of tissue to be resected. A sterile circular compressive dressing is placed, and the affected extremity is immobilized – especially in procedures close to joints. Temporary splinting or an external fixator for a few days serves the purpose here.

When mounting an external fixator to the affected lower extremity at the time of biopsy, care must be taken not to interfere with the later resection margins for definitive tumor resection. Preoperative findings of intraosseous skip lesions in bone sarcomas must be taken into consideration in this context. A fixator pin must never be set into an area for later resection, or the pin tract has to be included in the resection specimen.

Both incisional and excisional biopsies are not intended to adequately remove the tumor according to oncologic rules. Therefore, temporary vacuum-assisted closure techniques should be avoided and are rarely required anyway. Their angiogenetic potential and the risk of dissipation of tumor-cell containing wound secretions into the rest of the wound may negatively affect local oncologic safety. Larger studies are missing, however.

Re-operative biopsies and surgical revisions

Tumor centers frequently have to perform a surgical revision to confirm the diagnosis of sarcoma or to accomplish the correct surgical–oncological treatment. After previous attempts of inadequate biopsy or even after surgery that was intended to be definitive and curative, a re-operation is considered mandatory if at least one of the following situations is present:

- Only inadequate tissue material for definitive histology was gained at the first operation.
- Previous resections have not been performed according to current oncologic guidelines (see Case 4.2). Some indicators for a re-operation are incisions placed horizontally to the axis of the extremity and opening up several muscle compartments, intact nerve function after "resection of a malignant peripheral nerve sheath tumor", or normal leg motor function after "radical excision of extensor or flexor muscles".
- A clinically unsuspicious and presumably benign tumor was resected with the techniques of benign tumor surgery, but the postoperative histopathologic workup showed an unexpected malignancy.
- A tumor was resected during a non-oncologic surgery and detected in the postoperative workup ("unplanned excision").
- The tumor surface was visible intraoperatively.
- Previous operating room (OR) reports describe an "easy shelling-out from a capsule", but clinical and/or histologic and/or radiographic workup confirms a highly suspicious lesion or malignancy. A sarcoma resection out of its pseudocapsule results in local recurrences in up to 90% of patients.[6]
- The patient presents with early local tumor recurrence, despite a "radical resection" being stated in the previous OR report.
- Previous OR reports state a "compartment resection" in the axilla or around the elbow, popliteal fossa, or groin (which is anatomically not possible).
- OR and pathologic reports differ considerably in amount and integrity of the resected tumor.

Table 4.4 World Health Organization classification of tumor resection margins	
R_0	Resection with microscopically tumor-free specimen margins
R_1	Resection with microscopically tumor-positive specimen margins
R_2	Resection with macroscopically remaining tumor

- Any remaining tumor is present in any postoperative imaging (MRI).

In all these situations, at least an R_1-situation must be anticipated. The secondary resection should follow the exact principles of the surgical technique for definitive resection described below. The previous tumor bed should not be opened or visualized at all. If macroscopically visible remaining tumor is encountered during surgery (R_2-situation), the secondary revisional surgery may at least reduce the situation into an R_1-situation (Table 4.4). Following these revisional surgeries, radiotherapy is usually indicated for a reduction in the probability of local tumor recurrence.

Surgical technique for definitive resection

Soft-tissue sarcomas

As soon as the definitive histology is found and the tumor type, grading, and staging of the disease has been completed in the multidisciplinary workup, definitive surgery is initiated. If the tumor is deemed to be resectable and no neoadjuvant therapy was planned, the therapy of choice today is a wide excision with adequate margins. Before any definitive surgery is performed, the reconstructive strategy should be planned as meticulously as possible. It is necessary to fully inform the patient about the expected extent and length of the procedure and of possible donor sites of flaps, nerves, vessels, or skin grafts, etc. Furthermore, the anesthesiologic risk and invasiveness of monitoring should be explained to the patient and planned accordingly with the anesthesiologist. Also, placement of vascular access routes and regional pain catheters are important in that aspect. A well planned patient positioning on the OR table can allow a simultaneous team approach by oncologic and plastic surgeons and save a considerable amount of operative time.

Definitive sarcoma resection with a curative approach should be performed in a bloodless field with a pneumatic tourniquet or even temporary occlusion of the iliac or femoral artery by vascular surgery techniques. This reduces not only the risk for potential hemorrhage-induced contamination of the field with tumor cells but blood loss in general and is mandatory for a detailed dissection.

The resection must include all previous skin incisions, all previous stitch marks, and drain sites with a margin of 4 cm of healthy skin around them. This margin is also true for any ulcerated tumor locations. If the previous incision was performed properly, it creates an elliptical defect along the longitudinal axis of the leg. The advantages of this orientation are the preservation of the remaining subdermal lymph vessels and the ease in wound closure.

After adequate epifascial mobilization, the muscle fascia is opened and the sarcoma is resected with a no-touch/no-see

technique leaving a cuff of macroscopically unaffected tissue of 2–5 cm around it. Still there are no conclusive studies about the exact margins in sarcoma surgery, but many centers currently recommend a margin of 2 cm from the deep surface of the tumor and 4–5 cm laterally.[2,3,20,26] Any palpable pseudo-capsule of the tumor belongs to the tumor itself and should be resected but not opened or seen at all, otherwise the procedure is regarded as a R_1-resection. The tumor should not be retracted or manipulated with sharp or pointed-tipped instruments and should be resected in continuity with the skin island containing the previous incision.

The aforementioned margins are often difficult to maintain in the periphery of the lower extremity. Under these circumstances, ray amputations may suffice to achieve comparable local recurrence rates (<10%) if combined with local deperiostation and tenosynovectomy.[3]

Vascular involvement

Relevant deep vascular structures that are not directly infiltrated or encased in the tumor can usually be treated by longitudinal opening of the vascular adventitia opposite the tumor and subsequent microsurgical stripping of the adventitia under loupe magnification and en bloc with the tumor. Accompanying veins are usually ligated and included in this specimen if venous drainage of the extremity is still guaranteed in a different compartment. Preoperative MRI helps in this decision, otherwise the affected vessels have to be resected en bloc and replaced by a venous patch (less common), a vein graft, or, less commonly, an artificial vessel graft material (i.e., Gore-Tex). Any arterial side branches that do not lead into the tumor should be evaluated as possible recipient vessels for microvascular tissue reconstruction and be preserved. Preservation of septal branches or muscular vessels that are outside the tumor resection area may lifeguard local or regional muscle and skin flaps that can not only aid in postoperative dead-space elimination and wound closure but also in simple primary wound healing. Extraneous vessel ligation should therefore be avoided.

If the superficial venous systems (great and lesser saphenous veins) are not included in the resected sarcoma specimen, they should be preserved together with their subcutaneous branches if possible. This prevents venous congestion if the deep venous systems close to the tumor must be resected as mentioned above, adding to the radicality and safety. While there should always be an adequate arterial perfusion of the lower extremity after tumor removal, only the main arteries are reconstructed immediately. Interpositional vein grafts for large vein reconstruction in tumor patients have a higher risk of thrombotic failure than in traumatic cases and should be reserved for selected cases only.

Nerve involvement

The same dissection strategy applies to the main nerves in the lower extremity. Any affected epineural tissue or connective tissue around the nerve inside the safety margin around the tumor should be stripped or removed with careful microsurgical techniques. If only a few fascicles of an important main nerve trunk are adherent to the tumor, it is considered acceptable to resect these and leave the unaffected nerve bundles intact for some basic motor function and sensitivity. If a major nerve is encased completely, it must be resected and should be reconstructed primarily or secondarily (see Chapter 6).

Osseous involvement

For soft-tissue tumors in the lower extremity that are not primary osseous sarcomas and growing close to bone, the appropriate treatment has to be guided by clinical judgment and preoperative MRI and CT-scan. Real bony arrosion is relatively rare, and periosteal stripping, decortication, and partial bone resection are reasonable methods to comply with safe margins according to the principles of wide resection. However, these procedures weaken the bone mechanically in an area where later adjuvant radiotherapy further weakens the bone in the beam to an extent that may actually cause spontaneous fractures. Together with a systemically prevalent osteoporosis, this poses a considerable risk for spontaneous fractures.[3,27] Any resection of weight-bearing bones and joint segments should be balanced carefully against the complexity to reconstruct them. Frequently, the preservation of important skeletal structures permits quality of life to a degree that is comparable to an acceptable oncologic risk. Nevertheless, the full range of the plastic reconstructive operative armamentarium including bone flaps should be evaluated in providing the best outcome for the patient (see Chapter 6).

Primary osseous sarcomas

Primary osseous sarcomas may be diagnosed relatively accurately by plain radiographic imaging alone. The biopsy techniques are the same as in soft-tissue sarcomas, with the addition of opening up the bone cortex with a round burr hole under X-ray-assisted localization; gaining the biopsy; obtaining wound swabs for bacteria, fungi, and tuberculosis (differential diagnosis); and closing the hole with alloplastic hemostatic material.[25]

Wide surgical resection is also the treatment of choice for primary osseous sarcomas with comparable later reconstructive demands. Sometimes, the biopsy procedure may cause structural instability and external casts, splints, or external fixators are necessary. The method of choice for postresection leg stabilization should at best be determined before biopsy. If external fixators are planned for a definitive skeletal stabilization, the montage may already be applied during biopsy if the diagnosis is verified by a pathognomonic bone X-ray.

Specimen handling

If the resection is completed, the tumor and the tumor bed are photographed and the specimen is removed. It is extremely important to clearly mark the decisive anatomic landmarks and the topographic orientation of the tumor in its previous bed to allow unequivocal and exact determination of margins by the pathologist. Optimally, the examining histopathologist is present at this stage of the procedure. The surgeon has to ensure that any identifying orientation markings on the tumor are not shifted or torn off during transport.

Wound closure

Before wound closure, meticulous hemostasis and the placement of sufficient closed suction drains are necessary. Skin closure should be done in a multilayered fashion exerting detailed care for exact approximation of the wound edges in order to avoid any wound-healing disturbances that might hinder fast implementation of radiation therapy. Primary wound closure is dependent on the size of the tumor and the location in the leg. In the thigh, primary wound closure after wide resections is frequently possible, whereas around the knee and distally from it in the lower leg this is usually not feasible. The tumor resection bed should be narrowed by appropriate muscular and fascial sutures to prevent seroma and hematoma collection in it. Naturally, this usually applies for tumor locations at the thigh or proximal lower leg only.

Any wound closure must aim for a stable skin closure with only minor tension for fast primary wound healing and must avoid stretching of thinned-out, unsupported adipofascial skin flaps over empty wound cavities or bony protuberances. Wound closure must not be a trade-off against the appropriate radicality in tumor resection, especially in the context of available modern plastic surgical reconstructive options.

It is often quite useful to immobilize the operated leg with a splint for postoperative handling, analgesia, and aiding in hemostasis. A sterile circular compressive dressing is placed as well. However, in the case of a flap reconstruction, many surgeons defer from using this option because of the fear of compression forces onto the flap or the microvascular pedicle. An interim placement of external fixators is very useful in this context. They easily permit the bedside elevation of the operated extremity, especially in cases with free flaps that may not be dressed with circular bandages in the first postoperative days. External fixators may help in later daily wound care and aid in safe and fast flap healing, but may also be mounted in the proximal and distal metaphyses when a diaphyseal resection must be performed, or for interim stabilization until a surgical arthroplasty is healed or an orthopedic joint replacement is performed.

Depending on the patient and case profile, an immediate reconstruction may not be possible due to a variety of reasons. Cardiovascular instability, ventilation problems, a large blood loss, or unexpected surgical findings may render a continuation of the operation too dangerous, especially in patients with several comorbidities or advanced biologic age. In these cases, temporary vacuum-assisted wound closure may be used until final reconstruction. There is no evidence in the literature that these angiogenesis-promoting subatmospheric pressure devices have negative effects on oncologic safety *after a wide resection* that was intended to remove all neoplastic tissue including an appropriate safety margin.[28,29] This is in contrast to the situation after incisional or excisional biopsies where they are not recommended for use (see above).

Lymph node dissection

Less than 5% of all sarcomas spread in a lymphatic way. Therefore there is no indication for a standardized simultaneous dissection of the relevant lymph node areas (i.e., popliteal fossa/groin) if the region is not clearly involved clinically or radiographically. A lymph node dissection should always be performed, however, in sarcomatous tumor entities that are known for their lymphatic spread like the rhabdomyosarcoma, angiosarcoma, and epithelioid-like sarcoma subtypes. If regional lymph node metastases are present, a radical lymphadenectomy significantly improves median survival.[13,14]

Indications for amputation

In selected cases, amputation of the leg must be considered the best option for the patient despite very detailed imaging techniques, modern oncologic resection strategies, advanced sophisticated plastic reconstructions, and advances in radiologic and chemotherapeutic therapeutic regimens. Primary amputations for treatment of lower extremity sarcomas are necessary in less than 5% of all patients and in less than 15% in recurrences while demonstrating a comparable long-term survival.[2-4]

Amputations are chosen as an adequate primary therapy, if significant medical comorbidities prevent the safe completion of a major tumor resection with immediate defect reconstruction. Usually, these cases are very rare, and almost always the reconstruction can be deferred to a secondary operation. Modern advances in anesthesiology and intensive care medicine usually allow long procedures to be performed safely. The only exceptions where an immediate reconstruction must be performed are immediate revascularization procedures in cases with extensive main arterial involvement. Extensive lower limb reconstruction procedures also have to be balanced cautiously against amputation in para- or tetraplegic patients or patients with severe cerebral impairment who are bedridden for lifetime.

If the tumor demonstrates transmetatarsal growth, penetrates the interosseus membrane in the lower leg, already shows locoregional dissemination (for example with rhabdomyosarcomas), or the patient presents with a very large and extensively ulcerated tumor with circular leg involvement, an amputation may be inevitable. Primary multicomponent sarcomas in the proximal thigh may be treated best with an amputation as well as extensive tumor recurrences after exhaustion of all adjuvant or surgical modalities.

Uncontrollable chronic diseases that are not acceptable for major (microvascular) procedures or render the preservation of the sarcoma-infested extremity useless can make an amputation inevitable. Examples are open ulcers because of chronic venous insufficiency or atherosclerotic occlusive disease in the same leg, an ipsilateral unrelated tumor, or a history of previous trauma with subsequent subclinical osteitis. The latter could reactivate in the context of major surgery or adjuvant therapy.

Furthermore, the predictable inability to reconstruct a stable extremity and/or wounds that are not suitable for safe conservative wound care and patient handling are an indication for amputation, if the full reconstructive spectrum has been evaluated for leg salvage and a suitable solution was not found. This might include the unavailability of relevant donor sites for (microvascular) extremity reconstruction.

Lastly, patient preference in favor of amputation is very rare after thorough information about modern reconstructive possibilities but has to be respected in selected cases.

Reconstructive options for lower extremity preservation

Plastic surgical involvement in sarcoma treatment already begins during tumor resection. Several examples that demand plastic surgical and microsurgical knowledge during skin incision, tissue dissection, and neurovascular preparation

have already been mentioned above. In general, the plastic surgical reconstruction follows the reconstructive ladder with the lowest rung being the least invasive method (secondary healing) and the highest rung representing customized chimeric multicomponent free flaps. Like in many other reconstructive problems, the best option for the individual patient must be chosen regardless of whether it requires more complicated surgery ("reconstructive elevator").[30-32]

The following subsections demonstrate the vast diversity of plastic surgical methods, also found elsewhere in this book in detail. For sarcoma reconstruction, the surgeon has to keep in mind that pre- or postoperative radiation or previous chemotherapy can spoil his or her success rate, especially in complicated microvascular reconstructions. The use of large recipient vessels outside the radiation field, supple soft-tissue closure, and as little foreign material as possible are proven ways for successful surgery.

Soft tissue

Soft-tissue coverage for sarcoma reconstruction must always be seen in the context of preoperative and adjuvant radiotherapy. The goals are obliteration of dead space, closure of large skin defects with tension-free wound closure, preservation of thin but viable skin edges by supporting them with voluminous muscle flaps, and to cushion exposed bony prominences around the tibia, joints, or amputation stumps.

Local and regional fasciocutaneous flaps are slightly superior to skin-grafted muscle transposition flaps (i.e., medial or lateral gastrocnemius head or peroneus brevis) in terms of fast wound healing and radiation resistance. They might be of limited availability after large tumor resection. Local perforator flaps are very useful for primary reconstructions. However, if the area was irradiated, the perforators in the field are less reliable and extremely difficult to dissect due to fibrosis or became very small and fragile. Furthermore, the skin quality and elasticity is inferior for donor site closure in secondary reconstructions with local flaps.

Useful pedicled regional flaps to cover defects in the thigh may be harvested from the deep inferior epigastric artery system of the lower abdomen (i.e., transverse rectus abdominus myocutaneous, vertical rectus abdominus myocutaneous, deep inferior epigastric perforator, and rectus abdominis muscle) or from the buttock area (superior gluteal artery perforator and inferior gluteal artery perforator). The latter may have a suitable rotation radius if isolated on their respective perforators (Case 4.3).

Microvascular free flaps from all over the body may be used for lower extremity reconstruction and are chosen according to the defect geometry and depth, location, and functional requirements. For secondary reconstructions, recipient vessels are rare or fragile, if the area was irradiated and a preoperative angiogram is warranted. Sensate flaps (i.e., lateral arm flap) should be considered for weight-bearing areas at the foot or on amputation stumps.

Neuromuscular unit

Resected main nerves can be microsurgically reconstructed with multiple cable grafts from the sural nerve or other donor sites according to the cross-section of the recipient nerve.

Meticulous technique and the use of an operative microscope are paramount. In selected sarcoma resections that include bone and nerves, the bone may be restabilized with shortening of the extremity. This scales down the soft-tissue defect, facilitates wound closure, and can make primary nerve coaptation possible.

Depending on the muscular units that have to be resected, muscle or tendon transfers may be performed primarily. Biceps tendon or posterior tibial transfers are the most common transfers in the lower extremity to reconstruct knee extension and foot elevation, respectively (see Case 4.1). Tenodeses may preserve muscular power in partially resected compartments (i.e., adductors) and allow muscular stabilization of joints. Of course, free functional muscle transfers (i.e., mm. gracilis and gastrocnemius)[33] are very useful in young patients with high neuroregenerative potential as well.

Skeletal reconstruction

Reconstruction of the skeleton after resection of soft-tissue sarcomas involving bone secondarily and primary osseous sarcomas are the main interdisciplinary field of orthopedic and plastic surgeons. Expandable and non-expandable tumor prostheses, Van Ness or Borggreve rotationplasty,[34] resection arthroplasties, distraction osteogenesis, segment transport, or total joint replacements commonly belong to the orthopedic techniques. However, a combination of the above with pedicled or free vascularized bone may benefit the patient and augment the therapeutic armamentarium. Therefore this "orthoplastic approach"[35] does not only refer to post-traumatic reconstructions but is a fruitful strategy for oncologic plastic surgery as well.

In selected cases, a variety of traditional techniques like fibula-pro-tibia transfer require microsurgical dissection of the pedicle (Fig. 4.3) or an orthopedic osteosynthesis in the metaphyseal area may benefit from additional vascularized bone from a composite flap to augment the construction. Very useful flaps here are the latissimus-bone flap and the (para-)scapular bone flap with a lateral and or medial scapular bone segment of up to 11×3 cm that provides coverage or filling of extensive soft-tissue defects or prosthetic material. For smaller defects around the foot, composite flaps like the osteofasciocutaneous lateral arm flap are useful.[36]

Large defects of the long bones are more difficult to reconstruct with autologous tissue in the lower extremity than in the upper.[37] This is due to the geometrical and size mismatch of the largest human bone flaps, that is free fibula and vascularized iliac crest (deep circumflex iliac artery flap). However, vascularized bone is a vital, dynamic, growing, infection resistant, and relatively radiation resistant tissue. The various methods for single and double fibula reconstruction of extensive long bone defects in the lower extremity are discussed

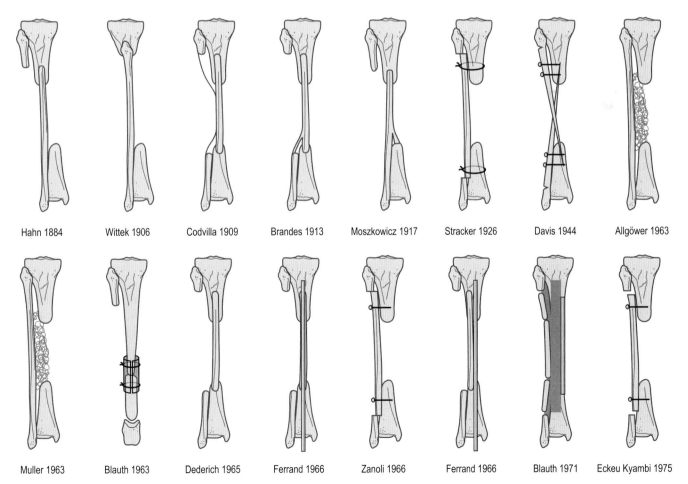

Hahn 1884   Wittek 1906   Codvilla 1909   Brandes 1913   Moszkowicz 1917   Stracker 1926   Davis 1944   Allgöwer 1963

Muller 1963   Blauth 1963   Dederich 1965   Ferrand 1966   Zanoli 1966   Ferrand 1966   Blauth 1971   Eckeu Kyambi 1975

Fig. 4.3 Historical overview of various fibula-pro-tibia techniques for lower leg reconstruction.

elsewhere in this book and apply to sarcoma reconstruction alike (Chapter 7).

In the context of adjuvant radiotherapy, avascular autologous or allogeneic bone grafts, with their high complication rate of fracture, infection, slow integration, and creeping substitution, should be used very carefully and only in selected cases. When using these grafts, there should be special emphasis on ample vascularization of the surrounding soft-tissue bed and obliteration of any dead spaces around the bone. This optimizes creeping substitution of the avascular allograft and reduces the probability of graft exposure after radiation.

Combination techniques using an avascular structural allograft with a vascularized free fibula inside, as described by Capanna, offer promising results especially for extensive skeletal defects in young tumor patients (see Case 4.7).[38,39] This hot-dog-like construct combines optimal vascularization of the vascularized autologous fibula with the structural stability of the geometrically matched allograft "shell". The osteosynthetic stabilization of this construct over the length of a long bone and in metaphyseal areas may be a compromise as the vascular pedicle and vascularization of the inner fibula must be preserved. Burring a trough into the allograft for guiding the peroneal pedicle through the allograft cortex to their recipient vessels has proven quite useful.[39,40]

Vascular surgery

Main arteries that need to be resected together with the tumor should be reconstructed immediately by interpositional vein grafts in the lower leg. Proximal to the knee, autologous vein grafts may be too small and alloplastic material may be considered as an alternative for vessel replacement or extra-anatomic bypasses. It is paramount to ensure a good soft-tissue coverage for these materials to prevent exposure, which is easier to achieve in the thigh than in the lower leg.

In selected cases, a temporary arteriovenous loop connected to large-bore vessels proximal to the recipient area offers large-diameter vascular access for microvascular anastomosis distant to any previously scarred or irradiated area. For the proximal thigh and groin area, even the contralateral femoral vessels can be used as recipients for a cross-over graft.[41] If available, autologous vein grafts should be used for vessel reconstruction. In selected cases with tumor-related resection of main arteries, a simultaneous defect coverage and vessel reconstruction can be provided by flow-through flaps (i.e., anterolateral thigh (ALT), radial forearm, and free fibula).

Due to the high rate of venous graft occlusion for vein reconstruction in oncologic patients, the procedure should be done only in selected cases.[42] One of the reasons for this might be the use of longer vein grafts in oncologic surgery than in trauma patients, which are more prone to thrombosis. Compared to trauma cases, venous outflow compromise by invasive tumor growth occurs more slowly and the dynamic nature of the lower leg venous system almost always allows the development of sufficient venous collaterals, if the affected deep veins are resected.

Complex approaches

For complex defects, free microvascular composite flaps from the subscapular, external iliac, or lateral circumflex femoral vessel systems provide large, multilobed transplants with a variety of different tissues for simultaneous soft-tissue and skeletal reconstruction.[49] Chimeric flaps further expand this enormous variability (i.e., free fibula with ALT).

In selected cases, where amputation or segment amputation is inevitable, the distal limb segments are viable and healthy. According to the spare-part principle of plastic surgery, the tissue may be transferred as a composite fillet flap, either pedicled or free microvascular, onto the amputation site providing length and suitable tissue quality for coverage. Preservation or coaptation of the contained nerves may achieve a sensate flap of excellent quality and skin texture.

Postoperative care

Immediate postoperative care

A firm concept of postoperative care is very important following biopsies, definitive sarcoma resection, and after any reconstructive surgical procedures for a variety of reasons. The postoperative protocol after incisional or excisional biopsies is focused on the prevention of hematoma and seroma formation and thereby possible tumor spread. While meticulous hemostasis and drainage placement is paramount (see techniques section), postoperative fluid collections in the resection bed and in tissue planes can be prevented effectively by bed rest, elevation of the affected lower extremity, and immobilization by external fixators or splints. Circular elastic bandaging and compressive dressings are also helpful.

Most reconstructive procedures in sarcoma surgery with larger lesions need defect closure with flaps of some kind. Lower extremities that were reconstructed with local, regional, or free flaps need to be positioned in a slightly elevated position for 5–7 days to accommodate the circulation rearrangements in the flap tissue and to prevent early venous congestion in the transplanted tissue. Frequent flap perfusion monitoring is paramount in the first days and ensures immediate intervention should a pedicle thrombosis or hematoma occur. Patients with neoadjuvant chemotherapy or preoperative intra-arterial perfusion are at high risk for vascular complications in this context.

Following this period of elevation, orthostatic "flap training" can be initiated with lowering the reconstructed extremity for 5 min t.i.d. associated with external compression by elastic bandaging. After this, the flap is clinically evaluated and the procedure can be extended in increments of 5–15 min daily over the next week until 1 h is accumulated. This allows reasonable intervals for early gait training and mobilization by stage-adapted physiotherapy.

Compressive bandaging should be replaced by custom-fit compressive garments worn for at least 6 months for all soft-tissue flap reconstructions of the lower extremity except pure osseous flap reconstructions. Usually, garment wearing is initiated when the sutures are removed and the wound is healed.

Postoperative weight-bearing depends on the bony resection and reconstruction procedures that were performed, the hardware used for osteosynthesis, and the bone quality. The mobilization schedule should be determined exclusively by the operating surgeon. Serial roentgenograms or CT-scans help in determination of the bone healing and regained functional stability of the extremity.

Oncologic postoperative care and follow-up

Patients after sarcoma resection with adequate margins and R_0-situation need postoperative adjuvant radiation therapy under most circumstances, especially in tumors that are classified as high-grade (G_2/G_3). Only superficial, low-grade lesions with tumor-free wide margins may be treated with wide resection only. The radiation oncologists start with the therapy according to the appropriate treatment protocols established by the tumor board decision as soon as the wound is healed. If any unexpected oncologically relevant factors occurred during resection or reconstruction (inappropriate or positive margins, vessel invasions, histology, etc.), the new findings should be presented in the tumor board as the treatment plan needs to be revised accordingly. This is also true for any late follow-up findings, which imply a change in the normal course of healing by emerging local recurrences or distant metastases.

The modalities or patient follow-up after completion of resection and possible adjuvant treatment are not clearly defined in the literature. The following investigations are well accepted in the current literature:

- Thoracic CT-scan. Distant metastases in lower extremity sarcomas almost exclusively occur through hematogenous spread into the lung with only a few exceptions (see above). It should be repeated every 3 months.
- Contrast-enhanced MRI of the primary tumor site every 3 months. This should always be evaluated by or together with the surgeons. MRI is also the diagnostic method of choice for evaluating lymphatic spread if applicable. However, MRI criteria of tumor stability or progression may not correlate with the tumor status correctly.
- Serial radiographs of the primary tumor location at least every 6 months if the skeleton was affected by the primary tumor or included in resection or reconstruction. The osteointegration of prosthetic material, bony healing, bone grafts, or transplants are controlled more frequently in the postoperative period anyway. A CT scan should be performed if the information by the plain radiograph is insufficient or suspicious findings occur.
- New imaging techniques evaluating the metabolic activity of tumor material like PET (or PET-CT) or magnetic resonance spectroscopy (MRS) are promising. While this is a fast developing field and the numbers of tracers are increasing, these methods are increasingly accurate in controlling preoperative response to adjuvant therapy and postoperative follow-up. No commonly accepted follow-up schedule exists for sarcomas so far, and patients should be integrated into suitable studies.

Secondary procedures

Early secondary procedures – soft tissue

After the initial tumor resection and extremity reconstruction is performed successfully and the wounds are healed, in the majority of cases plastic surgical therapy must continue during or after a possible radiotherapy to optimize the overall result.

Despite adequate healing during the primary reconstructive phase, wound healing disturbances, fistulas, and incision breakdowns may occur during the scheduled radiation cycles. If the initial soft-tissue closure was supple enough, early wound excision and secondary closure may suffice in minor cases. However, larger skin breakdowns may lead to exposure of functional structures like tendons, vessels, nerves, and bones, which need to be covered urgently to prevent radiation induced osteitis, vessel thrombosis, or tissue necrosis. Local flap solutions are only possible, however, if the appropriate vessels are still intact, as mentioned before.

With the radiation cycles completed, many patients experience fibrosis, scar formation, contractures, and tendon adhesions. Early function-improving procedures include tenolyses, contracture and scar releases, serial excisions, or tendon transfers that were not possible or justified primarily. It is often very difficult to evaluate during tumor resection, if any remaining musculature or nerves fascicles will suffice for an adequate basic motor function. A typical example for a secondary procedure like this is the posterior tibial tendon transfer for a clinical drop-foot caused by a muscular or neural insufficiency of the peroneal compartment. Neuroma formation or nerve entrapments in irradiated and fibrotic tissue should be approached with desensitization and conservative therapy first, but frequently may require early operative neurolyses.

Contour improving procedures of bulky transferred tissue should be performed not earlier than 6 months to be less independent from the vascular pedicle. They follow standard plastic surgical debulking techniques like direct sequential flap excision, tangential subcutaneous thinning, tangential thinning, and secondary resurfacing with split- or full-thickness skin grafts in muscle flaps or aspiration lipectomy. The same time frame applies to secondary procedures for forming amputation stumps. However, additive procedures on amputated legs like cushioning and stump lengthening by local and free flaps or sensitization by transfer of neurotized transplants can be planned earlier than 6 months after the amputation.

Early secondary procedures – skeleton

As mentioned above, skeletal reconstruction and stabilization should be performed as completely as possible during the primary reconstructive stage. Usually, orthopedic prosthetic joint or long bone replacements do not need any secondary surgery if the initial montage demonstrated uneventful osteo-integration. Prosthetic replacement is mostly used in primary osseous sarcomas with large skeletal defects after resection. However, infection, mechanical failure, and loosening are among the most common prosthetic complications in the context of radio- and chemotherapy. Major revision surgery is therefore needed, which is described in the pertinent orthopedic literature.

If plastic surgical reconstruction of the lower limb skeleton was performed by free autologous bone grafts, vascularized bone transplants, avascular allogeneic bone grafts, or combinations of the above, osseous healing is often slow in sarcoma patients, especially if the radiation field encompasses the zone of skeletal reconstruction. Therefore augmentation of previously inserted bone transplants or revision of pseudarthroses with corticocancellous bone packing is quite often necessary – especially in non-vascularized grafts. At this stage, the osteosynthesis may also be changed to a more stable and definitive method if the primary one has failed.

The microvascular medial femoral condyle corticoperiosteal flap may be a useful tool to provide vascularity and osteogenic potential for recalcitrant pseudarthroses in a previously irradiated field.[43,44]

Sarcoma-related partial joint resections in the weight-bearing lower extremity may be critical. Painless function with an acceptable range of motion must be the reconstructive goal. Especially after partial joint resections or resection arthroplasties, the functional outcome often cannot be adequately assessed until complete mobilization of the patient has taken place. If joint salvage surgery was not successful primarily, resulting in an unstable or painful joint with a severely impaired range of motion, secondary arthroplasties, joint replacement surgery, or arthrodeses may be necessary.

If the limb-preserving surgery consisted of a shortening of the limb, secondary distraction osteogenesis for extremity length adaptation can now be performed with all the soft tissue healed and the radiation therapy completed. However, docking failures are more frequent in irradiated patients. Corticocancellous augmentation is then needed to achieve stability.

Late secondary procedures

The number of patients that are long-term survivors after successful sarcoma therapy in the lower extremity is constantly increasing. A considerable number of them need late secondary reconstructions or surgical corrections of their reconstructed leg. The plastic surgical therapy at this stage aims to correct the sequelae of the previous interdisciplinary plastic surgical, radiologic, and orthopedic therapy. Though not life- or limb-saving anymore, these procedures are nevertheless important to help the patients complete their personal and social coping after the disease and to improve quality of life.

Scar releases and flap debulkings because of functional and aesthetic reasons that began in the early secondary stage frequently need revisions for several years. Irradiation may leave a hard, constrictive, and fibrotic soft-tissue integument behind, which may be painful in rest and in motion or while wearing clothing and shoes. If postirradiation ulcers and unstable scars further deteriorate the situation, the plastic surgeon must be aware of late local recurrences and secondary malignancies in the affected area. Excision of the lesions or the constricted scarred skin and transfer of unimpaired healthy tissue by local, regional, or free tissue transfer can improve the patient's quality of life considerably. Of course, any excised tissue from these areas must be evaluated histopathologically.

Peripheral neuropathies are less common after irradiation but more common after chemotherapy and may cause disabling chronic pain to the patient. Frequently, the nerve is relatively healthy, but entrapped and fixed by surrounding dense, fibrotic, and irradiated tissue. Adequate therapy consists of careful neurolysis, rerouting, and wrapping of the nerve in well-vascularized tissue by microsurgical methods.

Late secondary procedures after implantation of major hardware like modular prostheses or total joint replacements may include hardware exchange due to wear, mechanical failure, or loosening.

Long-term sarcoma survivors with a previous lower limb amputation may experience stump problems like retracted soft tissue with insufficient soft-tissue coverage of the bone, skin folds that impair proper wear of the prosthesis, painful neuromas, and trophic skin changes. Many patients are very experienced with their prosthesis and ask for specific plastic surgical stump corrections. In selected cases, this might include microvascular free flap transfers, preferably with sensate flaps.

Outcomes, prognosis, and complications

Outcomes and prognosis

Several specialized evaluation scores do exist (Musculoskeletal Tumor Society (MSTS),[45] Toronto Extremity Salvage Score (TESS),[46] European Organization for Research and Treatment of Cancer (EORTC QLQ-C30)) that rate various sets of subjective and objective parameters for functionality, quality-of-life, emotional, and social factors.[47,48]

Soft-tissue sarcomas

The current age-adjusted death rate for soft-tissue sarcomas is 1.3 per 100 000/year, based on data between 2001 and 2005.[1] A recent series, from the Memorial Sloan Kettering Cancer Center (MSKCC), of 1706 patients with primary and secondary soft-tissue sarcomas of the extremities with a mean follow-up of 55 months demonstrated a 5-year disease-specific survival rate of 85% in patients treated between 1997 and 2001. This number did not differ significantly from the survival rate in the previously treated patients from this group. The same was true for the subset of high-risk patients in this group with a 5-year disease-specific survival rate of 61% in those treated between 1997 and 2001. This indicates that the prognosis for patients with extremity soft-tissue sarcomas has not changed over the last 20 years. Throughout this period, tumor depth, size, grade, margins, presentation status, location (proximal vs. distal), and certain histopathologic subtypes as well as patient age remained significant prognostic factors (Table 4.5).[1]

Steinau et al. report about 85 soft-tissue sarcomas in the lower extremity among 744 sarcoma patients between 1980 and 1996. Mean age at presentation was 42.9 years (range 6–80 years), with 38 patients being previously operated elsewhere. Eighteen patients had 2–9 recurrences. Still, in 81 patients (95.3%) an R_0-resection with curative intention could be performed, whereas 4 patients underwent a palliative resection due to multilocular distant metastases. In 41/81 patients extensive tissue defects resulted after the resection and 17 local and 24 free flaps were needed for closure. Thirteen patients received a simultaneous tendon transfer with defect closure to improve their gait. In 18 patients with local skeletal infiltration, special plastic surgical bone reconstructions, conventional partial foot amputations, or atypical hindfoot amputations were done. All of these patients received

Table 4.5 Prognostic factors in soft-tissue sarcoma therapy

Factor	Distant recurrence-free survival	Local recurrence-free survival	Relapse-free survival	Disease-specific survival
Age >50 years	–	–	–	–
Recurrent sarcoma	–	–	–	–
Size >5 cm	–	–	–	–
Deep location	–			–
High–grade	–		–	–
Proximal position				–
Histology				
Fibrosarcoma		–		
Leiomyosarcoma	–		–	–
Positive microscopic margin	–	–	–	–
Time period of treatment				

Minus symbols indicate an independent adverse prognostic factor, and blank fields indicate a non-independent prognostic factor.
(Adapted from Weitz J, Antonescu CR, Brennan MF. Localized extremity soft-tissue sarcoma: improved knowledge with unchanged survival over time. *J Clin Oncol.* 2003;21:2719–2725.)

individualized orthopedic shoe and inlay adaptions and finally achieved (with and without these shoes) a better gait and ability to do sports, in comparison with patients who received lower leg prostheses. In 2 patients, a transtibial amputation was inevitable. In this group of 85 patients, a mean survival of 132 months and a 5-year survival rate of 62% was found.[3]

The Finnish experience, with 73 patients with lower limb soft-tissue sarcomas who received limb-salvage surgery, reports a 5-year local recurrence-free survival rate of 82%, a metastasis-free survival of 59%, a disease-free survival of 56%, and a disease-specific overall survival of 70% over a follow-up time of 65.9 months. Three-quarters of the patients were able to walk normally or had only minor walking impairment. They emphasize that microsurgery is an essential part of modern tumor surgery.[49] Long-term survivors have a higher probability of experiencing both sequelae of their primary plastic surgical treatment (i.e., contractures, bulky flaps, and unstable scars) and secondary malignomas (i.e., postradiation angiosarcomas).

A large study from an interdisciplinary sarcoma center in Germany had a mean follow-up of 36 months for 167 patients with extremity liposarcomas. Over this time, only 5 (3%) of the patients had to undergo amputation throughout this period. A clear margin R_0-resection could be achieved in 158 patients. The authors report an overall 5-year survival rate of 79%, though the study collective was biased in favor of extensive and previously operated cases due to the reference center status of the clinic. Patients with primary tumors had a 5-year survival rate of 90%, and an overall number of 37 local recurrences were found. The myxoid liposarcoma was responsible for most recurrences. Patients with recurrent tumors had a 5-year survival rate of 69%.[26]

Bone sarcomas

The European Osteosarcoma Intergroup reports a 57% 5-year survival rate in a patient group of 202 patients with a 49–85% limb salvage rate. An important finding of this study was that patients having undergone limb salvage surgery with later local recurrence had a slightly better survival rate than primarily amputated patients (37% vs. 31% at 5 years).[11,12] Marulanda et al. stated that for osteosarcoma patients there is no difference in survival between amputations and properly performed limb-salvaging procedures.[50]

Carty et al. reported their results after LSS of 20 intra-articular knee osteosarcoma patients and their reconstruction with endoprostheses. Evaluation was done by MSTS and TESS scores, and moderate to high function was achieved.[48]

A Norwegian study, involving 118 patients with osteosarcomas or Ewing's sarcoma in the extremities, evaluated the long-term functional outcome at a minimum of 5 years after treatment. The function was evaluated with the MSTS and TESS scores while quality of life was assessed using the Short Form-36 (SF-36). The mean age at follow-up was 31 years (15–57 years), and the mean follow-up was 13 years (6–22 years). A total of 67 patients (57%) initially had limb-sparing surgery, but 4 had a secondary amputation. The median MSTS score was 70% (17–100%), and the median TESS was 89% (43–100%). The amputees had a significantly lower MSTS score than those with limb-sparing surgery (p<0.001), but there was no difference for the TESS. Tumor localization above the knee level resulted in significantly lower MSTS and TESS scores. There were no significant differences in quality of life between amputees and those with LSS except in physical functioning. In a multivariate analysis, amputation, tumor location above the knee, and having muscular pain were associated with low physical function. Most of the bone tumor survivors managed well after adjustment to their physical limitations. A total of 105 patients were able to work and had an overall good quality of life.[51]

Complications – management of recurrent disease

If local tumor recurrences are present, they are usually found quite early if the patient is compliant according to his or her follow-up protocol. In many cases, this implies a heavy psychological burden to the patient, and careful and empathic communication and conjoint treatment planning are very important.

The surgical procedures in local recurrences do not differ in general from the initial tumor resection. However, previous surgery, flap transplantation with microvascular pedicles in a scarred and sometimes irradiated field, and extra-anatomic nerve and vessel grafts do make the resection much more difficult this time. Even so, a local recurrent tumor manifestation does not necessarily mean amputation. If local sarcoma recurrences can be re-excised and treated surgically, about two-thirds of the patients have a long-term survival benefit.

Depending on the previous protocol and overall radiation dose, secondary radiation therapy (brachytherapy) after resection of local recurrences should be evaluated together with the oncologic radiation specialist.

Case study 4.1 (Fig. 4.4) ○

A 35-year-old male presented with a growing tumor and painless swelling in his right quadriceps muscle. The patient referred this to a blunt trauma while playing soccer 6 months ago. Ultrasound and contrast enhanced MRI demonstrated a large intramuscular tumor suspicious for a liposarcoma (Fig. 4.4A & B). Histology was verified with incision biopsy. Staging with abdominal and thoracic CT-scan showed no distant metastases. The treatment protocol was discussed in the local tumor board and wide excision of the tumor was performed (Fig. 4.4C). As four-fifths of the quadriceps muscle had to be resected (Fig. 4.4D),

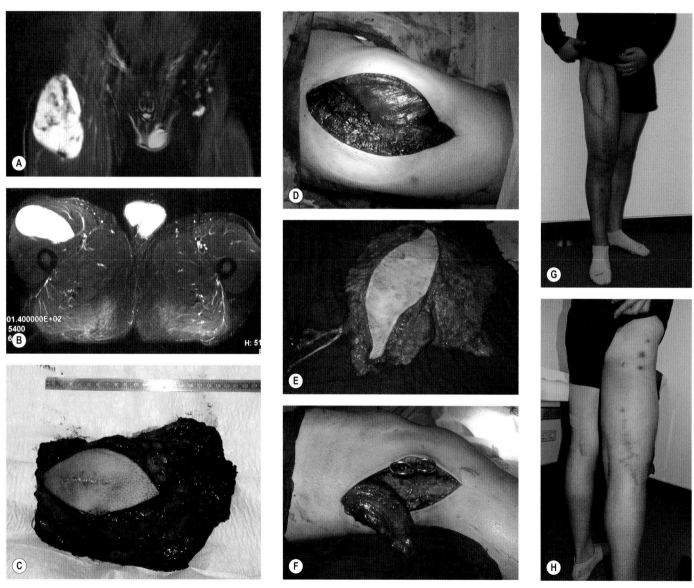

Fig. 4.4 (A,B) Contrast-enhanced magnetic resonance imaging demonstrating a large intramuscular tumor suspicious for a liposarcoma. **(C)** Tumor specimen after wide excision, including the incision biopsy scar. **(D)** The quadriceps muscle had to be resected subtotally. **(E)** This free functional musculocutaneous latissimus dorsi flap was harvested and revascularized to local vessels. Nerve coaptation was done to a branch of the femoral nerve close to the groin that could be spared from the resection. **(F)** To assist leg function this pedicled biceps femoris flap was rerouted around the distal lateral femur and woven into the new latissimus–quadriceps–tendon extensor apparatus. **(G,H)** Clinical result 3 months after resection.

a free functional musculocutaneous latissimus dorsi flap was harvested (Fig. 4.4E) and connected to local vessels. Nerve coaptation was done to a branch of the femoral nerve close to the groin that could be spared from the resection. The muscle transplant was fixed at the anterior superior iliac spine, and the remaining vastus medialis head and its tendon were woven into the quadriceps tendon and fixed securely with 1-0 non-resorbable sutures. To assist leg function until the latissimus muscle was reinnervated, we simultaneously also transferred a functional biceps femoris flap through a separate posterior incision (Fig. 4.4F) around the distal lateral femur and sutured it into the new latissimus–quadriceps–tendon extensor apparatus with an adequate pretension. The muscle bulk of the latissimus easily obliterated the space of the resected quadriceps muscle, while the skin island served for tension-free closure of the integument. For protection of the tendomuscular reconstructions, an external fixator across the knee was applied for 6 weeks. Healing was uneventful, the pathology showed clear and adequate margins (R0-situation). The fixator was removed in an outpatient procedure and physiotherapy begun. At 3 months after the resection and simultaneous reconstruction procedure, the patient showed an almost completely normal gait (Fig. 4.4G & H).

Case 4.2 (Fig. 4.5)

This 48-year-old male patient was referred to us with a horizontal (non-oncologic) incision of the right anterior lower leg (Fig. 4.5A & B) after a non-oncologic resection of an MFH leaving positive margins (R_1) elsewhere. Re-operation with a wide excision (9×8 cm) (Fig. 4.5C & D) was performed in our center and the defect closed with a pedicled medial gastrocnemius muscle flap (Fig. 4.5E) and split-thickness skin graft from the ipsilateral thigh. Histology now showed adequately wide and clear margins of this R_0 resection. Further healing was uneventful. Fig. 4.5G & I demonstrate follow-up results at 3 months after flap transposition and defect closure.

Case 4.3 (Fig. 4.6)

This 56-year-old male patient demonstrated a large intramuscular tumor highly suspicious of a soft-tissue sarcoma in the proximal left thigh close to the groin. His clinical complaints were swelling and pain over 6 months. MRI demonstrated close proximity to the superficial femoral vessels; however, the femoral nerve could not be identified in the MRI (Fig. 4.6A & B). The incisional biopsy showed a highly malignant synovial-cell sarcoma (G_3). After preoperative planning in the tumor board, a wide resection including most of the extensor muscles (Fig. 4.6C) was performed according to oncologic guidelines, yielding a 23×18×20 cm large tissue specimen including the tumor (Fig. 4.6D & F). The femoral nerve was encased by tumor tissue and required resection according to oncologic principles. From the contralateral abdomen, a pedicled vertical musculocutaneous rectus abdominis muscle (VRAM) flap (30×18 cm) was harvested and transferred into the defect (Fig. 4.6G & H). Additionally, the biceps femoris as well as the semitendinosus muscles where transferred to the

remnants of the patellar tendon to reconstruct knee extension. The postoperative course was uneventful with the exception of a small wound dehiscence applicable for conservative local wound care at the midabdomen flap harvest site. The patient underwent radiation therapy as well as chemotherapy due to metastases in the lung. Two years postsurgery the patient was able to extend his leg and had no recurrence of the tumor or the metastases in the lung (Fig. 4.6I).

Case 4.4 (Fig. 4.7)

A 6×7×5 cm large painless mass was detected in the right calf of this 31-year-old male patient. Contrast-enhanced MRI showed a lesion highly suspicious for a soft-tissue sarcoma. This diagnosis was confirmed by a longitudinal incision biopsy according to oncologic guidelines, and the definitive tumor resection was planned (Fig. 4.7A). The tumor resection was performed according to international standards for wide excision to leave a cuff of tissue surrounding the tumor of at least 2 cm to the depth and at least 4 cm to the sides (Fig. 4.7B & C). Due to encasement of the posterior tibial vessels and the tibial nerve by the tumor, they had to be resected as well (Fig. 4.7D). The tibial nerve was immediately reconstructed microsurgically by a free sural nerve harvested from the contralateral side (Fig. 4.7E & F). The sural nerve was doubled as a cable graft to allow cross-sectional matching to the tibial nerve and was set at 180° to improve neurotization. The resection defect was controlled for a perfect hemostasis, and drains were placed. As the tumor provided a "tissue-expansion-like" stretching of the calf, the wound could easily be closed primarily without having relevant dead spaces or skin "tenting" over unsupported wound cavities (Fig. 4.7G). Further follow-up showed uneventful healing and recurrence of sensation at the plantar side of the foot after 2 years.

Case 4.5 (Fig. 4.8)

A 70-year-old female complained of a painless mass in the lower extremity (Fig. 4.8A). The preoperative MRI imaging showed a tumor in the posterior and lateral compartment that also affects the fibula (Fig. 4.8B). Due to the overall age and the amount of resection, which included the peroneal vessels, a preoperative angiogram was done demonstrating a well-vascularized tumor as well as appropriate vessels for a free tissue transplantation and limb perfusion (posterior tibial vessels, Fig. 4.8C). After an incisional biopsy, which demonstrated a liposarcoma G_2, the planned resection was outlined (Fig. 4.8D) and a 13×11 cm specimen resected en bloc including a fibula segment (Fig. 4.8E & F). The defect was closed with a free fasciocutaneous parascapular flap, and radiation therapy was initiated. After 2 years, the patient was doing well without any metastases or local tumor recurrence (Fig. 4.8G).

Case 4.6 (Fig. 4.9)

Fig. 4.9A shows the foot of a 51-year-old-female with a mass 5×5 cm at the dorsum of the right foot. Diagnostic MRI demonstrated a tumor that encased the extensor tendons of the first ray (Fig. 4.9B). The incisional biopsy (Fig. 4.9C)

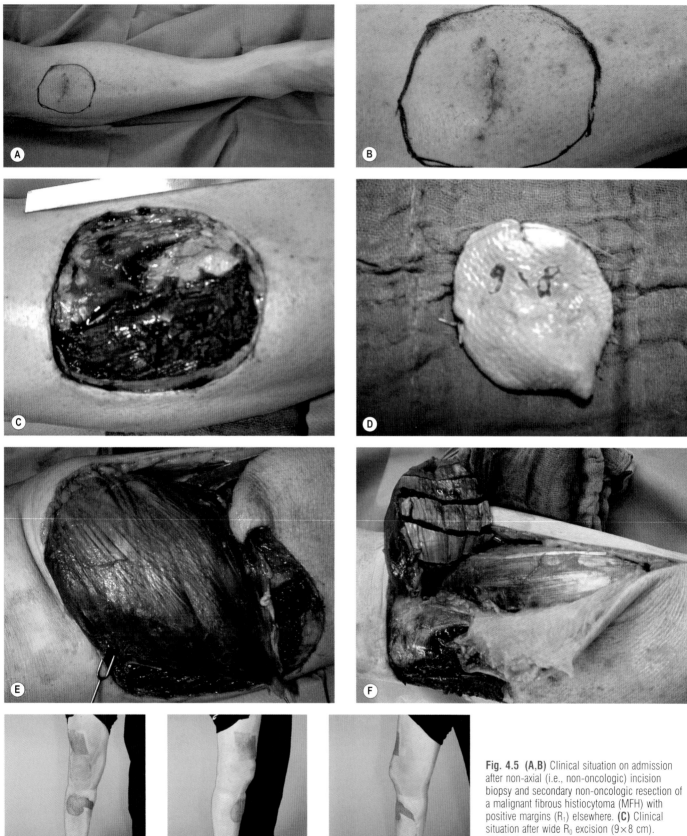

Fig. 4.5 (A,B) Clinical situation on admission after non-axial (i.e., non-oncologic) incision biopsy and secondary non-oncologic resection of a malignant fibrous histiocytoma (MFH) with positive margins (R_1) elsewhere. **(C)** Clinical situation after wide R_0 excision (9×8 cm). **(D)** Excised specimen including the scar of the former biopsy and primary resection. **(E)** A pedicled medial gastrocnemius muscle flap was used for closure. **(F)** Serial incision of the muscle tendon and fascia was performed to expand the reach of the flap and to allow supple wound closure. **(G–I)** Clinical result 3 months after resection and flap closure.

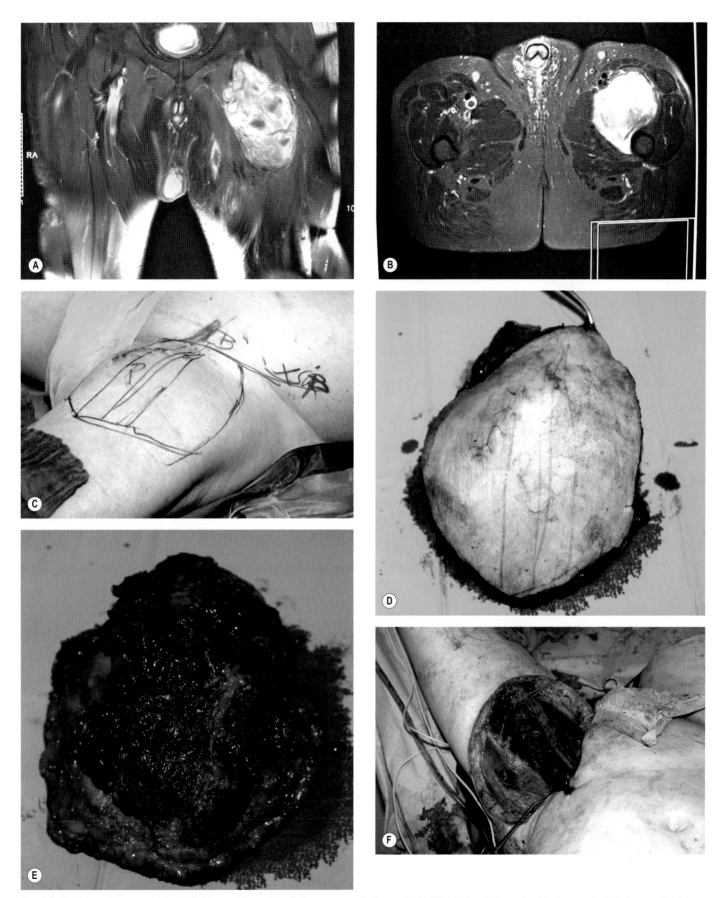

Fig. 4.6 (A,B) Large intramuscular tumor highly suspicious of a soft-tissue sarcoma in the proximal left thigh close to the groin with close proximity to the superficial femoral vessels; however, the femoral nerve could not be identified in the MRI. **(C)** After the incisional biopsy, wide resection including most of the extensor muscles was planned. **(D,E)** Resection specimen 23×18×20 cm including the tumor. **(F)** The femoral nerve was encased by tumor tissue and had to be resected according to oncologic principles.

Continued

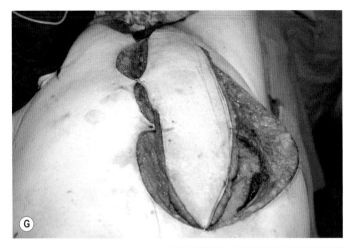

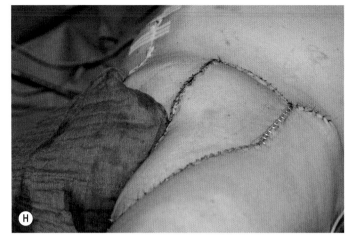

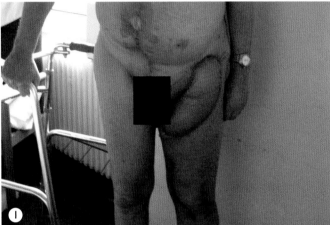

Fig. 4.6, cont'd **(G)** A contralateral pedicled vertical musculocutaneous rectus abdominis muscle flap (30×18 cm) was harvested. **(H)** Flap closure of the defect. **(I)** Clinical picture 2 years after surgery.

confirmed an MFH G₂. A wide excision including the extensor tendons of the first ray, the dorsal half of the first and second metatarsal bones, as well as the capsule of the metatarsophalangeal joint 1 was performed (Fig. 4.9D). Due to the resulting instability of this joint of the first ray an immediate arthrodesis was carried out and the defect covered with a free ALT perforator flap. One year after the operation and radiation therapy the patient was tumor free and able to walk and exercise (Fig. 4.9E).

Case 4.7 (Fig. 4.10)

The patient was a 12-year-old girl with an osteosarcoma of the right distal femur (Fig. 4.10A). She received four cycles of neoadjuvant chemotherapy consisting of doxorubicin and intra-arterial cisplatin. A total segment of 15 cm was then resected from the femur, with the distal transepiphyseal cut 3 cm proximal to the lateral joint line of the knee. A 2 cm fibula bone flap was harvested (Fig. 4.10B). The bone defect was repaired with an intercalary allograft and a vascularized fibula bone flap placed into the medullary canal of the allograft (Fig. 4.10C). The vascular pedicle of the fibula flap

was brought out through a side hole burred into the allograft. The allograft was fixed to the native bone with a 12-hole lateral locking plate (Fig. 4.10D). Proximally, 4 cm of vascularized fibula bone flap was inserted into the host femur; and, distally, 2 cm of fibula flap was inserted into the host femur (Fig. 4.10E). Microvascular anastomoses were performed end-to-end to branches of the femoral artery and vein.

Postoperatively, the patient received two additional cycles of chemotherapy. At 2 months, radiographs showed signs of healing with no complications, and touch weight-bearing was started. At 5 months, radiographs showed a small amount of callus formation and remodeling at the proximal and distal allograft-host junctions (Fig. 4.10F). The patient was allowed partial weight-bearing on the leg with a limit of 10–20 pounds. Another 6 months later, the patient progressed to full weight-bearing, with the restrictions of no running and no sports activity until full radiographic union (Fig. 4.10G).

(Case courtesy of David W. Chang, MD, MD Anderson Cancer Center, Houston, TX, USA).[39]

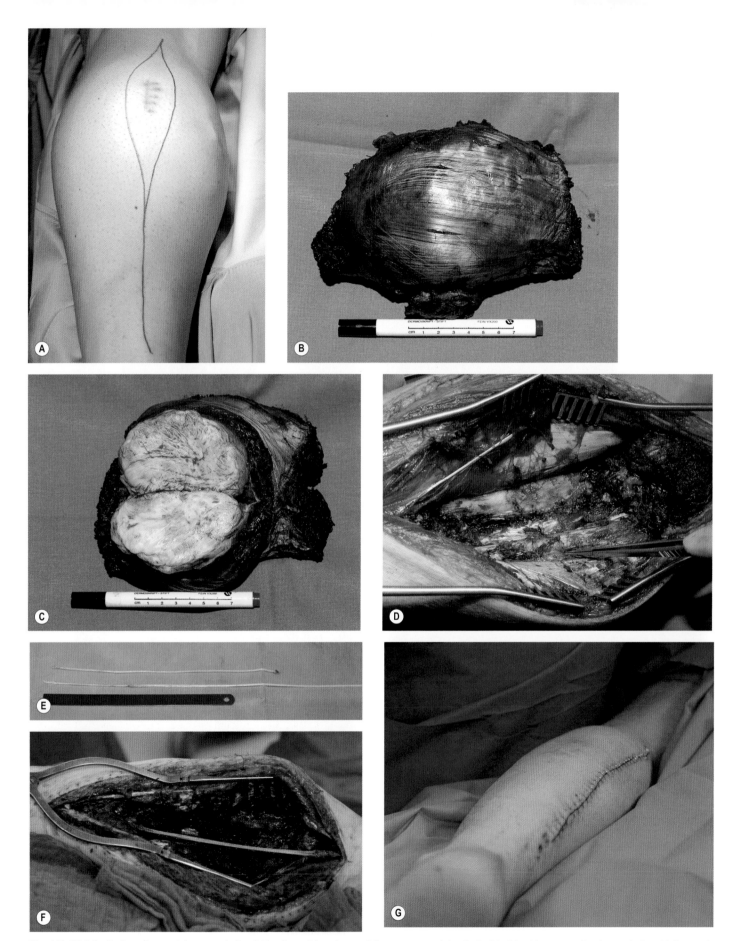

Fig. 4.7 (A) A 6×7×5 cm large painless mass in the right calf suspicious for a soft-tissue sarcoma. A longitudinal incision biopsy according to oncologic guidelines and the definitive tumor resection was planned. **(B,C)** The tumor resection was performed according to international standards for wide excision to leave a cuff of tissue surrounding the tumor of at least 2 cm to the depth and at least 4 cm to the sides. **(D)** Posterior tibial vessels and tibial nerve were encased and had to be resected as well. **(E,F)** The tibial nerve was immediately reconstructed microsurgically by a free sural nerve harvested from the contralateral side. The sural nerve was doubled as a cable graft to allow cross-sectional matching to the tibial nerve and was set at 180° to improve neurotization. **(G)** Postoperative view after primary closure without having relevant dead spaces or skin "tenting" over unsupported wound cavities.

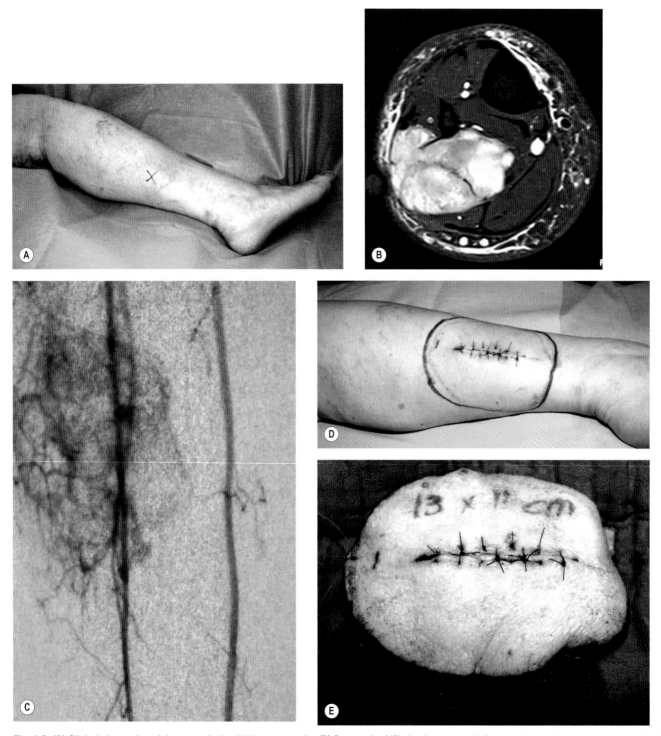

Fig. 4.8 **(A)** Clinical picture of a painless mass in the right lower extremity. **(B)** Preoperative MRI showing a tumor in the posterior and lateral compartment also affecting the fibula. **(C)** Preoperative angiogram demonstrating a well-vascularized tumor including the peroneal vessels. **(D)** After an incisional biopsy, which demonstrated a liposarcoma G_2, the planned resection was outlined. **(E)** En bloc resected, 13×11 cm large specimen including a fibula segment.

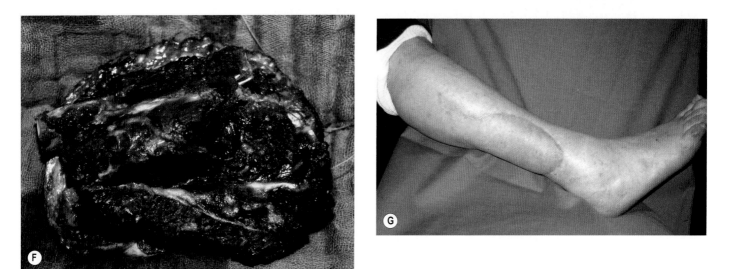

Fig. 4.8, cont'd (F) The tumor was not seen during surgery and was covered well with muscle according to adequate tumor margins. **(G)** Clinical picture 2 years after free parascapular flap closure.

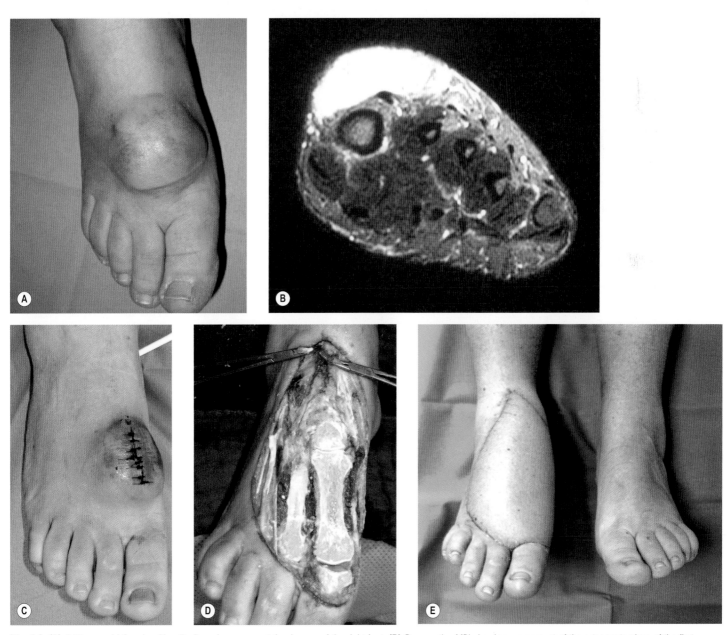

Fig. 4.9 (A) A 51-year-old-female with a 5×5 cm large mass at the dorsum of the right foot. **(B)** Preoperative MRI showing encasement of the extensor tendons of the first ray. **(C)** Clinical picture after incisional biopsy. **(D)** Clinical picture after wide excision including the extensor tendons of the first ray, the dorsal half of the first and second metatarsal bone, as well as the capsule of the metatarsophalangeal joint 1. **(E)** One year after the operation and radiation.

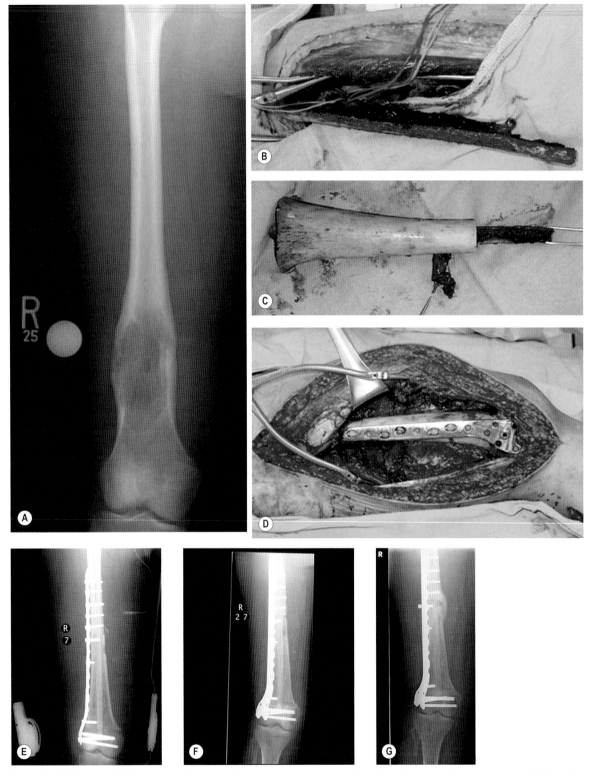

Fig. 4.10 **(A)** The right distal femur of a 12-year-old girl showing an osteosarcoma. **(B)** A 21 cm fibula bone flap was harvested. **(C)** The 15 cm long intercalary allograft and a vascularized fibula bone flap placed into the medullary canal of the allograft. **(D)** Fixation of the allograft with a 12-hole lateral locking plate. **(E)** Postoperative radiograph. Proximally, 4 cm of vascularized fibula bone flap was inserted into the host femur diaphysis and, distally, 2 cm of fibula flap was inserted into the host femur metaphysis. **(F)** Radiograph 5 months later, showing a small amount of callus formation and remodeling at the proximal and distal allograft–host junctions. **(G)** Radiograph after 11 months before progression to full weight-bearing. *(Fig. 4.10D: Courtesy of Dr. David W. Chang, Department for Plastic Surgery, MD Anderson Cancer Center, Houston, TX.)*

Access the complete references list online at **http://www.expertconsult.com**

1. Weitz J, Antonescu CR, Brennan MF. Localized extremity soft tissue sarcoma: improved knowledge with unchanged survival over time. *J Clin Oncol.* 2003;21(14):2719–2725. *This comprehensive single institution overview analyzes the risk factors of soft-tissue sarcoma treatment in 1261 patients.*

6. Enzinger FM, Weiss SW. *Soft Tissue Tumors.* 3rd ed. St. Louis: Mosby; 1995. *This comprehensive textbook still provides the basics of tumor biology and describes the vast majority of the soft-tissue tumors in great detail.*

12. Grimer RJ, Taminiau AM, Cannon SR. Surgical outcomes in osteosarcoma. *J Bone Joint Surg Br.* 2002;84(3):395–400. *This paper describes the outcomes of 202 patients treated in 3 different tumor centers of the European Osteosarcoma Intergroup. A very detailed paper that provides a comprehensive view of current osteosarcoma prognosis.*

13. Fong Y, Coit DG, Woodruff JM, Brennan MF. Lymph node metastasis from soft tissue sarcoma in adults. Analysis of data from a prospective database of 1772 sarcoma patients. *Ann Surg.* 1993;217(1):72–77. *This paper examines the natural history of lymph node metastasis in sarcomas and the utility of therapeutic lymphadenectomy in various tumor types. The data is based on a prospective sarcoma database including 1772 patients.*

22. Abraham JA, Baldini EH, Butrynski JE. Management of adult soft-tissue sarcoma of the extremities and trunk. *Expert Rev Anticancer Ther.* 2010;10(2):233–248. *This very recent paper summarizes the current treatment strategy in soft-tissue sarcomas seen from a single institution viewpoint but with a current and extensive reference list. It is more therapeutically oriented and serves well as an addendum and update to reference 3 above.*

5

Reconstructive surgery: Lower extremity coverage

Joon Pio Hong

SYNOPSIS

- Reconstructive surgery for the lower extremity has evolved from staged approach to proving best solutions for functional and cosmetic outcome.
- This chapter covers from the classical approach to the gradual change towards the principle that advocates a one-stage elevator approach.
- Special considerations are required to overcome the complexities of lower extremity reconstruction, such as diabetes and chronic infection.
- Finally, introduction of perforator flaps, the use of multiple flaps by combination, and supermicrosurgery will help you design and widen the reconstructive choices for the lower extremity.

 Access the Historical Perspective section online at
http://www.expertconsult.com

Introduction

Lower extremity reconstruction following severe trauma, cancer ablation, and chronic infections remains challenging. The involvement of multiple structures from bone, muscle, vessel, nerve, to skin makes it difficult to achieve the goals of lower extremity reconstruction where restoration of limb function, coverage for vital structures, and satisfactory appearance is achieved.

In the recent years, the management of the lower extremity has evolved with numerous new techniques and innovations and thus extremities are salvaged that would have been amputated in the past. Introduction of vascularized bone grafting, Ilizarov lengthening, bone matrix, and growth factors to manage the bone defects along with new ideas for coverage like perforator flaps, propeller flaps, and negative pressure therapy as well as increased knowledge for anatomy have led to successful management of lower extremity soft tissue and bone defects. If the extremity cannot be salvaged, the next goal would be to maintain maximal functional length with good soft-tissue coverage on the stump to bear the prosthesis for functional gait.

Extremity salvage is a long and complex process for the medical professionals as well as patients. Patients and family members must be educated and included in the decision-making process and made aware of the expected prognosis. Patient's motivation and compliance along with family's support will be critical during physical and psychological recovery.

Although early amputation and prosthetic treatment was thought to offer the potential for faster recovery and lower cost, recent reports have provided different views. A multi-center, prospective, observational study to determine the functional outcome of 569 patients with severe leg injuries resulting in reconstruction or amputation has provided information based on Sickness Impact Profile, a measure of self-reported health status.[1] Although reconstruction may be faced with more challenging processes, the Lower Extremity Assessment Project (LEAP) showed no significant difference in outcome at 2 years. Costs following amputation and salvage were also derived from data in a study that emerged from LEAP concluding that amputation is more expensive than salvage and amputation yields fewer quality-adjusted life-years than salvage.[2] Other reports have shown similar findings where projected lifetime healthcare costs for amputation may be as high as three times.[3,4]

Treatment of salvage evolves as with the coverage strategy. But still this process can be long and complicated. Despite that normal function and appearance can be difficult to achieve, it may be warranted to support successful reconstruction leading to successful salvage of the extremity.

Principles

The primary goal of surgical reconstruction of the lower extremity wound is to restore or maintain function. Function is addressed through a well-vascularized extremity, a skeletal structure able to support gait and weight-bearing, and an innervated plantar surface to provide protective sensation. Without proper function, the value of reconstruction will be reduced, which significantly increases emotional and financial burden to the patient.

An evaluation of the patient as a whole allows proper decisions to be made with regard to systemic conditions, socioeconomic status, and rehabilitative potential. Extremity injuries are best approached by teams of surgeons with knowledge of skeletal, vascular, neurological, and soft-tissue anatomy. Although evaluations such as the Mangled Extremity Severity Score (MESS), the Predictive Salvage Index, and the Limb Salvage Index can assist the team in making a decision for amputation, they must not be the sole criteria and the decision to amputate must be individualized for each patient.[19,25–28]

The value of autologous tissue

Whether acute or chronic, evaluation of lower extremity wounds and the eligibility for soft-tissue reconstruction begins with vascular status evaluation. If clinical and diagnostic examination reveals inadequate perfusion and the value of reconstruction is minimal, amputation should be individually decided. An amputated or avulsed tissue should never be disregarded, especially in acute traumas, unless severely contaminated or lacks vascular structure. Nothing can mimic the superiority of an autologous tissue, and all tissues from amputated parts should be considered as potential donor tissues for reconstruction. The skin harvested from the degloved or amputated part can be utilized as biologic dressings to permanent skin grafts (Fig. 5.1A–E).[29] The leg length can be preserved using soft tissue distal form the zone of injury as fillet pedicled or free flaps.[30–33] Amputated bones can be banked or used as a flap to reconstruct the leg.[34,35]

The reconstructive elevator

Once the wound is evaluated to have good vascular supply, stable skeletal structures, and a relatively clean wound, soft-tissue coverage is then considered. The concept of a reconstructive ladder was proposed to achieve wounds with adequate closure using a stepladder approach from simple to complex procedures (Fig. 5.2A). Although still valued and widely taught, the reconstructive ladder comes from the concept of the wound-closure ladder that dates back beyond the era of modern reconstructive surgery.[36] In the era of modern reconstructive surgery, one must consider not only adequate closures but also form and function. A skin graft after mastectomy can still provide coverage, but a pedicled TRAM (transverse rectus abdominis muscle) flap will provide superior results in addition to coverage. Now with the introduction of DIEP (Deep Inferior Epigastric Perforator) flaps the reconstructive ladder approach seems to show more flaws. Other techniques including tissue expansion, skin stretching, and vacuum-assisted closure have made new changes in approaching reconstructive options. A simpler reconstructive option may not necessarily produce optimal results. This is especially true for lower extremity coverage, where consequences of inadequate coverage will lead to complications such as additional soft-tissue loss, osteomyelitis, functional loss, increased medical cost, and even amputation. Thus to provide optimal form and function, we jump up and down the rungs of the ladder. The reconstructive elevator requires creative thoughts and consideration of multiple variables to achieve the best form and function rather than a sequential climb up the ladder (Fig. 5.2B). This paradigm of thought does not eliminate the concept of the reconstructive ladder but replaces it with a ladder of wound closure that makes its mark in the field where a variety of advanced reconstructive procedures and techniques is not readily available. Based on the reconstructive elevator, the method of reconstruction should be chosen based on procedures that result in optimal function as well as appearance.

Skin grafts and substitutes

Autologous skin grafts are used in a variety of clinical situations. They can be full or partial thickness and require a recipient bed that is well vascularized and free of bacterial contamination. The split-thickness grafts are usually used as the first line of treatment where wounds cannot be closed primarily or undue tension is suspected. In the extremity with complex wounds, bone exposure and/or avascular beds, infected wounds, and wounds with dead space and poorly coagulated beds, skin grafts should be avoided. Autologous cultured keratinocytes can be used where split-thickness donor sites are limited. However, the use of cultured epithelial autograft has been hampered by reports that show it to be more susceptible to bacterial contamination, have a variable take rate, and be costly.[37]

A skin substitute is defined as a naturally occurring or synthetic bioengineered product that is used to replace the skin in a temporary, semipermanent, or permanent fashion.[38] Temporary epidermal replacements may be beneficial in superficial to mid-dermal depth wounds. In deeper wounds, dermal replacements are of primary importance. Bioengineered products for superficial wounds are porcine products such as EZ Derm and Mediskin (Brennen Medical, LLC, Saint Paul, Minnesota), which help to close the wound, decrease pain, and improve the rate of healing.[38] Biobrane (UDL Laboratories Inc., Rockford, Illinois) is a bilaminate skin substitute that is used temporarily. The outer layer is formed with a thin silicone layer with pores that allow removal of exudates and penetration of antibiotics. The inner layer is composed of a 3D nylon filament weave impregnated with type I collagen to adhere to the wound. Bioengineered products that are used for deep wounds are allograft, Alloderm (Life Cell Corporation, Woodlands, Texas), Integra (Integra Life Sciences, Plainsboro, New Jersey), and Apligraf (Organogenesis Inc., Canton, Massachusetts). The gold standard for temporary skin coverage is cadaver skin or allograft. Allograft is used to cover extensive partial- and full-thickness wounds. It prevents tissue desiccation; decreases pain and insensible loss of water, electrolytes, and protein; suppresses the proliferation of bacteria; and decreases the hypermetabolic component of thermal injuries.[39,40] Alloderm is an acellular dermal matrix engineered from banked human cadaver skin. It can also provide single stage reconstruction when used with a split-thickness skin graft.[41] Alloderm is known to improve functional and cosmetic results in deep burn wounds (Fig. 5.3).[42] Integra is an acellular collagen matrix composed of type I bovine collagen cross-linked with chondroitin-6-sulfate and covered by

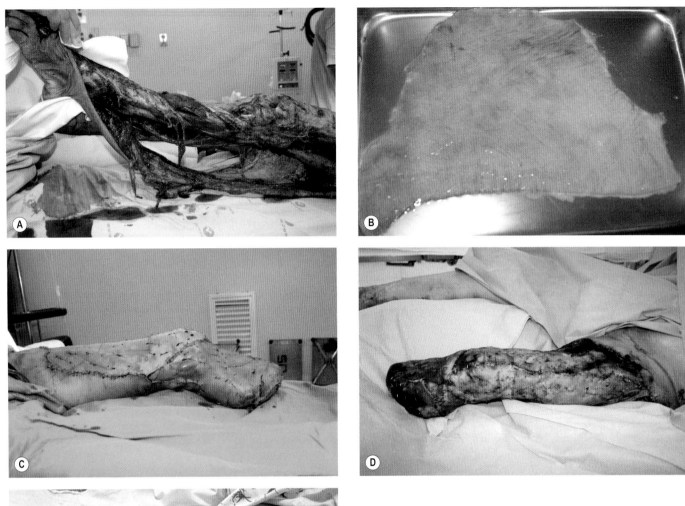

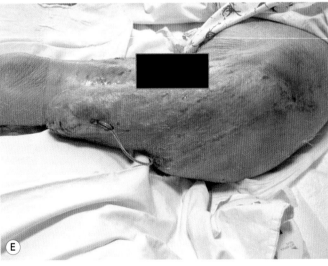

Fig. 5.1 (A) This 67-year-old patient was involved in a pedestrian traffic accident, which left her with ≈90% degloving injury of the entire left leg. **(B,C)** The injury involved major artery and nerve defects making salvage impossible and resulting in below knee amputation. The skin was harvested and defatted from the degloved tissues and grafted in hope for primary take as well as biologic dressings. **(D,E)** Only about 15% of the initial graft was taken, but healthy granulation was noted underneath the biologic dressing and made a favorable bed for secondary graft procedure.

a thin silicone layer that serves as an epidermis.[43] It is readily available, does not require a donor site, coverts open to closed wounds, and decreases metabolic demand on the patient. However, Integra must be used on clean wounds and requires a two-stage procedure later for the graft. Simultaneous use with negative wound pressure therapy may accelerate the vascularization. Apligraf is a bilaminate human epidermal and dermal analogue that can act as a permanent skin substitute. The epidermal layer is formed by human keratinocytes with a well-differentiated stratum corneum. The dermal layer is formed with bovine type I collagen lattice impregnated with human fibroblasts from neonatal foreskin. Apligraf is not antigenic, and the dermal layer incorporates into the wound bed. Apligraf has been shown to significantly decrease the time of venous ulcer healing compared to compression.[44]

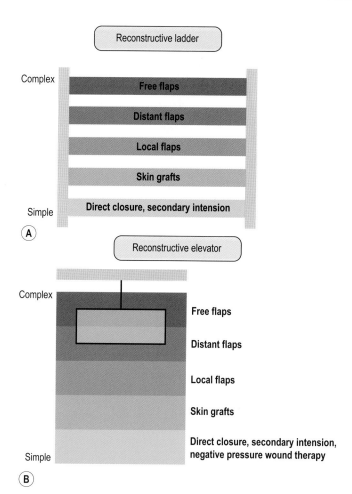

Reconstructive ladder (A)

Complex
- Free flaps
- Distant flaps
- Local flaps
- Skin grafts

Simple
- Direct closure, secondary intension

Reconstructive elevator (B)

Complex
- Free flaps
- Distant flaps
- Local flaps
- Skin grafts

Simple
- Direct closure, secondary intension, negative pressure wound therapy

Fig. 5.2 The reconstructive elevator requires creative thoughts and considerations of multiple variables to achieve the best form and function rather than a sequential climb up the ladder. This paradigm of thought does not eliminate the concept of a reconstructive ladder, but replaces it as a ladder of wound closure and makes its mark in the field where variety of advanced reconstructive procedures and techniques are not readily available. Based on the reconstructive elevator, method of reconstruction should be chosen based on procedures that result in optimal function as well as appearance.

Approach by location (local flaps)

Thigh

The thigh can be divided into 3 parts: proximal thigh, midthigh, and distal thigh (supracondylar knee). The proximal thigh wounds can result from various causes such as complications from hip fractures, infected bypass vascular grafts, after tumor resection, and trauma. The medial portion of the proximal thigh can be especially challenging due to location of vital structures and the likely formation of dead space. Local lower extremity muscle or myocutaneous flap options include using the flaps based from the lateral circumflex femoral artery such as tensor fascia lata, vastus lateralis, and rectus femoris flaps. Vertical rectus abdominis muscle or myocutaneous flap using the deep inferior epigastric artery can allow stable coverage of the proximal thigh. The gracilis muscle or myocutaneous flap based on the medial femoral circumflex artery may lack muscle bulk but is a good option when the dead space is not extensive. With the increased knowledge of perforator and perforator-based flaps, basically

any perforator can be chosen as a source of vascular supply to the skin flap and be rotated to cover a defect. This is known as the propeller flap.[45-47] When the use of local flaps is not feasible due to the complexity of the wound, free tissue transfer is indicated.

The midthigh wound, due to the anatomic character where femur is surrounded by a thick layer of soft tissue, rarely requires reconstruction using free tissue transfer and often is sufficiently reconstructed by skin graft or local flap. Local muscle or musculocutaneous flaps based on the lateral or medial femoral circumflex artery can be used when available. Also, any perforator can be chosen as a source of vascular supply to the skin flap and rotated to cover a defect. However, if the patient has undergone massive resection or has special considerations such as postoperative radiation therapy, it may warrant free tissue coverage.

The wounds of the distal thigh (supracondylar knee) can be very difficult due to the limit of rotation from previously described local muscle or musculocutaneous flaps from the thigh. Pedicled medial gastrocnemius muscle or musculocutaneous flap from the lower leg can be extended to cover this region. However, extensive or complex defects may require free tissue transfer or coverage using a perforator-based rotation (propeller) skin flap (Fig. 5.4).

Lower leg

The traditional planning for reconstruction of the lower extremity has been approached according to the location of the defect. Divided into thirds: gastrocnemius muscle flap for proximal third, soleus muscle flap for middle third, and free

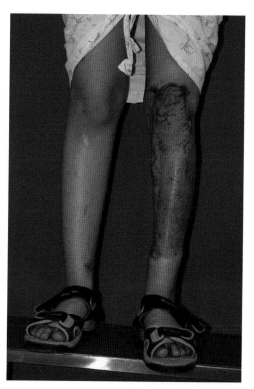

Fig. 5.3 A 10-year-old patient was seen 3 years after reconstruction of one-stage dermal allograft, an acellular dermal matrix engineered from banked human cadaver skin, and split-thickness skin graft. The patient is seen to have good elasticity and acceptable cosmetic results.

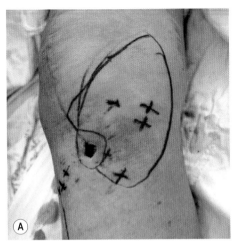
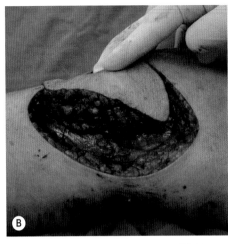
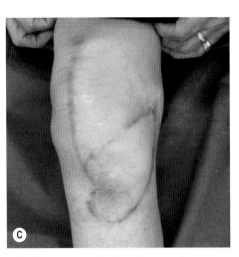

Fig. 5.4 **(A)** A 70-year-old patient is noted with chronic drainage after failed total knee replacement. **(B)** After complete debridement, a perforator-based flap was elevated and advanced using a perforator (dissected until just beneath the fascia) with visible pulse. **(C)** Long-term follow-up shows no recurrence of any infections, allowing her to undergo total knee replacement.

flap transfer for the distal third of the leg. Like the reconstructive ladder concept, this traditional approach can be useful, but the surgeon must individualize each wound and choose the initial procedure that can yield the best chance of success and avoid morbidity.

Microvascular free tissue transfer

One must choose a proper surgical plan to achieve optimal function and cosmesis. Flaps are selected based on accessibility of local tissue and donor morbidity. Frequently, lower extremity trauma due to high-energy impact results in extensive and complex wounds. Workhorse for soft-tissue coverage includes muscle or musculocutaneous flaps such as latissimus dorsi, rectus abdominis, and gracilis. The perforator flap where a skin flap is based on a single or multiple perforators, such as the anterolateral thigh flap or thoracodorsal artery perforator flap, can be added to the list.

Whichever flap you select, the guideline for lower extremity reconstruction using free flaps remains the same: anastomose the vessel outside the zone of injury, make end-to-side arterial anastomosis and end-to-side or end-to-end venous anastomosis, and reconstruct the soft tissues first and then restore the skeletal support.[48]

Treatment approach

Preoperative evaluation

The initial evaluation of the lower extremity wound involves visual and manual examination. An examination on the location, size, depth, and character of the wound is made. Neurological evaluation as well as vascular and skeletal evaluation is made to develop a plan for reconstruction. Also, presence of comorbidities including smoking, diabetes, obesity, and peripheral vascular disease should be accounted for. The initial evaluation enables assessment of the overall function and consideration of the possible outcome. One must not make the mistake of addressing the wound locally but rather approach the patient as a whole and take into consideration

socioeconomic status, rehabilitative potential, and patient's motivation and compliance.

After the decision is made to reconstruct the lower extremity, the first preoperative evaluation should start with vascular status. Physical examination of palpable pulse, color, capillary refill, and turgor of the extremity allows assessment of the initial status, and Doppler examination can provide additional information.[49] The use of preoperative arteriography for lower extremity reconstruction is considered when physical/Doppler exam reveals inconclusive vascular status or chronic vascular disease is suspected (Fig. 5.5). The use of computed tomography angiography may obtain vascular information of the recipient region without the risk of complications from arterial puncture of the groin and can also provide vascular information of the donor flap facilitating the planning and the

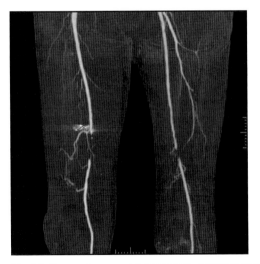

Fig. 5.5 Preoperative computed tomographic angiogram revealing collateral flows on bilateral femoral arteries for a patient with diabetes and poor pedal pulses. The use of computed tomography angiography may obtain vascular information of the recipient region without the risk of complications. The preoperative is selectively recommended in patients who have loss of one or more peripheral pulses, a neurological deficit secondary to the injury, or a compound fracture of the extremity that has undergone reduction and either external or internal fixation.

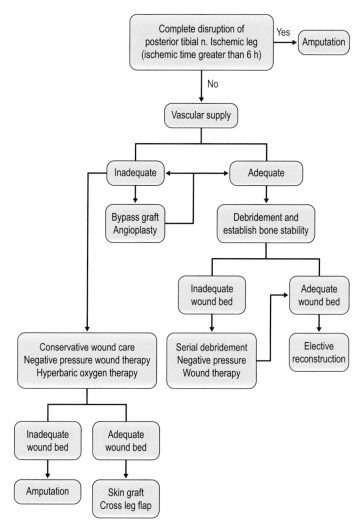

Fig. 5.6 Algorithm of approach for soft-tissue reconstruction of the lower extremity.

foot trauma, and anticipated protracted course to obtain soft-tissue coverage and tibial reconstruction.

In these cases where limb salvage is not possible, an attempt should be made to salvage as much limb length as possible. Every effort should be made to save the functional knee joint as below-knee amputation results in far superior ambulatory outcome and up to 2–3 times more full mobility compared to above knee amputation.[58] The energy consumption is far less for below-knee amputation, and this allows these patients to walk significant daily distances, thus maintaining good quality of life.[59] Though the ideal stump length below the knee is greater than 6 cm, any length of tibia should be preserved.[60] The stump may be closed primarily if adequate soft tissue exists, and where local tissue is inadequate then microsurgery enables preservation of the maximum length of the stump. If the tissue distal to the amputation is usable, a fillet flap can be performed. Other flaps, such as muscle, musculocutaneous, fasciocutaneous, and perforator, can be used for microsurgical reconstruction and achieve the same goal as well. Muscle flaps may have a tendency to heal slowly and to shrink due to muscle atrophy while skin flaps may provide better contours and sensibility.[61]

Debridement

Bony stability is first established using external or internal fixation devices. An external device is usually preferred if there is significant bone loss or bone revascularization and may facilitate coverage procedure. Debridement must cover devitalized soft tissue and bone and be performed until fresh bleeding is noted. Multiple stages of debridement may be needed to achieve adequate wound bed prior to soft-tissue coverage.

The vacuum-assisted closure can be used to optimize the wound bed and minimize dressing changes until definitive reconstruction. It must be used with caution and in conjunction with serial debridement. It does not replace surgical debridement and should not be used in heavily contaminated wounds with necrotic tissues. If a lower extremity wound is clean, bony stability is present, and no vital structures are exposed, application may be indicated.[54] This device facilitates dressing of the wound and often promotes healing.

Timing of reconstruction

Regardless of the degree of contamination and extent of injury when indicated for salvage, there is no need to delay definitive coverage provided that the general condition of the patient and the status of the wound are appropriate. General consensus favors early aggressive wound debridement and soft-issue coverage. Byrd *et al.* described acute, subacute, and chronic phases of an open tibial fracture.[62] Ideally, the wound is covered in the first 5–6 days after injury at the acute phase of the wound. In severe Gustilo type IIIB and type IIIC injuries, free muscle transplantation obtained the best results. At 1–6 weeks the wound enters the subacute phase where wounds have a higher tendency for infections and flap failures. Between 4 and 6 weeks, the wound enters the chronic phase and clear demarcation between viable and non-viable bone becomes apparent. Godina further demonstrated that radical debridement and coverage within 72 h results in the best outcome where only 0.75% of flaps fail, 1.5% are infected, and 6.8

surgical procedure.[50–52] In association with prior injuries to the lower extremity, the routine preoperative use of angiogram is controversial.[24,49,50,53–55] It is selectively recommended in patients who have loss of one or more peripheral pulses, a neurological deficit secondary to the injury, or a compound fracture of the extremity that has undergone reduction and either external or internal fixation.[54]

Nerve injuries that are irreversible may require special considerations. Peroneal nerve injury results in foot drop and loss of sensation of the dorsum of the foot. Thus lifelong splinting or tendon transfers may be required. Complete loss of tibial nerve function results in loss of plantar flexion and is an absolute contraindication for reconstruction.[56] The loss of plantar sensation can be devastating and may hinder the need for reconstruction but is not an absolute contraindication.[57] An algorithm of approach is outlined in Fig. 5.6.

Primary limb amputation

A study by Lange describes absolute and relative indications for primary amputation of limbs with open tibial fractures.[56] Absolute indications include anatomically complete disruption of the posterior tibial nerve in adults and crush injuries with warm ischemia time greater than 6 h. Relative indications include serious associated polytrauma, severe ipsilateral

months are needed for union of the bone.[11] The failure rate compares remarkably well to that of 12% when reconstructed from day 3 to 3 months and 9.5% when reconstructed after 3 months of injury. Yaremchuk *et al.* recommended early coverage between days 7 and 14 after several debridements to allow better identification of zone of injury.[63] The common idea behind early intervention is that it minimizes the risk for increasing bacterial colonization and inflammation leading to complications. Acute coverage by day 5–7 is generally accepted as having a good prognosis in terms of decreased risk of infection, flap survival, and fracture healing.[11,24,62,63] If the patient condition does not allow prolonged surgical procedures, then the wound should be debrided as early as possible and a clean and well-vascularized recipient bed maintained until conditions allow definitive reconstruction.[64]

Selection of recipient vessel

Many lower extremity wounds resulting from trauma are high-energy injuries with a substantial "zone of injury". This thrombogenic zone is known to extend beyond what is macroscopically evident, and failure to recognize the true extent of this zone is cited as a leading cause of microsurgical anastomotic failure. Within the zone, perivascular changes such as increased friability of vessels and increased perivascular scar tissue may lead to difficult dissection of recipient vessels and higher incidence of thrombosis after anastomosis.[65] The extent of this is very difficult to realize clinically. Thus Isenberg and Sherman demonstrated that clinical presentation of the recipient vessel (vessel wall pliability and the quality of blood from the transected end of the vessel) is more important than the distance from the wound.[66] Park *et al.* also concluded that site of injury and vascular status of the lower extremity are the most important factors in choosing a recipient vessel.[67] This was further supported by successful anastomosis of perforator to perforator adjacent to or within the zone of injury.[68] Based on these findings, one of the most important factors in selecting the recipient vessel may be the vascular quality itself.

Special considerations

Osteomyelitis

Osteomyelitis often follows severe open leg fractures with massive contamination or devascularized soft tissue and bone. Inadequate debridement or delayed coverage of the wound increases the chance for osteomyelitis, and early debridement remains the key to prevention.[69] Osteomyelitis should be seen as a spectrum of disease and should be individualized and managed accordingly. Factors known to be of prognostic significance include the duration of infection, the extent of bony involvement, the presence of associated fracture or nonunion, and overall immune status of the patient.[70] The wound is composed of exposed bone, infected bone, devitalized bone, and scarred tissue surrounding the bone. These components have diminished vascular supply making antibiotics difficult to reach. Thus to achieve the goal of infection control and the restoration of function, treatment principles for chronic osteomyelitis are debridement including the complete resection of involved bone, flap coverage with vascularized tissue, and a brief course of antibiotic treatment (Fig. 5.7). Local methods of antibiotic delivery can be used when complete debridement of bone is not possible. Although there has been controversy over selecting the type of flap for coverage, muscle flaps, rather than fasciocutaneous flaps, have been shown experimentally to have increased blood flow and antibiotics delivery, increased oxygen tension, increased phagocytic activity, and decreased bacterial counts.[71–73] Clinically, complete debridement and obliteration of dead space are the most important steps in treating osteomyelitis and the type of flaps seems less crucial.[74,75] Bone defects can be managed with vascularized bone flap, secondary bone grafting, bone distraction lengthening, or a combination of these techniques.

Not all chronic osteomyelitis can be salvaged. As with the indication for amputation, legs with nerves too damaged after osteomyelitis should not be salvaged. The general and

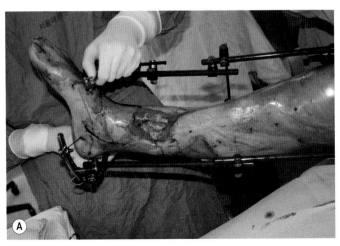
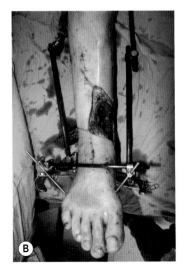
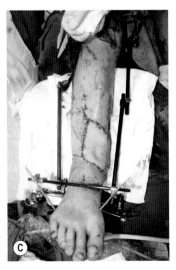

Fig. 5.7 (A) A patient with chronic osteomyelitis is noted with soft-tissue defect. **(B)** Complete debridement including resection of the involved bone was performed. **(C)** Flap coverage with well-vascularized anterolateral thigh flap combined with vastus lateralis muscle tissue was used with 6 weeks of antibiotic treatment.

socioeconomic condition of the patient should also be considered, and they should be offered the option of amputation and early rehabilitation.

Diabetes

Patients with diabetes provide additional concerns ranging from chronic renal failure, nutrition, to blood sugar control. These multiple issues are best approached by a multidisciplinary team.[76–79] Patients will frequently have chronic bacterial colonization, osteomyelitis, complex wounds, bone deformity, local wound ischemia, and vascular disease. The etiology behind these complicated wounds is from macrovascular angiopathy, bony deformities leading to pressure points, neuropathy, and poor metabolic control. When patients with diabetes are required to undergo a reconstructive procedure of the extremity, vascular status must be evaluated to ensure success.[80,81] Any vascular problems must be addressed first and corrected. If not correctable, the surgeon may be faced with a high risk of failure. One must consider the probability of successful reconstruction based on eliminating the underlying problems of the diabetic wound and also take into account long-term ambulation after reconstruction. In a retrospective study by Hong, only 71 patients out of 216 were deemed functionally salvageable using a microsurgical approach and a successful outcome was reported for 66 patients (Figs. 5.8 & 5.9).[80] Large and composite diabetic wounds must be aggressively debrided, including the necrotic bone, and covered with well-vascularized tissue.

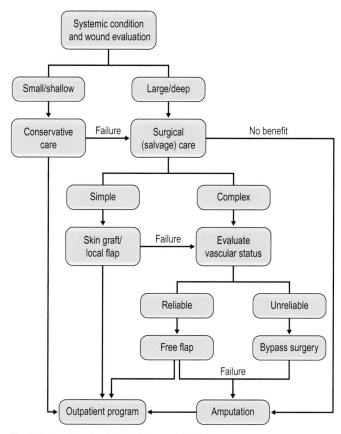

Fig. 5.8 Algorithm for diabetic foot reconstruction.

Coverage after tumor ablation

As with any reconstructive procedure, the aim of reconstruction after tumor ablation is to maintain quality of life by preserving function and achieving acceptable appearance. In addition, coverage must be able to withstand adjuvant treatment with radiation therapy and/or chemotherapy and play a role in achieving long-term local control of the disease. Surgeons should have close cooperation with the oncologists and must acquire adequate knowledge of tumor characteristics, behavior, and adjuvant treatment in order to plan and choose the type of reconstructive procedure. Knowing that reconstruction is feasible allows the oncologic surgeon to achieve a comfortable and satisfactory excision margin and may lead to a better outcome. Skin grafts are always an option especially for very extensive defects where flap coverage is not available. But for wounds scheduled for postoperative radiation therapy or located over joints and high friction regions, skin grafts should be avoided and reconstruction should be with a durable flap.[82] Special consideration should be given to preoperative radiation therapy where skin would become fibrotic and ischemic around the cancer and thus will not allow local coverage. Regarding adjuvant chemotherapy, free flap procedures will not interfere with chemotherapy nor will chemotherapy have an impact on free flap survival.[83,84] Overall success rate was shown to be 96.6% in a series of 59 free flaps in 57 patients undergoing lower extremity reconstruction after tumor ablation, with 12% major and 7% minor complications.[83] Various flaps such as omentum, muscle with skin graft, musculocutaneous, and perforator can be used for reconstruction depending on location, size, depth, adjuvant therapy, function, and cosmetic appearance (Fig. 5.10).

Exposed prosthesis

The traditional method to manage exposed hardware includes irrigation, debridement, antibiotics, and likely removal of hardware. However, several factors should be taken into account to manage exposed hardware before considering removal that may set back the treatment plan. Factors such as location of the hardware, infection (type of bacteria and duration of infection), duration of exposure of hardware, and hardware loosening should be considered as important prognostic factors for successful management of exposed hardware.[85] In the retrospective review by Viol *et al.* they concluded that if hardware is clinically stable, time of exposure is less than 2 weeks, infection is controlled, and the location of the hardware is for bony consolidation, then there is an increase in the likelihood that hardware can be salvaged using surgical soft-tissue coverage (Fig. 5.11).[85]

Exposed vascular grafts present life and limb threatening complications. They should be managed with early debridement and muscle flap coverage to salvage the graft. Synthetic grafts can be susceptible to bacterial colonization, and consideration should be given to replacement with an autologous graft. Local muscle flaps such as gracilis, sartorius, and tensor fascia lata are very useful in providing adequate coverage for exposed groin synthetic vascular prosthesis. If the defect is extensive, then an inferiorly based vertical rectus abdominis musculocutaneous flap can be considered. The management of exposed vascular grafts requires close cooperation with the

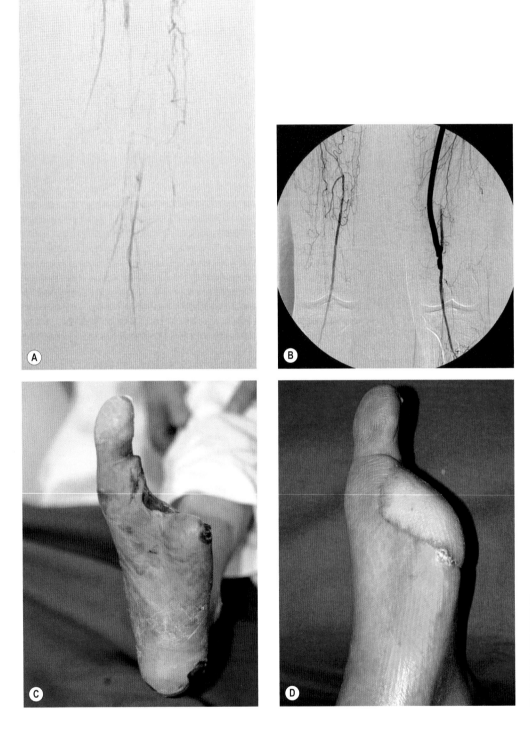

Fig. 5.9 A diabetic patient after partial amputation of the foot was noted with poorly healing stump. **(A,B)** The angiogram revealed poor flow to the lower leg, and femoral popliteal bypass was performed. **(C,D)** With improved circulation, the patient underwent reconstruction with anterolateral thigh perforator flap and the foot was salvaged.

vascular surgeon, aggressive debridement, and coverage with a well-vascularized tissue.

Soft tissue expansion

The use of tissue expansion in the lower extremity has not been as successful as in other areas of the body, such as the breast and scalp. The potential advantages of using expanded skin in the lower extremity include improved contours, coverage with like tissue, and improved aesthetic result. However,

use in the lower extremity has been associated with a high rate of infection and extrusion of the implant. Wound infection and dehiscence are the most common complications, but seroma, implant displacement, neurapraxia, hematoma, and contour defects can also occur. The technique can be reserved for unstable soft tissues or scars of moderate size. The implant is placed in a suprafascial position in the subcutaneous pocket of the lower extremity, and application on the ankle and foot region must be avoided. Transverse expansion has a lower failure rate compared to longitudinal advancement. For

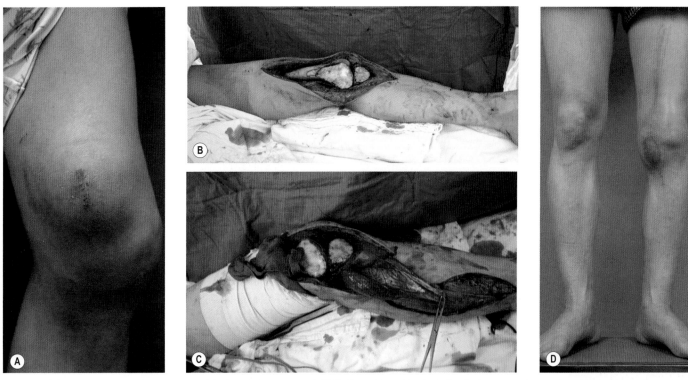

Fig. 5.10 (A) A patient with soft-tissue sarcoma of the knee region was noted. **(B,C)** After wide excision including the bone, a hemi-gastrocnemius muscle was elevated to resurface the knee joint. **(D)** Long-term results show good contour with acceptable function and appearance.

avoidance of wound dehiscence, neurapraxia, and fat necrosis, expansion should proceed slowly, stopping before the onset of pain or, if it is measured, before intraexpander pressure exceeds 40 mmHg.[86] Flap prefabrication with tissue expansion may have a role in select reconstructions of the lower extremity.[87]

Postoperative care

Monitoring

During the postoperative period the patient as a whole and the flap should be closely monitored. It is especially important to monitor hemodynamic and pulmonary function as adequate hydration and oxygenation are critical to flap survival. Input and output of fluid should be monitored closely as distal perfusion is primarily affected by hypotensive episodes. This can be a problem for patients with chronic renal failure who require dialysis that often removes large volumes of fluid. Limiting range of motion may be needed for flaps covering the joints as extension or flexion may increase the tension of the pedicle. Monitoring flaps, especially free flaps, in the first 24 h is essential as the majority of thromboses occur during this time. According to Chen *et al.*, up to 85% of the compromised flaps can be salvaged when the first sign of vascular compromise is clinically noted during the first 3 days after microsurgery.[88] There is no ideal method of flap monitoring, but recent techniques such as tissue oxygen measurement, implantable Doppler device, laser Doppler flowmetry, and fluorescent dye injections may assist the judgment made from clinical evaluation, which remains the golden standard of monitoring. Emergent re-exploration should be performed once pedicle compromise is noted.

Management of flap complications

Although there are no clinical reviews that conclusively show any agents that increase flap survival rate, about 96% of the 106 microsurgeons surveyed use some form of prophylactic antithrombotic treatment, such as heparin, dextran, and alone or in combination with other agents.[89–91] The routine use of dextran should be carefully approached due to allergic reaction and pulmonary edema, but aspirin, heparin, or low molecular weight heparin can be considered based on theory and related studies from different disciplines. Thrombolytics such as urokinase can be used when flow is not immediately reestablished after pedicle rearrangement or revision anastomosis.[91] But no agent can replace the meticulous surgical technique and early diagnosis of flap compromise.

Leeches have a role in the postoperative care of jeopardized flaps. In cases of venous congestion, by injecting a salivary component called hirudin, which inhibits platelet aggregation and coagulation cascade, leeches can decongest by extracting blood directly and by the oozing that occurs after it detaches. The use of leeches for 5–7 days can sometimes help salvage the flaps that do not resolve despite re-exploration of the venous flow.

Secondary operations

Bone grafts are usually placed 6 weeks after soft-tissue reconstruction to allow time for transferred tissue to settle in and sterilize the wound.[19] Cancellous autograft or vascularized

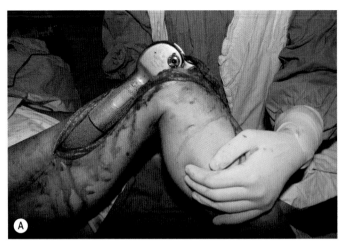

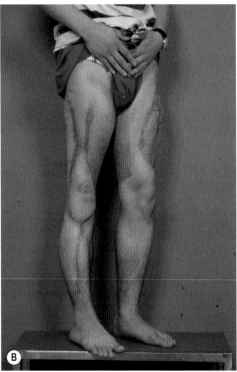

Fig. 5.11 A patient with total knee replacement, after contraction of the knee due to a traffic accident, presented with unstable skin and pending exposure of the knee implant for 1 month. **(A)** The unstable region of the skin was completely debrided and irrigated. **(B)** Upon debridement there were no apparent signs of infection. A large anterolateral thigh perforator flap including the deep fascia was taken to resurface the exposed prosthesis and showed stable recovery after 2 years.

bone transfers can be chosen depending on the length of the bone gap. In addition, the bone transfer mechanism can be an alternative to free bone transfer for bone defects longer than 6 cm.

To achieve optimal motion of tendons of the lower extremity, secondary tenolysis procedure may be needed. The risk for adhesion may increase when skin graft is performed over granulated tissue directly above the tendons and may warrant flap coverage.

The final stage to consider after reasonable functional recovery is appearance of the extremity. Patients after recovery frequently show scars, depression, bulky flaps, and donor site morbidities. Although complete restoration is nearly

impossible, a reasonable endpoint should be set and efforts to minimize scars and achieve good contours should be made. Debulking by surgical excision or liposuction can improve the contour of the flap, and fat grafts can be added to elevate depressed scars. Scar revision by Z-plasties or expanders can help to alleviate not only physical but psychological problems.

Muscle/musculocutaneous flaps

Tensor fascia lata

The tensor fascia lata is a small, thin, and short muscle with a long fascial extension from the iliotibial tract of the facia lata to the lateral aspect of the knee. The muscle originates at the anterior 5–8 cm of the external lip of the anterior superior iliac crest, immediately behind the satorius, and inserts to the iliotibial tract. It abducts, medially rotates, and flexes the hip, acting to tighten the fascia lata and iliotibial tract but is an expendable muscle. Its flat shape, excellent length, and reliable type I circulation pattern (dominant pedicle is the ascending branch of the lateral femoral circumflex artery and venae comitantes) make it useful in many reconstructive scenarios, both as a pedicled flap for local and regional coverage and as a free, composite unit that incorporates skin, muscle, and iliac bone. Motor innervation is from the superior gluteal nerve entering the deep surface between the gluteus medius and the gluteus maximus. Sensation is derived from T12, which innervates the upper skin territory, and the lateral femoral cutaneous nerve of the thigh (L2–3), which innervates the lower skin.

When based on the dominant pedicle, located 8–10 cm below the anterior superior iliac spine, the anterior arc of location will reach the abdominal areas, groin, and perineum while the posterior arc can reach the greater trochanter, ischium, perineum, and sacrum (Fig. 5.12).[92,93] The flap can also be advanced superiorly as a V–Y flap to cover trochanteric wounds.[94] The skin overlying the muscle and fascia lata can be harvested as a unit with the flap and can extend to within 10 cm above the knee.

The marking begins by identifying the major landmarks: the anterior superior iliac spine, lateral condyle of femur, and the pubic tubercle. A line from the anterior superior iliac spine straight down the thigh to a point 10–12 cm above the knee joint presents the anterior border of the flap, and a parallel line 12–15 cm posterior to the first line is drawn straight down the thigh, curving anteriorly as it crosses posterior to the lateral epicondylar area, to meet at the same point. The skin island can be designed within this long strip, according to the needs and distance to the recipient defect. The distal margin of the flap is entered, carrying the incision through the fascia lata and dissecting deep to the fascia lata and iliotibial tract. The pedicle is located approximately 10 cm below the anterior iliac spine along the line drawn. One must modify the flap when composite tissues are taken for reconstruction.

Rectus femoris

The rectus femoris is located superficially on the middle of the anterior thigh extending between ilium and patella. It is a central muscle of the quadriceps femoris extensor muscles

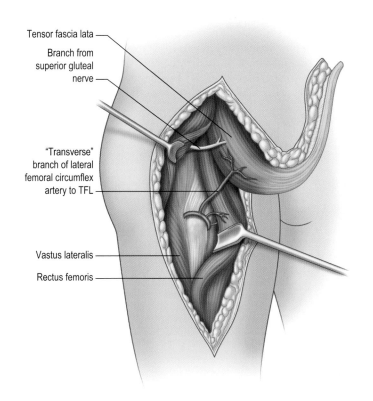

Tensor fascia lata

Branch from superior gluteal nerve

"Transverse" branch of lateral femoral circumflex artery to TFL

Vastus lateralis

Rectus femoris

Fig. 5.12 Tensor fascia lata flap elevation. When based on the dominant pedicle, located 8–10 cm below the anterior superior iliac spine, anterior arc of location will reach the abdominal areas, groin, and perineum while the posterior arc can reach the greater trochanter, ischium, perineum, and sacrum. TFL, tensor fascia lata.

group and acts to extend the leg at the knee. The muscle originates with two tendons, one from the anterior inferior iliac spine and one from the acetabulum, and inserts to the patella. It is a thigh flexor and a leg extensor that is important in stabilizing the weight-bearing knee and thus is not considered expendable. It has a type II pattern of circulation (the dominant pedicle is the descending branch of the lateral circumflex femoral artery with minor pedicles from the ascending branch of the same vessel, as well as from muscle branches of the superficial femoral artery) and can reach to cover the inferior abdomen, groin, perineum, and ischium.[95,96] Motor innervation is from the femoral nerve, and muscle branches enter adjacent to the dominant pedicle. The motor innervations and the adequate dimension of the flap allows it to be used as a functional muscle flap (Fig. 5.13).[97] In addition, the intermediate anterior femoral cutaneous nerve (L2–3) provides sensation. The skin perforators are most reliable over the midanterior two-thirds of the muscle itself in the central strip up to 12×20 cm.

A longitudinal incision is marked from 3 cm below the anterior superior iliac spine to just above the superior margin of the patella. With the anterior thigh muscle contraction, the lateral border of the vastus medialis and the medial border of the vastus lateralis are visualized creating a depression of skin. The tendon of the rectus femoris can be easily noted below the depression and above the patella. The skin island should be designed on the middle third of the thigh as the majority of the perforators are located in this region. Incision at the distal edge of the skin island, along the axis, allows the

rectus femoris muscle to be identified and separated from the vastus medialis and lateralis. The skin island is then incised circumferentially down to the fascia of the muscle. The rectus is elevated from distal to proximal and from medial to lateral so that the pedicle and nerve can be identified and protected medially along the underside of the muscle. The dominant pedicle enters the posterior medial muscle at a variable distance of 7–10 cm below the symphysis pubis and care must be given to preserve the motor branches from the femoral nerve to the adjacent vastus lateralis and tensor fascia lata. The donor area should be repaired by careful suturing together of the tendinous fascia of the vastus medialis and lateralis above the patella in an effort to preserve full knee extension.

Biceps femoris

This large, well-vascularized posterior muscle of the mid- and lateral thigh is useful for coverage of ischial pressure sores. The muscle has two heads; the long head originates on the ischial tuberosity and the short head originates on the linea aspera of the femur and both insert to the head of the fibula. The long head extends the hip, and both heads flex the leg at

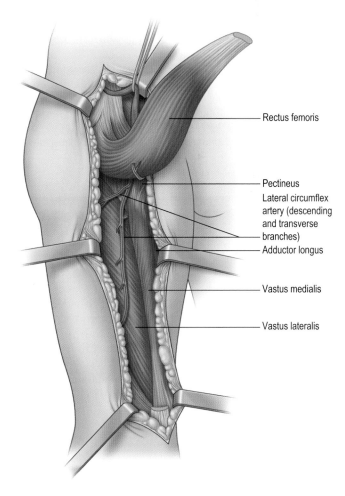

Rectus femoris

Pectineus

Lateral circumflex artery (descending and transverse branches)

Adductor longus

Vastus medialis

Vastus lateralis

Fig. 5.13 Rectus femoris muscle flap elevation. It is a type II pattern of circulation (the dominant pedicle is the descending branch of the lateral circumflex femoral artery with minor pedicles from the ascending branch of the same vessel as well as from muscle branches of the superficial femoral artery) and can reach to cover the inferior abdomen, groin, perineum, and ischium.

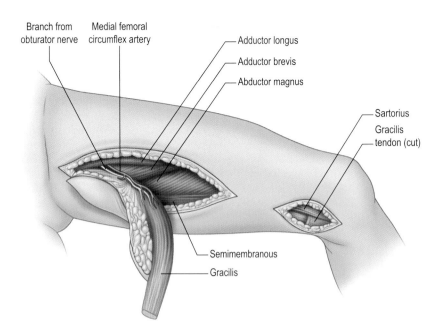

Fig. 5.14 Gracilis muscle flap elevation. It is a type II circulation pattern (the dominant pedicle is the terminal branch of the medial circumflex femoral artery and one or two minor pedicles arise as branches of the superficial femoral artery) and can reach to cover the abdomen, ischium, groin, and perineum as a muscle or musculocutaneous flap.

the knee and thus are not expendable. The pattern of circulation is type II (the long head has dominant and minor pedicles from the first and second perforating branches of the profunda femoris artery, respectively, and the short head receives the second (or third) perforating branch of the profunda and a minor source from the lateral superior geniculate artery) and can be turned over to cover the ischial regions based on the dominant pedicle.[98] The long head derives its motor innervations from the tibial division of the sciatic nerve, and the short head from the peroneal division of the sciatic nerve. The postcutaneous nerve of the thigh (S1–3) supplies the sensation.

The entire skin of the posterior thigh can be elevated and advanced in V–Y fashion as a musculocutaneous unit. The upper base of the skin flap is horizontally marked along the buttock crease and the apex just above the popliteal fossa. The relatively short pedicles make the flap unsuitable for wide rotation flaps but serve well in sliding the muscle proximally along the femur toward the pelvis. The medial thigh skin may also be left uncut, preserving skin as a rotation advancement modification of the flap.[99]

With the skin island isolated, the tendon is divided distally. The tendon is sectioned, and the dissection proceeds from the distal thigh toward the ischium, freeing the muscle on its deep aspect from the femur and from the adductor group of muscles medially until enough mobility is attained so that the defect can easily be filled. The flap should be inset and sutured with the patient in a jackknife position and the hips flexed to prevent dehiscence of the flap.

Gracilis

The gracilis is located on the medial thigh extending between the pubis and the medial knee. It is a thin, flat muscle that lies anteriorly bordered by adductor longus and sartorius and posteriorly by adductor magnus and semimembranosus muscles. It originates on the pubic symphysis and inserts onto the medial tibial condyle. The gracilis functions as a thigh adductor but is expandable from the compensation made

from abductor longus and magnus muscle. The muscle has a type II circulation pattern (the dominant pedicle is the terminal branch of the medial circumflex femoral artery and one or two minor pedicles arise as branches of the superficial femoral artery) and can reach to cover the abdomen, ischium, groin, and perineum as a muscle or musculocutaneous flap (Fig. 5.14). Motor innervation is from the anterior branch of the obturator nerve and enters the gracilis on its deep medial surface immediately superior to the entry of the dominant pedicle. The motor nerve allows gracilis to be used as a functional muscle flap for facial reanimation and upper extremity.[100] The sensory innervation is from the anterior femoral cutaneous nerve (L2–3) that provides sensation to the anterior medial thigh.[101]

When skin is harvested with the gracilis muscle, the flap is generally oriented longitudinally, centered over the proximal third of the muscle, where the majority of the musculocutaneous perforators are located. A proximal transversely oriented skin flap is optional, and the bulky fat of the medial thigh even makes this flap suitable for breast reconstruction.[102–104] The symphysis pubis and the medial condyle of the femur are major landmarks. The muscle extends the full length of the medial thigh and averages about 6 cm in width proximally and tapers to about 2–3 cm in the distal third of the muscle. Although the width may be narrow, the muscle can be fanned out to provide coverage over larger defects. With the patient in lithotomy position and slight extension of the knee will allow the gracilis to be seen and felt, and it tends to be more posterior than expected.

For muscle elevation, an incision is made 2–3 cm posterior to the line drawn connecting the symphysis pubis and medial condyle of the knee. The muscle is identified posterior to the adductor longus. If a skin flap is planned, the skin territory should be designed on the proximal part of the inner thigh. Usually the dissection is easily approached by a distal incision identifying the tendon of the gracilis posterior to the saphenous vein and the distal sartorius muscle. The tendinous insertion of semimembranous and semitendinosus muscle can be identified posterior to the gracilis. Traction on the

Figure labels:
Branch from obturator nerve
Medial femoral circumflex artery
Adductor longus
Adductor brevis
Abductor magnus
Sartorius
Gracilis tendon (cut)
Semimembranous
Gracilis

tendon will highlight the proximal outline of the muscle and allow accurate estimation of the location. This is an important step to minimize faulty elevation of the skin component as the medial thigh is mobile and makes it easy to incorrectly predict the skin position over the muscle. Dissection of the anterior and posterior skin borders then precedes proximally approximately half the length of the muscle, whereby the distal tendon is divided and the distal muscle elevated. During the elevation of the middle and distal third of the flap, one or two minor perforators from the superficial femoral artery will be identified and ligated. Retraction of the adductor longus muscle will expose the major pedicle passing over the deep adductor magnus approximately 10 cm below the pubic symphysis.

Soleus

The soleus is a very broad, large bipenniform muscle lying deep to the gastrocnemius muscle. The muscle has two muscle bellies, medial and lateral, separated by a midline intramuscular septum in the distal half. The lateral belly originates from the posterior surface of the head of the fibula and posterior surface of the body of the fibula, and the medial belly originates from the middle one-third of the medial border of the tibia. Both bellies of the soleus insert into the calcaneus bone through the Achilles tendon and contribute to the plantar flexion of the foot. The soleus is expandable taken that at least one head of the gastrocnemius is intact with function. The pattern of circulation is type II (with dominant pedicles from the popliteal, posterior tibial, and peroneal arteries and minor pedicles from the posterior tibial and peroneal arteries supplying the distal medial and lateral bellies, respectively) and can cover the middle and lower third of the leg (Fig. 5.15A). The motor nerve is derived from the posterior tibial and popliteal nerves.[105]

The arc of rotation for a proximally based soleus flap after division of minor pedicles and elevation of the distal two-thirds of the muscle can cover the middle third of the tibia. Hemisoleus flaps may improve the arc of rotation and preserve soleus function while sacrificing flap coverage area. The medial reversed hemisoleus pivots around the most superior distal minor perforator of the posterior tibial artery, approximately 7 cm above the malleolus; the lateral reversed hemisoleus has a tenuous blood supply through minor perforators from the peroneal and a shorter arc of rotation. The distal half of the muscle can be reversely transposed based on minor segment pedicles and cover the distal third of the leg.[106]

The medial border of the tibia is the landmark for medial exposure, and the fibula itself is the landmark for lateral exposure. A line can be drawn 2 cm medial to the medial edge of the tibia or laterally along the fibula. Subcutaneous neurovascular structures are identified and preserved, and the posterior compartment fascia is opened. The plane between the soleus and the gastrocnemius is usually well defined superiorly, but sharp scalpel dissection is needed to separate the tendons and maintain the gastrocnemius contributions to the Achilles tendon. For proximally based flaps, distal perforators are divided in the deep plane, and the tendon is divided distally. The dominant pedicle is usually located on the upper one-third of the muscle for both bellies of the soleus. Identification and dissection of the midline raphe allow a hemisoleus flap to be developed (Fig. 5.15B–D).

Gastrocnemius

The gastrocnemius muscle is the most superficial muscle of the posterior calf and has two heads, medial and lateral, that form the distal boundary of the popliteal space. Each head can be used as a separate muscle or musculocutaneous unit based on its own pedicle. The medial head originates from the medial condyle of the femur and the lateral from the lateral condyle of the femur, and both heads insert to the calcaneus through the Achilles tendon. It contributes to the plantar flexion of the foot, and either or both heads of the gastrocnemius are expandable if the soleus is intact. The pattern of circulation is type I (the medial muscle is supplied by the medial sural artery, and the lateral muscle is supplied by the lateral sural artery) and provides reliable coverage to the upper third of the tibia, suprapatellar thigh, and knee regions (Fig. 5.16). Both heads receive a minor source across the raphe that joins them as anastomotic vessels within the muscle substance. Motor innervation derives from branches of the tibial nerve. The sensation to the skin overlying the medial head is from the saphenous nerve and that to the lateral and distal skin overlying the lateral head is from the sural nerve.[107]

The arc of rotation of the medial head after complete elevation can cover the inferior thigh, knee, and upper third of the tibia. When the origin of the muscle is divided, an extended arc of rotation by 5–8 cm can be achieved to extend to the upper part of the knee. The lateral head can be elevated to cover the suprapatellar region, knee, and proximal third of the tibia. It can also be extended with the division of the muscle origin. Both heads can be inferiorly rotated based on the vascular anastomosis across the raphe between the two muscle heads to reach the middle third of the leg. A skin paddle can be designed, based on the perforating vessels, with the following dimension: 10×15 cm for the medial and 8×12 cm for the lateral head. But the use of a skin paddle leaves an unsightly donor scar.

A line is drawn either 2 cm medial to the medial edge of the tibia or along the posterior midleg. If the muscle alone is employed, a midline posterior incision affords excellent access to both heads. During elevation care is taken to protect the neurovascular structures, especially the more superficial saphenous and sural nerves. In the proximal third, the medial surface of the medial head is easily separated from the soleus. The dissection starts at the medial edge of the gastrocnemius muscle, and the plantaris can be easily noted below the gastrocnemius and above the soleus. The midline muscular raphe is located and, with finger dissection, the underlying soleus muscle is separated from the gastrocnemius proximally and distally. The musculotendinous raphe is then separated sharply. Distally, the thick tendinous layer is sharply dissected free from the remaining calcaneal tendon. The transaction of the origin of the muscle allows increased freedom. If a tunnel is made over the lateral proximal leg, care must be given not to violate the deep peroneal nerve.

Fasciocutaneous/perforator flap

A perforator flap is defined as a flap based on a musculocutaneous perforating vessel that is directly visualized and dissected free of surrounding muscles and an adequate pedicle length is achieved.[108] This concept may still be confusing

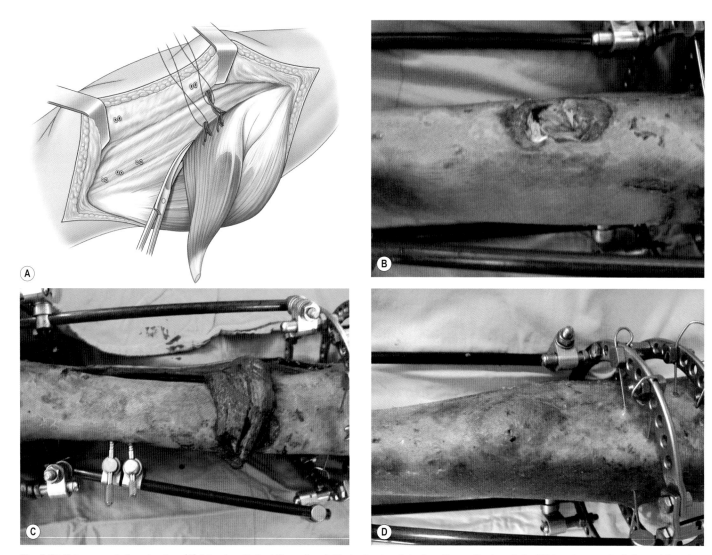

Fig. 5.15 Soleus muscle flap elevation. **(A)** It is a type II circulation pattern (with dominant pedicles from the popliteal, posterior tibial, and peroneal arteries and the minor pedicles rise from posterior tibial and peroneal arteries supplying the distal medial and lateral bellies, respectively) and can cover the middle and lower-third of the leg. **(B–D)** A patient with chronic osteomyelitis of the middle-third of the tibia is reconstructed using a hemisoleus flap.

because the same flap can be a septocutaneous flap when it is based on a vessel traveling intermuscular septum and becomes a perforator flap if the pedicle is from a direct musculocutaneous perforator. However, despite the confusion in nomenclature, this approach helps to achieve better accuracy by alleviating concerns of anatomic variations and minimizing donor site morbidity. This kind of flap that may be based on any perforator, "freestyle free flap", allows the freedom of flap selection from anywhere on the body.[108] This principle is used in local flaps as well where a flap can be rotated based on a single perforator to cover the defect as well as minimize donor site morbidity.[47] This flap can also be rotated based on the perforator to allow maximal arc of rotation and is also known as a propeller flap.[109] With the introduction of free style elevation of perforator flaps, different layers are now being used to elevate the flap. The classical fasciocutaneous flap is the elevation of flaps beneath the deep fascial layer. The subfascial elevation allows easiest dissection and clear identification of the perforator. However, elevation of the deep fascia may result in muscle herniation and suboptimal

aesthetic results. The report by Chang *et al.* showed that elevation can be made above the deep fascia on the radial forearm free flap.[110] Recent reports now show that elevation can be made safely between the layers of deep and superficial fat based on a perforator able to achieve harvesting thinner flaps for resurfacing (Fig. 5.17).[111,112] Thus the term fasciocutaneous flap can depict the flaps elevated with the deep fascia and the term skin flap or suprafacial perforator flap can be used for flaps elevated above the deep fascia. The natural evolution of skin flaps is now moving toward achieving minimal donor site morbidity. Koshima *et al.* showed that the flap and the pedicle can be taken above the deep fascia as a perforator flap allowing decreased donor site.[113,114] But anastomosis can be difficult with a vessel diameter of less than 1 mm, hence this technique is known as supermicrosurgery. Hong *et al.* have also stretched the boundaries of microsurgery by introducing the possibility of using perforators as recipient vessels and the concept of "freestyle reconstruction".[115] Since the basic approach may be similar, septocutaneous and perforator flaps will be discussed together when necessary.

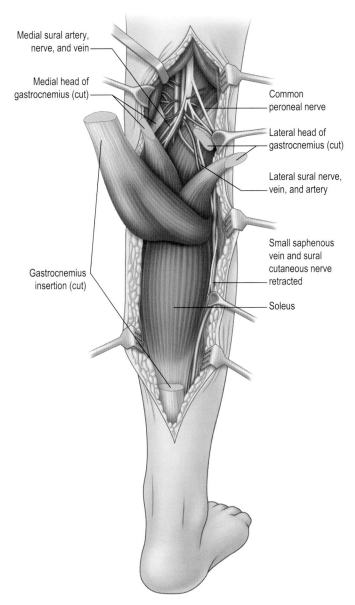

Medial sural artery, nerve, and vein

Medial head of gastrocnemius (cut)

Common peroneal nerve

Lateral head of gastrocnemius (cut)

Lateral sural nerve, vein, and artery

Small saphenous vein and sural cutaneous nerve retracted

Gastrocnemius insertion (cut)

Soleus

Fig. 5.16 Gastrocnemius flap elevation. It is a type I circulation pattern (the medial muscle is supplied by the medial sural artery, and the lateral muscle is supplied by the lateral sural artery) and provides coverage to the upper-third of the tibia, suprapatellar thigh, and knee regions.

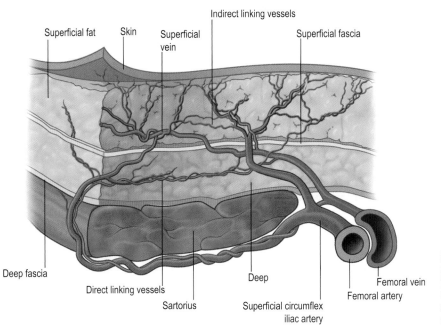

Indirect linking vessels

Superficial fat Skin Superficial vein Superficial fascia

Deep fascia

Direct linking vessels

Sartorius

Deep

Superficial circumflex iliac artery

Femoral vein

Femoral artery

Fig. 5.17 The elevation for fasciocutaneous flaps is made underneath (subfascial dissection) and including the deep fascia. The skin flap can be harvested over the deep fascia (suprafascial dissection) or between the deep and the superficial fat (superficial fascia dissection). Note the distinctive layers for elevation

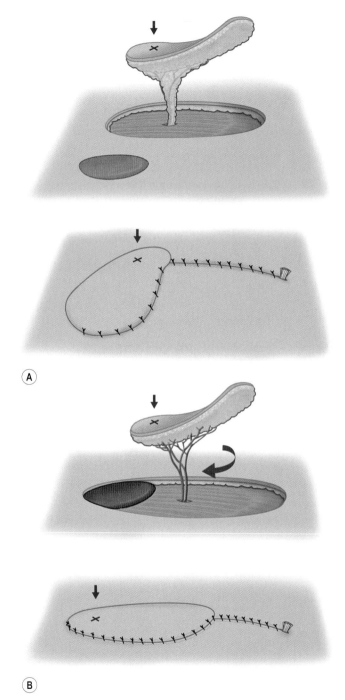

Fig. 5.18 Note the propeller flap rotated up to 180° based on the perforator.

Propeller flaps

A propeller flap can be defined as an "island flap that reaches the recipient site through an axial rotation". Every skin island flap can become a propeller flap. However, island flaps that reach the recipient site through an advancement movement and flaps that move through a rotation but are not completely islanded are excluded from this definition (Fig. 5.18).[109] When a perforator propeller flap is being elevated, the perforator is dissected free from the fascial and fat adhesions to minimize the chance of kinking. Although less rotation reduces the chance for kinking, the skin island may be safely rotated up

to 180°. In addition, although the extent of survival associated with the concept of angiosome is not clearly understood, venous charging of the flap may help to decrease the chance of congestion when the flap extends beyond two or three angiosomes.[109]

The propeller flap in the lower extremity is very useful. When the donor site is able to be closed after the rotation, it provides excellent coverage and a superb donor site. The thigh region can easily resurface moderate sized defects and close primarily. The use of the freestyle concept allows basing on any perforator around the defect (Fig. 5.19A–D).

Groin/superficial circumflex iliac perforator

The groin flap may be elevated extending between the femoral vessels and the posterior iliac spine. This flap was one of the early introduced fasciocutaneous flaps. The dominant pedicle is the superficial circumflex iliac artery, with venae comitantes and superficial circumflex iliac vein. A variation in anatomy with superior inferior epigastric artery have been reported, but Harii et al. conclude either source can supply the flap efficiently (Fig. 5.20).[116] The pedicle is very short: up to only 3 cm. Koshima defined that the superficial circumflex iliac perforator flap is different from the groin flap in that it is nourished by only a perforator of the superficial circumflex femoral system (Fig. 5.21).[117] The T12 sensory innervation is at the lateral margin of the flap away from the pedicle, precluding use as a sensate flap.

The long axis of the flap is centered over a line parallel and 3 cm inferior to the inguinal ligament with a flap width of 6–10 cm. The flap can be used as a free or pedicled flap. For pedicled flaps, the dissection should proceed from lateral to medial and distal to proximal. Elevation is begun in a plane superficial to the fascia lata and, when the sartorius muscle is visualized, the flap is elevated deep to the fascia and superficial to the muscle. The perforator flap is elevated suprafascially until a sizable perforator is located and is used either as a pedicled or free flap.

The groin flap as a septocutaneous flap may provide a large amount of skin and soft tissue and may need debulking where excess tissue is not needed. However, the perforator flap enables elevation with the thin skin above the fascia. The donor site is well tolerated and well hidden, but the pale skin and frequent hair growth of the donor site make for a poor match, particularly with head and neck reconstructions.

Medial thigh/anteromedial perforator and gracilis perforator

The medial thigh skin is supplied by musculocutaneous as well as septocutaneous perforators. The medial thigh flap is located at the midthigh, and the dominant blood supply for this fasciocutaneous flap is the anterior septocutaneous artery, and venae comitantes are from the superficial femoral artery and vein at the apex of the femoral triangle (Fig. 5.22).[118] The coverage extends to the abdomen, groin, and perineum. The saphenous vein may be elevated with the flap for improved venous drainage. The sensory innervations are from medial anterior cutaneous nerve of the thigh (L2–3). When the flap is based more anteriorly, it is termed the anteromedial thigh flap and is based on a branch of the lateral femoral circumflex artery emerging from the lateral border of the sartorius. Minor

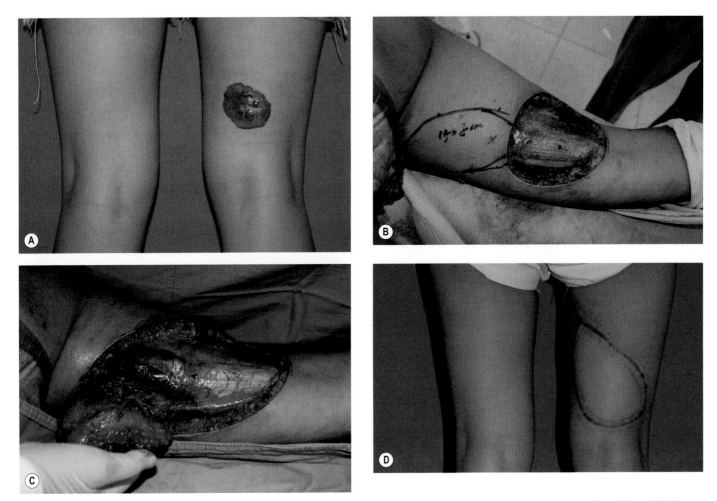

Fig. 5.19 **(A)** 45-year old patient with cancer on the thigh. **(B)** After the cancer resection, a perforator was found near the defect and enabled a free style propeller flap to be designed. **(C)** A near 180° rotation was made based on this perforator. **(D)** The patient at 2-year follow-up shows good contour and reconstruction results.

pedicles are contributed by musculocutaneous perforating vessels of the sartorius and gracilis muscles. When the flap is moved proximally to the groin, a perforator from the gracilis muscle is found originating from the profunda femoris vessel or the medial femoral circumflex vessel. All these flaps mentioned can be elevated as a perforator-based flap and named medial thigh perforator flap, anteromedial thigh perforator flap, and gracilis perforator (medial circumflex femoral artery perforator) flap, respectively.[119–122]

For the medial thigh septocutaneous flap, the dominant pedicle is typically located at the apex of the femoral triangle approximately 6–8 cm below the inguinal ligament and is bordered medially by the adductor longus and laterally by the sartorius. A proximal incision is made to locate the vessels at the apex of the femoral triangle. The remainder of the flap is then incised and elevated subfascially.

Lateral thigh/profunda femoris perforator flap

The lateral thigh flap located along the lateral aspect of the thigh between the greater trochanter and the knee can be based on the three perforating branches of the profunda femoris (Fig. 5.23).[118] The first perforator arises just below the insertion of the gluteus maximus, and flaps based on this perforator are used for proximally based flaps to reach the

trochanteric and ischial areas. The third perforator arises between the vastus lateralis and the biceps femoris muscles, midway between the greater trochanter and the lateral condyle of the femur, and the flaps based on second or third perforator are for use as microvascular transplantation because of the long pedicle. The flap is innervated from the lateral cutaneous nerve of the thigh (L2–3).

Anterolateral thigh perforator

The anterolateral thigh perforator flap is one of the most widely used perforator flaps. This flap was first reported as a fasciocutaneous flap by Baek and Song et al.[118,123] The skin can be elevated from a septocutaneous or musculocutaneous perforator. Numerous perforators are found along the region of intermuscular septum between the vastus lateralis and rectus femoris. These perforators usually drain into the descending branch of the lateral femoral circumflex artery, then proximally to the lateral circumflex artery, and then to the profunda femoris artery (Fig. 5.24). When perforators are traced to the source vessel, it allows the pedicle to have long length and thicker diameter. Innervation of the anterolateral thigh region is from the lateral femoral cutaneous nerve (L2–3). The perforator frequently dissected is usually located on the midpoint of the line drawn between the anterior

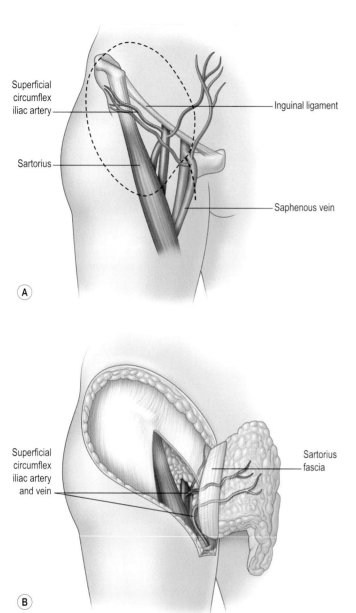

Fig. 5.20 Groin flap elevation. The dominant pedicle is the superficial circumflex iliac artery (**A**), with venae comitantes and superficial circumflex iliac vein (**B**).

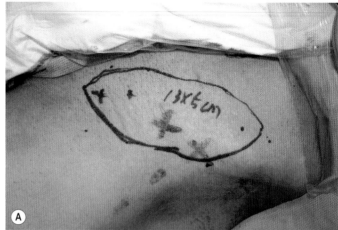

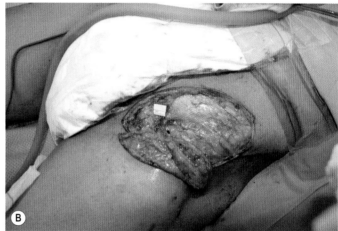

Fig. 5.21 The superficial circumflex iliac perforator flap is nourished by only a perforator of the superficial circumflex iliac system. A large dimension of skin from the inguinal region can be sufficiently supplied by a single perforator.

superior iliac spine and the superior lateral border of the patella. The perforator branches are identified with Doppler near the midpoint of this line. According to our clinical experience, about 90% of perforators are found within a 3 cm diameter drawn at the midpoint of the line. The skin flap is designed to include the perforator and is then elevated from the medial border. The flaps can be as large as 35×25 cm based on a single perforator.[124] The incision is made through the deep fascia and raised subfascially until the intermuscular septum between the rectus femoris and the vastus lateralis muscle is reached. Now with increased knowledge of the perforator flap anatomy, flaps can be easily elevated suprafascially taking just a small cuff of fascia. At that point, the descending branch of the lateral femoral circumflex is explored

along with the perforator to the skin flap. The flap can be harvested either as a perforator flap including only the perforator branch to the skin or combined with the vastus lateralis muscle as a musculocutaneous flap. According to the need, the skin paddle may be defatted up to a 3–4 mm thickness except for the portion that the perforator branch enters. The motor branch of the femoral nerve running medial to the

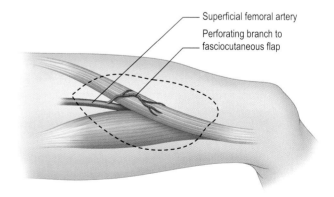

Fig. 5.22 The medial thigh flap located at the midthigh. The dominant blood supply for this fasciocutaneous flap is the anterior septocutaneous artery, and venae comitantes are from the superficial femoral artery and vein at the apex of the femoral triangle.

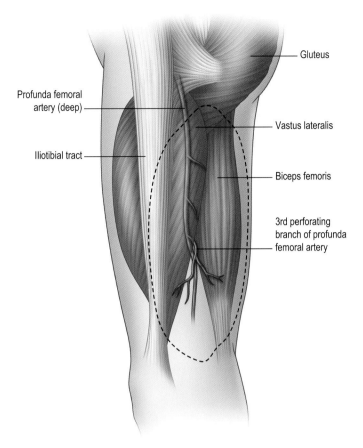

Fig. 5.23 The lateral thigh flap. This is located along the lateral aspect of the thigh between the greater trochanter and the knee and can be based on the three perforating branches of the profunda femoris.

descending branch of the lateral circumflex femoral artery should be preserved. To elevate as a sensate flap, a branch of the lateral femoral cutaneous nerve should be included. The donor site can be primarily closed depending on the laxity of the skin (Fig. 5.25).

Sural

The sural flap is located between the popliteal fossa and the midportion of the leg over the midline raphe between the two heads of the gastrocnemius muscle. It is one of the longest fasciocutaneous flaps of the lower leg based on the direct cutaneous artery (sural artery branch) in the upper central calf and extending to the Achilles tendon distally.[125,126] The lesser saphenous vein provides venous drainage. It can cover defects of the knee, popliteal fossa, and upper third of the leg. When used distally, based on a reverse flow through anastomoses between the peroneal artery and the communicating vascular network of the medial sural nerve, it can reach difficult defect areas in the lower leg, ankle, and heel region (Fig. 5.26).[127] It is innervated by the medial sural cutaneous nerve (S1–2).

The flap is raised from distal to proximal, in the plane beneath the deep fascia and above the gastrocnemius muscles. The sural nerve and lesser saphenous vein are divided distally and elevated with the flap. The pedicle should be visualized and protected in the popliteal fossa, with continued dissection of the pedicle for free tissue harvesting. For free

tissue transplantation, proximal superficial veins should be dissected and preserved for possible anastomosis because the venae comitantes are small.

Thoracodorsal artery perforator

This flap was first described by Angrigiani et al.[128] The vascular territory lies on top of the latissimus dorsi muscle. The main perforators are located along the course of the descending branch of the thoracodorsal artery or from the lateral branch. The most proximal perforator reaches the subcutaneous tissue at a point located 2–3 cm posterior to the lateral edge of the muscle and 8 cm below the posterior axillary fold.[129] The patient is positioned in a lateral decubitus position with the upper arm in 90° abduction and 90° flexion at the elbow. The lateral border of the latissimus is palpated and marked. Doppler can be used to identify potential perforators for the flap, and the most proximal perforator can be anticipated as mentioned above. Once perforators are identified, the flap can be designed based on the perforator. Although larger flap dimensions have been reported, flap dimensions under 255 cm² within its vascular territory are safe from partial necrosis.[130] Incision is made from the anterointerior border of the flap allowing the identification of the anterior border of the latissimus dorsi muscle. The dissection is performed between the fat and the deep fascia covering the muscle. This plane is easy to dissect as it is in a loose areolar plane. While dissecting for the perforator, care should be given when dissecting the proximal portion as direct

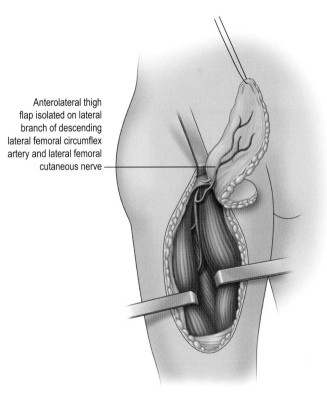

Fig. 5.24 The anterolateral thigh flap. Numerous perforators are found along the region of the intermuscular septum between the vastus lateralis and the rectus femoris. These perforators usually drain into the descending branch of the lateral femoral circumflex artery, then proximally to the lateral circumflex artery, and then to the profunda femoris artery.

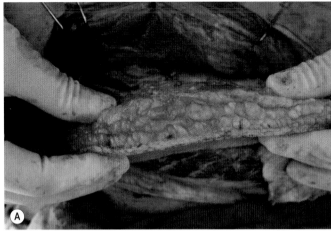

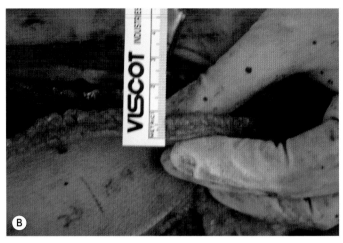

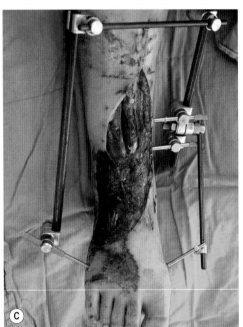

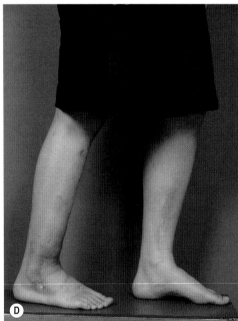

Fig. 5.25 **(A,B)** The deep fat portion of the anterolateral thigh can be debulked to obtain a thinner pliable flap. **(C,D)** The patient with soft-tissue defect of the ankle region is seen with excellent contour after reconstruction without further debulking.

cutaneous or perforators adjacent to the anterior borders are easily missed. After a suitable perforator is identified, the design of the flap in accordance with the defect and pedicle can be made. Perforators can be isolated or taken with a muscle cuff reaching down to the main pedicle. Total pedicle length depends on the location of perforator and the intramuscular course of the pedicle. Pedicle length can be acquired up to 14–18 cm (Fig. 5.27).

Compound flaps

The complexity of reconstruction has changed from simple coverage to addressing the issue of function and cosmetics. Frequently a simple flap can result in adequate reconstruction and may undergo several revisions until the final outcome becomes acceptable. A compound flap consists of multiple tissue components linked together in a manner that allows their simultaneous transfer.[131] These separate components can

be maneuvered and placed in a 3D manner to achieve an ideal one-stage reconstruction. Now as complex and complicated defects are challenged, reconstruction using these compound flaps is becoming routine for these cases.

According to Hallock's classification, the subdivisions of compound flaps are those with a solitary source of vascularization and those with combinations of sources of vascularization (Fig. 5.28).[132] Those with a solitary source include composite flaps, defined as multiple tissue components all served by the same single vascular supply, and thereby consisting of dependent parts. Those flaps with combinations of sources of vascularization include conjoined flaps and chimeric flaps. Conjoined flaps are defined as multiple flap territories, dependent because of some common physical junction, yet each retaining its independent vascular supply. Chimeric flaps are defined as multiple flap territories, each with an independent vascular supply, and independent of any physical interconnection except where linked by a common source vessel (Fig. 5.29).

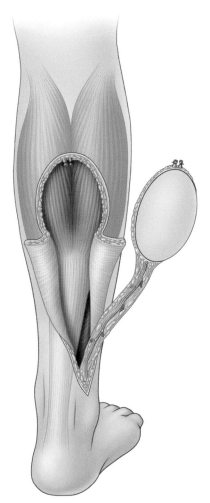

Fig. 5.26 The reverse sural artery flap is a fasciocutaneous flap based on the median superficial sural artery and its communication with the perforating branch of the peroneal artery situated in the region of the lateral malleolar gutter. Reverse flow is established after elevation of the flap and with division of the sural artery and the nerve proximally.

Supermicrosurgery

The supermicrosurgery technique is defined as microsurgical anastomosis of vessels, with a diameter <0.8 mm.[109,129] This technique, although reported frequently on lymphaticovenous shunting to treat lymphedema and sporadically in soft-tissue reconstruction with specific indications, is a relatively new concept for lower extremity reconstruction.[129–132] For the lower extremity soft-tissue reconstruction, one of the applications can be seen in the perforator-to-perforator anastomoses approach.[68,111] With an evident pulse on the perforating artery, it can be successfully used as a recipient vessel to supply a sizable flap. This approach will allow an increase in the selection of recipient pedicles. By using a perforator-to-perforator anastomosis approach, less time is consumed to secure the recipient vessel as the flap can be elevated by taking just a short segment of the perforator pedicle, which minimizes any risk for major vessel injury, or can utilize collateral circulation without apparent flow of major vessels while having acceptable flap survival (Fig. 5.30). Further, studies on physiology and anatomy will be needed to evaluate the extent of application.

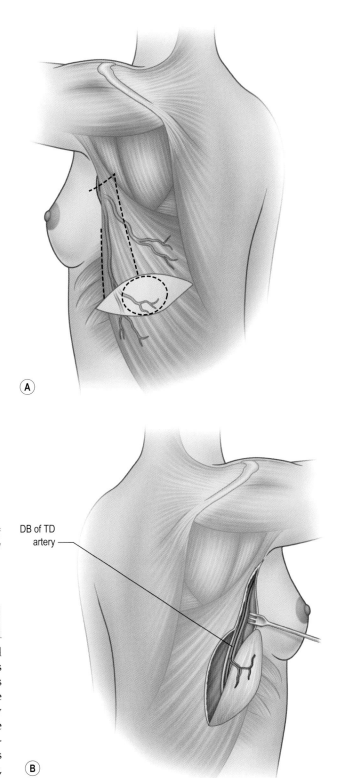

Fig. 5.27 Thoracodorsal artery perforator flap. The main perforators are located along the course of the descending branch of the thoracodorsal artery or from the lateral branch. The most proximal perforator reaches the subcutaneous tissue in a point located 2 or 3 cm posterior to the lateral edge of the muscle and 8 cm below the posterior axillary fold. DB, descending branch; TD, thoracodorsal.

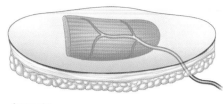

Composite

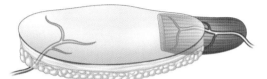

Conjoined

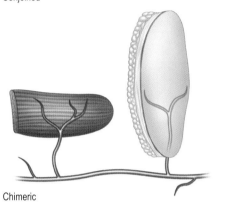

Chimeric

Fig. 5.28 Classification of compound flaps.

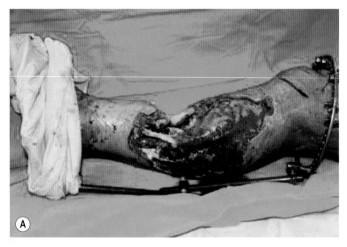

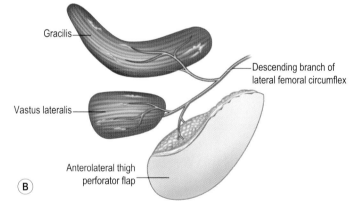

Gracilis

Descending branch of
lateral femoral circumflex

Vastus lateralis

Anterolateral thigh
perforator flap

(B)

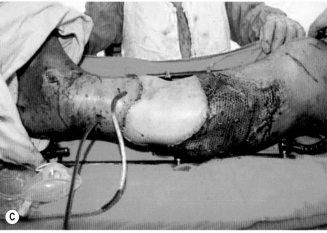

Fig. 5.29 The chimeric flaps defined as multiple flap territories, each with an independent vascular supply, and independent of any physical interconnection except where linked by a common source vessel. Example of complex extremity reconstruction is shown using a chimeric approach. The source vessel of the descending branch of the lateral femoral circumflex artery feeding the vastus lateralis and the anterolateral thigh perforator flap. A gracilis is connected using a branch from the source vessel.

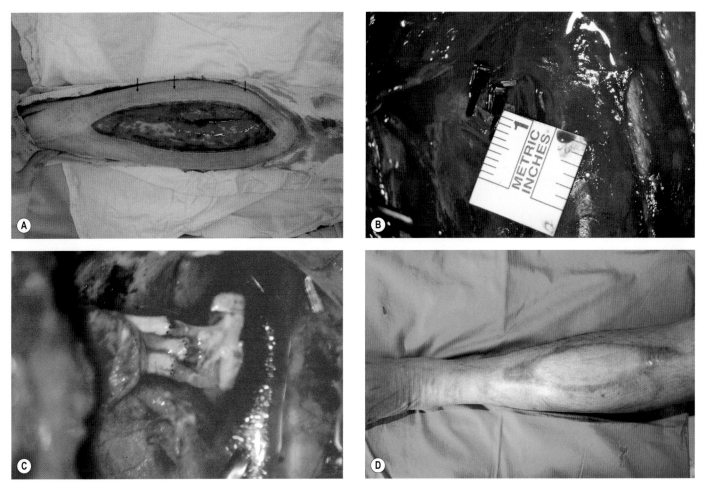

Fig. 5.30 (A) The application of supermicrosurgery (perforator-to-perforator anastomosis) on the lower extremity is shown. A patient with chronic osteomyelitis is seen after debridement. **(B)** A recipient perforator was located adjacent to the defect margin piercing the fascia with a good visual pulse. **(C)** After the elevation of anterolateral thigh with a short perforator pedicle segment, anastomosis is performed. **(D)** The flap is shown to have good contour without recurrence of infection.

Access the complete reference list online at **http://www.expertconsult.com**

1. Bosse MJ, MacKenzie EJ, Kellam JF, et al. An analysis of outcomes of reconstruction or amputation after leg-threatening injuries. *N Engl J Med.* 2002;347(24):1924–1931. *The authors from Carolinas Medical Center performed a multicenter, prospective, observational study of 569 patients with severe leg trauma and evaluated the sickness-impact profile: a multidimensional self-reported health status to determine the long-term outcomes after amputation or limb reconstruction. They report that at 2 years, there was no significant difference in scores for the Sickness Impact Profile between the amputation and the reconstruction groups. They advise that patients with limbs at high risk for amputation may undergo reconstruction and will have results in 2 years that are equivalent to those for amputation.*

2. Chung KC, Saddawi-Konefka D, Haase SC, et al. A cost-utility analysis of amputation versus salvage for Gustilo type IIIB and IIIC open tibial fractures. *Plast Reconstr Surg.* 2009;124(6):1965–1973. *The authors from the University of Michigan Health System evaluated the cost following amputation and salvage using the data presented in a study from the LEAP. The authors extracted relevant data on projected lifetime costs and analyzed them to include discounting and sensitivity analysis by considering patient age. They report amputation is more expensive than salvage, independently of varied ongoing prosthesis needs, discount rate, and patient age at presentation. Moreover, amputation yields fewer quality-adjusted life-years than salvage. Salvage is deemed the dominant, cost-saving strategy.*

11. Godina M. Early microsurgical reconstruction of complex trauma of the extremities. *Plast Reconstr Surg.* 1986;78(3):285–292.

19. Ong YS, Levin LS. Lower limb salvage in trauma. *Plast Reconstr Surg.* 2010;125(2):582–588. *The authors from the Duke University Medical Center review the approach to lower limb salvage. They state that the primary goal of limb salvage is to restore or maintain function based on proper patient selection, timely reconstruction, and choosing the best procedure that should be individualized for each patient. Aggressive debridement and skeletal stabilization, followed by early reconstruction, are the current standard of practice and give better results than the more traditional approach of repeated debridements and delayed flap cover. For reconstruction, they state that free tissue transfer remains the best choice for large defects, but local fasciocutaneous flaps are a reasonable alternative for smaller defects and cases in which free flaps are deemed not suitable.*

36. Gottlieb LJ, Krieger LM. From the reconstructive ladder to the reconstructive elevator. *Plast Reconstr Surg.* 1994;93(7):1503–1504.

56. Lange RH. Limb reconstruction versus amputation decision making in massive lower extremity trauma. *Clin Orthop Relat Res.* 1989;(243):92–99. *This study from the University of Wisconsin describes the absolute and relative indications for primary amputation of limbs with open tibial fractures. Absolute indications include anatomically*

complete disruption of the posterior tibial nerve in adults and crush injuries with warm ischemia time greater than 6 h. Relative indications include serious associated polytrauma, severe ipsilateral foot trauma, and anticipated protracted course to obtain soft-tissue coverage and tibial reconstruction. However, he states that individual patient variables, specific extremity injury characteristics, and associated injuries must all be weighed before a decision can be reached and further prospective studies are necessary before a well-defined protocol for primary amputation can be properly developed.

68. Hong JP. The use of supermicrosurgery in lower extremity reconstruction: the next step in evolution. *Plast Reconstr Surg.* 2009;123(1):230–235.

69. Kindsfater K, Jonassen EA. Osteomyelitis in grade II and III open tibia fractures with late debridement. *J Orthop Trauma.* 1995;9(2):121–127.

88. Chen KT, Mardini S, Chuang DC, et al. Timing of presentation of the first signs of vascular compromise dictates the salvage outcome of free flap transfers. *Plast Reconstr Surg.* 2007;120(1):187–195.

108. Wei FC, Celik N. Perforator flap entity. *Clin Plast Surg.* 2003;30(3):325–329. *The authors from the Chang Gung Memorial Hospital state that the perforator flap is not a new concept in microsurgery, but there is still confusion, and studies about the differences between these flaps and the conventional flaps, including donor site morbidity and long-term follow-ups, are increasing in literature. Better accuracy in reconstruction, including the use of only cutaneous tissue, minimization of the morbidity, and preserving the same survival rate in free flaps are reassurances to microsurgeons with regard to performing perforator flaps. He believes that in the near future, with refinements in the techniques and instruments, perforator flaps will be the first choice.*

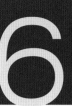

Diagnosis and treatment of painful neuroma and nerve compression in the lower extremity

Ivica Ducic, John M. Felder, and A. Lee Dellon

Access video content for this chapter online at expertconsult.com

SYNOPSIS

- Neuroma pain is due to regenerating axon sprouts trapped in the scar:
  - Nerve block may identify the peripheral nerve causing the pain
  - Remember that more than one peripheral nerve may be involved
  - If possible, a critical sensory nerve should be reconnected to its target
  - A non-critical sensory nerve should have the neuroma resected
  - It is OK to "lose your nerve": trade pain for anesthesia
  - The proximal end of the resected nerve must be placed into a "quiet place"
  - Implantation of a sensory nerve into a normal muscle is evidence-based
  - Choose an appropriate muscle for the location of the peripheral nerve
  - Remember that the painful neuroma may be in a painful joint
  - Postoperative rehabilitation to include water walking, not only massage.
- Chronic nerve compression is common in the lower extremity:
  - The most common site of entrapment is the distal tibial nerve
  - Next most common site is the peroneal nerve at the fibular neck
  - Next most common site is the deep peroneal nerve at the foot dorsum
  - Superficial peroneal nerve (SPN) can be entrapped too
  - Remember to look in both anterior and lateral compartments for SPN
  - Tarsal tunnel is not carpal tunnel, but analogous to the forearm
  - Must neurolyse medial and lateral plantar nerves distal to the tarsal tunnel
  - Must neurolyse calcaneal nerve in its tunnel distal to the tarsal tunnel
  - Postoperative rehab must include immediate ambulation.
- Standards of care:
  - Use of tourniquet, loupe magnification, and bipolar coagulation.

 Access the Historical Perspective section online at
http://www.expertconsult.com

Introduction

Though frequently ignored, misunderstood, or misdiagnosed, nerve injuries and nerve compression syndromes are a frequent occurrence in the lower extremity.

Painful neuromas, which occur following trauma or surgery to the lower extremity, may be an unremitting source of pain for affected patients, with detrimental effects on quality-of-life. As an entity, they are frequently missing from the diagnostic tree of many physicians. They may be mistaken for complex regional pain syndrome (CRPS) or other pain syndromes with which they share some clinical features, relegating patients to chronic medical pain management therapy rather than a direct, surgical approach to the problem. In this chapter we will discuss the pathophysiology of painful neuromas and then explain how to select and treat surgical candidates to achieve pain relief.

Lower extremity nerve compression syndromes are largely analogous to the well-recognized nerve compression syndromes of the upper extremity, yet they and the surgical approach to addressing them are often the subject of dispute or incredulity among medical practitioners without training in peripheral nerve surgery. These syndromes lead to loss of sensation or motor function and can be the source of significant morbidity for affected patients. In this chapter, we will discuss the pathophysiology of nerve compression and then explain how to select and treat surgical candidates to achieve nerve decompression. We will also discuss CPRS: how to distinguish it from neuromas or nerve compression and how to manage it.

The principles for surgical treatment of lower extremity neuromas and nerve compression syndromes were largely elucidated by Mackinnon and Dellon, in the 1980s and 1990s,[1] addressing, for example, the problems related to the tibial nerve at the level of the ankle and the problems related to the peroneal nerve at the knee, leg, and foot level, as well as the problems with the sural nerve and the interdigital nerve. Dr. Dellon also wrote extensively about these topics in the previous edition of this chapter, upon which this edition draws heavily.

Basic science/disease process

The painful neuroma

The cell body for a sensory neuron of the peripheral nervous system lies in a dorsal root ganglion and from the exit of this nerve from the vertebral foramen it is covered with Schwann cells (Fig. 6.1).

A painful neuroma develops following a discrete trauma to a peripheral nerve. Typically, complete transection divides the proximal and distal portions of the nerve. The axons of the proximal segment regenerate via growth cones and attempt to reach the axonal tubules of the distal segment (Fig. 6.2).[6–8,9] However, if this process is disrupted by misalignment, scar tissue, or other factors, the growing axons of the proximal segment may fail to reach their distal target and instead form a tangled mass of axonal sprouts, Schwann cells, and fibrous tissue. This tangled mass is known as a neuroma, and the nerve endings it contains are prone to spontaneous or ephaptic depolarization that is often centrally interpreted as pain. Physical tension on the neuroma with mechanical

deformation can further stimulate depolarization, and this is often seen when the neuroma is encased in a surgical scar or has healed in a superficial location prone to physical disruption, such as near a joint or subjacent to a weight-bearing surface.[10]

In concordance with these underlying pathophysiologic principles, treatment of an end neuroma focuses on separating the proximal nerve from the neuromatous bulb and placing it in an environment that will (1) discourage growth of another neuroma and (2) not produce tension or mechanical stimulation of the cut nerve end. Implanting the proximal transected nerve end securely within a bulky muscle has been shown experimentally to accomplish both of these goals.[11–13]

Chronic nerve compression

Chronic compression of a nerve has sequential effects on the anatomic subcomponents making up the peripheral nerve: the endoneurium, perineurium, Schwann cells, vasa nervorum, and axons are all involved in turn. As each of these components is involved, a corresponding sign or symptom becomes present in the patient presentation, permitting gradations in diagnosis and treatment that correspond to the degree of compression.

How the structure and function of the peripheral nerve are altered with increasing degrees of pressure and with increasing lengths of time have been investigated in rat, rabbit, and monkey models,[14–24] many of which have used the sciatic nerve.

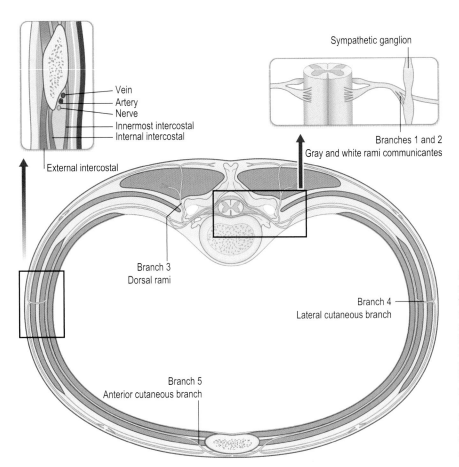

Vein
Artery
Nerve
Innermost intercostal
Internal intercostal
External intercostal

Sympathetic ganglion

Branches 1 and 2
Gray and white rami communicantes

Branch 3
Dorsal rami

Branch 4
Lateral cutaneous branch

Branch 5
Anterior cutaneous branch

Fig. 6.1 The spinal nerve is formed from a ventral (motor) root and a dorsal (sensory) root of the spinal cord. Note that the dorsal root is joined to dorsal ganglia that contain the cell bodies of the sensory neurons, whereas the cell bodies of the motor neurons are contained within the spinal cord itself. When the spinal nerve exits the vertebral foramen, it becomes ensheathed by Schwann cells and is termed a peripheral nerve. This particular peripheral nerve is illustrated as arising from the thoracic spine region, in which region its sensory branches directly innervate the skin without formation of a plexus, as occurs for the lower extremity from the lumbosacral plexus. Note that the dorsal ramus of the spinal nerve can be entrapped in its passage to the lower back, causing symptoms of chronic nerve entrapment termed "notalgia paraesthetica".

Peripheral Nerve   **Skeletal muscle**

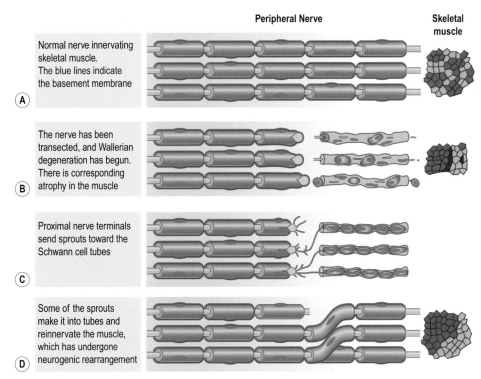

Normal nerve innervating skeletal muscle. The blue lines indicate the basement membrane

(A)

The nerve has been transected, and Wallerian degeneration has begun. There is corresponding atrophy in the muscle

(B)

Proximal nerve terminals send sprouts toward the Schwann cell tubes

(C)

Some of the sprouts make it into tubes and reinnervate the muscle, which has undergone neurogenic rearrangement

(D)

Fig. 6.2 (A) A transection injury to a peripheral nerve results in degeneration of the axon distal to the site of transection (Wallerian degeneration). **(B)** The Schwann cells along this distal segment of the axon survive, upregulate, and produce nerve growth factor, while the axons of the proximal segment produce sprouts for distal regeneration. **(C)** When neural regeneration proceeds unimpeded, the axons will return to their distal target organ, with the creation of an in-continuity neuroma. **(D)** When neural regeneration is impeded by scar tissue from the injury, distal regeneration does not occur and an end-bulb neuroma forms.

A review of this literature indicates that if there is a constriction of greater than 20% placed upon the diameter of the peripheral nerve, then acute axonal degeneration will occur. If there is a pressure of greater than 20 mmHg applied to the peripheral nerve, there will be a decrease in blood flow. In the acute situation, these conditions produce pain. If this degree of compression comes on over a gradual period of time, and over a length of the peripheral nerve that is several times the diameter of the nerve, then the conditions produce chronic nerve compression. After about 2 months of compression by a silicone tube that does not constrict the diameter of the nerve, the first changes in the pathophysiology occur. These are a weakening of the tight junctions of the endothelial cells in the perineurium, and this results in serum entering the endoneurial space. This creates endoneurial edema. When this occurs in the relatively tight confines of the perineurium, there is an increase in pressure that will decrease blood flow. The conscious perception of this is paresthesia. At this point in time, the only clinical findings will be related to the cutaneous sensory threshold for touch, which will first become elevated for static two-point discrimination, or will manifest itself as a change in perception of vibratory stimuli applied with a tuning fork or a vibrometer.[25,26] These pathophysiologic concepts provide a basis for staging chronic nerve compression (Tables 6.1–6.4).

After about 6 months of this degree of compression, the first histologic changes in myelin can be observed. This consists of thinning of the myelin. With progressive compression, there will be increasing loss of myelin, so that under slides in which a myelin stain has been used, it appears as if there has been a loss of the large myelinated, touch, fibers. They will not actually have begun to degenerate yet, as demonstrated by electron microscopy, in which the unmyelinated large fibers can be demonstrated still to be present. At this stage, the patient will have weakness in the motor system related to the muscles supplied by that nerve and increasing numbness in the territory (fingers) related to the sensory supply of that nerve. Pinch and grip strength can be measured directly. There will be no atrophy because without true loss of the motor axons, there will be no decrease in bulk of the muscles.

Table 6.1 Numeric grading scale for any peripheral nerve	
Grade	**Description**
0	Normal
1	Intermittent sensory symptoms
2	Increased sensorimotor threshold
3	Increased sensorimotor threshold
4	Increased sensorimotor threshold
5	Persistent sensory symptoms
6	Sensorimotor degeneration
7	Sensorimotor degeneration
8	Sensorimotor degeneration
9	Anesthesia
10	Muscle atrophy, severe

(Adapted from Dellon AL. A numerical grading scale for peripheral nerve function. *J Hand Ther.* 1993;4:152.)

Table 6.2 Numeric grading scale for the median nerve at the wrist level

Numeric score		Description of impairment
Sensory	Motor	
0	0	None
1		Paresthesia, intermittent
2		Abnormal pressure threshold (pressure-specified sensory device)
		<45 years old: ≤3 mm, at 1.0–20 g/mm^2
		≥45 years old: ≤4 mm, at 2.2–20 g/mm^2
	3	Weakness, thenar muscles
4		Abnormal pressure threshold (pressure-specified sensory device)
		<45 years old: ≤3 mm, at >20 g/mm^2
		≥45 years old: ≤4 mm, at 20 g/mm^2
5		Paresthesias, persistent
6		Abnormal innervation density (pressure-specified sensory device)
		<45 years old: ≥4 mm <8 mm, at any g/mm^2
		≥45 years old: ≥5 mm <9 mm, at any g/mm^2
	7	Muscle wasting (1–2/4)
8		Abnormal innervation density (pressure-specified sensory device)
		<45 years old: ≥8 mm, at any g/mm^2
		>45 years old: ≥9 mm, at any g/mm^2
9		Anesthesia
	10	Muscle wasting (3–4/4)

(Adapted from Dellon AL. A numerical grading scale for peripheral nerve function. *J Hand Ther.* 1993;4:152.)

At this stage of compression, the cutaneous pressure thresholds will be elevated increasingly for the quickly adapting fibers, measured either with vibrometry or moving two-point discrimination using the pressure-specified sensory device (PSSD),[27] and for the slowly adapting fibers, measured with static two-point discrimination using the PSSD. Although no longitudinal study using the Semmes–Weinstein nylon monofilaments has been published in patients with chronic nerve compression,[28] the analogous measurement, made with the PSSD, which is one-point static touch, is still normal at this stage of compression.[9] Two-point discrimination, measured in millimeters, is still normal because no nerve fibers have died. At this stage in chronic nerve compression, with myelin thinning, traditional electrodiagnostic testing may begin to detect increases in the distal sensory latency. Amplitudes will still be normal because no nerve fibers have died yet. In general, quantitative neurosensory testing is more sensitive than traditional electrodiagnostic testing (nerve conduction study/electromyogram), so it is more likely to detect this stage of nerve compression. Neurosensory testing is less expensive than nerve conduction study/electromyogram and will not cause the patient any pain.[29,30]

If either the length of time is increased for this degree of compression or the degree of compression increases, whether due to work or metabolic or rheumatologic disease, then neural degeneration occurs. As suggested in the preceding paragraph, this will be detected in the motor system by muscle wasting and in the sensory system by abnormal distance at which one from two points can be distinguished. Examples of these changes are given in Table 6.2 for median nerve compression at the wrist, Table 6.3 for ulnar nerve compression at the elbow, and Table 6.4 for tibial nerve compression in the tarsal tunnel.[23,25] Using the PSSD, this change occurs first for static two-point discrimination and then for moving two-point discrimination. This was demonstrated in a retrospective analysis of patients with carpal and cubital tunnel syndrome. The one-point static touch measurement will become abnormal some time after the change in two-point discrimination distance, and is therefore a relatively insensitive tool for detecting the onset of this stage. Vibrometry and tuning fork use can identify this stage but does not permit the therapist to identify correctly which nerve is being compressed without additional testing. It must be remembered that the vibratory stimulus travels as a wave, whereas the pressure stimulus remains localized to the applied test site.[19,20,27] For example, if the involved nerve is the tibial nerve and the hallux pulp is tested, there may still be relatively preserved sensation mediated by the peroneal nerve. Testing of both the dorsum of the foot and hallux pulp and medial heel may permit distinction of which nerve is involved.

Table 6.3 Numeric grading scale for the ulnar nerve at the elbow level

Numeric score		Description of impairment
Sensory	Motor	
0	0	None
1		Paresthesia, intermittent
	2	Weakness: pinch/grip (lb)
		Female: 10–14/26–39
		Male: 13–19/31–59
3		Abnormal pressure threshold (pressure-specified sensory device)
		<45 years old: ≤3 mm, at 1.0–20.0 g/mm^2
		≥45 years old: ≤4 mm, at 1.9–20.0 g/mm^2
	4	Weakness: pinch/grip (lb)
		Female: 6–9/15–25
		Male: 6–12/15–30
5		Paresthesia, persistent
6		Abnormal innervation density (pressure-specified sensory device)
		<45 years old: ≥4 mm <8 mm, at any g/mm^2
		≥45 years old: ≥9 mm, at any g/mm^2
9		Anesthesia
	10	Muscle wasting (3–4/4)

(Adapted from Dellon AL. A numerical grading scale for peripheral nerve function. *J Hand Ther.* 1993;4:152.)

Table 6.4 Numeric grading scale for the tibial nerve at ankle level

Numeric score		Description of impairment
Sensory	Motor	
0	0	None
1		Paresthesia, intermittent
2		Abnormal pressure threshold (pressure-specified sensory device)
		<45 years old: ≤5.6 mm, at 1.0–20 g/mm²
		≥45 years old: ≤7.8 mm, at 2.2–20 g/mm²
	3	Weakness, abductor hallucis
4		Abnormal pressure threshold (pressure-specified sensory device)
		<45 years old: ≤5.6 mm, at 20 g/mm²
		≥45 years old: ≤7.8 mm, at 20 g/mm²
5		Paresthesias, persistent
6		Abnormal innervation density (pressure-specified sensory device)
		<45 years old: ≥7 mm <10 mm, at any g/mm²
		≥45 years old: ≥9 mm <12 mm, at any g/mm²
	7	Intrinsic muscle wasting, clawing (1–2/4)
8		Abnormal innervation density (pressure-specified sensory device)
		<45 years old: ≥11 mm, at any given g/mm²
		≥45 years old: ≥15 mm, at any g/mm²
9		Anesthesia
	10	Intrinsic muscle wasting, clawing (3–4/4)

If there is some limitation on the gliding of the peripheral nerve through its site of anatomic narrowing, then, when the adjacent joint moves, there will be an increase in tension along the length of the nerve, which may manifest itself as a further increase in pressure upon the nerve. This limitation of gliding may come from some injury or anatomic variant that limits excursion of the nerves. This subject will be discussed in detail related to individual nerve compression syndromes.

Diagnosis/patient presentation (Videos 6.1, 6.2, 6.3 ⊙)

The painful neuroma

The patient with a painful neuroma will complain of an area of skin or a joint that causes pain either at rest or, more commonly, when the part is touched or moved. When an area of pain relates to the territory of a peripheral nerve, and the patient has had an injury or an operation in that area, then consideration must be given to the presence of a painful neuroma of that peripheral nerve. If there is no history of trauma or prior surgery, a "true" peripheral nerve tumor may be suspected instead.

Presentation and management of a single painful neuroma may be relatively straightforward. However, because multiple nerves may be injured and have neuromas, the distribution of pain may not follow that of a single nerve. Instead, the pain may correspond to a "region" of the limb. When this is the case, it is paramount to differentiate whether this "region of pain" is in fact caused by painful neuromas of adjacent nerves with overlapping innervation territories or is caused by another regional pain syndrome that is often treated nonsurgically: CRPS.

Classically, patients with painful neuromas will present with a discrete tender area with distal paresthesias or anesthesia at an old scar or area of injury, and the pain will be alleviated by local anesthetic blockade. If the symptoms are as described above and sequential blockade of adjacent nerves eliminates the pain, then multiple painful neuromas are likely responsible for creating the region of pain and surgical treatment is indicated. Patients with CRPS likewise have a region of spontaneous pain that may spread beyond the anatomic territory of a single nerve, but in contrast they will also present with edema, atrophy, vasomotor, and/or sudomotor abnormalities in the skin of the affected limb. Patients with CRPS may or may not have a history of obvious nerve injury. If there *is* a history of known or suspected nerve injury, the syndrome is called "CRPS type II" (formerly "causalgia") – in these cases, surgical treatment of the underlying nerve injury has potential to reverse the pain syndrome, although the physiology of this disease is complex and incompletely understood, and not all patients are helped by surgery. Undertaking surgery on such patients requires a more sophisticated approach to diagnosis and perioperative management that is discussed elsewhere in this book.[31] If a patient with CRPS *does not* have a known or suspected nerve injury, this is called "CRPS type I" (formerly reflex sympathetic dystrophy), and this syndrome is never treated with peripheral nerve surgery because there is no obvious peripheral pain generator that would be a target for surgical intervention. Instead, these patients are treated with multimodal care including physical therapy, sympathetic blocks, chronic pain management, and, at times, spinal cord stimulators.

One particular area of presentation that can become confusing is that of the painful joint. When a biomechanical abnormality has been ruled out and a patient complains of a painful joint after previous surgery or an injury, the diagnostic dilemma of multiple painful neuromas vs. CRPS again presents itself. Because most joints are innervated by multiple afferent nerves, and these nerves are small and often not found in textbooks, there is a temptation to consider the joint a "region" and label the patient with CRPS. However, it is mandatory for the peripheral nerve surgeon to exclude the possibility that multiple, treatable neuromas of joint afferents are causing the problem by first excluding the presence of the ancillary "sympathetic" features of CRPS on exam, and then performing sequential local anesthetic blockades of the joint afferents, looking for elimination of pain.

Anatomy books do not show nerves innervating joints, and this knowledge required cadaver dissections, which have been published for the knee (Fig. 6.3B & C)[32] and the ankle (Fig. 6.3A).[33] Clinical approaches and results for the lower extremity were reviewed in 2009.[5] Beginning with the knee and then extending this approach to the ankle, anatomic dissections were performed to identify joint innervation. With

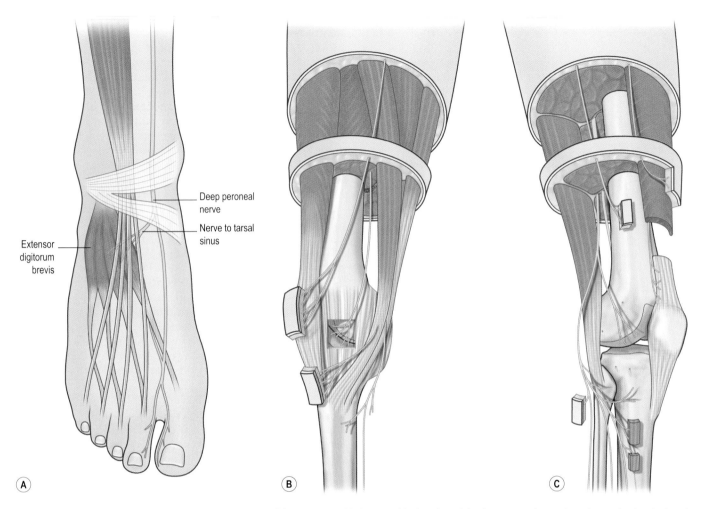

Extensor digitorum brevis

Deep peroneal nerve

Nerve to tarsal sinus

Fig. 6.3 Illustrations of the innervation of lower extremity joints. **(A)** The sinus tarsi is innervated by branches of the deep peroneal nerve that arise proximal to the lateral malleolus, just before the branch to the extensor digitorum brevis. **(B)** The medial aspect of the knee joint is innervated by a branch of the femoral nerve. After the femoral nerve innervates the vastus medialis, at which point anatomy books show the nerve terminating, the nerve continues distally and past the end of the muscle to innervate the medial knee structures. **(C)** The lateral aspect of the knee joint is innervated by a branch of the sciatic nerve, which, after it innervates the posterior knee capsule, travels anterior, deep to the biceps tendon, and then innervates the lateral knee structures. The medial and lateral retinacular nerves likely overlap anteriorly, although this has not been proven. *(With Permission from Dr. Dellon.)*

this knowledge, routes for the administration of local anesthetic were identified. Demonstrating that pain relief is possible by anesthetic blockade in patients who failed traditional musculoskeletal approaches led to the creation of surgical approaches to resect involved nerve(s).

A special category of patients with painful neuromas refers to those who have undergone lower extremity amputation and have developed painful neuromas of the amputation stump that prevent them from using their prostheses. Formation of such neuromas can be discouraged during the initial amputation by finding each major sensory or mixed nerve and implanting it to muscle or effectively doing so by cutting them on tension. However, many patients who undergo amputation will have painful stumps without a biomechanical or bony explanation and, if this pain can be localized and relieved with anesthetic block, they may be candidates for surgical treatment.[34]

In the patient with a painful neuroma, motor function should be normal physiologically with the exception of two considerations. Firstly, if there is ankle pain, then the patient

may not use muscles that cause ankle movement, leading to disuse atrophy of the muscles. Secondly, there is often wasting of the extensor digitorum brevis associated with ankle pain, since the nerve that innervates this muscle, the deep peroneal nerve, has been injured, usually with the stretch/traction associated with an inversion sprain.

Chronic nerve compression

The signs and symptoms of compression neuropathy are well known: the patient with chronic compression of a peripheral nerve will complain of numbness or paresthesias in the skin territory innervated by that nerve. The patient will complain of weakness in the muscles innervated by that nerve. However, just as multiple painful neuromas must be distinguished from CRPS, there is an analogous diagnostic overlap between multiple nerve compressions and metabolic neuropathies. For instance, if both the peroneal and tibial nerves have chronic compression at the same time, the patient will have numbness over the dorsal and plantar aspects of the foot that arises proximal to the ankle. This will give the same appearance as if the patient had a peripheral neuropathy, especially if the problem occurs in both legs. This type of situation occurs in patients who have sports injuries, or other injuries. As a contrast in etiology, but with the same clinical presentation, will be patients who do have a metabolic neuropathy, for example, those with diabetes, or chemotherapy-induced neuropathy, who have secondary chronic nerve compressions. These patients will present with a history of neuropathy and frequently will not have been examined to identify the presence of a chronic nerve compression.[35] If the nerve compression is diagnosed and treated in such patients, they will frequently experience sensory recovery despite the presence of diabetic neuropathy.[36,37]

The pathognomonic feature of chronic nerve compression on physical examination is the presence of a positive Hoffman–Tinel sign. With an understanding of the pathophysiology of chronic nerve compression (see above), it becomes clear that in the earliest stage there will be intermittent symptoms and there will be no physical findings present. This is often the situation with musicians, such as the pianist or violinist who complains of numbness in the little finger, from playing with the elbow bent, but has no Hoffman–Tinel sign over the ulnar nerve at the cubital tunnel. In the lower extremity, an analogous situation occurs with the soccer player whose leg may seem to give out, and who has received many a blunt trauma to the outside of the knee or repeated ankle inversion sprains, and has compression of the common peroneal nerve at the fibular neck. With further time and a greater degree of compression, axons will demyelinate and there will be an increase in the threshold required to produce a sensory response: a higher degree of vibration with the tuning fork, or a greater pressure required to discriminate one from two points when touching the big-toe pulp with the PSSD while two-point discrimination distance remains normal. In the motor system, this will correspond to weakness on manual muscle testing. At this point, the Hoffman–Tinel sign will become positive. With more time and a greater degree of compression, axons will die, there will be a decrease in two-point static touch discrimination (the distance before two points can be distinguished will increase), and muscle atrophy will occur. The Hoffman–Tinel sign will remain positive. With a very advanced degree of compression, the peripheral nerve seems to stop its attempt to remyelinate and regenerate, and the Hoffman–Tinel sign becomes negative. This variation in the presence of the Hoffman–Tinel sign over time is understandable in terms of progression of compression and changes within the peripheral nerve and should not be interpreted as a failure of the Hoffman–Tinel sign to be a valuable clinical examination technique.[38,39]

Patient selection

The painful neuroma

Selection of the patient for surgical treatment of the painful neuroma begins after the first 6 months of pain. During the first 6 months of the patient's pain, management will usually be done by the primary care physician and/or the original treating surgeon, often in conjunction with a therapist. Most often, the patient will have tried opiates, non-steroidal anti-inflammatory drugs, massage, ultrasound, and steroid injection. Once the pain has lasted 6 months, the patient enters the phase of chronic pain and is now traditionally referred to a pain management physician. At this point, the patient will usually be tried on neuropathic pain medication, such as nortriptyline, Neurontin, Cymbalta, or Lyrica, and often a combination of these.

A nerve block is critical in patient selection. In the management of the patient with chronic pain, the pain management physician will often do a nerve block with or without cortisone to identify and treat the peripheral nerve believed to be the source of the pain. If the pain resolves for a few hours and then returns, this block was actually a diagnostic block. If the pain partially resolves, then perhaps more than one peripheral nerve is the source of the pain. If the block fails to resolve, then the local anesthetic failed to achieve its effect either due to the presence of a second involved nerve or due to an anatomic variation in the peripheral nerve that was supposed to be blocked. If the block actually relieves pain for a prolonged period of time, then it was therapeutic, and it should be repeated by the pain management physician when or if the pain recurs. Failure of the repeat block to achieve pain relief signals an appropriate time for surgical intervention. A sequence of nerve blocks for a painful foot dorsum is given in Fig. 6.4.

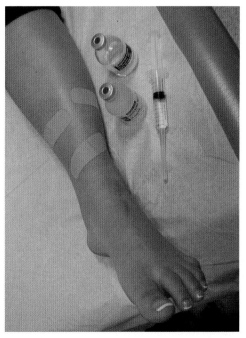

Fig. 6.4 Sequence of nerve blocks to identify source of dorsal foot pain. The nerve block is done using a sterile technique. After swabbing the skin with Betadine, a mixture is prepared that contains half 1% xylocaine and half 0.5% bupivacaine, each without epinephrine, is prepared. This is injected first next to the saphenous nerve, proximal to the medial malleolus. This is for a painful tarsal tunnel incision, a crushed foot, or a painful bunion incision. Then the deep peroneal nerve is blocked next, above the ankle, between the extensor hallucis longus and the extensor digitorum communis tendons. At this level, the block will also denervate the sinus tarsi. If sinus tarsi pain is only partially eliminated, then you must block the sural nerve, posterior to the lateral malleolus (not shown) as this nerve contributes to sinus tarsi innervation in 25% of patients. Finally, the superficial peroneal nerve is blocked next. This can be done as shown here at the site of a positive Tinel's sign, or just dorsolateral to the ankle joint. Following this the patient must attempt to walk, squat, and touch the top of the foot to determine the effect of the block on pain.

It is the goal of a nerve block to place the local anesthetic adjacent to, not into, the peripheral nerve. If the patient has immediate pain when the needle is inserted, and the pain radiates in the territory of that nerve, then the needle is in the nerve and you should not inject the anesthetic or you will cause a nerve injection injury. You should pull the needle slightly away and then inject. Success of the nerve block requires the patient to say that the pain has gone and, if it is a cutaneous nerve, that the expected area of skin has become numb.

Chronic nerve compression

Selection of the patient for surgical decompression of a peripheral nerve requires that at least four conditions are met:

1. The patient's symptoms fit with both the motor and the sensory distribution of the given peripheral nerve.
2. The impairment is documented by appropriate measurement of the motor and sensory function of that nerve.
3. There is a positive Tinel's sign at the known site of anatomic narrowing of that nerve.
4. All possible non-operative measures have been employed for 3 months without success in relieving the symptoms.

Note that it is not essential for an electrodiagnostic test to be performed and it is not essential that the results of that test demonstrate chronic nerve compression. This is because, even where traditional nerve conduction and electromyography are best for the median nerve at the wrist, the false-negative rate is 33%, and in patients with diabetes this type of testing cannot be relied upon to identify the presence of a chronic nerve compression in the presence of an underlying neuropathy.[40] In the lower extremity, in a patient over the age of 55, the false-positive rate for the medial plantar and electromyogram of the medial plantar-innervated muscles is 50%, and therefore, in the adult even without neuropathy, this testing is prone to error. Since traditional testing cannot identify nerve compression in the presence of neuropathy at the wrist, it certainly cannot identify it reliably at the ankle. Therefore the clinician must rely upon the presence of a positive Hoffman–Tinel sign to indicate the location of the chronic nerve compression.

Neurosensory testing with the PSSD is the most sensitive method of documenting sensibility in a piece of skin (Fig. 6.5). This has been documented to be valid and reliable for both the upper and lower extremity,[27,28,29,40–43] and to be essentially equivalent to the information obtained with traditional electrodiagnostic studies of the median nerve at the wrist in a level I study.[30] For the patient with heel pain, for example, the medial calcaneal nerve will have an abnormal pressure threshold with normal distance for distinguishing one-point from two-point static touch, with normal measurements for both the medial plantar (hallux pulp) and over the dorsum of the foot. When treatment for plantar fasciitis continues to fail after 3 months, and when the two-point static distance becomes abnormal, then it is appropriate to do a neurolysis of the calcaneal nerve. If the measurements for the hallux pulp are also abnormal, then tarsal tunnel syndrome is present. If the measurements for the dorsum of the foot are abnormal in addition to those for the tibial nerve, then the peroneal nerve

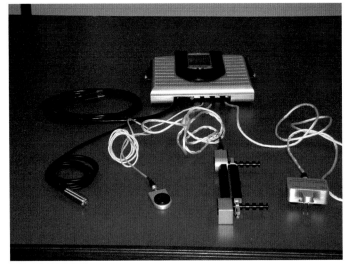

Fig. 6.5 The pressure-specified sensory device is shown with its components for grip and pinch strength, as well as the device with the two prongs, each of which is attached to a pressure transducer (silver attachment with prongs). The configuration shown is the PDA platform, which is portable between offices. No needlestick or electrical stimulation is used. Once the patient perceives the stimulus correctly, they can push a button that ends the digital signal acquisition, and therefore this is a subjective test of sensibility. *(With permission from Sensory Management Services, LLC, Towson, Maryland, USA.)*

is involved too. If the patient has back symptoms that radiate into the foot, then it is appropriate to obtain electrodiagnostic studies to be sure that there is not an L5 or L4 radiculopathy present.

Surgical technique

The painful neuroma (Box 6.1)

The common lower extremity neuromas of cutaneous nerves requiring surgical treatment are those of the SPN,[43] deep peroneal nerve,[43] saphenous nerve,[43] sural nerve,[43] and calcaneal nerve.[44] A Morton's neuroma is not a true neuroma, but a chronic nerve compression of an interdigital nerve caused by the intermetatarsal ligament, and the treatment is therefore neurolysis by division of the intermetatarsal ligament.[45] However, since most foot and ankle surgeons treat a Morton's neuroma by excision of the interdigital nerve, failure of that approach does create a true neuroma of an interdigital nerve, and this must be treated as a neuroma.[46,47] The most common lower extremity neuroma of a joint afferent is that of the deep

---

BOX 6.1 Successful treatment of the painful neuroma

Obtain complete relief of pain with a preoperative nerve block.

Remember that more than one nerve may be involved.

Remember that an afferent joint may be involved.

Remember that part of the pain may be from a compressed nerve.

Resect the painful neuroma.

Implant the proximal end of the divided nerve into a normal muscle.

BOX 6.2 Implantation of proximal end of nerve into a muscle

The proximal divided end of a cutaneous nerve will attempt to regenerate distally.

It has been demonstrated in non-human primates that a sensory nerve implanted into a normal muscle will not form a neuroma.

Choose a relatively large muscle that is proximal to a joint.

Choose a muscle with a relatively short excursion.

Implant a relatively long and loose loop of nerve into that muscle.

Do not suture the nerve into the muscle (suturing epineurium to fascia is OK).

the dorsum of the foot, either dorsomedial or dorsolateral, but not to the first webspace. The incision is centered on a vertical line that is about 10 cm proximal to the lateral malleolus (Fig. 6.6). Both the anterior and the lateral compartment must be opened since it has been demonstrated that about 25% of people will have a high division of this nerve, in either the anterior or both the anterior and the lateral compartment.[51] The branches of the SPN are injected proximally to shield the spinal cord from the pain signal associated with dividing this nerve. The nerve is cauterized distally to prevent bleeding. A segment can be sent to pathology, but this will be a normal nerve since the neuroma itself, in the scar, is not resected. Implanting the nerve proximally is done into the deep portion of the extensor digitorum communis, the largest muscle. Be careful to prevent kinking of the nerve across the intermuscular septum. The best way to do this is to excise the septum proximally for about 3 cm, being sure to cauterize the septum as it contains blood vessels. The edges of the fasciotomy of the anterior and lateral compartment are also cauterized to prevent postoperative bleeding. A suture of the epineurium into the muscle is not necessary since there is plenty of nerve length and the proximal joint (the knee) is extended during this procedure. Bupivacaine is then injected into the muscle and skin edges, and the wound is closed with 4-0 Monocryl

peroneal nerve to the sinus tarsi (Fig. 6.3A),[33,48] followed by neuromas of the medial and lateral retinacular nerves to the knee joint (Fig. 6.3B & C, Box 6.2).[49,50]

A neuroma of the SPN is most often caused by surgical procedures about the lateral ankle, either during open reduction and internal fixation of a fracture/dislocation or during a lateral ankle stabilization procedure. The physical examination usually demonstrates a painful scar with radiation into

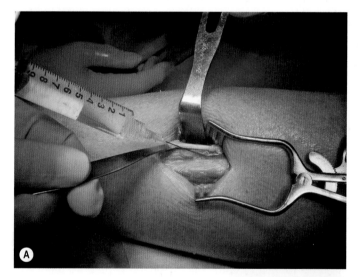

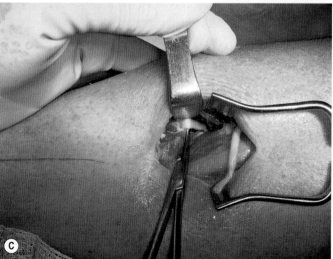

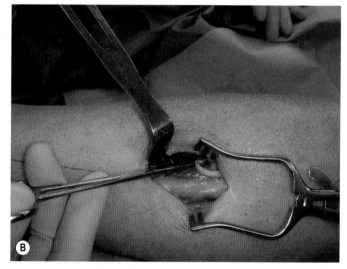

Fig. 6.6 Resection of the superficial peroneal nerve for a painful neuroma. **(A)** This is done at a distance of about 10 cm proximal to the lateral malleolus. Both the anterior and the lateral compartment must be opened, as shown here, since about 25% of people have a branch located in the anterior compartment. Note the nerve is blocked prior to dividing it to shield the spinal cord from the pain impulse. **(B)** The divided proximal end of the nerve is implanted into the underside of the extensor digitorum communis muscle, loosely, and without impinging upon the septum, a portion of which must always be resected to prevent recurrent pain. No suture is necessary. **(C)** Resection of the deep peroneal nerve requires a neurolysis of the superficial peroneal nerve and release of both the anterior and lateral compartments to prevent postoperative compartment pressure elevations related to the dissection. As is seen in this patient, sometimes this nerve and the superficial peroneal nerve must be resected in the same patient. The dissection proceeds along the interosseous membrane until the neurovascular bundle is identified against the tibia. The nerve is dissected as shown here, then injected, and a 3 cm section is resected, and the proximal end of the nerve allowed to drop back into the intermuscular space.

interrupted intradermal sutures, and 5-0 interrupted and continuous sutures to the skin.

A neuroma of the deep peroneal nerve can be due to injury over the dorsum of the foot or a stretch traction injury that causes problems with the nerve that innervates the sinus tarsi proximal to the ankle (Fig. 6.3A). In either situation, the surgical technique to resect the deep peroneal nerve is through an incision about 5 cm in length centered about 10 cm proximal to the lateral malleolus. Both the anterior and lateral compartments must be opened to gain access. A neurolysis of the SPN must be done to insure its safety. Then a dissection is done across the interosseous membrane, using the bipolar to lift the muscle origins from the membrane. The dissection continues until the tibia is reached. The retractor is then elevated, and the neurovascular bundle is visualized. The deep peroneal nerve is dissected from the artery and vein. Bupivacaine is injected into the nerve proximally (Fig. 6.6). A 2.5 cm segment of the nerve is resected, cauterizing the nerve proximally and distally with the bipolar coagulator first. The nerve proximally does not have to be implanted formally into muscle since it is surrounded by muscle. Bupivacaine is then injected into the muscle and skin edges, and the wound is closed with 4-0 Monocryl interrupted intradermal sutures, and 5-0 interrupted and continuous sutures of the skin.

A neuroma of the distal saphenous nerve is most often due to a previous surgical procedure, such as ankle arthroscopy, harvesting the saphenous vein, or a tarsal tunnel release. The incision for the neuroma resection must be proximal to the previous site of injury. Once the saphenous vein is identified, if it has not been harvested, you must explore both the sides of the vein, anteriorly and posteriorly for small (<1 mm) nerves. The saphenous nerve has often branched at this point to send the posterior branch into the region of the tarsal tunnel incision and the anterior branch into the region of the ankle arthroscopy. The nerves are each divided distally, dissected proximally, and a window opened into the fascia overlying the soleus muscle (Fig. 6.7). A tunnel is created into the muscle, and the nerves are loosely implanted. Bupivacaine is then placed, and the skin closed as above.[52]

A neuroma of the sural nerve is due to previous surgery about the ankle, most often during procedures to tighten the ankle from repeated inversion sprains, but often due to approaches used for open reduction and internal fixation of fractures. Somewhat more proximally, the nerve may have been injured during a sural nerve biopsy or excision of a skin lesion, or from a direct injury. The approach to the sural nerve must recognize that resecting the sural nerve in the leg, while technically easier, places the nerve at a location where shoes or boots will rub against the site into which the nerve is implanted, and if the nerve is implanted into the gastrocnemius muscle, then plantar flexion and extension may stimulate the nerve at the implantation site. From the practice of harvesting the sural nerve as a source of nerve graft material, there is considerable experience with leaving the proximal end of the nerve in the popliteal fossa. Therefore my preferred approach (Fig. 6.8) is to make an incision over the fibular neck, extending posteriorly into the popliteal fossa.

First, the common peroneal nerve is identified beneath the fascia then followed distally and a neurolysis completed by releasing the fascia of the peroneus muscle group and elevating these muscles to release a fibrous band, found in about 20% of normal cases.[53] Then, having safely identified and

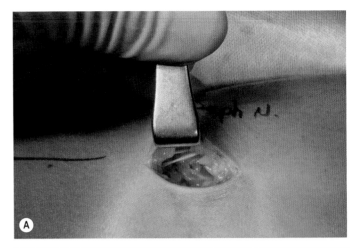

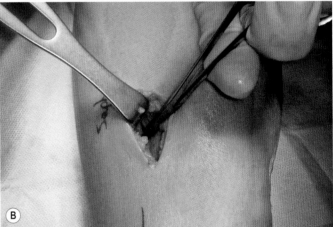

Fig. 6.7 The saphenous nerve innervates the skin of the proximal portion of the tarsal tunnel incision and can be the source of this scar hurting. Ankle arthroscopy can injure it as well. **(A)** The incision is made at the site of the Tinel's sign, and either one or two small branches will be identified, most commonly one on each side of the saphenous nerve. Each must be resected, dissected proximally, and then **(B)** a window created in the soleus fascia and the proximal ends of the nerves implanted into this muscle.

protected this nerve, the dissection proceeds into the popliteal fossa deep to this fascia. There is great variability in the sural nerve anatomy.[54] At the ankle, this is actually the common sural nerve. If the commonest variation is present, there will be one large sural nerve present with two fascicles and an artery, having been formed from a short medial sural branch from the tibial nerve and a short lateral sural nerve from the common peroneal nerve. A nerve stimulator is used to prove this is not an anomalous motor branch to a gastrocnemius or foot flexor. Then bupivacaine is infiltrated into the nerve proximally under very little pressure so that it is not forced proximally towards the sciatic nerve. The nerve is cauterized distally and proximally, the intervening 3 cm segment submitted to pathology, and the proximal end allowed to retract into the popliteal fossa proximal to the knee joint.

About 20% of the time, there will be a separate medial and a separate lateral sural nerve already present in the popliteal fossa, each going distally to join somewhere in the distal leg to form the common sural nerve. If the popliteal fossa exploration identifies a single fascicle, then you must continue the dissection into the medial part of the popliteal fossa to search for the second component. If the sural branches cannot be

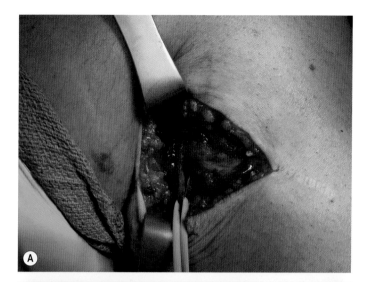

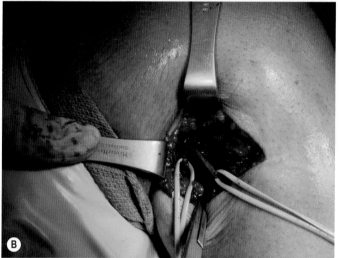

Fig. 6.8 The sural nerve ideally should be resected so its proximal end lies in the popliteal fossa. The sural nerve at the ankle is the common sural nerve. In the popliteal fossa there is one branch, the lateral sural nerve, arising from the common peroneal nerve and a second branch, the medial sural nerve, arising from the tibial nerve. **(A)** The common peroneal nerve is approached first, doing a neurolysis to protect it from harm. This large nerve is noted in the superior aspect of the incision. The incision has an extension into the popliteal fossa. The dissection goes beneath the deep fascia, and here the lateral sural nerve is usually found first, as seen in the vessel loop. **(B)** Two distinct fascicles should be identified, and a deeper dissection then demonstrates the medial sural nerve, shown in the second vessel loop. If the two branches have joined quite proximally, there may be one large nerve with two fascicles and one artery. Intraoperative electrical stimulation should be done to be sure these are not aberrant motor fascicles.

identified with certainty, then you must make an incision over the distal lateral leg, identify the common sural nerve, and gently put it under traction to identify the proximal components. In some patients, even after the proximal resection, there will still be some sensation and pain in the sural distribution. This is almost certainly due to the lateral sural nerve sending some axons along with the SPN. In this situation, there will be a posterior branch from the sural nerve that can be identified about 10 cm proximal to the ankle, and if pain is persistent after the proximal resection of the sural nerve, then a neurolysis of the SPN is indicated to identify and resect this branch.

A neuroma of the calcaneal nerve is due to an injury, most often during neurolysis of the tibial nerve during tarsal tunnel surgery or during an open or endoscopic plantar fasciotomy.[44] It is now appreciated that the posterior branch of the distal saphenous nerve innervates the part of the tarsal tunnel incision that is most proximal,[55] can be identified as a distally radiating sign anterior and proximal to this incision, and can be relieved with a block. Pain in the tarsal tunnel scar distal to this, or at the site of the medial plantar fasciotomy site, is due to a neuroma of one or more branches of the calcaneal nerve. This anatomy has been well defined.[56] For the most distal site of pain, this is a calcaneal branch that arises from the medial plantar nerve, crosses the vessels, and goes through the fascia of the abductor hallucis to enter the skin of the medial arch. This distal site is resected, and gentle traction will reveal the fascicle giving origin to it as the most anterior fascicle of the medial plantar nerve within the tarsal tunnel. This fascicle can be divided and implanted into the flexor hallucis longus muscle, the most distal muscle in the leg (Fig. 6.9). If the heel pain is more proximal, then it is due to a neuroma of one or more of the traditionally depicted branches of the lateral plantar nerve, or even the tibial nerve, arising on the posterior aspect of the tibial or lateral plantar nerve. This nerve is identified, divided, and implanted into the flexor hallucis longus muscle. This often requires microdissection, intraneural neurolysis, in order to preserve the distal sensory and motor branches of the lateral plantar nerve.

A neuroma of the interdigital plantar nerve is a true neuroma. The so-called Morton's neuroma, on the other hand, is not a true neuroma. It is a compression caused by the intermetatarsal ligament, and the treatment is neurolysis by division of this ligament.[45] If the Morton's neuroma is resected through the typical dorsal incision and pain returns, then there is a true neuroma of this plantar interdigital nerve. If there has been an injury, due to a penetrating foreign body or fracture fixation, then there is a true neuroma. The treatment of the true neuroma is to identify the correct interdigital nerve through a plantar incision in the non-weight-bearing surface of the foot.[46,47] First, the plantar fascia is split longitudinally and the flexor brevis muscle is dissected from this origin to permit inspection of both the medial and lateral plantar nerves as they exit the medial and lateral plantar tunnels. The branch to the medial side of the hallux and the branch to the lateral side of the fifth toe will not be seen as they originate more proximally. You must identify the branch to the first/second webspace and the fourth/fifth webspace and preserve these. The motor branches are identified with a nerve stimulator. The remaining branches, those to the second/third and third/fourth webspaces, can be resected if necessary depending upon the exact distal injury or previous surgery. These resected nerves then require microdissection, intraneural neurolysis, proximally until the point where they can be rotated and implanted into the arch of the foot without placing tension on the remaining intact nerves. These nerves must be implanted into the arch of the foot.

While it is hard to place a suture into the arch of the foot, this can be done, and the epineurium of the resected nerves can be attached loosely to that suture. My current preferred technique is to use a mini- (not micro-) Mitek anchor (Fig. 6.10). Remove the large suture that comes with it, and replace it with a 6-0 nylon. Suture the nerve loosely to the anchor, and then gently press the anchor into the fibrous structures of the

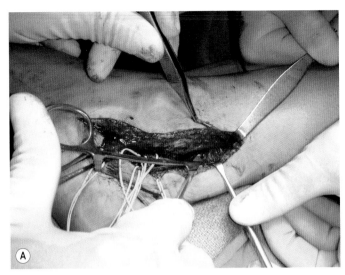
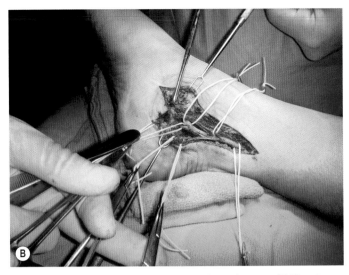

Fig. 6.9 The calcaneal nerve is resected whenever it has been injured by previous surgery, usually for plantar fasciitis, or in previous tarsal tunnel surgery. **(A)** There is often more than one calcaneal branch. Here there are branches related to the medial plantar nerve, held with vessel loops, and from the lateral plantar nerves, also held with vessel loops. The tibial nerve has had a neurolysis from the previous tarsal tunnel decompression scar. **(B)** The proximal end of the divided calcaneal nerve is ready to be implanted into the flexor hallucis longus muscle, just posterior to the tibial nerve.

arch. The nerve(s) are then suspended and covered with the plantar quadratus and the flexor brevis muscles. The plantar fascia is loosely closed with 4-0 Monocryl. The skin is closed with interrupted and continuous sutures of 4-0 nylon. Please note that about 75% of these patients also have tarsal tunnel syndrome, and this needs to be addressed at the same operation.[47]

A neuroma of the infrapatellar branch of the saphenous nerve is most often due to previous knee surgery with a midline incision. There is numbness over the lateral infrapatellar skin with a painful trigger over the insertion of the adductor muscles at Gerdy's tubercle. There can be two or three branches at this level. The surgical approach is through a longitudinal incision, identifying the branch or branches deep to the fascia, dissecting them proximally through their well-defined tunnel, injecting them with bupivacaine, dividing them distally after cauterization, and implanting them

proximally within their tunnel into one of the adductor muscles. This is done "blindly" without actually seeing the muscle (Fig. 6.11).[50]

A neuroma of the saphenous nerve in the adductor canal is are. Often, the adductor canal must be opened to identify branches of saphenous nerve at this level, especially if more distal resection failed to due to resolve the pain problem. This is often due to anomalous saphenous and/or obturator nerve branches. The nerves are first stimulated to prevent inadvertent vastus medial denervation, followed by implantation of proximal stump of resected nerve to the adductor magnus muscle (Fig. 6.12).

A neuroma of the innervation of the knee joint, the medial and/or lateral retinacular nerve is due to previous surgery, whether to reconstruct the ligaments, or endoscopy, or to total knee replacement. The innervation of the knee joint has been described and is constant (Fig. 6.3).[32] Depending upon the

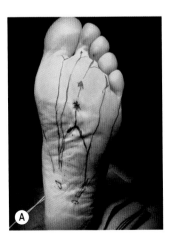
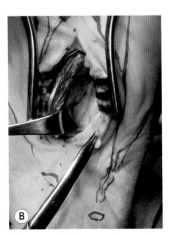
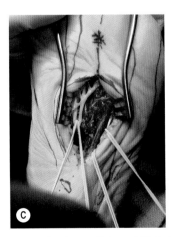
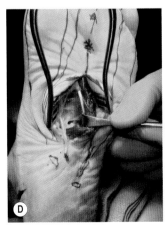

Fig. 6.10 True neuroma of the plantar interdigital nerve. **(A)** After resection of the nerve compression, incorrectly termed Morton's neuroma, a true neuroma will form. If it becomes symptomatic, it must be approached plantarly, and the presumed anatomy is drawn. **(B)** After making an incision on the non-weight-bearing skin and incising the plantar fascia, the flexor brevis is retracted laterally to dissect the medial plantar nerve. **(C)** Then the lateral plantar nerve is dissected and the branches to the neuroma, in this case, one from each, are encircled with the vessel loop. **(D)** The divided nerves have been dissected proximally, brought into the wound, and inserted onto a mini-Mitek metal suture to be implanted into the fibrous structures of the arch of the foot.

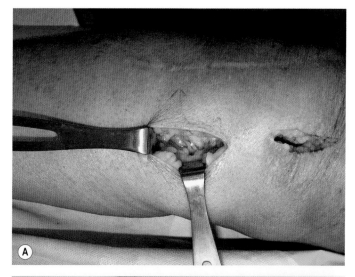

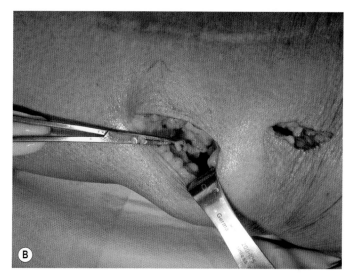

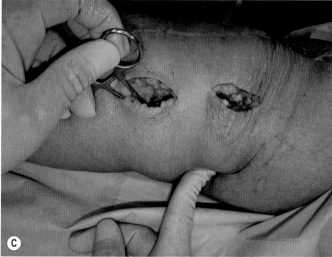

Fig. 6.11 The infrapatellar branch of the saphenous nerve is most often injured proximally during total knee arthroplasty, as shown here. **(A)** The incision is made over Gerdy's tubercle and is distal to the incision for the medial knee denervation (shown). While the leg is exsanguinated, the knee is left with some blood still present, and this helps identify the nerve adjacent to the vein. **(B)** The nerve is divided distally, cauterized to prevent bleeding from its end, and its tunnel is dissected. **(C)** The proximal end of the nerve is then pushed backwards into the tunnel with a clamp that is used to implant the nerve into an adductor muscle proximal to the knee joint.

nerve block, these nerves, usually both of them, must be resected. If the patient has had a total knee arthroplasty, the implant is not exposed. Longitudinal incisions are made midmedial and midlateral. Medially (Fig. 6.13), the medial retinaculum is opened, and just distal to the vastus medialis, the medial retinacular nerve will be identified next to the recurrent geniculate vessels. The nerve is blocked proximally, cauterized distally, and then dissected proximally where its proximal end is implanted into the vastus medialis muscle. Laterally (Fig. 6.14), the iliotibial tract is incised longitudinally, at which location it has become the lateral retinacular, and just distal to the vastus lateralis and adjacent to the recurrent geniculate vessels is the lateral retinacular nerve. It is blocked proximally with bupivacaine, cauterized distally, dissected proximally to where it goes deep to the biceps femoris insertion, cauterized again, and resected under tension and dropped into the popliteal fossa, since it originates from the sciatic nerve.[5,49,50,57]

Patients with amputation stump pain should be approached with a surgical technique analogous to those described above. The nerves most commonly involved are the saphenous, medial and lateral sural, tibial, and superficial and deep peroneal in below-knee amputation stumps. In above-knee stumps, the posterior femoral cutaneous, anterior femoral cutaneous, and sciatic nerves are most commonly involved. In all cases, the suspected nerve is approached from proximal to the site of the scar to avoid distortion of the anatomy and surgical field. Once identified, the nerve is transected and implanted into locally available muscle.[38]

A study of 100 neuroma specimens submitted to pathology revealed that in no case was there evidence of occult malignancy or anything beyond "expected" traumatic neuroma tissue. Thus we no longer routinely submit typical-appearing resected neuromas to pathology.[58]

Chronic nerve compression (Box 6.3)

The diagnosis and treatment of lower extremity chronic nerve compression are the same as that for upper extremity chronic nerve compression: only the anatomy differs. To begin treating patients with lower extremity peripheral nerve compression, it is advisable to review your anatomy and to do a cadaver dissection.

The fact that many patients with chronic nerve compression syndromes are not referred is due to many issues, not least of which is an ignorance on the part of the primary care physician of the various nerve compressions and the symptoms associated with them. There is also a degree of ignorance

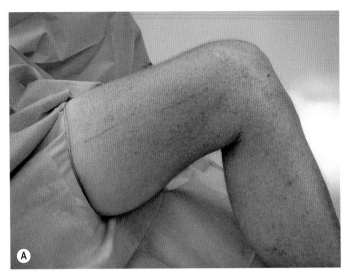

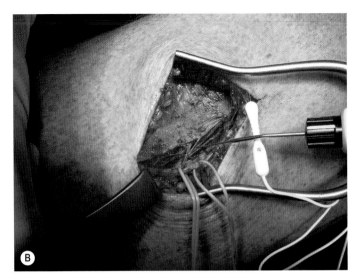

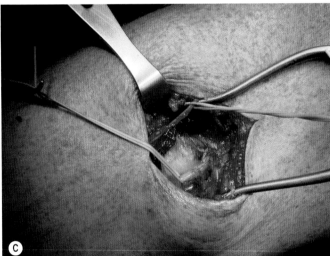

Fig. 6.12 The adductor canal should contain the saphenous nerve. Distal to the canal, this nerve divides into the infrapatellar and distal branches, but these divisions may exist within the canal already. **(A)** The incision for either decompression of the saphenous nerve or resection of the nerve is the same and is located at about the junction of the middle and distal third of the medial thigh at the site of the maximum tenderness. This patient had seven previous attempts to resect the infrapatellar branch at more distal sites. **(B)** A femoral nerve motor branch is often in the canal to the vastus medialis, and here electrical stimulation is used before resecting a nerve to be sure that just a sensory nerve is being resected. **(C)** Two distinct nerves are apparent in this patient. Each will be resected and implanted proximally into an adductor muscle.

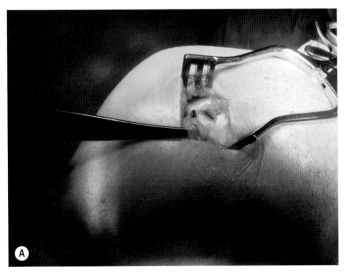

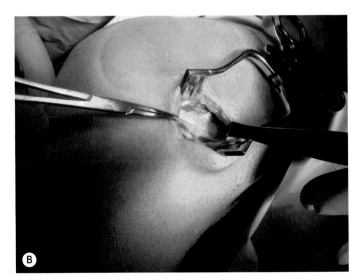

Fig. 6.13 Medial knee denervation **(A)** is approached through an incision just distal to the vastus medialis, where the medial retinaculum is opened. The medial retinacular nerve is adjacent to the recurrent geniculate vessels, which are visible because the knee region has not been exsanguinated by the tourniquet. **(B)** The medial retinacular nerve is dissected proximally from its origin beneath the vastus medialis muscle and implanted deep into this muscle.

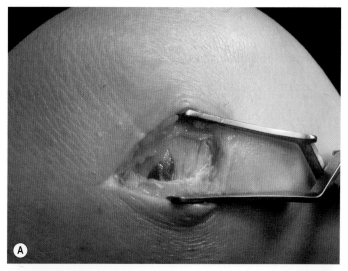

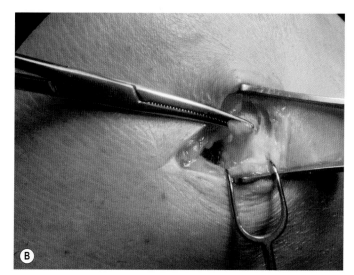

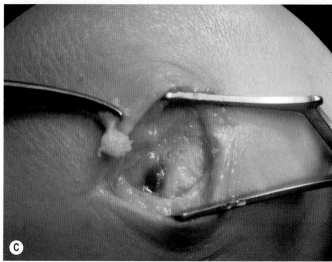

Fig. 6.14 Lateral knee denervation **(A)** is approached through an incision just distal to the vastus lateralis, by incising the iliotibial band, which is the lateral retinaculum. The lateral retinacular nerve is adjacent to the recurrent geniculate vessels, which are visible because the knee region has not been exsanguinated by the tourniquet. **(B)** The lateral retinacular nerve is dissected proximally from its origin beneath the biceps tendon and **(C)** is resected so it drops into the popliteal fossa.

to the fact that there are subspecialists who are interested in conditions of the peripheral nerve. Towards these ends, the American Society for Peripheral Nerve was initiated in 1990 and includes surgeons from plastic surgery, orthopedic surgery, and neurosurgery. Compression of the tibial and peroneal nerves were among the first to be recognized.[1] The principles used to evaluate and treat these nerves were the same as those developed to treat the upper extremity nerves and relied upon detailed neurosensory and motor evaluation and careful attention to surgical technique. Without much change, the approach today should be the same as the approach recorded then.

The most common nerve entrapment is the tibial nerve and its branches at the tarsal tunnel region. The next most frequent is entrapment of the common peroneal nerve at the fibular neck. The third most common is the deep peroneal nerve over the dorsum of the foot. The fourth most common is the SPN. Interdigital plantar nerve compression may be treated more commonly than many of the above, but most of these are treated conservatively. Calcaneal nerve entrapment may be common but often goes misdiagnosed as plantar fasciitis (Box 6.4).

Decompression of the four medial ankle tunnels has been described in detail.[1,2,35,40] An incision is made proximal and posterior to the medial malleolus extending to the end of the tarsal tunnel. If there has been no previous injury, edema, or surgery, the deep fascia is thin and immediately subjacent is the thicker, but usually loose, flexor retinaculum that used to be called the lanciate ligament. Once this has been divided the tarsal tunnel is officially released. If there is no space-occupying lesion, the surgery is done, and it is appreciated that not much has been decompressed. It is appropriate to elevate the tibial artery and veins from the tibial nerve, and evaluate if there is intraneural fibrosis or not, if there is a high division of the tibial nerve or not, and the number of calcaneal nerves originating within the tarsal tunnel. It has been demonstrated that the pressure within the tarsal tunnel of patients with neuropathy is no different than in the tarsal tunnel of cadavers.[59] The pressure here does increase with ankle plantar flexion and pronation, and this is no longer occurs after release of the flexor retinaculum. With the realization that the tarsal tunnel is analogous to the carpal tunnel in the human forearm, an operation was developed that decompressed the medial and lateral plantar tunnels and the calcaneal tunnel(s) and

Take time listening to patients' complaints: diagnosis often comes from the history.

Document the sensory and motor exam for the peripheral nerves in question.

Localize site of entrapment with your own physical diagnosis: use the Tinel's sign.

Remember that more than one nerve may be compressed in the same extremity.

Remember that the same nerve can be compressed at more than one site along its path.

Remember: an underlying systemic disease, a neuropathy, predisposes to compressions.

External neurolysis separates the peripheral nerve from surrounding structures.

Intraneural fibrosis, determined intraoperatively, requires intraneural neurolysis.

Segmental blood flow can be disrupted: respect longitudinal blood flow of the nerve.

Postoperative mobilization is a critical aspect of neurolysis.

Don't become a wrapper!

removed the septum that is between the medial and lateral plantar tunnels in order to create a larger volume for these nerves (Fig. 6.15). To accomplish this in surgery, an incision is made towards the plantar aspect of the foot and proximally to join the incision for the tarsal tunnel release (Fig. 6.16). Of course, these two incisions can be drawn and made at the same time, but it is important conceptually to appreciate that these distal tunnels are at the foot level, and the entrapment sites are not within the tarsal tunnel. The tarsal tunnel ends at the origin of the abductor hallucis. The fascia superficial to the abductor is incised, taking care not to injure the branch from the medial plantar nerve, often through this fascia, and into the skin of the medial arch. This little nerve remains unnamed, after its initial description.[53] The abductor muscle is then retracted to reveal its ligamentous origin, which forms the roof of the medial and lateral plantar tunnels. Each roof is incised. The septum between them is cauterized and then longitudinally released and excised. This septum is of variable size. Sometimes the medial, sometimes the lateral, and sometimes both plantar tunnels are small and constricting of the nerves within them. Intraoperative pressure measurements in patients with neuropathy demonstrate that these are the sites of elevated pressures, even with the ankle in the neutral position, and these pressures increase dramatically with plantar flexion and pronation. It is necessary to release each of these tunnels and excise the septum to get maximum reduction of these pressures.[59] If the patient has had complaints of heel pain and has not responded to treatment for plantar fasciitis, it is likely that the source of heel pain is compression of the calcaneal nerve(s). Often there are more than one of these and more than one tunnel. Each must be decompressed to relieve the heel pain.

Neurolysis of the common peroneal nerve at the fibular head is well known[60] (Fig. 6.17). However, it is an operation that is usually deferred by orthopedic surgeons as their literature supports expectant waiting once a foot drop develops after a hip or knee procedure, or a sports injury. From a peripheral nerve perspective, the position can be defended to do the neurolysis at 3 months or earlier.[61] In addition to foot drop, neurolysis is indicated to relieve chronic pain related to this compression. The incision does not have to be longer than 4–5 cm in a normal-sized leg. The incision is oblique in case you must extend the surgery into the popliteal fossa or distally in the leg (Fig. 6.18). There is sometimes a cutaneous nerve in this location, the lateral cutaneous nerve of the calf, and this should be preserved. The deep fascia, in the absence of trauma, will not be adherent to the common peroneal nerve. This nerve is white in the absence of glucose intolerance, in which case it is swollen and infiltrated by yellow fat, giving it almost the appearance of a lipoma. This is not a lipoma, so it is important not to excise it! The nerve is released into the popliteal fossa, but the entrapment site, again in the absence of trauma, is completely between the neck of the fibula and the overlying structures related to the peroneus muscles. Begin by releasing the superficial peroneus fascia transversely, proximally, and distally in a stellate fashion. There is often a septum between muscles that should be released, taking care not to extend the scissor tips too deeply and injure the nerve. Then retract the muscle. In cadavers, there is a fibrous band of fascia deep to the muscle in 20% of cases, but this is present to some extent in 80% of those coming to surgery,[55] and this band must be carefully released to reveal the compressed,

Intraoperative tibial nerve pressures have documented the necessity to decompress four medial ankle tunnels for the treatment of tarsal tunnel syndrome.*

Superficial peroneal neurolysis requires fasciotomy of both anterior and lateral compartments: 25% of people have a branch in the anterior compartment,† and, rarely, it can be within the septum itself.‡

Deep peroneal neurolysis almost never requires release of the anterior tarsal tunnel.

Common peroneal neurolysis potentially requires release of several structures.§

In the diabetic, there can be multiple peripheral nerve entrapments in the same limb.¶,‖

The proximal tibial nerve can be entrapped at the soleal sling – soleal sling syndrome.**,††

(Adapted from *Rosson GD, Larson AR, Williams EH, et al. Release of medial ankle compartments reduces pressure upon tibial nerve branches in patients with diabetic neuropathy. *Plast Reconstr Surg.* 2009;124:1202–1210. †Ducic I, Dellon AL, Graw KS. The clinical importance of variations in the surgical anatomy of the superficial peroneal nerve in the mid-third of the leg. *Ann Plast Surg.* 2006;56:635–638. ‡Williams E, Dellon AL. Intra-septal superficial peroneal nerve. *Microsurg.* 2007;27:477–480. §Aszmann OC, Ebmer JM, Dellon AL. The cutaneous innervation of the medial ankle: an anatomic study of the saphenous, sural and tibial nerve and their clinical significance. *Foot Ankle.* 1998;19:753–756. ¶Dellon AL. The Dellon Approach to neurolysis in the neuropathy patient with chronic nerve compression. *Handchir Mikrochir Plast Chir.* 2008;40:1–10. ‖Dellon AL. The four medial ankle tunnels; a critical review of perceptions of tarsal tunnel syndrome and neuropathy. *Clin Neurosurg.* 2009;19:629–648. **Williams EH, Dellon AL. Anatomic site for proximal tibial nerve compression: a cadaver study. *Ann Plast Surg.* 2009;62:322–325. ††Williams EH, Williams CG, Rosson GD, et al. Combined peroneal and tibial nerve palsy. *Microsurgery.* 2009;29:259–264.)

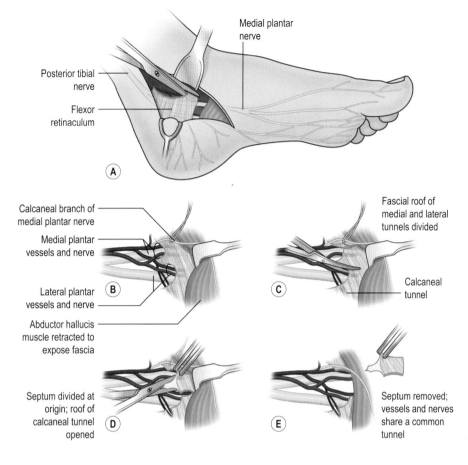

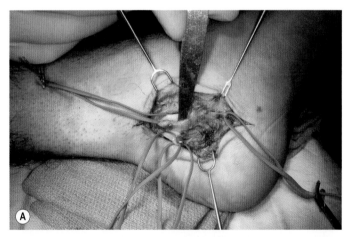

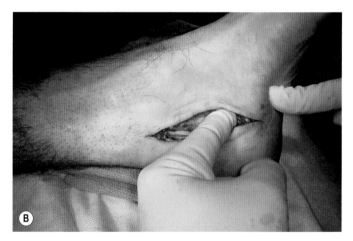

Fig. 6.15 Release of the four medial ankle tunnels. **(A)** The tarsal tunnel is opened. **(B)** The abductor hallucis is retracted, protecting the calcaneal branch from the medial plantar nerve to the arch. **(C)** The roof of the medial and the lateral plantar tunnels is incised. **(D)** The calcaneal tunnel is incised. **(E)** The septum between the medial and lateral plantar tunnels is excised. *(With Permission from Dr. Dellon.)*

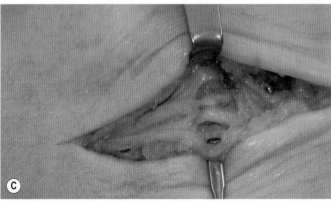

Fig. 6.16 Intraoperative views of tarsal tunnel surgery. **(A)** Left tarsal tunnel opened to demonstrate a high division of the medial and lateral plantar nerves, proximal to the tunnel, encircled with vessel loops, with the distal medial plantar nerve identified with a loop just entering the medial plantar tunnel, and from the lateral plantar nerve, a high originating calcaneal nerve, also encircled with a loop. **(B)** After release of the distal tunnels and resection of the septum, a finger can pass into the plantar aspect of the foot. **(C)** Variation in which the medial and lateral plantar nerves exchange fascicles within the tarsal tunnel. The calcaneal branch originating from the medial plantar and one from the lateral plantar are also noted.

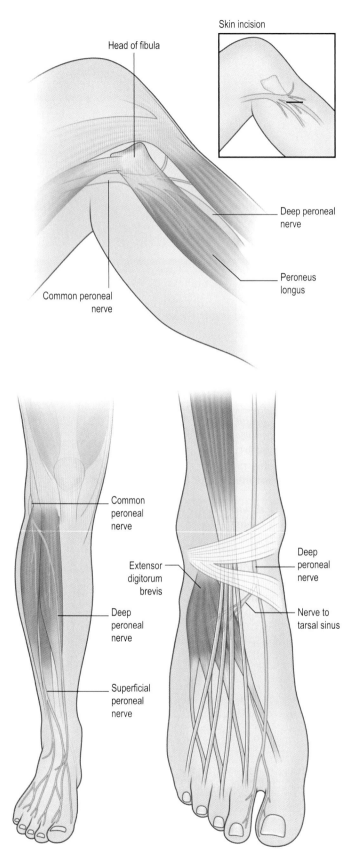

Skin incision

Head of fibula

Deep peroneal nerve

Peroneus longus

Common peroneal nerve

Common peroneal nerve

Extensor digitorum brevis

Deep peroneal nerve

Superficial peroneal nerve

Deep peroneal nerve

Nerve to tarsal sinus

Fig. 6.17 Illustration of the sites of compression of the peroneal nerves. Common peroneal nerve entrapment at the fibular neck. Superficial peroneal nerve entrapment as it exits the fascia in the distal leg. Deep peroneal nerve entrapment beneath the tendon of the extensor hallucis brevis. *(With permission from Dellon. com.)*

flattened, ischemic soft nerve below. Then the nerve is gently elevated. In about 15% of patients there will be a fibrous origin on the lateral head of the gastrocnemius.[55] This must be cauterized and divided. In a few patients the opening into the anterior compartment also needs to be widened by releasing some of the fibrous muscle origins. If there is intraneural fibrosis, a very gentle intraneural dissection can be done. Intraoperative electrical stimulation that demonstrates motor function is very useful in giving the patient with a foot drop a good prognosis upon awakening from surgery. Be sure not to get any bupivacaine on the nerve during the infiltration of the skin edges in order to avoid the patient awaking with poor motor function.

Neurolysis of the SPN is misleadingly simple. Despite all anatomy books illustrating the location of this nerve in the lateral compartment, the author has had the experience of resecting this nerve in this location, only to find that the patient still had sensation over the dorsum of the foot that could be relieved by a local block at the anterior ankle. The paradox is resolved by realizing that 25% of people have either the entire SPN in the anterior compartment, or, instead of this nerve dividing into its dorsomedial and dorsolateral branches at the level of the ankle, it has a high division and will have a branch not only in the lateral compartment but also in the anterior compartment or a subcutaneous location (Fig. 6.19).[51] Therefore it is critical that when you make an incision over the site of the Tinel's sign, which is often where there is a slight bulge as the nerve exits the fascia accompanied by some fat, that you take care not to injure a small branch to the skin at this location, and also plan to do a fasciotomy of both the anterior and the lateral compartment. This location is on average centered 10 cm proximal to the lateral malleolus but can range from 4 to 20 cm, so be prepared to lengthen your incision if you cannot find the entrapment (exit) point. This fascia is well vascularized and can lead to postoperative bruising or hematoma, and therefore each incised side/edge should be cauterized. The SPN must be released proximally until it is surrounded by muscle, and if it is pressed up against the septum, a section of septum should be cauterized and removed. If there is no nerve identified in either compartment, it may be in the septum itself, so care should be taken when dividing this septum.

Neurolysis of the deep peroneal nerve does not require opening the anterior tarsal tunnel. The anterior tarsal tunnel is a relatively large space, and unless there has been a crush injury to the ankle, or previous surgery in this region, the usual site of compression of the deep peroneal nerve is over the dorsum of the foot, not the ankle. In this location, electrodiagnostic testing will not be helpful because the sensory nerve is small and too distal. Neurosensory testing can document this sensory loss in the dorsal first webspace, and there will be a Tinel's sign beneath the extensor hallucis brevis tendon where it compresses the nerve against the underlying prominence of the junction of the first metatarsal and the cuneiform bone. This is often the site of an exostosis, and the most common site for a ganglion. The common LisFranc fracture/dislocation can also cause this compression, as will wearing high heels or tight sports shoes, such as in ice-skating. If there has been direct trauma or antecedent surgery, then it may be more appropriate to resect this nerve in the lower leg, but if not, then neurolysis is the appropriate choice. A 2 cm oblique incision is made between the first and second

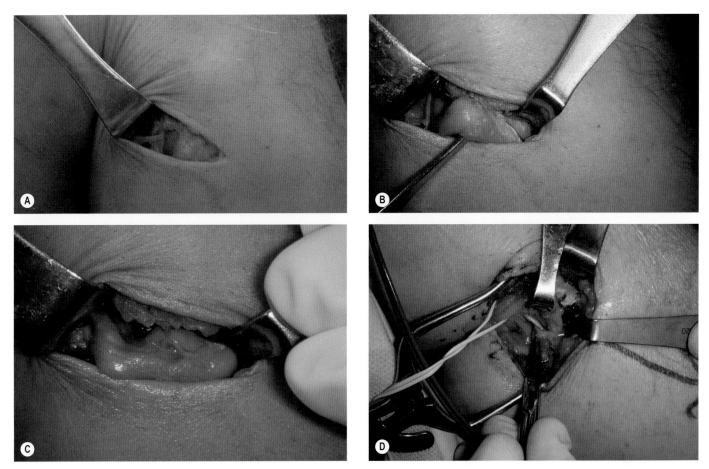

Fig. 6.18 The common peroneal nerve is **(A)** approached through an oblique incision over the fibular neck. In this location, the lateral cutaneous nerve of the calf should be protected. **(B)** The deep fascia is opened to identify the common peroneal nerve, and then the fascia of the peroneus muscles is released and these muscles are retracted. The site of compression is the fibrous band just deep to the retracted muscles. This band is carefully divided. **(C)** The swollen proximal nerve is noted. The discontinuation of the longitudinal blood supply along the nerve is noted. The flattened, compressed nerve beneath the band is noted. The deep from the superficial peroneal nerve divisions is apparent. **(D)** This view, in another patient, shown after release of the steps above, demonstrates a white fibrous band present deep to the common peroneal nerve, part of the gastrocnemius fascia, which, when present, also must be released.

metatarsals and the cuneiform bone. The SPN is protected. The deep fascia is opened overlying the visible oblique tendon or muscle belly of the extensor hallucis brevis. This tendon is resected, and the nerve is elevated from its adherence to the underlying bone.[62] There is often a clear indentation of the nerve. Proximally, the nerve is released until it is loose at the inferior extensor retinaculum. Distally, there is often a second site of compression beneath a thin fibrous band just before the nerve becomes subcutaneous in location. A small branch innervating the metatarsocuneiform joints can be observed here.

A new site of compression of the proximal tibial nerve beneath the soleal sling has been described anatomically.[63] Compression at this site is best termed "soleal sling syndrome". As the tibial nerve travels beneath the fibrous origin of the soleus muscle, it can become compressed. The sensory complaints are similar to those of tarsal tunnel syndrome except that they are not present at night. The sensory findings are the same as tarsal tunnel syndrome. The physical findings can differ in that there is weakness of toe flexion, particularly weakness in flexion of the big toe (Fig. 6.20A). The innervation of the flexor hallucis longus occurs at the level of the soleal sling, causing this finding. Neurolysis at this anatomic site can recover toe flexion.[64,65] The incision is made from the medial

popliteal fossa laterally and then inferiorly. The distal saphenous nerve travels in this location and is preserved. The fascia is released to bluntly dissect and posteriorly retract the medial head of the gastrocnemius muscle. The tibial nerve will be noted to be just beneath the soleal sling and just posterior (in front for the surgeon) of the popliteal vein (Fig. 6.20B–D). The safest approach is to cauterize the soleus overlying the course of the tibial nerve and then lift up on the deep posterior compartment fascia and release it. The tibial nerve can be separated from the popliteal vein, and the fascicles in this location can be stimulated to demonstrate recovery of toe flexion (Fig. 6.20E). Movement in the big toe can be restored.

Finally, compression of the lateral femoral cutaneous nerve (LFCN) is occasionally seen, particularly amongst those who wear heavy belts (security guards and carpenters) and kickboxers. Although some advocate division of this nerve with retraction into the retroperitoneum for treatment of meralgia paresthetica, the most sensible treatment is to begin treatment of this compression neuropathy with decompression. Neurolysis of the LFCN is accomplished by making a longitudinal incision over the proximal origin of the Sartorius muscle. Dissection is carried down to the Sartorius sheath, where the nerve is usually identified within or adjacent to the sheath. The nerve is freed from surrounding compressive structures

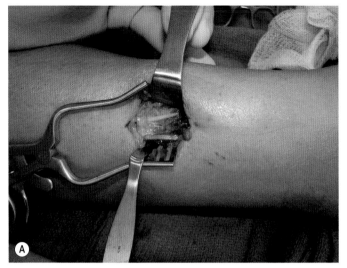

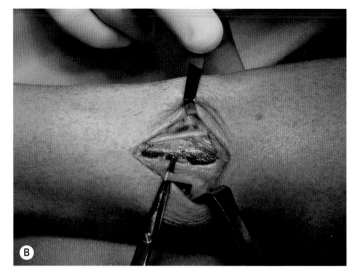

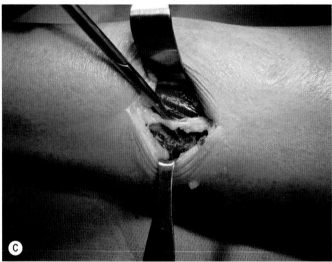

Fig. 6.19 Neurolysis of the superficial peroneal nerve must begin with the knowledge that, although this nerve is supposed to be in the lateral compartment, there is considerable variation and both the anterior and the lateral compartment must be opened. **(A)** Note a branch of this nerve in each compartment. If no nerve is found in either compartment, carefully open the septum **(B)** as the nerve can be intraseptal. **(C)** In some patients, one of the two branches may already be subcutaneously located.

proximally up to and beneath the inguinal ligament, taking care to avoid the deep circumflex iliac vessels at the most proximal portion of the dissection.[66,67]

Postoperative care/rehabilitation

The painful neuroma

The patient is allowed to ambulate immediately after surgery. The patient is instructed to change chairs and walk around the bed every 2 h to minimize the risk of postoperative venous thrombosis. A cane or walker can be utilized. In general, crutches are discouraged, as the patient may fall, and hurt the hands and armpits. Walking should not be for distances longer than about 50 feet (15.25 m). For distances greater than that, a wheelchair is encouraged. Following final suture removal, the patient begins a "water walking program", beginning with 10–15 minutes a day, working up to about an hour a day, doing this 4–6 times a week (Fig. 6.21B). This is a form of desensitization for the lower extremity. A therapist should not touch the leg. The patient should not touch the

place where the nerve proximally has been implanted. That site remains tender in about half of patients. The water walking will send new stimuli to the cortex to cause reorganization of the cortex, and facilitate learning about the new sensation, or lack thereof, following the denervation of that skin territory. Water therapy will help the 50% of people in whom collateral sprouting from the adjacent intact nerve (e.g., from the sural and deep peroneal and saphenous if the SPN has been resected) causes paresthesias during the 3rd–12th week postoperatively. Once the water walking and swimming have been accomplished, progression to the stationary bicycle and the elliptical machine can begin. Treadmill use is discouraged. By the fourth or fifth postoperative week, the patient can resume usual exercises again. At this point, if the patient had been habituated to narcotics, a withdrawal program can be initiated under the care of a certified pain management specialist.[28]

Chronic nerve compression

The same time sequence for dressing change and suture removal is used for these procedures as for the painful

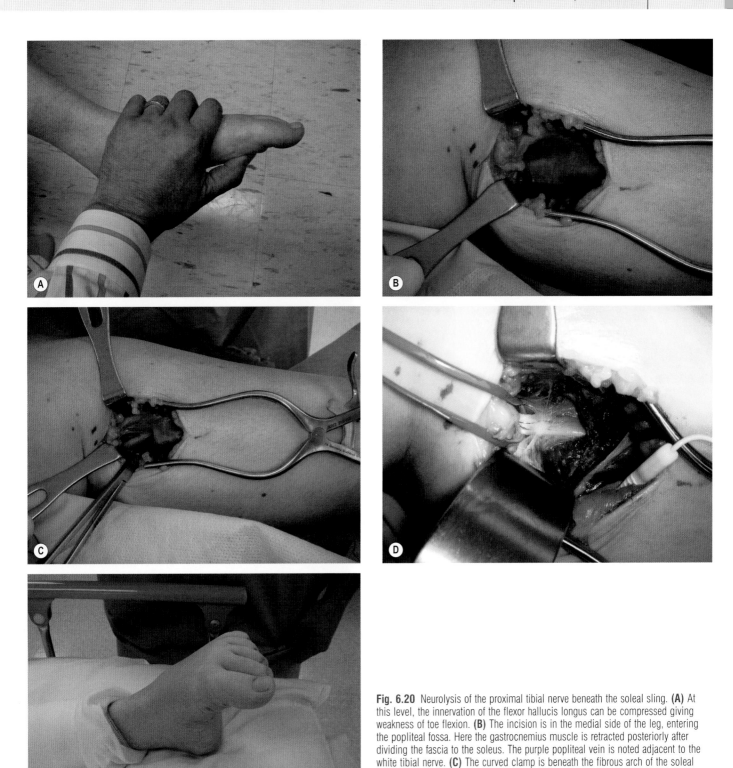

Fig. 6.20 Neurolysis of the proximal tibial nerve beneath the soleal sling. **(A)** At this level, the innervation of the flexor hallucis longus can be compressed giving weakness of toe flexion. **(B)** The incision is in the medial side of the leg, entering the popliteal fossa. Here the gastrocnemius muscle is retracted posteriorly after dividing the fascia to the soleus. The purple popliteal vein is noted adjacent to the white tibial nerve. **(C)** The curved clamp is beneath the fibrous arch of the soleal sling that is compressing the tibial nerve. **(D)** After bipolar cauterization of the soleus, the fibrous arch can be divided along with the posterior compartment fascia to release the nerve and, if needed, the posterior compartment. Note the difference in color and vascularity of the tibial nerve proximal and distal to the compression site. **(E)** Note flexion of the big toe has been achieved postoperatively.

neuroma procedures. Since it is critical that the peripheral nerve, which has been neurolysed, gets immediate mobilization, it is imperative that the patient walks immediately after the operative procedure. A walker is recommended so that the patient can hold on with both hands, carry some weight on the foot that had the surgery, and not lose balance and fall

(Fig. 6.21A). For walking, on the side that had the surgery, the operated extremity begins its step by lifting from the knee and then leaning forward. The ankle is often prevented from moving too much, especially in those patients who have had tarsal tunnel decompression, so that ankle movement does not pull out the sutures. This is so critical in the patient with

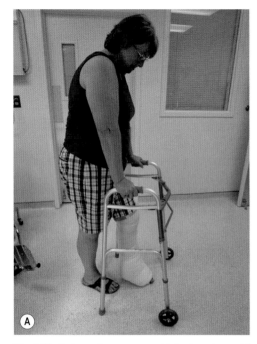
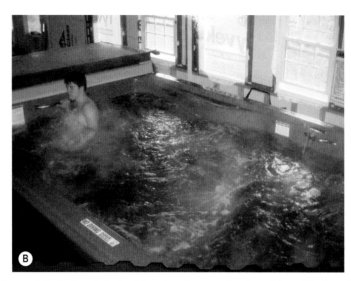

Fig. 6.21 Postoperative management following release of the four medial ankle tunnels for tarsal tunnel syndrome requires immediate mobilization of the tibial nerve and its branches, but sufficient support so that the sutures do not pull out. **(A)** The extensive soft bulky supportive dressing applied to the foot and ankle permits immediate ambulation with a walker, with the patient being reminded to lift from the knee and hip. This is continued for 3 weeks. **(B)** Following removal of the sutures at 3 weeks, a water therapy program is begun and progressed. This is helpful not only for those patients having nerve decompressions but, and perhaps even more importantly, for those patients following neuroma resection for complex regional pain syndrome.

neuropathy who usually cannot tell that ankle movement is tearing out the sutures. It is precisely for this reason that the large Robert Jones, bulky, ankle dressing is used to protect the ankle suture line in patients with insensitive feet.

The walker is used for 3 weeks. Once the sutures are out, then the same rehabilitation with water therapy is used with the same schedule as given above for the patient who has had a painful neuroma excised (Fig. 6.21B).[28]

Outcomes, prognosis, and recurrence

The painful neuroma

As a general rule, if the patient responds with pain relief after a nerve block of the suspected nerve, or nerves, whether cutaneous or joint afferent, then the prognosis is 90% that the patient will achieve good to excellent relief of pain.[4,5,43,44,46–50,52] Failure to obtain the desired result is usually due to the presence of another injured nerve, whose presence was masked by the severity of the original pain. A clue to this is the original pain level of 8–10 not being reduced to 1 or 2 after the block. Of course, not all surgery can be 100% successful, but neuroma resection with muscle implantation is highly predictable and successful. It is "OK to lose your nerve". The historic concern over "anesthesia dolorosa" is unfounded today if the nerve block is successful, and if the muscle implantation is maintained. The most common nerve to require repeat surgery is the SPN, which may pull from the extensor digitorum communis muscle during vigorous athletic jumping or repeat ankle injury. If this occurs, the nerve must be resected at a more proximal level, additional septum resected, and the nerve implanted again into the same muscle.

Failure to treat a painful neuroma also carries a risk of poor outcome. Untreated chronic pain may sensitize the peripheral and central nervous system, leading over time to wind-up and centrally-mediated pain that can no longer be effectively treated by surgery of the peripheral nervous system.[68,69] Untreated painful neuroma may in fact result in CRPS type II. Patients who are not treated and continue to live with chronic pain that they cannot effectively cope with also risk marginalization, psychological sequelae such as depression, and long-term dependence on pain medications. For all of these reasons, it is important that patients with chronic postoperative or post-traumatic pain lasting beyond the expected time course be evaluated in a timely fashion by a peripheral nerve surgeon after other potential causes for the pain have been ruled out.

Chronic nerve compression

Success for neurolysis approaches 90% in the lower extremity,[45,51,60,64,62–71] as it does in the upper extremity. Table 6.5 contains a review of the results for tarsal tunnel decompression. Prognosis is based upon the degree of axonal loss. If there is just demyelination, with primarily intermittent symptoms and some weakness, the success can be above 90%, and recovery of function can occur in the early postoperative period. Sometimes motor function recovers dramatically in the recovery room. If there is severe axonal loss, with loss of two-point discrimination, with muscle wasting or paralysis, then the success may not only be much lower, but recovery of function may extend over 1 year, and the nerve regeneration may be painful. If there are comorbidities, like diabetes or another form of neuropathy, the same general guidelines apply, but the expected recovery is 80% relief of pain, 80%

Table 6.5 Results of tarsal tunnel decompression

Clinical study (n)*		Excellent	Good	Poor	Failure	Worse
Tarsal tunnel syndrome						
Byank*	(51)	26%	53%	12%		8%
Pfeiffer and Crachhilo†	(32)	15%	29%	18%		32%
Mullick and Dellon‡	(88)	82%	11%	5%		2%

*n = number of tarsal tunnel decompressions in study.
(Adapted from *Byank RP, Curtis MJ. Diagnosing tarsal tunnel syndrome. *Compl Orthoped*. 1992;7:202–206. †Pfeiffer WH, Cracchiolo A. Clinical results after tarsal tunnel decompression. *J Bone Joint Surg*. 1994;76:1222–1230. ‡Mullick T, Dellon AL. Results of treatment of four medial ankle tunnels in tarsal tunnels syndrome. *J Reconstr Microsurg*. 2008;24:119–126.)

recovery of sensation, plus prevention of ulceration and amputation.[35,40,72] Unless there has been a new trauma, recurrence of symptoms is unusual once successful recovery has occurred. For patients in whom the first neurolysis was not successful, repeat surgery can be done, but with a reduced expectation for success[73] and with an increased risk for complications.

The prognosis for recovery of untreated chronic compression neuropathy is invariably poor. Delay of intervention leads to progressive irreversible changes that combine to inhibit nerve regrowth, including atrophy of the muscle and neuromuscular junction as well as a reduced capacity of the Schwann cells to support regenerating axons.[74–76] Currently, timely surgical decompression is the only means of preventing these degenerative changes.

Complications

Complication rates in peripheral nerve surgery are typically very low. A retrospective review of 5219 procedures found an overall complication rate of 2.91%, with a minor complication rate of 2.47%, an intermediate complication rate of 0.44%, and a major complication rate of 0%. Minor complications included seroma, superficial wound dehiscence, or localized wound infection. Intermediate complications include full wound dehiscence or infection, hematoma, or DVT. Severe complications such as unintentional nerve injury, injury to adjacent structures, limb loss, or mortality should never occur with proper knowledge of anatomy and careful technique.[77]

🌐 Access the complete reference list online at **http://www.expertconsult.com**

2. Dellon AL. *Pain Solutions*. Lightning Source Publications: Dellon. com; 2007. *A comprehensive review, told as patient vignettes, with historical background, anatomic illustrations, intraoperative photos of real patients with problems related to neuropathy, joint pain, Morton's neuroma, pain stimulators, and much more. Only available online.*

4. Dellon AL. Partial joint denervation I: wrist, shoulder, elbow. *Plast Reconstr Surg*. 2009;123:197–207.

5. Dellon AL. Partial joint denervation II: knee, ankle. *Plast Reconstr Surg*. 2009;123:208–217. *Partial joint denervation is the concept of preservation of joint function and relief of joint pain by interrupting neural pathways that transmit the pain message from the joint to the brain. This review article focuses on the application of these principles to the knee and ankle and demonstrates that the results obtained for partial joint denervation of the upper extremity can be successfully applied to the knee and ankle joints.*

30. Weber RA, Schuchmann JA, Albers JH, et al. A prospective blinded evaluation of nerve conduction velocity versus pressure-specified sensory testing in carpal tunnel syndrome. *Ann Plast Surg*. 2000;45:252. *A level I study comparing neurologists' use of the classic electrodiagnostic test (using painless, non-invasive neurosensory testing) with the Pressure-Specified Sensory Device, demonstrating that the same*

information is obtainable without pain (p <0.001), yet with the same sensitivity and specificity. This approach is used in the lower extremity.

35. Dellon AL. The Dellon Approach to neurolysis in the neuropathy patient with chronic nerve compression. *Handchir Mikrochir Plast Chir*. 2008;40:1–10. *A systematic review of the literature demonstrating 80% relief of pain, 80% recovery of sensation, prevention of ulceration and amputation when the Dellon triple nerve decompression is done in patients with neuropathy plus superimposed compression of the tibial nerve in the tarsal tunnels and compression of the peroneal nerves.*

41. Dellon AL. Neurosensory testing. In: Slutsky D, ed. *Master Skills in Nerve Repair; Tips and Techniques*. Elsevier; 2008:575–586.

43. Dellon AL, Aszmann OC. Treatment of dorsal foot neuromas by translocation of nerves into anterolateral compartment. *Foot Ankle*. 1998;19:300–303.

45. Dellon AL. Treatment of Morton's neuroma as a nerve compression: the role for neurolysis. *J Am Podiatr Med Assoc*. 1992;82:399.

47. Wolfort S, Dellon AL. Treatment of recurrent neuroma of the interdigital nerve by neuroma resection and implantation of proximal nerve into muscle in the arch. *J Foot Ankle Surg*. 2001;40:404–410.

7

Skeletal reconstruction

Arash Momeni, Stephen J. Kovach III, and L. Scott Levin

 Access video content for this chapter online at expertconsult.com

SYNOPSIS

- The reconstruction of defects of the appendicular and axial skeletal structures has been an evolving clinical endeavor that has mirrored our understanding of the basic science of bone biology.
- This chapter serves as an overview of the basic tenets of bone biology and the methods of skeletal reconstruction, and a discussion of the most common skeletal defects and how the reconstructive surgeon can reasonably approach them.
- Perhaps no other clinical tool has had as much of an impact on the ability to reconstruct skeletal defects as the microsurgical transfer of bone. Thus no chapter on skeletal reconstruction would be complete without a review of the microsurgical principles of bony reconstruction.
- The reader should understand how to approach skeletal defects and the algorithm for their reconstruction upon reading this chapter.

 Access the Historical Perspective section and Figs. 7.2, 7.3, and 7.6 online at
http://www.expertconsult.com

Introduction

Skeletal reconstruction remains a challenging problem for both orthopedic and plastic surgeons. While skeletal defects may be encountered in isolation, such as after oncologic resection, more commonly coexisting soft-tissue defects complicate the clinical picture, such as after trauma or chronic infections. Additionally, traumatic injuries that have been treated with definitive fixation may subsequently develop a nonunion (either aseptic or septic) requiring bony debridement and subsequent reconstruction of the skeletal defect. The majority of these skeletal defects are of the appendicular skeleton, but the reconstructive surgeon may also be called upon to reconstruct defects of the axial skeleton or pelvis. Successful reconstruction requires not only a comprehensive assessment of the patient and existing defect as well as meticulous technical execution of the surgical procedure, but also demands a thorough understanding on the underlying biology of osseous healing. This chapter will serve as an overview regarding skeletal reconstruction.

Biology of bone healing and bone grafts

While tissue *repair* is the mode by which most other tissues and organs heal, bone has an incredible restorative capacity that allows true *regeneration* with return to its pre-injured state.[1] Understanding the basic requirements necessary for uninterrupted bone healing to occur is critical. Although the importance of adequate immobilization has been known for thousands of years, we are beginning to understand other biologic components critical to successful bone healing, such as the importance of progenitor cells and establishment of a favorable scaffold, as well as adequate perfusion. Disruption of any of these components invariably results in impeded bone healing.

Bone healing is a complex process that requires a coordinated interplay of local and systemic progenitor cells (i.e., mesenchymal stem cells [MSCs]), production of an extracellular matrix for support and proliferation of MSCs, as well as secretion of a variety of growth factors.[2-7] The most thoroughly investigated group of growth factors are certainly members of the transforming growth factor beta (TGF-β) superfamily known as bone morphogenetic proteins (BMPs).[8-13]

Understanding these biologic principles is important as they have direct therapeutic consequences. An example is the patient presenting with a nonunion after osteosynthesis. Using radiographic imaging a nonunion may be classified as hypertrophic, oligotrophic, or atrophic. While the presence of hypertrophic nonunion is indicative of excessive motion as a result of inadequate fixation, the diagnosis of atrophic nonunion poses greater therapeutic challenges. The former clinical scenario reflects adequate healing capacity and is best treated by rigid fixation, while the latter requires additional measures to augment local bone healing, such as bone grafting.[14,15]

A profound understanding of the mechanisms by which bone grafts and bone substitutes facilitate bone healing is mandatory to allow the reconstructive surgeon to make the correct choices when attempting reconstruction. Bone grafts heal through a variety of mechanisms known as osteoconduction, osteoinduction, and osteogenesis.

Osteoconduction represents the ingrowth of MSCs, capillaries, and perivascular tissues from the recipient site into the transplanted graft, i.e., scaffold. Osteoinduction is the recruitment of MSCs with subsequent differentiation to chondroblasts and osteoblasts. This process is modulated by growth factors, e.g., BMPs. Osteogenesis is synthesis of new bone by viable cells within the graft.[15,16]

Autologous bone grafting is considered the gold standard as it allows osteoconductive, osteoinductive, and osteogenic mechanisms to augment bone healing. Differences exist, however, as to the distribution of these various mechanisms, based on the type of graft chosen for reconstruction. Autologous bone grafts may be classified as non-vascularized (i.e., conventional cancellous and cortical bone grafts) and vascularized bone grafts.

Cancellous bone grafting is certainly the most commonly used mode of bone grafting and is characterized by a remarkable osteogenic potential, which is due to the large number of osteocytes and osteoblasts that remain viable due to the rapid revascularization that occurs as long as the graft is placed in a well-vascularized wound bed. Its drawback, however, is its limited structural integrity. In contrast, cortical bone grafts are strong constructs. However, the density of the cortex results in slower revascularization of the graft. As such, these grafts incorporate by a process known as "creeping substitution", which represents gradual resorption of the graft with subsequent deposition of new bone (i.e., osteoconduction).

Vascularized bone grafts are segments of bone that are harvested with their vascular pedicle. Thus after successful transfer and revascularization at the recipient site, cells within the graft survive and heal to the surrounding bone by primary and secondary bone healing, rather than by "creeping substitution". Advantages of vascularized bone grafts include the fact that these are live constructs that are capable of growth and hypertrophy in response to stress, load bearing (Wolff law), vascularity, and additional environmental signals.

The perfusion pattern of any given bone determines the technique of flap harvest. The blood supply to long bones is derived from multiple sources. The nutrient artery supplies the marrow and inner cortex, while the periosteal vessels supply the outer cortex of the diaphysis. Additional metaphyseal and epiphyseal vessels traverse the cortex and have an anastomotic arcade with the nutrient artery.[17] For example, a long-bone free flap, such as the fibula, can remain viable with its periosteal blood supply only.

The dual blood supply of long bones is contrasted by the predominantly periosteal blood supply of membranous bone. An example is the free iliac crest flap, which is based on a periosteal pedicle derived from the deep circumflex iliac artery (DCIA) and was first described by Taylor.[18,19]

In contrast to autologous bone, the reconstructive surgeon has the option to use allografts for the purpose of skeletal reconstruction. Drawbacks of autologous bone, such as limited autogenous supply of bone and donor site morbidity, are thus averted. Allografts are functionally strong, but their incorporation remains questionable, due to the fact that they exhibit merely osteoconductive properties. As they do not contain viable cells they are not osteogenic; however, they may have osteoinductive properties when combined with growth factors, e.g., BMPs. Also, they have been associated with relatively high complication rates that include nonunion, fracture, and infection, all of which necessitate their removal.[20–22] There are methods to combine the initial structural integrity of the allograft with a vascularized autograft to take advantage of both methods.[23,24] This will be discussed in a subsequent section.

In summary, the decision regarding the mode of bone grafting depends on a variety of different factors, including the anatomic location and 3D configuration of the defect, soft-tissue envelope, limb vascularity, overall patient condition, as well as availability of donor bone. An ideal reconstruction is characterized by rapid bone healing and minimal donor site morbidity, ultimately resulting in functional restoration of the extremity.

Patient evaluation

It is the reconstructive surgeon's responsibility to apply these basic science principles to the specific clinical situation that is encountered in treating patients with skeletal defects. Injuries to the appendicular and axial skeleton are commonly encountered at most major medical centers. Both plastic and orthopedic surgeons are called upon to treat these challenging patients on a routine basis. These patients are best served with the "orthoplastic" approach in a multidisciplinary setting.[32,33] Members of this multidisciplinary team supporting the orthopedic and plastic surgeons include prosthetists, physical therapists, vascular surgeons, infectious disease physicians, musculoskeletal radiologists, and nursing staff well-versed in patients undergoing extremity and skeletal reconstruction and convalescence.

As with any clinical problem, the approach begins with the clinical assessment of the patient. One must consider the nature of the defect, including its anatomic position, length of bony defect, associated injuries of the ipsilateral and contralateral extremity, concomitant traumatic injuries, potential for a functional recovery, patient compliance, and cost associated with reconstruction, both financial and social. Furthermore, potentially available donor sites for vascularized and non-vascularized bone grafts should be determined. While this may seem straightforward, numerous injured patients, e.g., polytrauma patients, may have limited donor sites. Both form and function must be considered when establishing a reconstructive plan.

One of the key concerns in reconstruction of the appendicular skeleton is the blood supply to the bone graft. In non-vascularized bone transfer the condition of the wound bed, i.e., its vascularity, determines the likelihood of bone graft survival. If there is poor blood supply to the wound bed, the likelihood of success of a non-vascularized bone graft is poor despite meticulous surgical technique. It is important to determine, however, if the poorly vascularized wound bed is secondary to a reversible, i.e., treatable, flow-limiting lesion.

An intervention by vascular surgery may successfully address the underlying problem in these cases, thus allowing converting the local environment into a more favorable one. As such, a thorough vascular exam should be part of every extremity examination. In patients with an abnormal vascular exam, angiography is indicated to discern the vascular anatomy and to determine if there is a reversible flow-limiting lesion. Furthermore, evaluation of the vascular anatomy is critical prior to performing a vascularized bone graft, as adequate inflow and outflow vessels are mandatory to achieve success.

In patients with an abnormal vascular exam with weakly palpable or non-palpable pulses, it is the authors' preference to obtain a formal arteriogram to aid in preoperative planning. It has been the convention to obtain an invasive arteriogram to delineate the vascular anatomy.[34] However, invasive arteriograms are not a morbid-free procedure, and computed angiography has become widely available. CT angiography has the advantage of concomitantly assessing the venous system, skeletal defect, as well as surrounding soft tissues.[35] Patients with known vascular disease and limited inflow with soft-tissue defects can be successfully reconstructed with free tissue transfer with acceptable flap success rates if patient selection is appropriate.[36,37]

Perhaps the most challenging question when evaluating patients with skeletal defects, particularly in the acute traumatic setting, is who should be offered salvage versus amputation. Much of the data regarding the utility of limb salvage has been derived from the Lower Extremity Assessment Project. Functional outcomes of amputation versus limb salvage for limb-threatening injuries have been extensively studied.[38–47] Outcomes between patients undergoing reconstruction and those receiving amputation are equivalent. Those patients who elect to undergo reconstruction for traumatic skeletal defects will require an increased number of operative interventions compared to those patients undergoing amputations, but if patients are carefully selected, they have the potential to have a superior functional outcome. Obviously, the overwhelming majority of patients desire to keep the injured extremity if at all possible.[39,48] Ultimately, the decision to proceed with complex extremity reconstruction must be individualized to the patient and his or her potential for recovery.

Methods of skeletal reconstruction

Patients requiring skeletal reconstruction are frequently readily identified, such as those with traumatic skeletal defects, osteomyelitis, or neoplasms requiring osseous resection. More challenging clinical situations involve patients who have bone loss, e.g., osteoradionecrosis, as a result of prior oncologic treatment or those with recalcitrant nonunion following a fracture. What is not always straightforward is how to achieve a stable skeletal reconstruction within the available means. To maximize the potential for skeletal stability, one must have a thorough understanding of the methods of skeletal reconstruction and the limitations of each approach.

A variety of treatment modalities exist. These include conventional, i.e., non-vascularized, cancellous or corticocancellous bone grafts, non-vascularized allografts, pedicled or free vascularized bone grafts (with or without associated soft-tissue component), and distraction osteogenesis. These modalities are not mutually exclusive and may be combined to extend the capability of one approach alone.

Bone grafting

Traditionally, corticocancellous bone grafts had been used for bone defects that are 5 cm or less in length. The main tenets of bone grafting were put forth by Kazanjian in 1952 and still hold true today.[49] These principles include adequate blood supply to the recipient site to ensure survival of the graft, establishment of bone-to-bone contact, immobilization at the fracture/defect site through the use of rigid fixation, and absence of infection. For defects greater than 5–6 cm in length, graft resorption typically prevents complete healing.[50,51]

Interestingly, Masquelet described a technique that has been used with success for intercalary defects ranging from 5 to 24 cm.[52] This two-stage approach involves inducing a bioactive membrane that permits reconstruction of large defects with non-vascularized autograft.[52,53] The principles of reconstruction with this technique begin with the basic tenets of wound preparation that include radical debridement of devitalized tissue and delineation of the intercalary defect. Next, a cement spacer is inserted into the bony defect and, in cases of a deficient soft-tissue envelope, soft-tissue reconstruction performed with a muscle or skin flap. In a second stage, approximately 6–8 weeks later, the spacer is removed and the membrane that is induced by the spacer is left in place. The resultant cavity is then packed with cancellous bone graft derived from the iliac crest. The induced membrane is then closed over the autograft, resulting in a contained system. The induced membrane has been shown to have biologic properties, including a rich vascular network, a synovial-like epithelial lining, as well as biologic activity as evidenced by its ability to secrete growth factors such as vascular endothelial growth factor (VEGF) and transforming growth factor beta-1 (TGF-β-1). Additionally, extracts from the membrane have been shown to stimulate bone marrow cell proliferation and differentiation to osteoblastic cell lines.[54]

Donor sites for bone grafts have evolved over time. In the early 20th century, the tibia was the preferred site for cortical as well as cancellous bone grafts. However, large grafts cannot be obtained from the tibia without a significant donor defect and the risk of chronic pain at the donor site as well as secondary pathologic fractures. Non-vascularized autografts are now harvested routinely from the iliac crest. The iliac crest contains an abundant source of cancellous corticocancellous bone for grafting that may be harvested from an anterior or posterior approach depending on the positioning needs of the patient. In general, 50 cc of bone graft can be obtained from either the anterior or posterior approach, which is typically adequate for defects amenable to reconstruction with cancellous grafts.

Vascularized bone transfer

Intercalary defects that are larger than 5 cm typically require reconstruction with vascularized bone. Vascularized bone grafts have significant advantages over their non-vascularized counterparts.[55] Additionally, composite osteocutaneous flaps permit single-stage microsurgical reconstruction of both bone and soft-tissue defects. A variety of parameters influence the decision-making when choosing a free vascularized graft.

These include pedicle length, available bone stock, graft dimension, its osteogenic potential, and ease of harvest at the time of surgery if concomitant orthopedic procedures are to be performed.

Since it was first described in 1975, the fibula has become the preferred source for vascularized bone in reconstruction of defects of the axial and appendicular skeleton.[56] The fibula is well suited for use as a free vascularized bone graft given the length of bone that can be harvested, the ability to perform multiple osteotomies, its reliable anatomy, as well as its acceptable donor site morbidity.[56] Up to 26 cm of vascularized bone can be harvested from the fibula in the typical adult patient (Fig. 7.1). The fibula is triangular in shape and primarily a cortical bone with a small medullary component. These anatomic characteristics allow it to resist angular and rotational stress and to remodel with graduated weight-bearing in the postoperative period after reconstruction of intercalary defects. The blood supply to the diaphysis of the fibular is based on an endosteal and musculoperiosteal component, which is provided by the peroneal artery and vein. In a small number of patients the peroneal artery is the dominant supply to the lower extremity.[57] Peroneus magnus may not be evident on preoperative clinical exam, but if it is encountered intraoperatively, the fibular harvest should be abandoned so as not to render the foot ischemic. If the patient has an abnormal pulse exam or has a traumatized extremity that suggests possible underlying vascular injury, preoperative vascular imaging is indicated. A skin paddle may be harvested with the fibula to reconstruct associated soft-tissue defects concomitantly. Perforators supplying the skin paddle exit through the posterior crural septum and are found in greatest concentration between the middle third and the distal third of the fibula (Fig. 7.2 ⊙).[58]

Fig. 7.2 appears online only.

The blood supply to the epiphysis of the fibular head is derived from the anterior tibial artery.[59] If epiphyseal growth, i.e., longitudinal growth, of the fibula is needed for skeletal reconstruction in the immature skeleton, the epiphyseal blood supply needs to be included in the graft.[60] However, there is no need to harvest both pedicles if only a small, proximal diaphyseal segment is needed for reconstruction as survival of this segment is ensured via small musculoperiosteal branches. If a significant length of the fibular diaphysis is needed, then both the anterior tibial and peroneal arteries must be included with the graft to ensure adequate survival of the segments (Fig. 7.3 ⊙).

Fig. 7.3 appears online only.

Several important technical aspects must be followed during the harvest. A thin cuff of muscle (1 mm) is usually left attached to the graft in order to preserve the periosteal circulation to the bone segment. Furthermore, the distal 6 cm of the fibula should be preserved in adults in order to maintain ankle stability. If there is a question of ankle stability following fibular harvest in children, a syndesmotic screw should be placed for additional stability of the ankle joint and to prevent hindfoot valgus deformity with growth.

Harvest of the fibula is not without consequences. Large series have demonstrated persistent long-term morbidity, including pain, ankle instability, and weakness, after free fibula harvest. In fact, up to 11% of patients may have persistent pain in the donor leg.[61] In a prospective cohort study, 17% of patients were found to have long-term morbidities postoperatively. These included ankle instability (4%), leg weakness (8%), great toe contracture (9%), and decreased ankle mobility (12%).[62] While leg weakness rarely causes a disability in the patient's postoperative functioning, comparative isokinetic testing does demonstrate a significant decrease in strength at the knee and ankle after fibula harvest.[63] Despite these potential complications, however, the combination of surgical experience, meticulous surgical technique, and comprehensive postoperative care minimize the potential for untoward long-term sequelae.[64]

A variety of additional flaps are available to the reconstructive surgeon. While this will not serve as an exhaustive review of vascularized bone flaps, there are additional flaps worth mentioning due to their common use in vascularized bone reconstruction.

The scapular vascular axis is a well-established source of expendable skin, fascia, muscle, and bone for use in microsurgical reconstruction of defects requiring bone and soft tissue in complex 3D relationships. Composite bone and soft-tissue flaps derived from the subscapular vascular axis include the osteocutaneous scapular flap (based on the circumflex scapular artery), the "latissimus/bone flap", and the thoracodorsal artery perforator-scapular osteocutaneous flap. The osseous segment in the latter two flaps is based on the angular artery, which derives either from the thoracodorsal artery or the serratus branch.[65–69]

The radial forearm flap provides for a thin fasciocutaneous skin paddle and can be harvested with a segment of the distal radius approximately 8–10 cm in length and 1–1.5 cm in width. The available bone stock is of reasonable length but by virtue of its thickness does not permit use for larger intercalary defects, with the exception of metacarpal or metatarsal reconstruction. Its chief advantage is a long reliable vascular pedicle and fasciocutaneous component. Bone harvest exposes the radius to fracture postoperatively. Thus avoidance of stress risers is important when performing osteotomies for harvest of the bone segment.

The free osteocutaneous lateral arm flap is a fasciocutaneous flap that is supplied by the posterior radial collateral artery. The vascular pedicle length can be up to 8 cm but is more typically 4–6 cm. The external arterial diameter of the posterior radial collateral artery is small, with an average diameter of 1.5 mm. This flap can be raised with an osseous segment up to 1 cm in width and 10 cm in length that is harvested from the lateral cortex of the humerus along a line parallel to the attachment of the lateral intermuscular septum. Much like the radial forearm, the bone stock available with this flap does not permit reconstruction of large intercalary defects, with the exception of metatarsal or metacarpal defects.

The vascularized iliac crest bone flap was popularized in the 1980s and is based on the DCIA. It has the advantage of allowing the harvest of a large segment of bone as well as skin. A segment of vascularized bone up to 4×11 cm can be harvested with a skin paddle measuring 8×18 cm. Limitations of this flap include the curve of the native ileum, which limits its usefulness in intercalary defect reconstruction, as well as the fact that the skin/soft-tissue component is rather bulky and not mobile, thus not allowing independent inset from the bone segment. In general, reconstruction of intercalary defects with the free iliac crest flap is limited to 10 cm. If defects are more than 10 cm, then osteotomies are required to account for the curvature of the graft. Further disadvantages of this flap

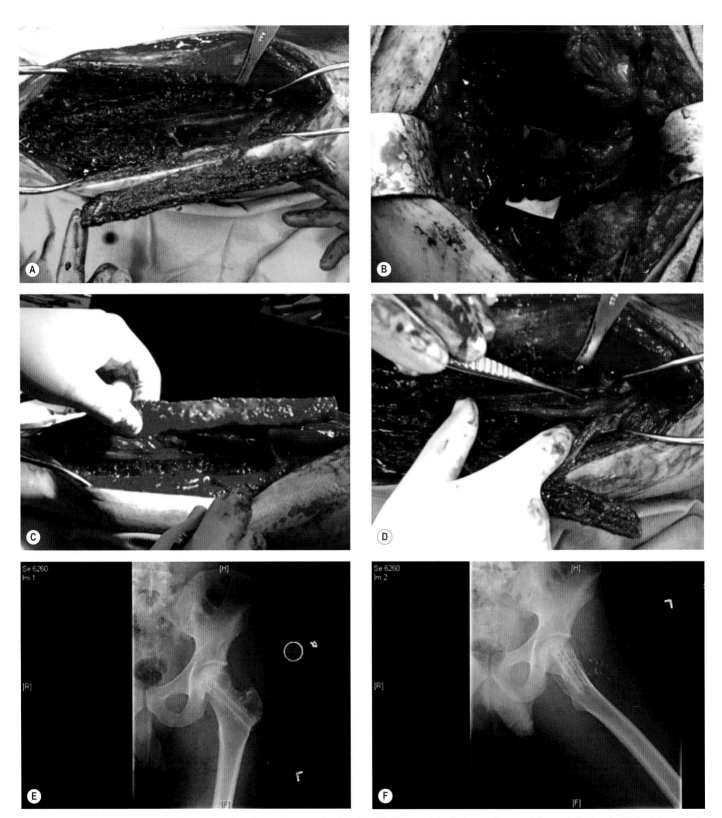

Fig. 7.1 Free vascularized fibula graft for reconstruction of avascular necrosis of the hip. **(A)** Harvest of the fibula as a "bone-only" vascularized graft. **(B)** Recipient vessel dissection, i.e., ascending branches of the lateral femoral circumflex system. **(C)** Fibula graft isolated on peroneal vessels. **(D)** Demonstration of peroneal vessel take-off at the tibioperoneal trunk. **(E,F)** Follow-up radiograph at 2.5 years following core decompression of right femoral head and reconstruction with free vascularized fibula graft.

include the potential for hernia formation postoperatively as well as anesthesia in the distribution of the lateral femoral cutaneous nerve. In a large series it was noted that 9.7% of patients developed a hernia after flap harvest. These donor-site hernias are challenging to repair secondary to their anatomic location. Also, persistent pain is a problem and was reported in 8.4% of patients at 1 year after harvest.[70]

Periosteal and other bone flaps (Video 7.1 ○)

Periosteum has long been known to have significant osteogenic activity.[71,72] In addition, it is suggested that periosteum provides a major source of osteoblast precursor cells.[1] The osteogenic properties of the periosteum can be utilized by harvesting a vascularized periosteal flap. The clinical correlates of this concept are the periosteal and osteoperiosteal grafts that are raised from the medial femoral condyle. These were first used as pedicled flaps and subsequently as free flaps.[73,74] The free vascularized MFC flap has a constant blood supply via the descending genicular artery (1.5–3.5 mm in diameter at its origin) and is ideal for treatment of smaller nonunions.[75] It may be harvested as an osteogenic periosteal, an osteoperiosteal, or a cutaneous osteoperiosteal flap depending on the needs of the reconstruction. The versatility of this flap is reflected in its numerous clinical applications, ranging from reconstruction of scaphoid nonunions[76] to mandibular and midface reconstructions,[77–79] as well as a variety of other indications involving the axial and appendicular skeleton (Figs. 7.4 & 7.5).[80–85]

The MFC flap is harvested via a medial longitudinal incision along the posterior border of the vastus medialis muscle. Upon visualization of the muscle fascia, the vastus medialis muscle is retracted anteriorly, thus exposing the descending geniculate artery. If reconstruction of a composite defect is required, perforators to the skin can be spared, thus adding a skin component to the MFC flap (Fig. 7.2 ◉). Once the pedicle is traced towards the medial femoral condyle, an osseous segment is harvested with a sagittal saw or osteotomes.[85]

Distraction osteogenesis

The Ilizarov technique, developed in the 1950s by Gavril A. Ilizarov, has profoundly changed our ability to treat fractures, nonunions, segmental bone loss, malrotation, and congenital abnormalities.[86,87] While it was initially developed for management of lower extremity pathology, it is now widely used for a variety of indications, including craniofacial disorders.[88,89] The basic principle of the Ilizarov technique is that osteogenesis can occur at an osteotomy site given the appropriate degree of retained vascularity, fixation, and quantified distraction. As such, it becomes evident that therapeutic success is dependent on a variety of factors that may be categorized into biologic, clinical, and technical factors.[90] The postoperative period is characterized by (1) a period of latency, defined by the period between corticotomy and distraction, followed by (2) a period of distraction, during which the Ilizarov frame is adjusted to allow for a distraction rate ranging between 1 and 2 mm per day, and finally (3) the period of consolidation.

Interestingly, it is not just bone that expands but rather muscles, nerves, blood vessels, and skin and soft tissues, which similarly expand in response to the tension applied by

virtue of tissue proliferation at the cellular level.[91,92] In many patients, however, coexisting soft-tissue defects preclude the use of the Ilizarov method as the sole treatment modality. In these complex cases of composite defects the Ilizarov method may be combined with conventional soft-tissue reconstruction, i.e., flaps. Furthermore, an existing bony defect may be reconstructed primarily with a free vascularized bone graft, which is subsequently distracted. The Ilizarov technique has been used successfully for reconstruction of defects up to 17 cm and may be combined with free vascularized bone grafts in order to achieve reconstruction.[93,94] The utility of this combined approach was first elucidated by Fiebel et al. in 1994 and subsequently expanded upon by numerous authors.[95–97]

Despite the impressive outcomes that can be achieved by means of the Ilizarov technique, a subset of patients will still require an amputation. An overall limb salvage rate of 84% has been reported, with the only predictor of amputation being the inability to achieve primary bony union.[93] Given these encouraging clinical results along with a lifetime cost benefit over amputation,[98] an aggressive approach to achieving bony union seems justified.

In addition to combining various surgical modalities with the Ilizarov technique, advances in the construct of the frame itself are noteworthy. The Taylor spatial frame has shown promise in the treatment of traumatic injuries with acute bone loss as well as tibial nonunions with associated bone defects.[99–102] The spatial frame differs from the standard Ilizarov construct in that it is a thin wire frame with virtual hinges and computer software support to facilitate fine corrections of bone length, angulation, and rotation. The spatial frame allows the reconstructive surgeon to have control over multiple variables through utilization of a hexapod construct and sophisticated computer algorithms to correct underlying deformities without frame modification, as is the case with a standard Ilizarov frame. Additionally, the spatial frame allows for potential early weight-bearing and range of motion, which may lead to improved rates of union.

Allograft reconstruction

Bone allograft is sterilely processed bone from human cadavers that is readily available in a variety of different forms. Its main advantage is the lack of donor site morbidity associated with its use. Allografts may be used as cortical grafts for support, osteochondral grafts, cancellous grafts, or as demineralized bone matrix (DBX). They are cataloged and selected based on their specific anatomic characteristics and reconstructive needs.[103] Given their acellularity, they do not have osteogenic potential and merely display osteoconductive capability. As such, incorporation is a rather slow process and typically incomplete. This is reflected by a nonunion rate of up to 35%.[104]

Time to bony union can vary considerably depending on the anatomic position and size of the allograft. While union times for allografts placed in the intercalary position may be as long as 23 months, time to union in the osteoarticular position takes up to 12 months.[105–108] Time to union, however, is influenced by a variety of additional factors. The need for chemotherapy, for example, can contribute to a delay in healing time. Despite their widespread use and availability, the avascular nature of these grafts predisposes them to

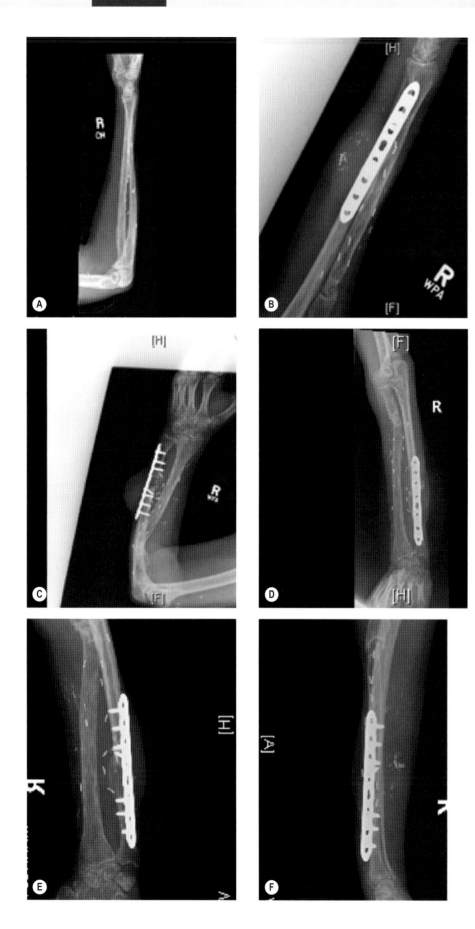

Fig. 7.4 Sequential images demonstrating bony callus formation and hypertrophy after reconstruction of an ulnar nonunion with a vascularized osteocutaneous medial femoral condyle graft based on the medial geniculate artery. **(A)** Preoperative image; **(B–D)** 2 months postoperatively; **(E–F)** 14 months postoperatively.

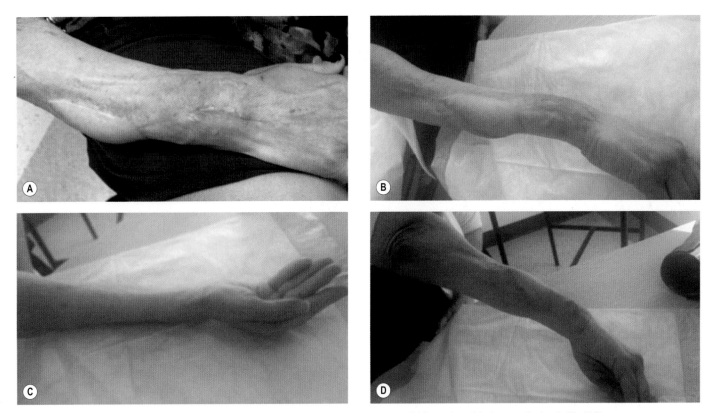

Fig. 7.5 Postoperative appearance after reconstruction of ulnar nonunion with osteocutaneous medial femoral condyle (same patient as in Fig. 7.2).

complications, including infections and fractures in addition to the need for surgical revisions.[109,110] Successful outcome is furthermore dependent on the condition of the surrounding soft tissues. Allograft placement in the setting of a compromised soft-tissue envelope, e.g., post-traumatic or radiation-induced, is certainly associated with a higher complication rate, including infections, fractures, and nonunions.[22,111–115]

When looking at a large series of long-bone reconstructions with allografts, a failure rate of 14% for intercalary grafts, a significantly longer time to union (compared to autografts), as well as a wide-ranging complication rate are reported, e.g., a complication rate of up to 35% and failure rate of 37%.[116–118] The majority of these failures occur within the first 3–4 years following reconstruction, with return to function being much better for allografts in the intercalary position than when combined with a prosthesis or when used in an allograft arthrodesis.[103] Data, however, suggest that intercalary allograft reconstruction fares much better than any other.[114,119–121] This fact has bearing on the current discussion, as most reconstructive surgeons will be primarily involved in reconstruction of intercalary defects, with most osteoarticular or reconstructions combined with a prosthesis being performed by an orthopedic surgeon.

The combination of allograft and vascularized autograft, i.e., Capanna technique, merges the favorable characteristics of both and is particularly suitable for reconstruction of massive skeletal defects.[24,122–125] The intercalary allograft provides initial stability and mechanical strength, while the free vascularized bone allows integration, the capacity for bony remodeling, and long-term viability of the construct and bony union.[126] The technique involves cutting the cortical allograft to the appropriate size to fit the skeletal defect. Next, the medullary portion of the allograft is enlarged to facilitate

placement of the free fibula bone graft within the medullary canal. Typically, the ends of the free fibula are left longer than the allograft so that they will overlap with the proximal and distal ends of the native bone. A canal or trough is cut within the allograft for the vascular pedicle and to facilitate microvascular anastomoses. This method can be used to reconstruct defects of the femur, tibia, and humerus. It may be used in the immediate setting after tumor resection, or in a delayed setting for nonunion of a previously placed allograft. For patients undergoing resection for sarcoma and immediate reconstruction, the allograft will provide mechanical stability and allow for earlier ambulation without the requisite delay for hypertrophy of the free fibula graft. Using this technique, a mean time for bony union of 8.6 months has been reported in addition to a limb salvage rate of up to 94%.[124,127]

The authors have modified the method and have incorporated an approach we call the "hemi-Capanna" in which the cortical allograft is bisected. This simplifies not only positioning of the fibula free flap and vascular pedicle but also further facilitates microvascular anastomosis. Yet, it still takes advantage of the mechanical strength provided by the allograft. Furthermore, the authors believe that the additional space provided by the "hemi-Capanna" allows the fibula graft to hypertrophy without facing restrictions from the surrounding allograft.

Reconstruction by anatomic area

Clavicle

Clavicular defects most commonly result from tumor resection, chronic infection, or trauma.[128,129] In fact, fractures of the clavicle represent one of the most common fractures of the appendicular skeleton, constituting 5–10% of all fractures.[130,131] Despite the common occurrence of clavicular fractures, the nonunion rate, defined as an ununited fracture 16 weeks after injury, is surprisingly low and reported to be less than 1%.[130,131] While the initial treatment of a clavicular nonunion is repeat open reduction and internal fixation, this approach is associated with a failure rate of 8%. These patients may suffer from persistent pain and restricted shoulder motion.[132–134] A symptomatic nonunion can even result in a space occupying pseudoarthrosis, with resultant neurovascular compromise and gross deformity.[135]

Although the importance of the clavicle for full shoulder motion is well known, controversy exists regarding whether bony reconstruction of the clavicle is indeed indicated. A small case series in the pediatric population demonstrated comparable shoulder function following total clavicular resection in patients with and without reconstruction. Li *et al.* similarly reported favorable functional outcomes in patients undergoing total claviculectomy without reconstruction.[136] Despite these reports it is agreed upon that some loss of shoulder function ensues subsequent to loss of clavicular integrity, i.e., clavicular resection. As such, bony reconstruction is recommended, particularly in patients with high functional demands as well as those with cosmetic concerns.[135]

Given the hostile wound environment, which is typically present secondary to chronic inflammation, infection, and scarring, non-vascularized bone grafts are not suggested for the purpose of clavicle reconstruction. The use of vascularized bone grafts is strongly recommended if bony reconstruction of the clavicle is desired. The free vascularized fibula and MFC graft are particularly suitable for this indication.[137–139]

Humerus

Skeletal reconstruction of any upper extremity defect must be tailored to the specific reconstructive needs of the patient. Many younger patients with osseous malignancies will require a functional reconstruction due to the high functional demands of the extremity. Although reconstructions of the upper extremity are not considered weight-bearing *per se*, a high degree of physiologic stress is placed on any reconstruction. Small (<6 cm) defects in well-vascularized, non-radiated, non-articular defects may be reconstructed with conventional bone grafting. If the defect is articular, prosthetic reconstruction or a composite of prosthesis and allograft may be considered.

The established treatment of segmental bone defects of the upper extremity greater than 6 cm is with the vascularized fibula graft. Its application to large defects of the humerus, with and without a skin paddle, has become routine for the reconstruction of defects after recalcitrant nonunion, tumor extirpation, hardware infection, or failure of conventional bone grafting.[33,94,125,140] The fibula is well suited for intercalary reconstruction of the humerus given its size, length, and ease of harvest.

A two-team approach allows an efficient and expeditious reconstruction. While one team establishes the humeral defect by resecting any non-viable bone and prepares the recipient site, a second team harvests the fibula. The approach to the humerus is determined by previous incisions as well as existing soft-tissue defects; however, the medial approach is

preferred whenever possible due to easy access to the brachial vessels, thus, facilitating microvascular anastomosis. It is important to maintain an intact circumferential cortex at the proximal and distal end of the bone defect, as this facilitates inset of the vascularized fibula graft into the intramedullary canal of the residual humerus proximally and distally. Ideally, about 1–2 cm of fibula should be impacted proximally and distally within the humerus. The entire construct can then be stabilized with dynamic compression plates, transcortical screws, Kirschner wires, or external fixators. The ability to harvest the fibula as a skin–muscle–bone composite graft is particularly helpful in cases in which overlying scars need to be replaced or soft-tissue contractures need to be corrected.

Using this technique, primary osseous union was achieved in 11 of 15 patients (73%). Three patients were noted to have early failure of graft fixation at the proximal or distal fixation site. These patients subsequently underwent open reduction and internal fixation with compression plates as well as cancellous bone grafting for augmentation at the graft junction with the native humerus. One patient in the series required a second free fibula graft for graft resorption. In three patients who achieved primary union, a secondary fracture of the fibula was noted. These patients were also subsequently treated with open reduction and internal fixation with compression plating as well as additional bone grafting. They went on to achieve union within 4 months.[141]

In patients who have an existing construct with an underlying atrophic nonunion or a pathologic fracture associated with a prior allograft reconstruction, the fibula graft may be placed in an onlay fashion as a strut that spans the nonunion. There have been encouraging reports in the literature of this technique in salvage of pathologic fractures associated with allografts of the humerus and other long bones.[142–144] In the largest series in the literature on the use of the free fibula graft for salvage of pathologic fractures, 4 of the 25 patients never obtained union, for a failure rate of 16% of the attempted fibula salvage of the allograft. The overall limb salvage rate was 90%; however, the limbs that were salvaged after failure of the fibula were done so with an endoprosthesis.[145]

Reconstruction of the humerus with the vascularized fibula graft is a well-recognized modality. Interestingly, the outcome of reconstruction of the humerus is worse when compared to the use of the fibula for radial forearm reconstruction. The relatively high rate of fracture of the fibula when used for humeral reconstruction seems to be consistent across multiple studies.[141,146] Certainly, there is an inherent rate of complication associated with complex reconstructions of the humerus. In patients who underwent oncologic resection followed by vascularized fibula reconstruction in the form of glenohumeral arthrodesis, intercalary autograft, or onlay for pathologic fracture, a mean of 2.8 operations per patient was required to achieve the desired outcome. This included 3 of the 15 patients requiring the use of their contralateral fibula for a second vascularized fibula transfer. Fracture and infection were the most common complications, all of which were treated successfully for limb salvage.[125]

Forearm

The free osteoseptocutaneous fibula graft is well suited for reconstruction of the radius or ulna due comparable osseous dimensions. Furthermore, in many cases of composite defects of the forearm, the skin and soft tissues associated with the fibula can be used for reconstruction.[147] The dynamic nature of the forearm and the ability of the forearm to perform supination and pronation are crucial in the function of the upper extremity. Reconstruction of the forearm and restoration of length with osseous union may not completely provide for the restoration of forearm rotation.[148,149] Any associated contracture of the interosseous space from loss of bony length can result in decreased forearm rotation and disability. It is therefore crucial to reconstruct the radius and ulna with the kinematics of the forearm in mind.[150]

Forearm defects are typically the result of trauma, oncologic resection, or nonunion after a prior traumatic injury. However, with modern methods of internal fixation the nonunion rates of diaphyseal fractures of the radius and ulna are typically less than 5%.[151-154] The reconstruction of diaphyseal defects less than 6 cm is amenable to cancellous autograft as long as there is no underlying infection or prior radiation therapy. In a large series of patients with diaphyseal atrophic nonunions, all patients were healed in 6 months after conventional cancellous bone grafting and compression plating. The diaphyseal defect averaged 2.2 cm and involved both bones in approximately 4% of patients.[155] This study demonstrates that excellent results can be achieved in reconstruction of diaphyseal defects with conventional, time-honored means in appropriately selected patients.

The vascularized free fibula graft remains the gold standard for reconstruction of large segmental defects of the forearm (e.g., the setting of defects longer than 6 cm) or of diaphyseal defects in the setting of infected nonunion, and prior to radiation therapy within the anticipated field of reconstruction.[147,156,157]

One should plan for excess length of the fibula graft in order to achieve the ideal final length. Having an appropriately sized fibula graft is crucial to ensure that the distal radioulnar joint is in alignment.[158] During the course of reconstruction, the fibula graft is temporarily placed in its anticipated final position and a radiograph is obtained with the wrist in neutral position. This allows for verification of the appropriate anatomic position of the fibula as well as the forearm length, ulnar variance, and congruity of the distal radioulnar joint. Microvascular anastomoses are done either to the distal brachial artery or to the radial or ulnar artery, ideally in an end-to-side fashion to preserve maximal flow into the distal extremity. Venous anastomoses may be performed to the venae comitantes or to a subcutaneous vein.

The outcome following forearm reconstruction with the free fibula graft is well documented. A survey of the literature regarding time to union of the fibula graft to the native bone reveals a mean time to union ranging from 3.8 to 4.8 months, with the majority of patients able to achieve a primary union.[147,159-165] A small subset of patients will require a secondary procedure such as adjunctive cancellous grafting to achieve union.

An interesting application of the vascularized fibula for forearm reconstruction is the "double-barrel" technique. This allows reconstruction of both the radius and ulna with or without an associated soft-tissue defect with a single vascularized flap.[149,166,167] However, the issue of decreased range of motion secondary to limited pronation and supination remains.

Scaphoid

The scaphoid is the most commonly fractured carpal bone, accounting for 50–80% of all carpal fractures.[168] Despite high union rates, approximately 10% of all scaphoid fractures progress to nonunion.[169] Risk factors for the development of scaphoid nonunion include proximal fracture location, avascular necrosis, instability, displacement, and delay in treatment.[170] While conventional bone grafting such as the Matti–Russe inlay graft technique may result in union rates of 70–90%, reconstructions based on the use of non-vascularized bone grafts are typically not successful in cases of proximal nonunion or avascular necrosis (AVN) of the proximal pole.[171,172] In these more challenging cases, reconstruction with vascularized bone grafts should be strongly considered. The objectives for treatment of scaphoid nonunion include restoration of scaphoid anatomy (e.g., correction of humpback deformity), primary osseous union, pain relief, improvement of range of motion and grip strength, as well as prevention of future arthritis.[173,174]

A variety of bone graft donor sites have been proposed for the purpose of scaphoid reconstruction; however, the distal radius and medial femur have become the most popular in recent years. This is related to the favorable profile of these graft sites with respect to donor site morbidity. In a recent systematic review, harvest of a non-vascularized iliac crest bone graft was associated with an overall incidence of complications of 9% vs. only 1% in patients with distal radius bone grafts.[175]

The distal radius as a source for a pedicled vascularized bone graft was first reported in 1991.[176] Perfusion to this flap is provided by the 1,2 intercompartmental supraretinacular artery (ICSRA).[170,177] Despite initial enthusiasm, a critical review of the literature reveals a rather heterogeneous success rate with this treatment modality. High success rates of greater than 90% have indeed been reported.[170,176,178] However, a union rate of only 12.5% in cases of nonunion with avascular proximal poles portends the limitations of this treatment modality.[179] The advantages of using a pedicled vascularized bone graft from the distal radius are quite evident and include ease of dissection, minimal donor site morbidity, and avoidance of microsurgical technique. It certainly represents a valuable tool for treatment of scaphoid nonunion in carefully selected patients. A disadvantage, however, is related to the limited degrees of freedom when attempting to inset the graft.

An alternative to the pedicled vascularized radius bone graft is the MFC corticoperiosteal flap (Figs. 7.3 & 7.6 ●). The versatility of the MFC flap is reflected in the wide range of reported applications, ranging from use for reconstructions of the cranio-maxillofacial skeleton, radius, ulna, humerus, and clavicle, to lower extremity reconstructions. However, it has most commonly been used for treatment of scaphoid nonunion.[78,83,139,180-188] Its malleable quality and osteogenic potential have made it particularly suitable for this indication. This flap is based on either the descending articular genicular or the superomedial genicular artery, thus allowing harvest of an osteoperiosteal or corticoperiosteal flap. The flap has a consistent vascular supply that has been studied extensively and allows inclusion of a skin island as well.[75,189,190] Superior outcomes with the free MFC flap have been reported when compared to the pedicled vascularized distal radius graft in the setting of scaphoid nonunion with carpal collapse and avascular necrosis. Furthermore, an improvement in carpal alignment and architecture has been associated with the use of the MFC flap.[140,186,191]

Figs. 7.3 and 7.6 appear online only.

An elegant solution for the treatment of proximal pole scaphoid nonunions with inadequate proximal fragment bone quality to permit pole-preserving reconstructions is the use of the medial femoral trochlea (MFT) flap.[192,193] The similarities between the convex surface of the MFT and the greater curvature of the proximal scaphoid make this osteocartilaginous flap an ideal solution for this challenging problem. In a series of 16 patients, computed tomography confirmed healing in 15 patients, with all patients experiencing either complete or incomplete pain relief.[193] A pedicle length of 8 cm with an arterial diameter of 1.2 mm facilitates pedicle positioning and microsurgical anastomosis. Of note, reported donor site morbidity with this procedure is minimal.[193]

While favorable outcomes with the various vascularized bone grafts have been reported, a recent systematic review concluded that there continues to be no optimal treatment of scaphoid nonunion. As this is related to a paucity of clinical series that are comparable, standardized reporting is recommended to facilitate comparability of clinical findings.[175]

Pelvis and spine

The use of bone grafts as an adjunct in spinal surgery is indicated after tumor resection, traumatic defects, failed spinal fusions, and kyphoscoliosis. Historically, thoracic spinal defects were reconstructed with pedicled rib grafts. Anterior placement of a vascularized pedicled rib graft has demonstrated the ability to achieve bony union but is limited in its applicability to the thoracic spine.[194,195] The use of conventional cancellous bone grafting is indicated for small defects with a suitable wound bed. Non-vascularized bone strut grafts have also been described for defects greater than 4 cm. However, these grafts have a high fracture rate and may result in nonunion, loss of spinal height, and potentially neurologic compression.[194,196] For larger defects, free vascularized bone grafting is indicated. Both the iliac crest as well as the free fibula flap have been described as surgical options.[197] The versatility of the free fibula flap is evidenced by its use for reconstruction of defects along the entire spine.[197–208]

Vertebrectomy defects can be reconstructed with prostheses. However, if the underlying hardware is involved in infection or osteomyelitis is present, hardware removal is mandatory. Vascularized bone grafting of spinal defects after removal of hardware represents a salvage procedure. Several options are available for vascularized bone grafting. Vascularized rib grafts can be utilized and rotated on their vascular pedicle to facilitate reconstruction of the thoracic spine. However, one is limited by the pedicle length and proximity to the thoracic cage.[194,209] In most instances free vascularized bone grafting is required, and most of these cases are effectively treated with the free fibular vascularized graft. Recipient vessels in the cervical region are branches of the external carotid artery for inflow and tributaries to the internal jugular vein for outflow. For defects in the thoracic, thoracolumbar, and lumbar defects, segmental intercostal vessels may be used in an end-to-end fashion for inflow and outflow. However, if there are no suitable intercostal vessels for inflow, an end-to-side anastomosis to the aorta can be performed. An aortic punch that is commonly used in cardiac surgery may be used to facilitate the anastomosis.[210] For reconstructions of the lumbar spine or pelvis the iliac vessels may be used in an end-to-side fashion.

The use of free vascularized bone reconstruction for spinal defects is a relatively rare procedure. Most reports in the literature are small series or technique papers and lack long-term outcomes data. In a large case series, 12 patients underwent vascularized free fibula grafting after multilevel resection of the spine. Two of these patients underwent bilateral simultaneous reconstruction with a free fibula graft after resection of one or more vertebral bodies or a partial or total sacrectomy. Successful outcome was defined as bony union between the fibula and the native bone. All patients required posterior fixation, and 7 of the 12 patients had additional autologous bone grafts placed at the junction of the fibula and native bone at the time of reconstruction. All patients who underwent surgery for tumor or infection were able to achieve bony union, with a mean time to union of 4.5 months. While there was a relatively high complication rate associated with these reconstructions, these are difficult, complex cases without other alternatives for reconstruction.[211] The authors of this series are to be commended for their reconstructions in this very difficult patient population.

Resections of the lumbosacral skeleton have significant functional implications as they result in discontinuity between the bony pelvis and the spine. As such, patients are unable to bear weight without reconstruction. Any resection of the bony pelvis which involves the sacroiliac joint will need restoration of its mechanical continuity in order to distribute the weight to the lower extremities.[212] It is imperative to reconstruct this defect and give patients undergoing this complex surgical procedure the best opportunity to achieve bony union and weight distribution through their axial and appendicular skeleton with the functional goal being return to ambulation. In instances of large defects, there is little choice other than large vascularized bone transfers to span the significant bony gap. These large bone defects have been successfully reconstructed with vascularized fibula grafts. A multidisciplinary approach, however, is mandatory for optimal outcomes.[211,213–217]

Femur

The femur is the longest bone in the human body and is subject to large amounts of axial loading as well as significant rotational angular stresses. Skeletal defects of the femoral shaft typically result from tumor resection, traumatic loss, chronic osteomyelitis, failed allografts, infected nonunion, and congenital anomalies. The principles of bony reconstruction as outlined above are applied to the clinical problems that are encountered. In defects of 6 cm or less, conventional bone grafting can be performed if the wound bed is clean, adequately vascularized, and free of infection. While the Masquelet technique has been successfully used for defects greater than 6 cm in length, the most common mode of reconstruction is vascularized bone transfer. Iliac crest may used, but its utility is limited given its curvature that necessitates osteotomy when used for reconstruction of intercalary defects. Hence the vascularized fibula graft has established itself as the gold standard for reconstruction of large femur defects.

The maximum length of the fibula that can be harvested for reconstruction of the segmental defect is about 26 cm in a typical adult patient and depends on the body habitus of the individual patient. If the defect is longer than the available fibula length, an option is to combine free fibular reconstruction of the femoral shaft with subsequent distraction osteogenesis in order to correct any limb length discrepancy and rotational abnormality.[218] Additional cross-sectional strength may be obtained with the free fibula graft by making a "double-barrel" fibula segment, while taking care to protect the vascular pedicle. This "double-barrel" reconstruction allows the construct to bear more force in the early postoperative period and may aid in postoperative stabilization, as it is inherently a more structurally stable construct.[219,220] However, there is a requisite period of non-weight-bearing until there is adequate hypertrophy of the fibular segment as well as union to the native femur. There is adequate evidence to demonstrate that vascularized fibula grafts have superior strength when compared with avascular bone grafts. This observation is explained by the inevitable loss in strength as the graft undergoes creeping substitution.[221–223] For most patients, after demonstration of bony incorporation of the fibula into the native femur as well as healed soft-tissue envelope, graduated weight-bearing may begin. This typically starts at approximately 6 months postoperatively, at which time the patient is followed though plain radiographs every several months to ensure ongoing hypertrophy of the fibula.

Successful microsurgical reconstruction requires adequate arterial inflow and venous drainage. Depending on the approach to the femur, pedicle length, and quality of recipient vessels, interposition vein grafts may be needed. The saphenous vein is the most commonly used for this purpose. The authors have previously reported a modification for the use of the ipsilateral fibula in microvascular reconstruction of the femur that allows a reduction in the number of microsurgical anastomoses. The ipsilateral greater saphenous vein is transposed for the purpose of establishing venous outflow, while arterial inflow is created by means of a conventional interposition graft. Thus the number of anastomoses is reduced from four to three.[224] Alternative recipient vessels to consider include the descending branch of the lateral femoral circumflex artery and its venae comitantes. Using these vessels obviates the need for interposition vein grafting altogether.

Overall, the outcome of long bone reconstruction using the vascularized fibula graft is favorable. Within large series of extremity reconstruction, the functional outcome is good and there is a high rate of bony union.[161,225–227] Hence the fibula should be considered the first choice for autologous vascularized reconstruction of the femur.

Knee

The knee is a common site for osseous neoplasms. Reconstructive options following resection are numerous and include endoprostheses, osteoarticular allografts, and knee arthrodesis with intercalary allografts, non-vascularized, or vascularized autologous bone grafts.[228–231] Despite advances in implant technology, knee arthrodesis remains a valuable reconstructive option, particularly in young patients as well as those with large bony defects and avascular segments of infected bone.[232] Furthermore, arthrodesis may be a salvage procedure in cases of failed prosthetic-based reconstructions and may represent the only alternative to amputation. The oncologic safety of tumor resection and knee arthrodesis for management of malignant knee tumors has been demonstrated, with local disease control being comparable to thigh amputation.[233]

Knee arthrodesis is a time-honored procedure after extensive resections around the knee joint with initial reports by Lexer in the first half of the past century.[27] The first large case series documenting functional outcomes following resection arthrodesis with segmental autologous bone grafts was published by Enneking and Shirley in 1977.[233] Since then a variety of different approaches have been proposed for knee arthrodesis, including variations in the mode of fixation as well as material for bone reconstruction.[228,233,234] Over time, however, vascularized fibula grafts have proven to be particularly suitable for this indication. Reasons include the ability of the fibula graft to bridge a large bony defect, its osteogenic potential, as well as its ability to hypertrophy.[235] High rates of bony consolidation have been reported with this technique.[232,236] However, challenges remain and are related to the morbidity of the procedure. The complication rate is rather high with septic complications and mechanical failure being the most common complications encountered postoperatively.[231] Infection rates and graft fracture rates up to 53% have been reported.[231] Additional complications include peroneal nerve palsy and deep venous thrombosis.[231,232]

In light of existing concerns regarding the mechanical stability of the fibula in the setting of knee arthrodesis, techniques have been introduced that overcome this limitation. One option is the technique proposed by Capanna et al. in which a vascularized fibular graft is combined with an allograft.[24] In addition to the stability provided by the bone graft, the issue of fixation has been a focus of investigation. While the use of a centromedullary nail has been quoted to represent the best way of securing knee arthrodeses, rigid assemblies, which exclude mechanical graft loading, are made responsible for weakening the bone graft with resultant high rates of postoperative stress fractures.[235,237,238]

Surgical treatment of neoplasms around the knee joint is not the only indication for performing a knee arthrodesis. Additional clinical scenarios in which this procedure might be indicated include failed knee arthroplasty secondary to recurrent infections as well as extensive trauma involving the tibial plateau with destruction of the knee joint and loss of soft tissue.[237,239] These cases are particularly challenging and represent a patient population distinctly different from tumor patients. In patients undergoing oncologic resection the bone defect is created in a controlled fashion with minimal compromise to the surrounding soft-tissue envelope. As such, reconstructive attempts with non-vascularized bone grafts may be successful. In contrast, post-traumatic defects are not only characterized by large bony gaps but also display a deficient, scarred, or colonized soft-tissue envelope. As such, reconstruction with vascularized bone grafts is almost mandatory to ensure success. Despite these challenges, the pedicled vascularized fibula graft provides for a reliable reconstruction in these patients. Given the compromised soft-tissue envelope, however, the vascularized fibula graft is ideally harvested as an osteoseptocutaneous graft for simultaneous reconstruction of the soft-tissue envelope.[239]

From a technical standpoint it is important to highlight that in the majority of cases of knee arthrodesis the vascularized fibula graft may be transferred as a pedicled graft, thus avoiding microsurgical anastomoses. While technical expertise in microsurgical vessel dissection is mandatory, the ability to avoid microsurgical anastomoses undoubtedly simplifies the procedure. However, in cases where the femoral defect is larger than 10 cm then free transfer of the fibula becomes mandatory.[232] This is an important point to consider when planning the reconstruction.

Tibia

Segmental tibial defects are common and typically seen after trauma or after tumor resection. The use of the fibula for tibial reconstruction is a time-honored approach. Tibiofibular synostosis was described as early as 1941 and persisted as a means for tibial reconstruction into the 1960s. This approach, however, had significant limitations, including the need for large amounts of interposed cancellous bone grafts in addition to taking a long time for consolidation. Despite advancements in microsurgical techniques in the 1970s that permitted transfer of vascularized fibula grafts, small series of pedicled vascularized tibial reconstructions with ipsilateral fibula persisted in the literature with overall good results and union.[240,241] Use of the pedicled, ipsilateral fibula flap for tibial shaft reconstruction remains a reasonable choice. However, most reconstructive surgeons prefer a free ipsilateral or contralateral vascularized fibula for tibial shaft reconstruction. Harvesting the fibula as a free flap allows an additional degree of freedom regarding mobility, positioning, and inset of the graft that is not afforded with a pedicled flap.

Diaphyseal tibial defects can be quite challenging to reconstruct, particularly when associated with overlying tissue loss. Those gaps associated with soft-tissue loss, such as are seen in complex tibia fractures, may require concomitant soft-tissue reconstruction. Patients with a segmental tibial defect greater than 6 cm with associated soft-tissue loss are ideal candidates for reconstruction with an osteocutaneous vascularized free flap, such as the free vascularized fibula graft. The concept of reconstruction of the tibial shaft with a vascularized fibular graft was first suggested in 1981 when Chacha and colleagues utilized the ipsilateral fibula as a vascularized pedicle graft for nonunion of the tibia.[242] The use of the ipsilateral vascularized fibula for tibial reconstruction has been shown to be a reliable technique.[243] Hertel et al. used a pedicled ipsilateral fibula for tibial shaft reconstruction and were able to achieve full, unprotected weight-bearing at a mean of 5.5 months. However, the majority of these patients required additional soft-tissue reconstruction in the form of a free or pedicled soft-tissue flap either pre- or postoperatively in addition to the tibial shaft reconstruction. Additionally, two of these patients required cancellous bone grafting. Since that time, microvascular reconstruction has evolved and become a reliable means for diaphyseal tibial reconstruction.

Patients undergoing segmental tibial resection for limb-sparing, oncologic surgery are candidates for the adjunctive use of an allograft in conjunction with the free fibula graft via the Capanna technique. While an allograft provides for significant mechanical strength initially via its strong cortical bone, it is associated with a risk of nonunion at the allograft–host junction as well as fracture of the allograft itself. The addition of vascularized fibula adds osteogenic capacity to the construct, thus providing the potential for revascularization and remodeling. The use of autologous bone that can grow and remodel with the patient is a particularly attractive option in younger patients requiring oncologic resection of their tibial shaft. Most authors utilize the Capanna technique with a free fibular graft, but it has also been reported with a pedicled fibular graft as well.[244,245] Utilization of the Capanna technique allows more rapid weight-bearing without the requisite time to allow fibular hypertrophy, and takes advantage of both allograft and free vascularized bony reconstruction. When one considers the anatomic location of tibial diaphyseal defects, they are more challenging than other long-bone reconstructions within the appendicular skeleton. The tibia is subject to large physical loads and has a relatively thin soft-tissue envelope, which makes it more prone to complications compared to other skeletal defects. If the tibial defect involves the articular surface, the reconstruction may be combined with an endoprosthesis. A comprehensive discussion of reconstructive options of the joint in conjunction with a diaphyseal defect is beyond the scope of this chapter.

Foot and ankle

The vascular anatomy of the foot predisposes certain anatomic areas to be prone to complications subsequent to trauma or operative intervention. The blood supply to the navicular bone and talus is particularly tenuous in this regard. Similar to the scaphoid, these bones have a large cartilaginous surface with limited entry points for nutrient vessels.[246] As such, it is not surprising that any insult, be it iatrogenic or post-traumatic, predisposes patients to develop complications such as AVN and nonunion.[247] It is important to understand that even anatomic reduction of fractures in this region does not reliably prevent AVN. Untoward sequelae include nonunion, subsidence, and degenerative joint disease that ultimately require arthrodesis.[248] While primary arthrodesis is associated with high success rates, nonunion rates up to 40% have been reported in patients with comorbidities.[249–252] In the setting of failed arthrodesis, particularly after non-vascularized bone grafting, the transfer of vascularized bone should be considered.

These patients pose several challenges, including the fact that they have typically undergone numerous previous attempts at surgical correction prior to being referred to the reconstructive surgeon. Furthermore, a history of osteomyelitis as well as coexisting peripheral vascular disease is not uncommon in this patient population.[248]

Options for vascularized bone transfer for the purpose of foot and ankle reconstruction include iliac crest, fibula, MFC, and scapula. In the authors' practice, however, the fibula and MFC have established themselves as routine vehicles for skeletal reconstruction of the foot and ankle. While the iliac crest allows harvest of adequate bone stock, the donor site morbidity can be problematic. Additionally, the skin component, when raised as a composite flap, is unreliable at times.[175,253] A sound treatment algorithm was recently published outlining the indications for the fibula vs. MFC flap for foot and ankle reconstruction.[248]

The main parameter influencing flap choice is the size of the bone defect. In isolated cases of tarsal bone AVN as well as nonunion, reconstruction with a free MFC flap is recommended. Similarly, an osseous defect less than 3.5 cm is ideally reconstructed with a free MFC flap (Figs. 7.7 & 7.8). In a recent

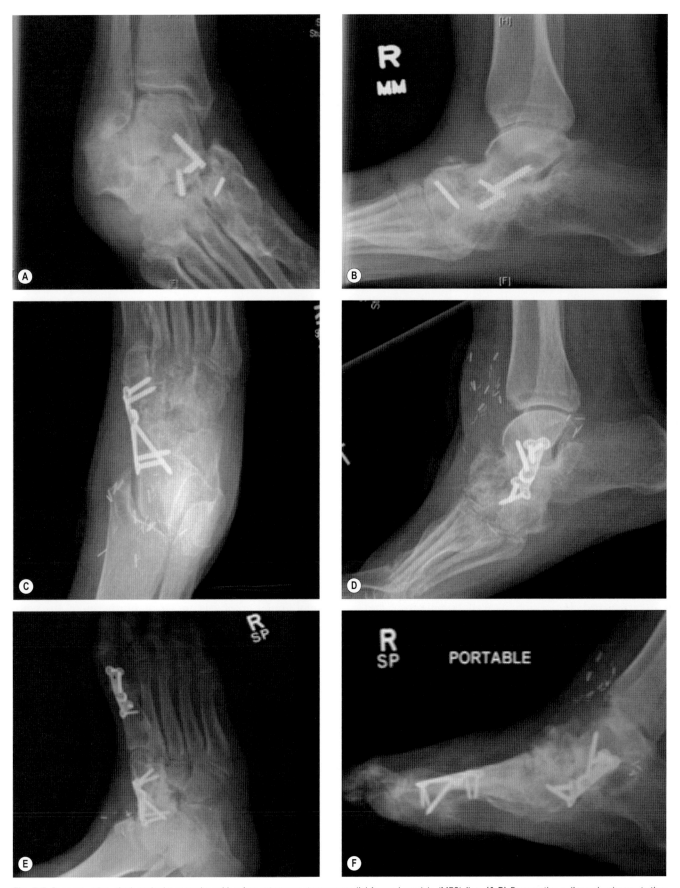

Fig. 7.7 Reconstruction of talonavicular nonunion with a free osteomyocutaneous medial femoral condyle (MFC) flap. **(A,B)** Preoperative radiographs demonstrating talonavicular nonunion; **(C,D)** 1-month postoperative radiographs; **(E,F)** 6-month postoperative radiographs demonstrating successful talonavicular fusion.

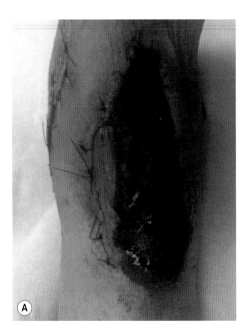
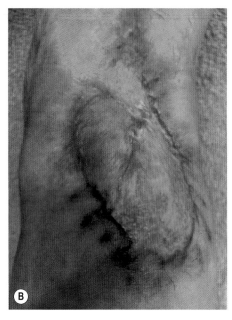

Fig. 7.8 Postoperative appearance of free osteomyocutaneous medial femoral condyle (MFC) flap (same patient as in Fig. 7.6). **(A)** Immediate postoperative appearance with exposed vastus medialis muscle. **(B)** Final postoperative appearance after flap revision and split-thickness skin grafting.

retrospective analysis of post-traumatic patients with complex foot and ankle pathology, a 100% union rate was achieved with the free MFC flap. Given the favorable clinical outcomes obtained the authors concluded that the MFC flap has become the ideal donor location when reconstructing small bone defects.[85] Advantages of the MFC flap include ease of harvest, reliable anatomy, minimal donor site morbidity, as well as ability to include a skin island that can be inset fairly independently from the osseous component.

Bone defects greater than 3.5 cm and pantalar degenerative joint disease are best treated with vascularized fibula transfer.[248] Procedural aspects to consider include which fibula to use (i.e., ipsilateral vs. contralateral) as well as how to revascularize the fibula without compromising perfusion to the foot. Options include transferring the fibula as a pedicled graft based on retrograde perfusion. While the authors have done this successfully, the technical difficulties, as they relate to flap rotation, pedicle position, as well as bone inset and fixation, cannot be underestimated.[248] Hence the authors prefer to use the fibula as a free vascularized bone graft. The ipsilateral fibula is preferred so as to limit the procedure to one extremity. The free fibula graft may be revascularized by the anterior tibial vessels when using an anterior approach to the ankle. A more elegant solution, however, particularly when a lateral approach is chosen, is to use the proximal peroneal vessels to revascularize the fibula via extension interposition vein grafts. Hence vascularity to the foot is preserved to the greatest extent possible. Radiographic and clinical outcome after ankle arthrodesis for management of talar AVN using a free fibula graft is shown in Figs. 7.9 and 7.10.

Vascularized epiphyseal reconstruction

Vascularized epiphyseal reconstruction has a capacity to restore joint function as well as growth potential of the reconstructed limb. If the epiphysis is resected or lost secondary to tumor or trauma, respectively, growth potential can be restored in a child with skeletal immaturity through vascularized epiphyseal transfer. The restoration of growth potential is not possible with non-vascularized autografts, allografts, prostheses, or vascularized bone grafts without an epiphysis. Only through epiphyseal transfer is the potential for longitudinal growth maintained.[254] The donor site for a vascularized epiphyseal reconstruction is the proximal fibular epiphysis with its adjacent diaphyseal shaft. The proximal epiphysis of the fibula is supplied by an epiphyseal branch from the anterior tibial artery that also supplies the proximal two-thirds of the diaphysis through small, musculoperiosteal branches.[59] Initially, it was thought that the diaphysis was perfused via the peroneal artery, thus necessitating harvest of both anterior tibial and peroneal arteries to ensure survival of the epiphysis and the diaphysis. It has been demonstrated, however, that adequate perfusion of the proximal diaphysis is maintained without the need to harvest both pedicles. The dissection can be challenging, as the branches that supply the proximal fibular epiphysis are small. Furthermore, the peroneal nerve is at risk for iatrogenic injury. Innocenti *et al.* have provided a beautifully illustrated dissection technique of this challenging flap.[254,255]

The proximal fibular epiphysis has several advantages over other vascularized bone grafts. The proximal head of the fibula has an articular surface and provides for a true physis and epiphysis as well as a proximal diaphysis, which facilitates bone fixation and diaphyseal reconstruction. The anatomic structure of the fibula and its proximal epiphysis lends itself to reconstruction of the long bones of the forearm as well as the humerus in the growing child. The addition of a true physis and epiphysis with the proximal fibular graft provides for growth in addition to being capable of adapting to the new functional requirements as the immature skeleton grows. CT studies of children who underwent reconstruction of their distal radius with a vascularized proximal fibular epiphyseal graft revealed progressive remodeling of the articular surface to adapt to the proximal carpal row, which translated into improvement in function of the reconstructed joint.[255] This ability to provide a vascularized articular surface, and to preserve the capacity for longitudinal growth and adaptation,

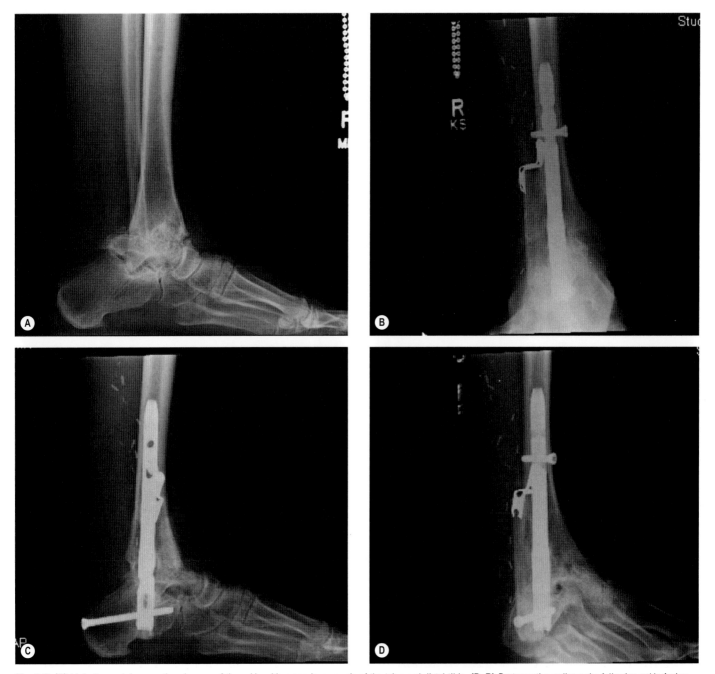

Fig. 7.9 (A) Malunion and degenerative changes of the ankle with avascular necrosis of the talus and distal tibia. **(B–D)** Postoperative radiographs following ankle fusion with intramedullary rod fixation and free osteocutaneous fibula flap transfer. The proximal peroneal vessels were used to revascularize the fibula via extension interposition vein grafts. Hence vascularity to the foot was preserved to the greatest extent possible.

is unique to vascularized epiphyseal reconstruction. In patients with an immature skeleton who require the capacity for growth to prevent limb length discrepancy or deformity, vascularized epiphyseal transfer from the proximal fibula should be considered (Fig. 7.9).

Postoperative care

Postoperative monitoring

A multitude of options exist for postoperative monitoring following free vascularized tissue transfer.[256] While clinical evaluation represents the gold standard of postoperative flap monitoring, this mode of monitoring is not possible after transfer of vascularized bone alone, unless a skin or other soft-tissue component is included and exposed to permit clinical evaluation. In osteoseptocutaneous flaps, for example, the skin island is evaluated clinically as well as with a Doppler probe. In order to facilitate Doppler examination the site of the skin perforator is marked with a 5-0 non-absorbable suture.

The ideal method of monitoring should allow an objective evaluation of the transferred tissue, be promptly reactive to changes in blood flow, and allow continuous monitoring even by nursing and ancillary staff. In light of these criteria, the

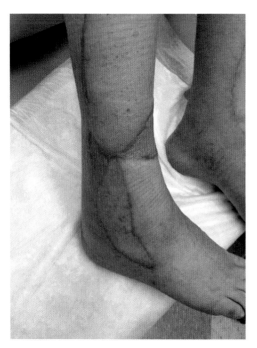

Fig. 7.10 Clinical appearance of right ankle after reconstruction with osteocutaneous fibula flap (same patient as in Fig. 7.9).

authors believe that the inherent characteristics of the implantable Doppler probe allow this device to replace clinical monitoring in the appropriate setting.[257] As such, the authors routinely use the implantable Cook Doppler for postoperative monitoring.

While monitoring the vascular status is critical in the early postoperative period, the critical long-term outcome measure after skeletal reconstruction is osseous union. This is typically assessed through serial conventional radiographs or cross-sectional imaging, such as CT or MRI. An additional technique for assessing viability of the skeletal construct is by means of technetium-99 bone scans.[258]

Postoperative aesthetic considerations

Many patients who undergo skeletal reconstruction will be left with a significant scar burden or contour deformity of the reconstructed extremity. While functional considerations are most important, it is prudent to provide the patient with the aesthetically most appealing reconstruction possible. Adjunctive measures, such as scar revisions, contouring procedures, etc., should be offered liberally. A variety of treatment options exist to improve the appearance of a reconstructed limb.

The scar burden may be reduced through serial excision. Another method that has long been recognized as a valuable adjunct to soft-tissue reconstruction of the extremity is tissue expansion.[259–261] Placement of an expander in the fascial cleft of the extremity allows recruitment of additional soft tissue, thus allowing excision of disfiguring scars and coverage with regional tissue. Expanders may be placed through a minimally invasive approach, which shortens the time needed for reconstruction and yields a similar, more compliant flap.[224] The final result of this treatment modality is a linear scar in the affected extremity. One must be careful not to place the scar over the flexor surface of the joint, however, as this may result in scar contracture with resultant functional compromise, i.e., decreased joint mobility.

Erythematous scars may be treated with laser resurfacing to improve their appearance and aid with blending into the surrounding soft tissue. This may be performed in the office under topical or no anesthesia. The authors use the Candela Vbeam laser for vascular scars with acceptable results.

Patients who have had prior extremity reconstruction with a soft-tissue free flap or an osteocutaneous free flap with a bulky soft-tissue component may benefit from a contouring procedure. This can be achieved by direct excision of excess tissue or via liposuction. Any attempt at contouring, however, is delayed until a stable reconstruction is achieved and the long-term results are evident, typically after a minimum of 3–6 months from the time of the initial reconstruction. If patients who have had a prior reconstruction require revision or adjunctive bone grafting, the stable soft-tissue portion of the flap may be raised and thinned at the time of the revision.

Conclusion

Reconstruction of the skeleton remains a challenging task. There are several modalities to accomplish reconstruction of the skeleton. The optimal means of skeletal reconstruction for any existing defect is at the discretion of the reconstructive surgeon. This chapter cannot be an exhaustive review but rather an outline of the general principles to consider when approaching these complex patients. One must be familiar with all the available techniques and the associated outcomes, as well as the risks and benefits of each method of skeletal reconstruction. With most reconstructive procedures there is not only the defect to consider but also the donor site morbidity associated with the proposed reconstructive plan. The goal of skeletal reconstruction is to achieve osseous union along with a stable and aesthetically appealing soft-tissue reconstruction. This endeavor mandates a multidisciplinary approach in order to achieve an optimal outcome. One needs a dedicated multidisciplinary team to facilitate efficient and optimal care of patients undergoing skeletal reconstruction and rehabilitation.

 Bonus images for this chapter can be found online at
http://www.expertconsult.com

Fig. 7.2 Reconstruction of scaphoid nonunion with osteocutaneous medial femoral condyle (MFC) flap. **(A,B)** Dissection of recipient site with establishment of intercalary defect. **(C–E)** Harvest of osteocutaneous MFC flap.

Fig. 7.3 Reconstruction of scaphoid nonunion with free medial femoral condyle (MFC) flap. **(A,B)** Preoperative radiographs demonstrating scaphoid nonunion with avascular proximal pole. **(C,D)** Postoperative radiographs at 8 weeks. **(E,F)** Postoperative radiographs at 2 years postoperatively with successful union of the scaphoid.

Fig. 7.6 Postoperative appearance after reconstruction of scaphoid nonunion with free medial femoral condyle (MFC) flap.

11. Friedlaender GE, Perry CR, Cole JD, et al. Osteogenic protein-1 (bone morphogenetic protein-7) in the treatment of tibial nonunions. *J Bone Joint Surg Am.* 2001;83-A(suppl 1 Pt 2): S151–S158.

24. Capanna R, Campanacci DA, Belot N, et al. A new reconstructive technique for intercalary defects of long bones: the association of massive allograft with vascularized fibular autograft. Long-term results and comparison with alternative techniques. *Orthop Clin North Am.* 2007;38(1):51–60, vi. *This paper describes the use of an allograft combined with a vascularized fibula for the reconstruction of intercalary defects. It details the advantages and power of this technique, which takes advantage of the strong mechanical properties of the allograft with the ability of the vascularized fibula to hypertrophy and remodel as a living graft of bone.*

25. De Long WG Jr, Einhorn TA, Koval K, et al. Bone grafts and bone graft substitutes in orthopaedic trauma surgery. A critical analysis. *J Bone Joint Surg Am.* 2007;89(3):649–658.

39. Bosse MJ, MacKenzie EJ, Kellam JF, et al. An analysis of outcomes of reconstruction or amputation after leg-threatening injuries. *N Engl J Med.* 2002;347(24):1924–1931. *This prospective study examined the functional outcomes of patients with severe lower extremity trauma who underwent amputation or limb salvage. Patients were rated on a self-reported health scale. This study demonstrated equivalent outcomes between amputation and limb salvage, and lends credence to attempts at limb salvage if medically feasible.*

40. MacKenzie EJ, Bosse MJ, Kellam JF, et al. Factors influencing the decision to amputate or reconstruct after high-energy lower extremity trauma. *J Trauma.* 2002;52(4):641–649.

52. Masquelet AC, Fitoussi F, Begue T, Muller GP. Reconstruction of the long bones by the induced membrane and spongy autograft. *Ann Chir Plast Esthet.* 2000;45(3):346–353. *This paper elucidates the Masquelet technique of inducing a bioactive membrane for the reconstruction of skeletal defects. It demonstrates that the scope of conventional bone grafting can be greatly improved by allowing the formation of a bioactive membrane to consolidate bony defects that would typically be reconstructed with vascularized bone grafting.*

86. Ilizarov GA. The tension-stress effect on the genesis and growth of tissues: part II. The influence of the rate and frequency of distraction. *Clin Orthop Relat Res.* 1989;239:263–285.

87. Ilizarov GA. The tension-stress effect on the genesis and growth of tissues. Part I. The influence of stability of fixation and soft-tissue preservation. *Clin Orthop Relat Res.* 1989;238:249–281. *These are seminal papers for distraction osteogenesis as initially elucidated by Ilizarov. The principles of distraction as they relate to extremity reconstruction are found in these papers. In addition, these papers demonstrate the power of distraction to generate additional soft tissue and bone length and to correct rotational deformities.*

102. Feldman DS, Shin SS, Madan S, Koval KJ. Correction of tibial malunion and nonunion with six-axis analysis deformity correction using the Taylor Spatial Frame. *J Orthop Trauma.* 2003;17(8):549–554.

105. Bauer TW, Muschler GF. Bone graft materials. An overview of the basic science. *Clin Orthop Relat Res.* 2000;371:10–27.

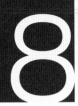

8

Foot reconstruction

Michael V. DeFazio, Kevin D. Han, and Christopher E. Attinger

SYNOPSIS

- Successful wound healing is dependent upon accurate determination of wound etiology, biomechanical optimization, establishment of adequate blood supply, and proper identification/eradication of infection.
- Functional limb salvage mandates a multidisciplinary team approach comprising, at the very least, a vascular surgeon, foot and ankle surgeon, plastic surgeon, infectious disease specialist, endocrinologist, pedorthotist, and prosthetist.
- Planned surgical incisions and flap design should be based on a detailed knowledge of anatomy, angiosomes, and vascular status.
- Adequate debridement of the wound, prior to closure, is critical and may require the implementation of a staged reconstructive approach.
- The reconstructive plan must be individually tailored to provide the best biomechanical result given the patient's age, goals, and functional capacity. This may involve local wound care, grafting, local–regional flaps, free tissue transfer, and/or amputation for similar wounds presenting in different hosts.
- Postoperative wound care and biomechanical offloading are essential to ensure successful reconstruction and prevent unnecessary complications such as wound breakdown and delayed healing.

Introduction

The distal lower extremity has unique structural and functional significance, serving as a dynamic platform for posture and ambulation that is subject to repetitive trauma from large stress loads. Considering the complex anatomic variations and functional demands of the foot and ankle, restoration of defects in this region poses a significant reconstructive challenge. Trauma, infection, oncologic resection, and alterations in blood supply, sensation, and mechanical alignment can compromise skeletal stability and increase the likelihood of soft-tissue breakdown. Inability to salvage the injured foot often results in major amputation, which carries its own physical, psychological, and socioeconomic morbidity, including

a lifetime dependence on prosthetic devices. Still, even with adequate resources and rehabilitation, a significant percentage of patients never regain their capacity for ambulation and instead are condemned to a wheelchair-bound existence. In diabetics, major amputation is associated with a 5-year mortality rate as high as 78%, with a 50% risk of contralateral lower extremity amputation within 2 years.[1–4] Therefore a reconstructive strategy that incorporates measures to mitigate risk, restore biomechanical function, and promote successful wound healing is paramount and has significant implications with respect to patient survival, functional prognosis, and quality-of-life.

Successful foot/ankle reconstruction and functional limb salvage begins with a multidisciplinary team approach that includes collaboration between a vascular surgeon skilled in endovascular and open vascular bypass, a foot and ankle surgeon competent in internal/external skeletal stabilization techniques, a plastic surgeon familiar with principles of modern wound healing and soft-tissue reconstruction, and an infectious disease physician specializing in surgical infections. For the at-risk or biomechanically unstable foot, a podiatrist and pedorthotist specializing in routine foot care and orthotics/shoe wear are critical in preventing recurrent wound breakdown. In the setting of major amputation, a skilled prosthetist is necessary for the creation of a customized prosthesis capable of optimizing the biomechanical potential of the residual limb. In addition, endocrinology, nephrology, cardiology, hematology, rheumatology, and dermatology consultations may be indicated to address the patient's comorbid medical conditions.

The reconstructive plan must be individualized to provide the best biomechanical result given the patient's age, goals, and functional capacity. This may involve local wound care, grafting, local–regional flaps, free tissue transfer, and/or amputation for similar wounds presenting in different hosts. Surgical goals in foot and ankle reconstruction center on the "3 Bs": (1) blood supply, (2) bioburden, and (3) biomechanics. Ensuring adequate local blood flow, aggressive debridement to a clean wound base, and correction of biomechanical/

structural abnormalities prior to reconstruction offers the best opportunity for durable, efficient, and uncomplicated wound healing. Following adequate preparation and subsequent wound closure, effective offloading and graduated postoperative rehabilitation are essential to prevent relapse and optimize long-term functional outcomes, respectively. With these considerations in mind, most reconstructions can be successfully accomplished utilizing simple techniques (90%), whereas only a minority of cases will require complex flap reconstruction (10%). This chapter will focus on the critical aspects of foot and ankle reconstruction including anatomy, evaluation, diagnosis, and treatment with commonly used reconstructive modalities.

Anatomy

Angiosomes of the foot

G. Ian Taylor first introduced the concept of "angiosomes" in human anatomy to describe a 3D unit of tissue supplied by a single source artery.[5] Attinger et al.[6] further developed this principle as it applies to the foot and ankle, eventually illustrating six specific angiosomes of the foot originating from three primary source arteries. All vascular supply to the foot and ankle enters through the popliteal fossa as the three terminal branches of the popliteal artery: (1) the anterior tibial artery, (2) the posterior tibial artery, and (3) the peroneal artery (Fig. 8.1).

Above the ankle, the peroneal artery bifurcates into (1) the anterior perforating branch and (2) the calcaneal branch. The anterior perforating branch pierces through the distal anterior intermuscular septum and sends a branch superiorly overlying the intermuscular septum (this encompasses the area from which the lateral supramalleolar flap[7] can be harvested). The anterior perforating artery then connects directly with the anterior lateral malleolar artery (anterior tibial artery) and supplies the anterolateral ankle angiosome. At the level of the lateral malleolus, the lateral calcaneal artery emerges laterally between the Achilles tendon and the peroneal tendons. It curves with the peroneal tendons 2 cm distal to the lateral malleolus and gives rise to four or five small calcaneal branches. The lateral calcaneal artery terminates at the level of the fifth metatarsal tuberosity, where it connects with the lateral tarsal artery (dorsalis pedis). The lateral calcaneal branch supplies the lateral and plantar heel angiosome.

The posterior tibial artery has three terminal branches: (1) the calcaneal branch, (2) the medial plantar artery, and (3) the lateral plantar artery. The medial calcaneal artery arises inferiorly and arborizes into multiple branches that travel in a coronal direction to supply the medial and plantar heel. Thus the plantar heel receives dual blood supply form the calcaneal branches of the posterior tibial and peroneal arteries, which ensures adequate flow to an area regularly traumatized during ambulation. Development of heel gangrene, on the other hand, usually implies severe vascular disease involving both the peroneal and posterior tibial arteries. The posterior tibial artery then enters the calcaneal canal, underneath the flexor

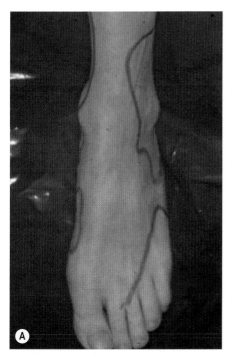 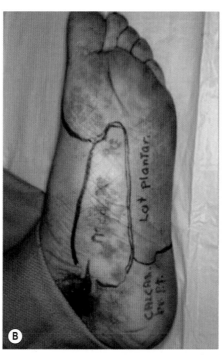 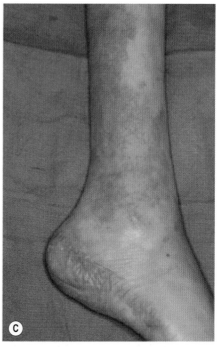

Fig. 8.1 This injection study demonstrates the angiosomes of the foot and ankle. **(A)** The anterior tibial artery supplies the anterior ankle and continues distally as the dorsalis pedis artery to supply the dorsum of the foot. **(B)** The peroneal artery supplies the anterolateral ankle and the lateral heel via the anterior perforating and lateral calcaneal branches, respectively. **(C)** The medial plantar heel, instep, and lateral plantar midfoot and forefoot are fed by the calcaneal, medial plantar, and lateral plantar branches of the posterior tibial artery, respectively. Note that the heel receives dual blood supply from the medial calcaneal (posterior tibial artery) and lateral calcaneal (peroneal artery) angiosomes. Depending on anatomic variability, the blood supply to the hallux may be derived from either the plantar or dorsal circulation. *(From: Attinger CE, Evans KK, Bulan E, et al. Angiosomes of the foot and ankle and clinical implications for limb salvage: reconstruction, incisions, and revascularization. Plast Reconstr Surg. 2006;117(7 Suppl):261S–293S.)*

retinaculum, and bifurcates into the medial and lateral plantar arteries at the level of the transverse septum between the abductor halluces longus and flexor digitorum brevis muscles. The medial plantar artery's angiosome encompasses the instep, while the lateral plantar artery supplies the lateral plantar surface as well as the plantar forefoot.

At the level of the lateral malleolus, the anterior tibial artery gives off (1) the lateral malleolar artery that joins with the anterior perforating branch of the peroneal artery. At the same level, the medial malleolar artery arises and anastomoses with the posteromedial artery of the posterior tibial artery. The anterior tibial artery then emerges under the extensor retinaculum of the ankle to become the (2) dorsalis pedis artery, which supplies the entire dorsum of the foot.

Clinical relevance of the angiosome model

In the absence of vascular anomalies or disease, blood flow to the foot and ankle is redundant with multiple arterial–arterial connections that provide a margin of safety in the setting of distal source vessel occlusion. For example, the anterior perforating branch (peroneal artery) connects with the lateral malleolar artery (anterior tibial artery) at the ankle. At the Lisfranc joint, the dorsalis pedis artery dives into the first interspace to connect directly with the lateral plantar artery (posterior tibial artery). This vascular loop is critical in determining the direction of flow within the anterior and posterior tibial arteries, which can be antegrade, retrograde, or both. Furthermore, the plantar and dorsal metatarsal arteries are linked to one another at the Lisfranc joint by proximal perforators and at the webspace by distal perforators. The posterior tibial and peroneal arteries connect via one to three perforators crossing deep to the distal Achilles tendon.

Using a Doppler ultrasound probe and selective occlusion, it is possible to determine the patency of these interconnections as well as the direction of blood flow. This is critical to optimize the success of any planned treatment or procedure. Incision placement along the boundary of two adjoining angiosomes ensures optimal blood flow from either side, thereby facilitating safe exposure of underlying skeletal structures as well as the design of vascularly reliable flaps. Among patients with infrapopliteal disease, angiosome-directed revascularization has manifested higher rates of healing (91% vs. 38%) and fewer amputations (9.1% vs. 38.1%) than indirect revascularization through arterial connections in the foot and ankle.[8] Similar findings have also been confirmed for infrapopliteal lesions treated with endovascular techniques.[9] This detailed knowledge of vascular anatomy further aids the surgeon in determining the likelihood of limb salvage for a given wound and existing blood supply. When salvage is not possible, early recognition and effective design of amputations minimizes the risk of distal tissue necrosis and spares the patient needless, costly, and potentially dangerous procedures that have little chance of success.

Innervation

Proximal to the popliteal fossa, the sciatic nerve bifurcates into the tibial and common peroneal nerves. The tibial nerve continues distally within the deep posterior compartment of the leg where it innervates muscles of the deep and superficial posterior compartments (except gastrocnemius muscle).

Distal to the tarsal tunnel, the tibial nerve trifurcates into the calcaneal (S1, S2), medial (L4, L5), and lateral plantar nerves (S1, S2), which supply motor branches to the intrinsic muscles of the foot (except the extensor digitorum brevis [EDB] muscle). Additionally, the calcaneal branch supplies sensibility to the plantar heel pad; the lateral plantar nerve supplies the lateral two-thirds of the sole and the fifth and lateral fourth toes; and the medial plantar nerve supplies the medial one-third of the sole as well as the first, second, third, and medial fourth toes.

The common peroneal nerve passes around the lateral aspect of the fibular head before splitting into the superficial (L4–S1) and deep (L4–S1) branches. The deep peroneal nerve innervates the extensor muscles of the anterior compartment, passing deep to the extensor retinaculum to innervate the EDB muscle in the foot. It provides sensory innervation to the ankle and midfoot joints, sinus tarsi, and first webspace. In the leg, the superficial peroneal nerve innervates the everting peroneal muscles of the lateral compartment. The nerve pierces the fascia, 10–12 cm proximal to the lateral ankle, to become subcutaneous and provide sensibility to the lateral lower leg, dorsum of the foot, and skin of all toes except the lateral fifth toe (sural nerve) and first webspace (deep peroneal nerve).

The sural nerve (L5, S1), derived from both the tibial and common peroneal nerves, descends distally in the posterior subcutaneous plane of the calf along the course of the lesser saphenous vein. It provides sensibility to the posterior and lateral skin of the distal third of the leg, prior to passing between the anterolateral border of the Achilles tendon and the lateral malleolus to supply the dorsolateral skin of the foot and lateral fifth toe. The skin of the medial half of the distal leg and dorsomedial foot is innervated by the saphenous nerve (L5, S1) – a cutaneous branch of the femoral nerve. The dorsum of the foot has communicating branches between the saphenous, sural, and superficial and the deep peroneal nerves; thus there is often an overlap in their respective sensory distributions. The same is true for the medial and lateral plantar nerves, which often overlap in their territories with the saphenous and sural nerves, respectively.

Wound comorbidities

The etiology of foot and ankle wounds is commonly traumatic, with the patient's underlying systemic pathophysiology complicating the healing process. Significant comorbid disease processes include diabetes, infection, ischemia, neuropathy, venous hypertension, lymphatic obstruction, immunologic abnormalities, hypercoagulability, vasospasm, neoplasm, self-mutilation, or any combination of the preceding. The more frequent of these comorbidities, including diabetes, neuropathy, peripheral vascular disease, connective tissue disorders, and venous hypertension, are discussed in greater detail below.

Diabetes mellitus

In the USA, approximately 29.1 million (9.3%) people have been diagnosed with diabetes.[10] Nearly 15% of the healthcare budget in the USA goes toward the management of diabetes, with 20% of hospitalizations and 25% of diabetic hospital days for the treatment of diabetic foot ulcers.[11] In patients with diabetes, the estimated annual and lifetime risk of developing a foot ulcer is in the range of 1–2 % and 15%, respectively.[11–14] Once an ulcer develops, the risk of amputation increases to 1% per year. Indeed, 1 in every 4 patients who present to the emergency room with diabetic foot ulceration or gangrene undergo immediate amputation, which in itself carries devastating prognostic implications.[15] Following major amputation in the diabetic, the risk of a second amputation in the contralateral limb approaches 50% within the first 2 years. Furthermore, 3-year postamputation mortality rates range from 20–50% and have been reported as high as 78% after 5 years.[1,12] Despite widespread strategies to improve glucose control and monitor for impaired sensibility, the number of diabetes-related amputations in the USA continues to rise from 54 000 in 1990 to 73 000 in 2010.[10]

Diabetic peripheral polyneuropathy is the major culprit behind non-healing diabetic foot wounds – accounting for 80–85% of amputations in diabetic patients.[16] Elevated intra-neural concentration of sorbitol, a glucose byproduct, is thought to be a principle mechanism mediating peripheral nerve damage. Resultant swelling of the injured nerve within anatomically tight confines (i.e., tarsal tunnel) leads to the "double crush syndrome", which may be partially reversible with early surgical release.[17] Unregulated glucose levels elevate advanced glycosylated end products that induce microvascular injury by cross-linking collagen molecules. Decreased insulin levels, along with altered concentrations of neurotropic peptides, may interfere with the maintenance and/or repair of damaged nerve fibers. Other factors implicated in the development of peripheral polyneuropathy include altered fat metabolism, oxidative stress, and abnormal levels of vasoactive substrates, such as nitric oxide.

Although peripheral neuropathy is generally considered the primary cause of diabetic foot wounds, the presence of infrapopliteal arterial occlusive disease significantly increases the risk of ulceration, reconstructive failure, and amputation in diabetic patients.[18] However, the lack of a PO_2 gradient between arterial blood and foot skin among diabetic patients (with and without ulceration) and non-diabetic patients (with normal transcutaneous oxygen tension) implicates a non-ischemic etiology for the majority of diabetic foot ulcers.[19] Previous misconceptions regarding an increased prevalence of "small-vessel" disease and intimal hyperplasia as the primary etiology of foot ulceration in diabetics have not been corroborated by findings from more recent prospective studies.[20–24] Nevertheless, the detrimental effects of hyperglycemia on capillary blood flow and tissue perfusion are significant. Erythrocyte aggregation and stiffness as well as the increased oxygen affinity result from non-enzymatic glycosylation of spectrin (red blood cell membrane protein) and hemoglobin, respectively, and contribute to reduced blood flow and relative tissue ischemia in diabetics. The altered flow characteristics that result trigger a compensatory rise in perfusion pressure, with increased transudation across capillary beds further perpetuating a rise in blood and plasma viscosity (Fig. 8.2 ⬤).

Fig. 8.2 appears online only.

In general, the importance of tight glycemic control in the promotion of wound healing and prevention of infection cannot be overemphasized. Hyperglycemia itself can impair the body's ability to combat infection. Chronic hyperglycemia diminishes the ability of polymorphonuclear leukocytes

(PMNs), macrophages, and lymphocytes to destroy bacteria. In addition, the diabetic's capacity to coat bacteria with antibiotics is diminished, which further shields bacteria from phagocytosis. As a result of this immunocompromised state, diabetics are especially prone to *Streptococcal* and *Staphylococcal* skin infections. Deeper infections tend to be polymicrobial, with gram-positive cocci, gram-negative rods, and anaerobes frequently detected on culture. Postoperative complication rates also correlate directly with the degree of chronic and perioperative glycemic control. At our institution, a perioperative blood glucose level less than 200 mg/dL and hemoglobin A1C level less than 6.5% (48 mmol/mol) serves as the preferred threshold for minimizing complications and dehiscence after wound closure in high-risk diabetic patients.[25]

Neuropathic changes

Neuropathic changes observed in the diabetic foot result from abnormalities in the motor, sensory, and autonomic nervous systems. The loss of pseudomotor function from autonomic neuropathy leads to anhidrosis and hyperkeratosis. Fissuring of the desiccated skin facilitates bacterial entry and subsequent infection. The lack of sensibility over bony prominences and between the toes often delays detection of skin barrier disruptions. In addition to the nerve changes discussed previously, diabetic patients are unusually susceptible to peripheral nerve compression as evidenced by histologic similarities between chronically entrapped nerves and those seen in diabetic neuropathy.[26,27] When a Tinel's sign is present on exam, early peripheral nerve release, at known anatomic sites of compression, may prevent the progression of neuropathy and subsequent loss of protective sensibility.[28] Currently, however, there are no randomized studies to substantiate the benefits of this approach over medical therapy alone.

Charcot neuroarthropathy is a destructive process of the bones, joints, and soft tissues of the foot, occurring in 0.1–2.5% of diabetic patients.[29,30] When present, the tarsometatarsal joints (30%), metatarsophalangeal joints (30%), intertarsal joints (24%), and interphalangeal joints (4%) are commonly involved. Etiologically, these degenerative changes are thought to be mediated by the interplay between sensorimotor and autonomic neuropathy, repetitive trauma, and abnormal bony metabolism.[31] The process likely begins with a ligamentous soft-tissue injury accompanied by synovitis and joint effusion. In the absence of pain perception, continued use of the extremity exacerbates the inflammatory process. Eventual distension of the joint capsule leads to ligament attenuation and joint instability. The destructive changes that occur result in collapse of the medial longitudinal arch, which alters gait biomechanics. The normal calcaneal pitch becomes distorted, causing severe strain to the ligaments that bind the metatarsal, cuneiform, navicular, and other small bones that form the long arch of the foot.

Motor neuropathy further contributes to Charcot deformities as the intrinsic foot musculature atrophies and becomes fibrotic. The resulting metatarsophalangeal joint extension and interphalangeal joint flexion produces excessive pressure on the metatarsal heads and the distal phalanges. Loss of both the transverse and longitudinal arches of the foot exacerbates the unfavorable weight distribution across the midfoot and metatarsal heads. Patients who continue to ambulate abnormally load weight over new bony prominences – precipitating

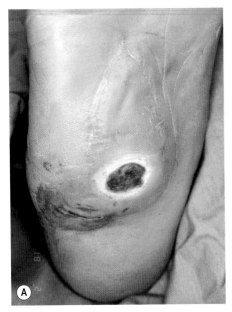

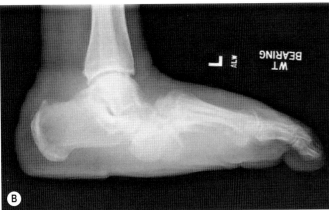

Fig. 8.3 Charcot arthropathy. **(A)** Chronic plantar foot ulceration in a patient with Charcot deformity and altered gait biomechanics. **(B)** Lateral weight-bearing plain film of the foot demonstrating severe architectural distortion of the midfoot skeleton with dorsal dislocation at the Lisfranc joint and collapse of the medial longitudinal arch.

the development of chronic ulceration, infection, gangrene, and eventual limb loss if the process is not halted in its early stages (Fig. 8.3).

Ischemia

Atherosclerotic disease is a common cause of non-healing foot ulcers, particularly in the setting of diabetes. Hypercholesterolemia, hypertension, and tobacco use are also considered major risk factors for atherosclerosis. Ischemic ulceration in the distal lower extremity may result from small-vessel disease, including thromboangiitis obliterans (i.e., Buerger's disease), vasospastic disorders (i.e., Raynaud's phenomenon/disease), vasculitis, and/or thromboembolic disease (Fig. 8.4 ●). In any case, the etiology of distal limb ischemia must be accurately diagnosed in order to determine the need for revascularization, as well as the appropriate sequence and timing of soft-tissue reconstruction.

Fig. 8.4 appears online only.

In the presence of distal limb ischemia, successful reconstruction mandates the establishment of uninterrupted blood

flow to the region of soft-tissue loss. Intuitively, achieving this goal through directed, antegrade inflow is more likely to affect healing than reliance upon non-specific, collateral circulation.[5] Indeed, angiosome-directed revascularization increases the rate of wound healing by 50% and reduces the risk of major amputation four-fold.[8] For ulcers on the dorsum of the foot or ankle, the anterior tibial artery or dorsalis pedis provides an ideal target for revascularization when possible. If the connection between the dorsalis pedis and the lateral plantar artery is intact, then bypass to the posterior tibial artery offers a potential alternative. For ulcers involving the heel, either the posterior tibial artery or peroneal artery should be targeted. The posterior tibial artery should also be chosen in the setting of mid- and/or forefoot plantar wounds; although, revascularization of the dorsalis pedis can be effective if its connection with the lateral plantar artery remains intact. In situations where the ideal target is not amenable to endovascular intervention or open vascular bypass, indirect revascularization should proceed with an understanding that the risk of failure and ultimate limb loss approaches 15% or more.

When patients with severe vascular disease present with gangrene, the timing of revascularization and wound debridement is critical. In the presence of stable dry gangrene without cellulitis or infection, revascularization takes priority and should proceed promptly, as premature debridement of a devascularized wound may promote loss of potentially salvageable tissue. In contrast, immediate and aggressive debridement is appropriate when wet gangrene, ascending cellulitis, or necrotizing fasciitis is present. Revascularization should then proceed on an urgent basis thereafter, as progressive gangrene and necrosis will ensue in the absence of newly established blood flow. Following adequate revascularization, soft-tissue reconstruction is often delayed until signs of infection and inflammation have resolved and the wound bed is manifesting initial signs of healing (i.e., granulation). In our experience, this frequently occurs between 5 and 10 days after targeted reperfusion of an affected angiosome. In the setting of indirect revascularization, however, healing may be delayed by 3–4 weeks.

Venous ulcers

Venous stasis ulcers are 3–4 times more prevalent than arterial ulcers and are caused by local venous hypertension. The leg has low-pressure superficial and high-pressure deep venous systems that directly communicate through interconnecting perforators. Venous return is largely facilitated by muscle contraction, which compresses the veins and propagates blood flow back to the heart. The direction of flow within the veins is controlled by the presence of unidirectional valves that prevent backflow. These valves can become incompetent after thrombus formation or with advanced age.

Venous testing should assess for valvular competence and thrombosis. A history of prior thrombus warrants further evaluation for coagulopathy. The mainstay of venous ulcer therapy centers around compression and exercise to increase venous return to the heart. Unna boots are often effective in the active patient, while multilayer compression dressings (2 to 4-ply) are more effective in patients who are more sedentary. Chronic ulcers may benefit from absorptive dressings, aggressive wound debridement, and/or application of cultured skin derivatives (recalcitrant cases) once edema has improved. Surgical treatment of incompetent saphenous or lesser saphenous veins or of incompetent perforators can help relieve local venous hypertension sufficiently to allow healing. To remain healed, lifetime compression therapy is often mandatory.

Connective tissue disorders and thrombophilia

Connective tissue disorders (i.e., systemic lupus erythematosus, rheumatoid arthritis, and scleroderma) are frequently associated with Raynaud's disease – a vasospastic condition that causes intermittent cutaneous ischemia and distal ulceration. Treatment of these disorders frequently includes the use of immunosuppressive medications (i.e., steroids and/or chemotherapeutic agents) to mitigate immune-mediated destruction of local tissue. Although the wound retarding effects of steroids can be partially reversed with oral vitamin A (10000 U/day while the wound is open), high systemic doses may counter the therapeutic immunosuppressive effects of steroids, which would be undesirable in the setting of autoimmune disease. The use of topical vitamin A (1000 U/g of ointment) offers a safe and effective alternative to promote wound healing in these patients. Nevertheless, close coordination with a rheumatologist is imperative as treatment of inflammatory and/or vasculitic wounds is principally medical in nature. Once underlying abnormalities have been identified and corrected, wound-healing adjuncts such as cultured dermis/skin equivalents, maggot debridement therapy, and/or hyperbaric oxygen can be used to stimulate the formation of healthy granulation tissue. Patience is often required as these wounds can take in excess of 18 months to heal completely.

To complicate matters further, nearly 50% of patients with vasculitic wounds are thrombophilic and have an underlying propensity for pathologic thrombus formation. The more common of these hypercoagulable states include factor V Leiden, anomalous factor II (G202010A mutation), hyperhomocysteinemia, antiphospholipid syndrome (lupus anticoagulant, anticardiolipin, anti-B$_2$-glycoprotein 1), plasminogen activator inhibitor (PAI)-1 mutation, and deficiencies in antithrombin III, protein C, and/or protein S. The presence of single or multiple hypercoagulable traits can be particularly troublesome for patients who may require microvascular reconstruction, as thrombotic events in these patients tend to occur more frequently, present later, and are often refractory to conventional salvage techniques.

A recent review of our institutional data revealed a high prevalence of subclinical thrombophilia (61%) among patients undergoing non-traumatic lower extremity reconstruction. This observation is not entirely surprising given that limb salvage patients often present with disproportionately higher rates of comorbidities known to potentiate thrombosis (i.e., systemic lupus erythematosus).[32] Sixteen percent of these patients ultimately experienced a thrombotic complication resulting in flap loss, despite multiple attempts at conventional flap salvage. Indeed, salvage rates following postoperative thrombosis as low as 0% have been reported in the setting of undetected hypercoagulable states.[33] Therefore the importance of identifying thrombophilic patients preoperatively and counseling them regarding the poor prognostic

implications associated with microvascular thrombosis cannot be over emphasized. If a diagnosis of thrombophilia is either known or suspected based on historical information, referral to a hematologist and/or laboratory screening for commonly encountered hypercoagulable traits is recommended.[34]

Patient evaluation and diagnosis

Clinical history

Effective management of foot and ankle wounds is predicated upon an accurate determination of wound etiology, previously administered therapies, host comorbidities, and baseline biomechanics. The origin and age of the wound should be determined. Traumatic wounds should be defined in terms of acute versus chronic; high versus low impact; and mechanism of injury (i.e., biomechanical, thermal, caustic, radiation-induced, etc.). The patient's tetanus immunization status should be obtained and updated as indicated. In chronic wounds, the age of the wound is important as long-standing wounds have the potential for malignant transformation (i.e., Marjolin's ulcer). Previous topical therapies must be elucidated, as caustic agents (i.e., hydrogen peroxide, 10% iodine, Dakin's solution, etc.) may contribute to wound chronicity.

A careful medical history should be obtained to identify disease states that negatively affect wound healing (i.e., diabetes mellitus, peripheral vascular disease, autoimmune conditions, immunocompromise, hematologic disorders, malnutrition, and so on). The presence of rheumatologic autoimmune conditions such as rheumatoid arthritis, pyoderma gangrenosum, systemic lupus erythematosus, and scleroderma are frequently associated with inflammatory wounds that initially necessitate medical rather than surgical management. Optimizing coagulopathies (i.e., factor V Leiden, protein C deficiency, protein S deficiency, anti-thrombin III deficiency, anomalous factor II, etc.) in patients with vasculitic wounds is critical for progression of normal wound healing. A complete list of medications and drug allergies should be obtained, as medications used in the treatment of autoimmune disease (i.e., steroids and/or chemotherapy) frequently impair healing. Nutritional status must also be optimized to promote healing (albumin >3.5 g/dL and/or total lymphocyte count >1500). Smoking significantly decreases local cutaneous blood flow and should be documented and addressed with each patient. Given the complexity of various disease processes, multiple specialties are often called upon to assist in optimizing the patient's medical condition in order to improve the chances of successful wound healing.

Limb function

Assessment of the patient's current and anticipated level of activity is important to determine if the leg should be salvaged and to what extent it should be reconstructed. A poorly functional limb in a young, otherwise active, patient may be counterproductive, and the patient may in fact do better with a modified below-knee amputation (Ertl) and a well-adapted prosthetic. For the less active or non-ambulatory patient, if the limb is functional or can at least facilitate simple transfers, salvage – if medically tolerable and technically feasible – is usually indicated. In contrast, if the limb is non-functional and the patient is non-ambulatory, strong consideration should be given to performing a knee-disarticulation or above-knee amputation to cure the problem and minimize the risk of recurrent breakdown and/or development of a life-threatening infection.

Similarly, the complexity of the reconstruction is largely influenced by the patient's health and functional goals. For the younger patient or athlete who can tolerate a prolonged microsurgical procedure, restoration of normal function is the goal. However, a complex reconstruction for a marginally functional leg is often worse than a well-designed below-knee amputation with an athletic prosthesis. For the patient who only uses the leg to transfer, the simplest solution that will achieve this goal should be pursued, even if it entails sacrificing part of the foot.

Wound assessment

The complete physical exam starts with a careful 3D wound measurement (length, width, and depth), as well as evaluation of involved tissue types (i.e., epidermis, dermis, subcutaneous tissue, fascia, muscle, tendon, joint capsule, and/or bone). A metallic probe can be used to assess underlying skeletal involvement. Direct palpation of bone at the base of the wound is highly sensitive (87%) and specific (91%) for the presence of osteomyelitis.[35] Diabetic ulcers with an area greater than 2 cm^2 have a 90% chance of harboring osteomyelitis, regardless of findings on the probe-to-bone test.[36] The level of tissue necrosis and potential avenues for the spread of infection (i.e., flexor and/or extensor tendon surfaces) must be determined. The presence and extent of cellulitis must be noted and differentiated from dependent rubor by direct leg elevation above the level of the heart. If cellulitis is present, the erythema will not resolve with elevation and its border should be delineated with a marker, and dated and timed accordingly. This permits the clinician to accurately monitor the progress of infection and/or response to initial treatment.

Vascular workup

The vascular status of the foot must be accurately evaluated. The presence of palpable pulses (i.e., dorsalis pedis and/or posterior tibial artery) signals that blood flow is likely adequate to promote healing. If pulses are not palpable, however, the Doppler signal over the posterior tibial artery, dorsalis pedis artery, and anterior perforating branch of the peroneal artery should be assessed. Doppler ultrasound allows the surgeon to evaluate both the quality and direction of flow through major and minor arteries in the foot, which aids in the design of reliable local flaps and amputations. In the setting of vascular obstruction, the normal triphasic waveform may deteriorate distally to a biphasic waveform with a reversed flow component, which will become biphasic, monophasic, and ultimately aphasic as the obstruction becomes more significant. All patients with aphasic waveforms and foot wounds should undergo revascularization before attempts at advanced reconstruction are made. Triphasic or biphasic flow along the artery being evaluated indicates normal and adequate blood flow, respectively. These patients generally do not require vascular reconstruction. On the other hand, limbs with monophasic flow warrant further investigation and possible referral to a vascular surgeon, depending on the location of the wound

and complexity of the proposed reconstruction. A monophasic signal, however, does not necessarily reflect inadequate blood flow; rather, it can also indicate a lack of vascular tone with absent distal resistance, as is often seen in calcified vessels.

If non-palpable pulses are monophasic, then formal non-invasive arterial Doppler studies are indicated. It is important to obtain pulse volume recordings (PVRs) and segmental pressures at each level along the lower extremity (high and low thigh, calf, ankle, metatarsal, and digital cuffs), as both ankle/brachial indices and absolute pressure measurements are often unreliable in patients with calcified vessels (Fig. 8.5).[37] Non-compressible arterial walls are seen in 5–30% of diabetics and are caused by mural calcification, which falsely elevates the values for both tests. A PVR amplitude less than 10 mmHg indicates that ischemia may be present. As digital arteries are less likely to be calcified, absolute toe pressures provide an alternative, more accurate prediction of healing potential in the diabetic foot.[38–40] Values less than 30 mmHg are indicative of severe ischemia and the potential need for vascular intervention.[41] Tissue oxygen pressure levels are also helpful in determining whether extremity blood flow is sufficient, with levels less than 40 mmHg suggestive of inadequate local perfusion. For patients with known vascular disease and/or those undergoing microvascular reconstruction, duplex imaging generates useful information. Real time B-mode imaging and pulsed Doppler provide anatomic, geometric, and velocity data, as well as blood flow measurements from various locations within the vascular system.

If any of the aforementioned non-invasive tests suggest ischemia, an arterial imaging study should be obtained to help evaluate whether a vascular inflow (absent femoral pulse) and/or outflow (absent distal pulse) procedure is required. With advances in endovascular techniques, revascularization with dilatation, recanalization, and atherectomy of stenosed/obstructed arteries can be performed in patients who would otherwise be poor candidates for open vascular bypass.[42,43] As part of our algorithm for planned microvascular reconstructions, we obtain a diagnostic angiogram for patients with non-palpable pulses and absent or monophasic Doppler signals, in order to provide an accurate assessment of flow to the distal lower extremity. In situations where intervention is deemed necessary, targeted percutaneous transluminal angioplasty (PTA), with or without stent placement, is employed in the same setting to restore both direct and peripheral inflow – thereby obviating the need for separate diagnostic (i.e., computed tomographic angiography) and therapeutic procedures. Beyond the more obvious advantage of augmenting arterial inflow to the recipient site, we utilize targeted PTA to improve recipient vessel caliber in locations where calcifications, occlusions, and stenoses often complicate microvascular anastomosis. Our early results with this protocol have been encouraging for patients with multi-vessel disease and may indicate a role for targeted endovascular therapy, as an adjunct to free tissue transfer, in regions of compromised distal blood flow (Fig. 8.6 ⊕).[44]

Fig. 8.6 appears online only.

Sensorimotor examination

Sensibility is evaluated with a 5.07 Semmes–Weinstein filament that represents 10 g of pressure. If the patient cannot feel the filament, protective sensation is absent and the risk of

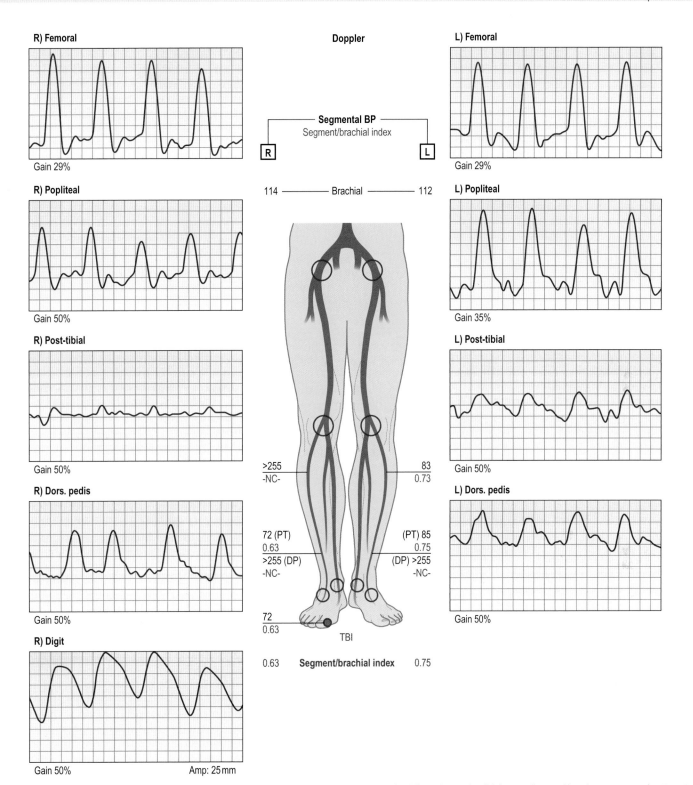

Fig. 8.5 Example of a pulse volume recording and segmental pressures readout demonstrating bilateral posterior tibial artery disease. Note the more severely attenuated, irregular, and low amplitude waveforms on the left side of the readout (patient's right lower extremity) as compared to the right (patient's left lower extremity). BP, Blood Pressure; DP, Dorsalis Pedis Artery; NC, Non-Compressible; PT, Posterior Tibial Artery; TBI, Toe-Brachial Index.

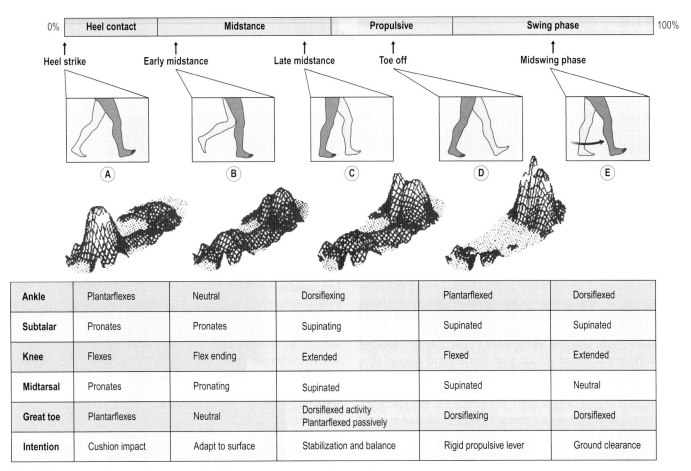

	Heel strike	Early midstance	Late midstance	Toe off	Midswing phase
Ankle	Plantarflexes	Neutral	Dorsiflexing	Plantarflexed	Dorsiflexed
Subtalar	Pronates	Pronates	Supinating	Supinated	Supinated
Knee	Flexes	Flex ending	Extended	Flexed	Extended
Midtarsal	Pronates	Pronating	Supinated	Supinated	Neutral
Great toe	Plantarflexes	Neutral	Dorsiflexed activity Plantarflexed passively	Dorsiflexing	Dorsiflexed
Intention	Cushion impact	Adapt to surface	Stabilization and balance	Rigid propulsive lever	Ground clearance

Fig. 8.8 The normal gait cycle with phase-specific F-Scan pressure mapping and joint motion.

breakdown and/or ulceration is significantly increased. Motor function is assessed by looking at the resting position of the foot and by testing the strength and active range of motion of the ankle, foot, and toes.

Gait analysis

Gait abnormalities resulting from musculoskeletal imbalances are frequently detected in patients evaluated for chronic wound management. Preoperative assessment of gait, therefore, is critical and should include a measure of ankle dorsiflexion as well as an F-scan analysis or pressure mapping. Evaluation for equinus deformity should occur with the leg held first in complete extension, to keep the gastrocnemius muscles at their full resting length, and then with the knee flexed (which reduces stretch/tension on the gastrocnemius) to assess the soleus muscle (Fig. 8.7 ⊙). If the ankle only dorsiflexes when the knee is flexed, then the gastrocnemius muscles are responsible for the equinus posture of the foot and can be released by performing a gastrocnemius recession. If the ankle remains tight during knee extension and flexion, then both gastrocnemius and soleus contributions to the Achilles tendon have to be released, usually percutaneously.

Fig. 8.7 appears online only.

The F-scan gait analysis uses multiple pressure-sensing surface probes that record pressures on the sole of the foot during all phases of gait. Areas of excessive compression during weight-bearing are displayed graphically and help

plan the biomechanical components of the required reconstruction as well as the customized design of subsequent orthotic devices (Fig. 8.8). Furthermore, this tool can be used to document and monitor biomechanical changes that occur following tendon transfer and/or lengthening procedures.

Skeletal assessment

The bony architecture is evaluated by looking at whether the arch is stable, collapsed, or disjointed. Bone prominence can occur with collapsed midfoot bones (i.e., Charcot destruction of the midfoot), osteophyte formation, and/or abnormal biomechanical forces (hallux valgus, hammer toe, etc.). Three-view plain films of the foot (anteroposterior, oblique, and lateral) help delineate underlying osseous abnormalities to guide the formation of an operative plan. Lateral views should always be weight-bearing to assess the stability and contour of the bony arch. Calcaneal, sesamoid, and metatarsal head views may be indicated if local pathology is suspected in those areas.

It is important to remember that radiographic signs of osteomyelitis lag behind clinical appearance by up to 3 weeks. Thus the presence of a normal radiograph in the setting of an infected foot wound does not rule out the diagnosis of osteomyelitis. A magnetic resonance imaging (MRI) scan can aid in earlier detection, as well as the differentiation of osteomyelitis from Charcot collapse. In general, bone scans are of no value in the setting of an open wound. The underlying bone will show increased uptake, regardless of the presence of osteomyelitis. A negative bone scan, however, can be useful in ruling out the proximal spread of infection along the surface of a long bone. Ultimately, if osteomyelitis is suspected, then a bone biopsy is indicated (i.e., "gold standard"), utilizing a separate approach other than through the ulcerated wound. Most often, however, bone is sampled through the operative site because it is often present at the base of the debrided wound. In these instances, unexposed medullary tissue should be obtained with a previously unused curette and submitted for both decalcification (in formalin) and culture (in a few drops of normal saline solution), which is used to guide sensitivity-directed antibiotic therapy.

Management

Trauma and crush injuries

Crush injuries or ischemic insults to the foot can elevate pressures within myofascial compartments; and, like that in the leg, compartment syndrome in the foot must be evaluated and treated if necessary. The signs and symptoms of compartment syndrome of the foot are similar to those found elsewhere in the body (i.e., 6 Ps: pain, paresthesia, pallor, paralysis, pulselessness, poikilothermia). Pain out of proportion to the clinical examination is often the first symptom. Weakness of the toe flexors/extensors and pain with passive dorsiflexion of the toes represent important physical signs. Pallor, paresthesia, a palpably tense compartment, and absent digital pulses on Doppler assessment eventually occur. Compartment pressure recordings should be obtained by a physician who understands the compartmental anatomy of the foot.

When measuring pedal compartment pressures, it may be difficult to determine the compartment in which the pressure is actually being recorded. If clinical indications are present, a four-compartment release should be performed.[45] The medial approach to the foot, as advocated by Henry, allows decompression of all four compartments through a single incision.[46] Mubarak and Hargens advocate two longitudinal incisions on the dorsum of the foot through which the interosseous compartments may be decompressed (analogous to that in the hand).[47] Whitesides anecdotally described compartment syndrome of the foot, secondary to burns and direct trauma, and recommended decompression using the medial approach of Henry.[48]

For adequate compartment decompression, a curvilinear incision is made along the medial glabrous junction of the foot, beginning at the first metatarsal head and extending to the heel. The skin and fascia are divided, and the incision is carried down to release the abductor hallucis muscle and its tendon – thus decompressing the medial compartment. Retraction of the abductor hallucis towards the plantar surface exposes the medial intermuscular septum, which is divided to release the central compartment. The small toe compartment is released next utilizing a linear incision along the lateral glabrous junction that extends from the fifth metatarsal head to the calcaneus. Through this incision, the fascia enveloping the small toe compartment is released. Decompression of the interosseous compartment is best achieved through two linear, dorsal incisions overlying the second and fourth metatarsals. The fascia overlying the four interosseous spaces is then opened (Fig. 8.9).

Wound infection and directed antibiotic therapy

Wound infection is characterized by the presence of replicating microorganisms within a wound, resulting in a subsequent host response such as erythema, warmth, swelling, pain, malodor, and purulent drainage. If not recognized and treated early, the infection will spread systemically leading to fever, leukocytosis, and possibly sepsis. The line between colonization and infection may be minute, so prompt identification is critical to healing wounds and minimizing complications. For most microorganisms, a bacterial count (bioburden) of 10^5 bacteria/g of tissue or greater has been defined as the quantitative threshold for wound infection and inhibition of the wound healing process.[49]

When managing infected foot wounds, it is important to determine the source and extent of infection. The erythematous border surrounding the wound should be delineated, timed, and dated for serial comparison. The original mark is used as a reference point for determining the effectiveness of antibiotics and/or prior debridement. Radiographic evaluation of the affected area will help identify skeletal involvement as well as the presence of soft-tissue gas. If gas is visualized radiographically within the tissue planes, beyond the immediate location of an open ulcer, gas gangrene is most likely present and the wound becomes a surgical emergency. Gas is usually a byproduct of anaerobic bacteria (i.e., *Clostridium perfringens*); it tends to be foul smelling and travels along the fascial planes. Compartment pressures in the affected area should be assessed, as high pressures in the diabetic foot with gas gangrene are frequently missed secondary to neuropathy. If a deep abscess is in question, ultrasound imaging or computed tomography can be very useful to ascertain its size and location.

If the wound is acutely infected with purulent drainage, malodor, and/or proximally ascending erythema, immediate and aggressive debridement is indicated to prevent sepsis, possible limb loss, or death. The involved compartments of the extremity should be released if there is any suspicion of elevated compartment pressures. Wounds with foul-smelling odors should be debrided sufficiently to get rid of the odor. Persistent malodor signals the need for further debridement and excision of any remaining necrotic or infected tissue. It is important to remember that the presence of gas gangrene is not an absolute indication for amputation. Aggressive serial debridement±adjunctive hyperbaric oxygen can often salvage enough of the limb to preserve functional integrity. Hyperbaric oxygen has been shown to be particularly effective in the control of anaerobic infections.[50]

Aerobic and anaerobic cultures of the wound should be obtained during each debridement by taking samples deep to the surface of the infected tissue and purulence. Superficial swabs and tissue cultures are of limited use, as they usually reflect surface flora rather than the underlying bacteria that are responsible for infection. Broad spectrum antibiotics should be started after deep tissue cultures are obtained and subsequently narrowed based on culture results and sensitivities. It is important to be aware that deep cultures may miss up to two-thirds of the bacteria species present within a wound.[51] Therefore persisting signs of infection after 48 h of antibiotic therapy signal a need to reconsider

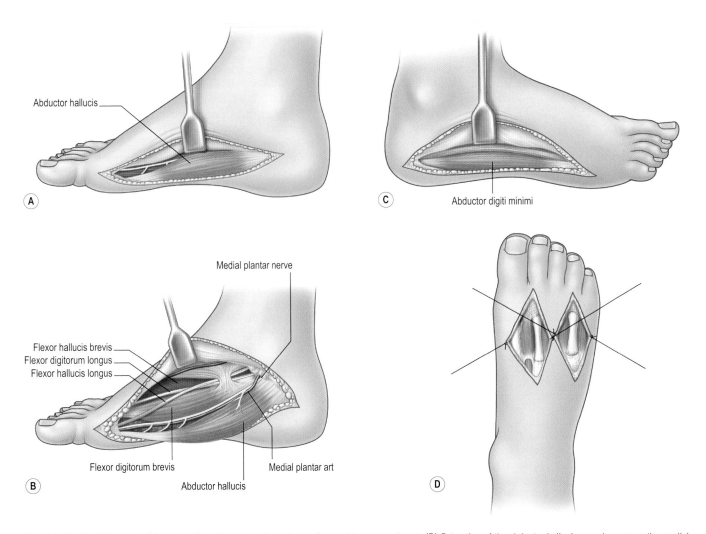

Fig. 8.9 **(A)** Medial instep incision along the glabrous junction releases the great toe compartment. **(B)** Retraction of the abductor hallucis muscle exposes the medial intermuscular septum, which is incised to release the central compartment (retracted). **(C)** Lateral incision along the glabrous junction releases the small toe compartment. **(D)** Decompression of the interosseous compartment is best achieved through two linear dorsal incisions overlying the second and fourth metatarsals.

the choice of antibiotics as well as the necessity of further debridement.

For suspected osteomyelitis, cultures of both debrided bone and normal proximal bone should be obtained. It may be helpful to label the osteomyelitic bone culture as "dirty" and the normal proximal bone culture as "clean" so that the quality of debridement can be assessed and the length of antibiotic treatment determined. If a wound is closed and the "clean" culture is showing no growth (i.e., only healthy bone remains at the base of the wound), then a 1-week course of appropriate antibiotic therapy is often sufficient. In contrast, if the "clean" culture is positive for bacterial growth, then re-resection of bone or a 6-week course of antibiotics may be necessary. If the surgeon suspects that the bone left behind still harbors osteomyelitis despite negative cultures (i.e., calcaneus or tibia), then a 6-week or longer course of antibiotic therapy may be needed to eradicate the infection.[52,53] The appropriate antibiotic choice and duration is best determined and monitored by an infectious disease specialist, who is also adept at managing the untoward side effects of prolonged antibiotic therapy.

Biofilm

By definition, open wounds are contaminated, meaning that the bed contains planktonic bacteria and biofilm. Acute wounds have only 6% biofilm present, whereas chronic wounds have biofilm in excess of 90%. Biofilm is characterized as a microbial community embedded within an extracellular polymeric matrix that is irreversibly adherent to both living and non-living surfaces.[54] This structurally heterogeneous matrix promotes enhanced cell-to-cell signaling between bacteria (i.e., quorum sensing), allowing biofilms to grow and act as independent organisms.[55–57] Biofilms require highly specific growth media that are not commonly found in the hospital setting, and, as a result, typical specimen cultures are often inadequate for the positive characterization of bacteria.[58] Polymerase chain reaction (PCR) technology, however, permits rapid identification of causative organisms within a matter of hours. PCR studies of biofilm have identified over 60 different bacterial species, more than 60% of which are anaerobes. These multi-species colonies coexist at a far lower energy state and serve as a medium for extrachromosomal

DNA plasmids that confer antibiotic resistance up to 1000 times greater than that of planktonic bacteria alone. Within 48 h, the biofilm matures and becomes resistant to both topical and systemic antibiotic penetration as well as phagocytosis by the host immune response.[59] The colony then spreads passively through fragmentation (70%) or by active individual seeding of undifferentiated planktonic cells (30%). Biofilm causes inflammation of the surrounding tissue, and, while classic signs of infection may not predominate, increased pain/tenderness, exudate, abnormal odor, and/or friable granulation tissue often signal its presence, as well as the need for aggressive mechanical debridement to stimulate healing of healthy underlying tissue.

Acute vs. chronic wounds

The goal of treating any wound is to promote healing in a timely fashion. The first step toward realizing this objective is to establish a clean and healthy wound base. An acute wound is defined as a recent wound that has yet to progress through the sequential stages of wound healing. In the setting of adequate blood flow, a clean base can be established with simple debridement techniques and the wound closed either immediately or following application of a local dressing to facilitate healing by secondary intention or closure at a later date. In contrast, a chronic wound is one that is arrested at some stage of healing (usually the inflammatory stage) and cannot progress on its own. Converting a chronic wound to an acute wound mandates the correction of underlying medical comorbidities (i.e., hyperglycemia, coagulopathies, changing or modifying drug therapy, etc.), restoration of adequate blood flow, administration of appropriate antibiotics when indicated, and aggressive wound debridement. If the wound has responded appropriately, healthy granulation will appear, edema will decrease, and neo-epithelialization of the wound edges will occur. Measuring the wound area weekly is a useful means to monitor progress, as the normal rate of healing equates to a 10–15% decrease in wound surface area per week. Assuming any underlying abnormalities have been corrected (i.e., infection, ischemia, coagulopathy), a healing rate below that expected may necessitate the incorporation of adjuncts, such as negative pressure wound therapy (NWPT), topical growth factors, cultured skin/dermal substitutes, and/or hyperbaric oxygen.

Surgical preparation of the wound bed

Necrotic tissue, foreign material, and bacteria/biofilm impede the body's attempt to heal through the production of proteases, collagenases, and elastases that overwhelm the local healing process.[60] Aggressive mechanical debridement, therefore, is essential to overcome these barriers and stimulate normal healing. Nevertheless, surgical debridement is the single most underperformed procedure in treating foot and ankle wounds, secondary to concern over resultant defect closure.[61] Leaving dead or infected tissue or bone behind, however, leads to subsequent infection and possible amputation. Tissue with clotted veins or arteries in the dermis or subcutaneous tissue, liquefied fascia or tendon, and nonviable bone should all be debrided. Debridement should be considered complete only when normal bleeding tissue remains. By the same token, any viable tissue should be preserved as it may prove useful at the time of definitive reconstruction.

The most effective debridement technique consists of tangential excision of all grossly contaminated and devitalized tissue, until only normal tissue is present. This minimizes the amount of viable tissue sacrificed while ensuring that only healthy tissue remains. Gentle tissue handling, sharp dissection, skin hook retraction, and pinpoint cauterization of bleeding vessels serve to minimize trauma and promote tissue viability. One should avoid harmful maneuvers such as crushing skin edges with forceps or clamps, burning tissues with electrocautery, and/or suture-ligating healthy perivascular tissues.[62] Useful surgical tools include a scalpel blade, Mayo scissors, curettes, rongeurs, sagittal saw, power burr, and hydro-surgical debrider (Versajet, Smith & Nephew, Hull, UK). Serial debridement is performed regularly, and as often as necessary, until the wound is deemed clean and ready for closure.[61,63,64]

Three technical adjuncts can be used in combination to ensure adequate debridement of the entire wound: (1) topical staining of the wound with methylene blue, (2) utilizing color to guide debridement, and (3) tangential excision of senescent wound margins. Prior to debridement, methylene blue is liberally applied to the wound base using a cotton tip applicator. This allows the surgeon to adequately address all portions of the wound by ensuring complete removal of all visibly stained tissue from the wound base (Fig. 8.10). In addition, the surgeon must be familiar with normal tissue colors (i.e., red, white, and yellow). Using these colors as a guide provides an endpoint to debridement and helps prevent removal of healthy tissue.[65] Finally, excision of 3–5 mm of marginal tissue during initial debridement removes senescent cells from chronic wound edges and permits healthy underlying cells to progress through the stages of normal wound healing.[66]

Biomechanical considerations

Biomechanics are a critical part of the reconstructive plan and may involve bone rearrangement, partial joint removal/fusion, or tendon lengthening/transfer. Charcot deformities of the midfoot are often heralded by mild effusions, joint instability, crepitus, and swelling. If these symptoms are identified early, conservative treatment with offloading and casting may prevent the evolution of a fixed midfoot deformity.[67]

Ulcers under the metatarsal head(s) occur because biomechanical abnormalities place excessive or extended pressure on the plantar surface of the forefoot during the gait cycle. Although hammertoes, sesamoids, long metatarsals, and joint dislocations can be contributing factors, the principle cause of abnormal weight dispersion is a tight Achilles tendon that prevents ankle dorsiflexion beyond the neutral position. If dorsiflexion remains poor with the knee bent or straight, either the gastrocnemius and soleus contributions to the tendon or the posterior capsule of the ankle joint may be tight. If percutaneous release of the Achilles tendon fails to improve dorsiflexion, then a posterior capsular release of the ankle joint should be performed. Alternatively, if the ankle only dorsiflexes when the knee is flexed, then the gastrocnemius muscles are responsible for the equinus posture of the foot and a gastrocnemius recession should correct the problem. Lengthening or release of the tight Achilles tendon results in

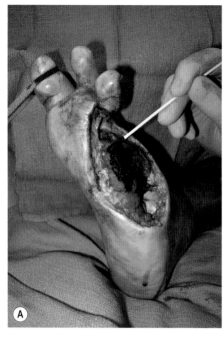
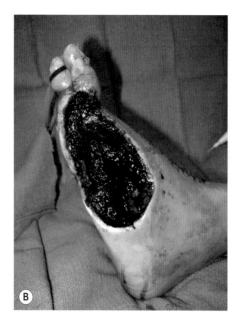
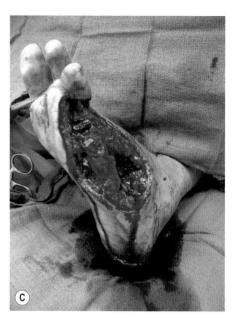

Fig. 8.10 Topical staining of a wound with methylene blue to ensure adequate debridement and removal of surface biofilm. Methylene blue dye is applied liberally to the wound base using a cotton swab applicator. After debridement, there should be no residual dye left in the wound.

rapid healing and long-term protection, decreasing ulcer recurrence rates by 75% at 7 months and 52% at 25 months, when compared with contact casting alone (Fig. 8.11).[68,69]

Patients with prior transmetatarsal amputations and recurrent forefoot ulceration are another group whose wounds are attributable to biomechanical disturbances. Recurrent ulceration following distal amputation results from musculotendinous imbalance within the foot, which leads to abnormal posturing (equinovarus deformity), instability, and altered weight distribution during ambulation. These patients often

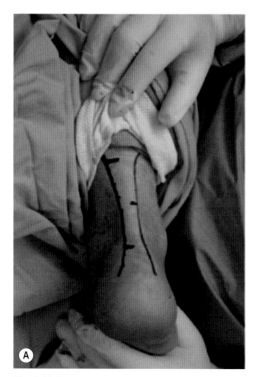
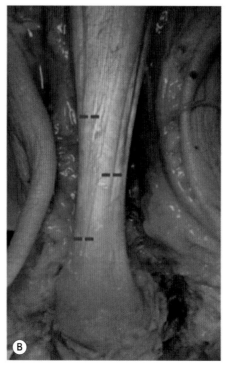
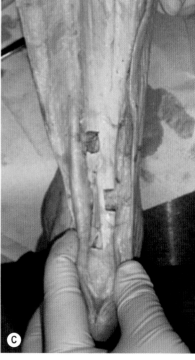

Fig. 8.11 Percutaneous Achilles tendon lengthening. If both the gastrocnemius and the soleus portions of the Achilles tendon are tight, the tendon can be released percutaneously by making three alternating stab incisions at 3 cm, 6 cm, and 9 cm proximal to the insertion of the Achilles into the calcaneus. A No. 15 blade is inserted into the central raphe of the tendon and the scalpel turned so that half of the tendon is cut at each site. The ankle is gently dorsiflexed until the tendon releases and immobilized to promote healing in a lengthened position. This technique provides an increase in Achilles tendon length by approximately 2 cm. *(Courtesy of John Steinberg, DPM; Center for Wound Healing, MedStar Georgetown University Hospital, Washington DC.)*

require Achilles tendon lengthening and/or tibialis anterior tendon transfer to restore proper biomechanical balance.[70] Alternatively, chronic heel ulceration may occur following a previously undetected injury to the Achilles or from overcorrection during a prior Achilles tendon lengthening procedure. Reconstruction mandates some form of shortening and/or strengthening of this important musculotendinous unit.

For patients with normal dorsiflexion and ulceration caused by metatarsal head prominence, the affected metatarsal head(s) can be elevated superiorly (2–3 mm) with "floating" neck osteotomies and internal fixation.[71] The resultant pressure relief is usually sufficient to promote healing by secondary intention. When forefoot ulceration occurs over the fifth metatarsal head, resection through the metatarsal neck is recommended. This may be accomplished either through the debrided wound (in deeply penetrating ulcers) or through a longitudinal, tendon-splitting, dorsal incision. The first metatarsal is debrided only if it is exposed at the ulcer base. Complete resection of the first metatarsal is not recommended as it destabilizes the medial column, resulting in excessive weight transfer to the adjacent metatarsal head. Instead, resection of the plantar flare of the first metatarsal head is preferred to minimize bony prominence while preserving biomechanical stability.

Wound healing adjuncts

After initial debridement to clean, healthy tissue, it is important to prevent subsequent build up of metalloproteases that destroy naturally produced growth factors. Bacterial biofilm and proteinaceous debris that form on the wound surface must be removed at regular intervals. This can be done by scrubbing the wound daily with soap or using wet-to-dry dressings. In between debridements, topical antibiotics can help reduce the bacterial load. Bacitracin is most useful for minimally infected wounds, mupirocin for methicillin-resistant *Staphylococcus aureus* (MRSA) contamination, and silver sulfadiazine or gentamicin ointment for *Pseudomonas* infections. For most contaminated wounds, antibiotic beads, 1% acetic acid, silver sulfadiazine, mafenide acetate, and Iodosorb work well. Short-term use of quarter- or half-strength Dakin's solution may be appropriate for temporizing heavily contaminated and/or necrotic wounds in patients who require medical optimization prior to operative debridement. An absorbent dressing (i.e., alginate, hydrofiber, foam, hydrocolloid, etc.) with bactericidal ingredients (silver or iodine) is effective for heavily exudative wounds.

For patients who are poor operative candidates, maggot debridement therapy (MDT), using larvae of the blowfly *Phaenicia sericata*, is a proven, cost-effective alternative for treating drug-resistant, chronically infected wounds.[72] MDT serves to enhance healing through selective debridement of necrotic tissues and reduction of bacterial burden. A recent meta-analysis evaluating the safety and effectiveness of MDT revealed significant improvements in both the rate and efficiency of chronic wound healing, longer antibiotic-free intervals, and a lower amputation risk among patients with diabetic foot ulcers.[73] Nevertheless, the prospect of maggot escape, failure to control secretions, and use of tenuous/labor-intensive dressings often precludes the use of maggots in geometrically complex locations. For circumferential lower extremity wounds and/or those complicating the foot/ankle,

we utilize a ventilated, closed-system dressing that permits unrestricted migration of maggots in a well-oxygenated, sanitary, and low-maintenance environment (Fig. 8.12 🌐). The dependent portion of the construct is suspended freely for 48–72 h to prevent mechanical crush and promote free-range debridement of necrotic tissues.

Fig. 8.12 appears online only.

Once the wound is clean and adequately vascularized, NPWT using a vacuum-assisted closure (VAC) device can help expedite healing by secondary intention. NPWT increases local blood flow, reduces tissue edema, controls bacterial proliferation, and catalyzes the formation of granulation tissue.[74,75] Level-one data demonstrate the ability of NPWT to hasten healing and reduce amputation rates in the setting of diabetic foot wounds.[76] Furthermore, because the VAC is changed every 48–72 h, the wound is less susceptible to cross contamination when compared to the normal level of contamination that occurs when the dressing is changed two or three times each day. NPWT with instillation (NPWTi) represents an important evolution in the management of complex acute/chronically infected wounds, those with underlying osteomyelitis, and wounds with exposed orthopedic hardware and/or joint implants, among others.[77] NPWTi is a novel therapy that combines negative pressure (−125 to −150 mmHg) with automated, intermittent instillation of a topical wound solution (antimicrobial vs. saline) of set volume (until sponge is visibly saturated), dwell time (10–20 min), frequency (every 1.5–2 h), and duration (2–10 days). In a retrospective, historical, cohort-controlled trial examining the impact NPWT with (n=68) and without (n=74) instillation, NPWTi was shown to reduce the total number of operative procedures, expedite the time to wound closure, and shorten the length of hospital stay when compared with NPWT alone. The percentage of wounds closed prior to discharge and a qualitative improvement in Gram-positive cultures were also observed with NPWTi.[78] Future questions that remain to be answered pertain to the optimal volume and solution for instillation, dwell time, and duration of therapy, which should be assessed through appropriately conducted, high-powered, randomized controlled trials.

If the wound fails to show signs of healing despite being clean and having adequate blood flow, providing biologically active coverage, such as platelet-derived growth factor (Regranex, Ortho-McNeil-Janssen Pharmaceuticals, Raritan, NJ, USA) or cultured skin substitutes (Apligraf, Organogenesis Inc., Canton, MA, USA; Dermagraft, Advanced Tissue Sciences, La Jolla, CA, USA), may facilitate more rapid healing.[79–82] The formation of new tissue over exposed healthy bone or tendon can also be stimulated through the application of a dermal regenerative template (Integra, Integra LifeSciences, Plainsboro, NJ, USA), with or without VAC support, and allowing it to revascularize over the course of 2–3 weeks. The newly incorporated dermis can then be skin grafted with a thin autograft to provide coverage. Finally, level-one evidence has demonstrated the ability of systemic hyperbaric oxygen therapy (HBOT) to reduce amputation rates and promote granulation of certain complicated, non-healing wounds.[83,84] HBOT stimulates local angiogenesis in the wound bed, promotes collagen cross-linking and extrusion from cells, and potentiates the ability of macrophages/granulocytes to kill bacteria. Any and/or all of these modalities may prove valuable when used in concert with more traditional reconstructive strategies.

External fixation

Postoperatively, strict offloading and elevation of the extremity are critical to eliminate edema, promote healing, and help control infection. For many patients, however, 100% compliance with offloading and immobility is unrealistic, and the temptation to prematurely ambulate or bear weight – even for simple transfers – leads to repetitive shear and torque about mobile joints with ultimate wound breakdown. Furthermore, decubitus pressure from prolonged immobility may result in delayed healing and/or new ulceration. External fixation has an established role in the treatment of fractures and osteomyelitis.[85–87] The ability to immobilize the skeletal framework without utilizing internal hardware – which is contraindicated in the setting of infected/contaminated wounds – has led to the salvage of limbs that previously required amputation.[88] The Ilizarov frame, in particular, provides superior immobilization and has been shown to shorten healing times, decrease pin track infections, and promote early weight-bearing through the addition of a protective plantar foot plate.[89]

In addition, motion along a joint underlying a soft-tissue reconstruction is often responsible for dehiscence or delayed wound healing. A 6-year review of our own institutional data identified 24 consecutive patients in whom external fixation was utilized solely for protection following soft-tissue reconstruction. For patients placed in multiplanar vs. monoplanar fixation, the overall limb salvage rates were 83% and 73%, respectively.[90] Soft-tissue reconstructions in our series included primary closure, skin grafts, and local flaps. For larger reconstructions involving either a free flap or sural artery perforator flap, an Ilizarov frame is ideal as it not only suspends the foot and heel in good skeletal alignment but also protects the flap from external pressure and/or any potential trauma. As patient compliance with alternative offloading schemes averages approximately 20% at our institution, we have found external fixation to be a useful adjunct to ensure adequate healing of complex soft-tissue reconstructions involving the foot and ankle (Fig. 8.13 ⊕).

Fig. 8.13 appears online only.

Surgical techniques for soft-tissue reconstruction

Options for wound closure

Although the vascular anatomy of the foot and ankle was discussed in detail previously, it is worth re-emphasizing the critical significance of the angiosome model and its implications for guiding successful reconstruction. Understanding the boundaries of each angiosome as well as the vascular interconnections between source arteries provides the basis for logically, rather than empirically, designed incisions for tissue exposure and/or planned reconstructions or amputations that preserve maximal blood flow to promote healing of surgical wounds. Aside form hemodynamic considerations, the timing of reconstruction plays an equally important role in ensuring successful outcomes and minimizing complications after wound closure. Aggressive attempts at premature closure lead to increased rates of incisional

dehiscence, infection, flap failure, and progressive tissue necrosis. Therefore, prior to closure, it is essential to ensure that the patient's medical comorbidities and abnormal wound parameters have been corrected and signs of inflammation have resolved. Negative postdebridement cultures along with resolution of pain, wrinkled skin edges, healthy granulation, and neo-epithelialization signal that a wound is ready for reconstruction.

Options for closure are numerous and depend on the patient's health, size and location of the wound, presence of exposed vital structures (i.e., tendon, bone, joint space, and neurovascular structures), surgeon experience, and availability/quality of local tissues. These options include (1) healing by secondary intention, (2) delayed primary closure, (3) skin graft, (4) local flap(s), (5) pedicled flap(s), (6) free tissue/composite tissue transfer, or any combination thereof. In the absence of exposed vital structures, certain wounds (i.e., large, irregular, and/or potentially contaminated) can be left to heal by secondary intention through the application of daily dressing changes, wound healing adjuncts, HBOT, and/ or NPWT. If surgical closure is indicated and feasible, the freshly debrided wound should be pulse lavaged and new sterile instruments brought into the field to avoid recontamination of the wound bed. Quantitative cultures of the instruments used to debride the wound yield up to 10^3 bacteria, and their use during closure would needlessly increase the risk for postoperative infection.

Delayed primary closure is easier to accomplish when tissue edema and induration have resolved. The VAC device can be very helpful in this endeavor. After primary closure, it is important to ensure that relevant arterial pulses have not diminished due to an excessively tight closure. If the closing tension is too high, the wound can be closed serially, or the residual gap can be left to heal secondarily with the aide of NPWT. For larger wounds, internal VAC – utilizing a partially buried sponge and tension sutures to gradually approximate the skin edges – collapses the wound cavity and facilitates tension-free closure at a later date (Fig. 8.14). An adequate soft-tissue envelope can also be created by removing underlying bone. This occurs in partial foot amputations where just enough bone is removed to facilitate delayed primary closure (Fig. 8.15 ⊕). Correcting a Charcot midfoot collapse by removing the arch and fusing the metatarsals to the hindfoot also allows for loose approximation of plantar soft-tissue defects. In all cases, use of deep sutures during closure should be avoided as they could potentiate re-infection. Simple vertical mattresses with monofilament suture (i.e., nylon, polypropylene, etc.) are least likely to harbor bacteria.

Fig. 8.15 appears online only.

Skin grafting can be used to close most foot and ankle wounds that possess a healthy granulating surface (Fig. 8.16 ⊕). In the setting of inhospitable wound beds (i.e., tendon or bone), a collagen lattice framework, such as Integra (Integra Lifesciences, Plainsboro, NJ, USA), can be used to generate a healthy, vascularized neodermis capable of accepting a graft. Recipient bed preparation is optimized by shaving off the superficial granulation tissue to remove any residual bacteria within the interstices of granulating buds. The skin graft can be meshed at a 1:1 ratio or pie crusted to prevent build up of fluid that could preclude graft adherence. The use of low continuous suction NPWT (−75 mmHg), as a dressing for the first 3–5 days, will maximize skin graft take.[91] On the

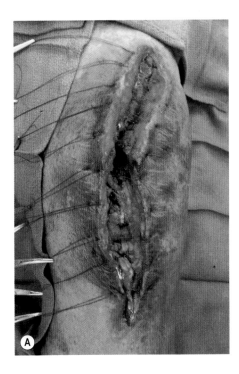
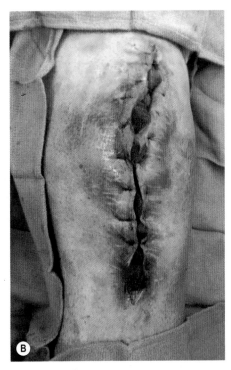
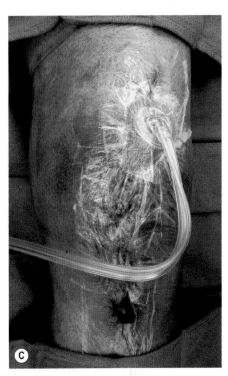

Fig. 8.14 Use of the internal vacuum-assisted closure technique to enable delayed primary closure of a large anterior knee wound following removal of infected hardware, debridement, and placement of an antibiotic spacer in a patient with a failed total knee arthroplasty. Negative pressure wound therapy, using a partially buried sponge, minimizes soft-tissue edema and accelerates wound contraction. Gradual approximation of the skin edges is achieved through use of vertical mattress polypropylene tension sutures, placed along the entire length of the wound, to facilitate soft-tissue creep. The dressing is changed every 3–5 days until tension-free approximation of the wound margins is possible.

weight-bearing plantar surface of the foot, glabrous skin grafts, harvested at 30/1000 of an inch, provide a thicker alternative that can better resist the shear forces applied during ambulation.[92,93] The instep provides an ideal donor site and should, itself, be grafted with a thin autograft (10/1000 of an inch) to speed up healing following graft harvest. If compliance is an issue, consideration should be given to placing an Ilizarov frame with a protective footplate until the plantar graft has healed completely. Innervated full-thickness skin grafts have also been employed in select patients utilizing defatted skin flaps from the sural nerve territory, great toe, and/or forearm.[94]

Fig. 8.16 appears online only.

Local random flaps consist of tissue with an unidentified blood supply that is either rotated about a pivot point, transposed, or advanced into an adjacent defect. They comprise various sizes and shapes (square, rectangular, rhomboid, semi-circular, or bilobed) as well as tissue compositions (skin, fat, fascia, etc.). Only exposed bone, tendon, and/or joint need flap coverage, while skin grafts are often sufficient to cover the remaining soft-tissue deficit. The combination of limited local flap and skin graft frequently obviates the need for larger pedicled flaps or free tissue transfer. An appropriately designed local flap can improve surgical exposure of underlying tissues, bone, joints, and tendon – obviating the need for additional incisions. Furthermore, local flaps can provide coverage of wounds within the tight confines of an external fixator.

The ratio of length-to-width is critical for the survival of random pattern flaps.[95] Because the capillary beds supplying the skin of the foot and ankle are not as dense as in the face, this ratio should not exceed 1:1 to 1:1.5 in dimension. If a cutaneous perforator can be Dopplered at the base of, or within, the planned flap, the length-to-width ratio may be increased. To ensure tension-free coverage, the flap should be designed in the area of maximal tissue mobility and slightly larger than the defect to be covered. A force of 25 mmHg causes enough venous congestion for flap necrosis unless the tension is released within 4 h.[96] If the flap remains pale at inset, it should be rotated back into its bed and delayed for 4–7 days while it develops more robust blood supply. During that time, NPWT can be used to cover the open wound in order to minimize edema and ensure that wound edges remain malleable. Finally, we have found that the application of incisional NPWT, for 3–5 days postoperatively, helps to ensure local flap viability by decreasing venous congestion.[97]

Pedicled flaps of the foot and ankle require more sophisticated anatomic knowledge to dissect and have higher perioperative complication rates, although equivalent long-term success as free tissue transfer. Free flaps to the foot and ankle, however, carry the highest failure rate in the microsurgical literature and must be planned carefully.[98,99] Vascular calcification and large zones of injury in the lower extremity often contribute to flap failure. Whenever possible, end-to-side anastomosis to the recipient artery and two-vein anastomoses should be performed to preserve maximal blood flow to the distal limb and optimize venous drainage from the flap, respectively.

The free flap donor site is chosen based on the size and location of the wound, the length of pedicle needed, and the functional and aesthetic demands of the region to be reconstructed. Levin and colleagues reviewed the Duke experience with lower extremity free tissue transfer and proposed a subunit principle to guide donor site selection.[100] The authors noted that ill-conceived flap designs may be subject to breakdown, interfere with proper foot wear, and/or prevent efficient ambulation. True to all free flap reconstructions, emphasis should be placed on creating a biomechanically stable framework (i.e., removal of bony prominences, arch reconstruction, etc.) followed by meticulous flap inset under appropriate tension (i.e., height should be level with surrounding tissue). Patient education and close longitudinal monitoring will help identify complications that may jeopardize flap integrity and permit early intervention to improve the likelihood of functional flap salvage.

Regardless of the type of flap used for a given defect, an accurate assessment of blood flow is mandatory. For local flaps, a Dopplerable perforator should be included in the base of the flap. With pedicled flaps, the dominant branch supplying the flap should be patent. For free flaps, there should be an adequate recipient artery and vein(s). If there is any question, a duplex scan, magnetic resonance angiogram, or conventional angiogram must be obtained prior to surgery.

Reconstruction by anatomic location

Given that the reconstructive options for foot and ankle wounds vary by location, it is best to differentiate between five distinct anatomic regions: (1) anterior ankle and dorsal foot, (2) plantar forefoot, (3) plantar midfoot, (4) plantar hindfoot and medial/lateral ankle, and (5) Achilles region. The following discusses some of the key biomechanical considerations, workhorse flap options, and salvage amputations specific to each region.

Anterior ankle and dorsal foot

Soft tissue around the foot and ankle is sparse and has limited flexibility. In the presence of healthy granulation tissue, defects in this region can be successfully treated with simple skin grafts. If the paratenon covering the extensor tendons is absent or insufficient, a dermal regenerate template (i.e., Integra) can be used with or without NPWT. Local flaps (i.e., rotation, rhomboid, bilobed, or transposition) may be useful for small defects. For larger wounds, however, pedicled flaps are often necessary. The most useful of these are the EDB muscle and lateral supramalleolar flaps. The dorsalis pedis flap, which can be proximally or distally based, is rarely used because the skin-grafted donor site is often problematic for ambulatory patients who wear shoes.

Extensor digitorum brevis muscle flap

The EDB is a type II muscle that may be transposed proximally to cover anterior ankle, proximal dorsal foot, and/or lateral malleolar wounds. Its dominant blood supply is derived from the lateral tarsal artery, which branches off the dorsalis pedis artery at the distal extensor retinaculum. Exposure is obtained through a dorsal curvilinear incision that communicates with the wound to be closed. As long as the dorsalis pedis has antegrade blood flow, it can be divided distal to the lateral tarsal artery to increase the arc of rotation for muscle transposition; however, this is not recommended in diabetics with peripheral vascular disease. The lateral minor tarsal branches are ligated as the dissection proceeds proximally. The lateral

tarsal vessel should be elevated with the muscle as its origin is divided off the lateral calcaneus. The four slips of muscle are broad and thin (4.5×6 cm in adult), making the flap useful for relatively small wounds (Fig. 8.17).[101] If need be, the EDB muscle can also be raised as a distally-based reverse-flow muscle flap supplied by a distal branch of the dorsalis pedis receiving retrograde flow from the lateral plantar artery. However, its arc of rotation in this direction is rather limited.

Lateral supramalleolar flap

The lateral supramalleolar flap is most useful for coverage of bony defects that accompany loss of soft tissue over the lateral malleolus and anterior ankle. The flap should be distally based as the blood supply is derived from skin perforators off the anterior perforating branch of the peroneal artery as it pierces the interosseous membrane 5 cm proximal to the tip of the lateral malleolus. Cutaneous vessels then course proximally, anterior to the fibula, and anastomose with the vascular network that accompanies the superficial peroneal nerve. The perforating branch of the peroneal artery is located with a hand-held Doppler, and the base of the flap should be centered at this point. Flap width includes the fasciocutaneous tissue between the fibula and the tibia. The length should be adequate to reach the lateral malleolus (6–8 cm) or more distally as dictated by wound location (Fig. 8.18).[7]

Most often, the flap is developed as a distally based fascial flap, and its surface is then skin grafted. The incision is made centrally over the space between the fibula and the tibia so that skin flaps may be elevated off the deep fascia. The fascia is then incised along its medial margin and progressively reflected until the perforating branch is seen. Branches of the superficial peroneal nerve course within the fascia and must be divided to permit safe elevation and rotation. Final release of the flap requires an incision through the lateral margin and release of its attachments to the septum that separates the anterior and lateral muscular compartments. When harvested in this manner, the donor site may be closed directly.

For more distally based wounds of the anterior ankle/proximal dorsal foot, the anterior perforating branch is ligated proximally to increase flap reach. The flap then becomes dependent on retrograde flow from the lateral malleolar artery to the anterior perforating branch, and thus patency of this vessel as well as the anterior tibial artery must be confirmed prior to flap harvest. Donor site healing with this approach, however, can be problematic and may require the use of neo-dermis, subsequent skin grafting, and ankle immobilization to ensure successful graft take.

Free tissue transfer

Large dorsal foot and ankle wounds with exposed tendon and/or bone require thin, pliable tissues for proper shoe fitting. In addition, these wounds have the highest aesthetic demand, and thus replacement of tissue with flaps that possess a cutaneous component will provide durable coverage and improved overall appearance when compared to those that require skin grafting.[100] Vascularized tendon or bone can be incorporated to accommodate specific reconstructive demands. Flaps that have proven to be very successful in this region include the lateral arm, radial forearm, and parascapular fasciocutaneous flaps. Perforator flaps, such as the

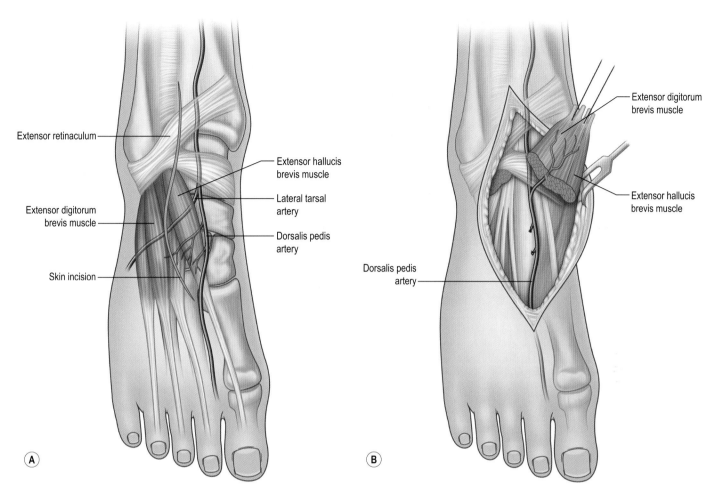

Fig. 8.17 Extensor digitorum brevis muscle flap. This type II muscle derives its dominant blood supply from the lateral tarsal artery, which is a branch off the dorsalis pedis artery. The dorsalis pedis can be divided distal to the origin of the lateral tarsal vessels to increase the arc of rotation for muscle transposition. The four slips of muscle are broad and thin, measuring 4.5×6 cm in the adult, making the flap useful for relatively small wounds.

anterolateral thigh (ALT) flap, have also been utilized with excellent functional and aesthetic results (Fig. 8.19). This flap is based on perforators originating from the descending branch of the lateral circumflex femoral system and can supply large quantities of fasciocutaneous tissue on a safe and reliable pedicle with minimal donor site morbidity.[102] In patients who are overweight, bulky fasciocutaneous and/or perforator flaps may necessitate secondary flap debulking 3–4 months after the initial procedure. Alternatively, the use of a thin fascial flap, surfaced with a skin graft, may be more effective at facilitating single-stage reconstruction in obese patients.

The radial forearm flap (Fig. 8.20) is an excellent option for dorsal foot wounds.[103,104] The flap is thin, pliable, and can be harvested with a sensory nerve (lateral antebrachial cutaneous nerve). The palmaris longus can also be included to reconstruct missing extensor tendons if necessary. Furthermore, the radial artery with its venous comitantes provides an excellent vascular pedicle of up to 14 cm in length. If inset properly at the time of transfer, the flap rarely needs to be tailored. Despite these favorable qualities, the donor site can be problematic, and an Allen's test must be performed to ensure adequate ulnar-based perfusion to the hand prior to

flap harvest. The lateral arm flap, based on the posterior radial collateral vessels, can be harvested as a sensate flap (lower lateral cutaneous nerve) with a relatively long vascular pedicle (up to 14 cm).[105] For larger defects, the flap can be extended to include the skin overlying the elbow. The parascapular flap (Fig. 8.21) is supplied by the circumflex scapular artery and is an adequate choice for large defects.[106,107] The flap is insensate and often requires secondary debulking. It can also be harvested as an adipofascial flap and skin grafted to yield a thinner, more pliable soft-tissue construct.[108]

Plantar forefoot

The area distal to the midshaft of the metatarsals is referred to as the forefoot. Local flaps play a major role in reconstructing deep wounds of the distal third of the foot. Toe ulcers and gangrene are best treated with limited amputations that preserve viable tissue so that the remaining toe will be as long as possible when closed. Attempts to preserve at least the proximal portion of the proximal phalanx of the second, third, and fourth toes should be made so that it can serve as a spacer to prevent central collapse of adjacent toes into the empty space. If the hallux is involved, maximal length preservation should

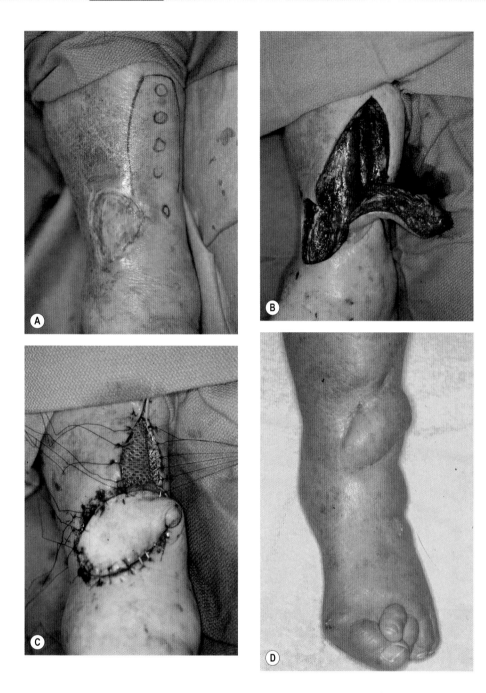

Fig. 8.18 Lateral supramalleolar flap. **(A)** Full-thickness anterior ankle wound with outline of a supramalleolar flap. The anterior perforating branch of the peroneal artery is located with a hand-held Doppler, and the base of the flap should be centered at this point. Flap width includes the fasciocutaneous tissue between the fibula and the tibia. **(B)** Harvest of the lateral supramalleolar flap. **(C)** Rotation and flap inset. The donor site is surfaced with a split-thickness skin graft. **(D)** Final appearance 1-year postoperative.

be the goal given its critical role in ambulation. Most often, plantar and dorsal flaps of the proximal toe remnant can be fashioned for simple closure. If additional soft tissue is needed an adjacent toe may be filleted and transposed. Some of the more reliable options for forefoot repair include local fasciocutaneous flaps, the fillet of toe flap, and the neurovascular island flap.[109,110]

Local fasciocutaneous flaps

Vertical perforating vessels located throughout the plantar aspect of the foot facilitate the design of many different local flaps. Forefoot skin, fat, and fascia may be elevated and advanced (i.e., V-Y), rotated, or transposed – either singly or in pairs – to close wounds as large as 4–5 cm³ with exposed bone, joint, and/or tendon. Preferably, the flap is harvested from the side that is most mobile and that has a definable perforator at its base. Thus four possible designs exist: proximally or distally based and medial or lateral to the wound. The plantar fascia along the edge of the flap must be completely incised and care taken to divide the septal attachments to the underlying metatarsals in order to maximize flap mobility. Occasionally, the defect is large enough such that tissue from opposing sides is needed for closure. Whatever is not covered by the flap(s) is then skin grafted. NPWT can be placed on the entire construct for 3–5 days to ensure both

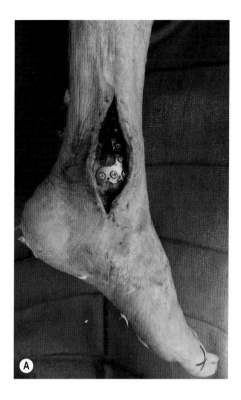
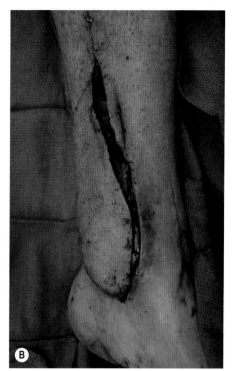
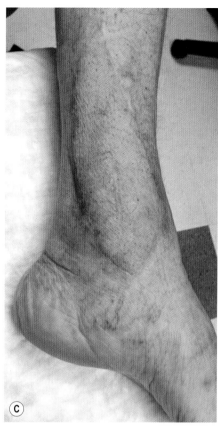

Fig. 8.19 Anterolateral thigh flap. A 71-year-old male with a left total ankle arthroplasty presented 6 weeks after deltoid tendon allograft reconstruction with an infected open wound and exposed underlying hardware. **(A)** Intraoperative photograph following serial debridement of infected soft tissue, bone, and tendon allograft. Exposed hardware is seen fixated to the distal tibia and medial malleolus along with a large overlying soft-tissue deficit. **(B)** Transfer of an anterolateral thigh fasciocutaneous free flap to the recipient site defect. End-to-side anastomosis was performed between the posterior tibial artery and the descending branch of the lateral circumflex femoral artery. **(C)** Evaluation at 1-year follow-up demonstrating durable coverage and excellent aesthetic contour of the medial malleolus.

optimal graft take and flap survival. These flaps can also be applied to the plantar midfoot, hindfoot, malleoli, and dorsum of the foot for defect coverage (Fig. 8.22).

Fillet of toe flap

The fillet of toe flap is useful for small webspace ulcers and distal forefoot wounds (Fig. 8.23). Under tourniquet control, the flap is elevated, beginning distally, by removing the entire nail complex. Depending on the desired arc of rotation, a dorsal, medial, or lateral incision is made to expose the underlying phalanges, which are subsequently removed with care taken to preserve the plantar digital vessels. The volar plates and flexor/extensor tendons are removed to improve flap pliability. A connecting incision is made to permit transposition of the flap into an adjacent defect. If necessary, more proximal dissection of the plantar neurovascular structures may extend the flap's arc of rotation to more proximal locations. The flap works best with the first or fifth toes; however, the reach of this flap is frequently less than anticipated.

Neurovascular island flap

An alternative, more elegant variation is the neurovascular island flap, where part of the toe pulp and its digital artery is raised without having to sacrifice the entire toe. This flap is

frequently centered over the lateral neurovascular bundle of the hallux. Elevation occurs distal to proximal at the level of the plantar phalangeal periosteum. Identifying the digital neurovascular bundle in the webspace permits a more proximal dissection for increased mobility. A connecting incision is made from the webspace to the debrided wound in order to transpose the flap. Depending on the flap size, the donor site is closed either directly or with a skin graft.[111,112] Both the fillet of toe flap and the neurovascular island flap are effective for wounds up to 2–3 cm in diameter. A complete preoperative vascular assessment of the extremity is mandatory to ensure adequate distal perfusion prior to flap harvest.

Free tissue transfer

The most controversial area of reconstruction centers on the weight-bearing surfaces of the foot (i.e., plantar forefoot and heel). There is still some debate as to whether plantar fasciocutaneous flaps or muscle flaps with skin grafts better withstand the stresses imposed by ambulation. Fasciocutaneous flaps offer the advantage of durable skin coverage with preserved tendon glide and easier re-elevation to access antibiotic spacers and/or underlying hardware. On the other hand, muscle flaps provide a more robust blood supply to the recipient site, making them better suited for coverage of previously

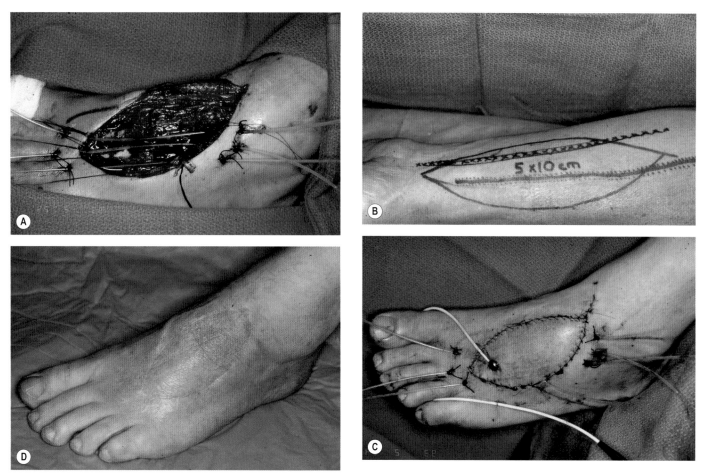

Fig. 8.20 Radial forearm free flap. **(A)** Dorsal foot defect following wide resection of a soft-tissue sarcoma including partial excision of the extensor digitorum longus tendon. **(B)** Innervated radial forearm free flap with palmaris longus tendon outlined on the volar distal forearm. **(C)** Transfer and inset of the composite flap into the recipient-site. End-to-end anastomosis between the radial artery and dorsalis pedis artery was performed along with sensory nerve coaptation between the lateral antebrachial cutaneous and the superficial peroneal nerves to establish protective sensibility to the flap. The palmaris longus graft was used to reconstruct the extensor tendon defect. **(D)** Evaluation at 1 year demonstrating excellent aesthetic contour of the dorsal foot.

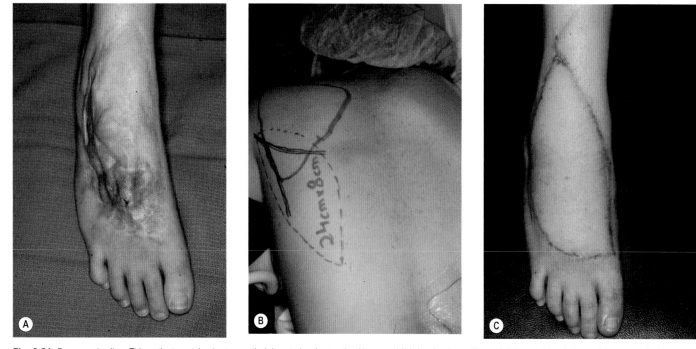

Fig. 8.21 Parascapular flap. This patient sustained a traumatic injury to her foot and ankle as a child, leaving her with a painful, unstable platform. Adequate soft-tissue cover was needed before ankle fusion could be performed. **(A)** Chronic, unstable soft-tissue scarring. **(B)** A parascapular flap was harvested from her left back. The descending branch of the circumflex scapular artery was anastomosed end-to-side into the anterior tibial artery. **(C)** Secondary flap debulking with liposuction was performed after 6 months.

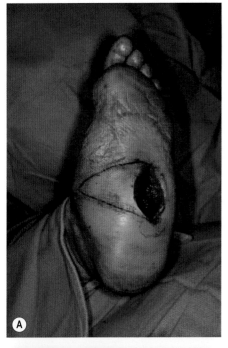

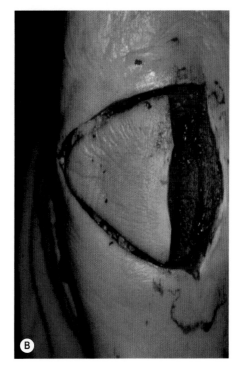

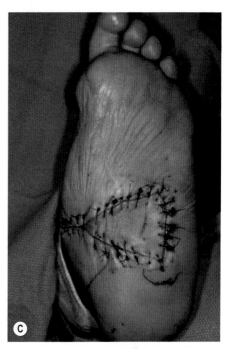

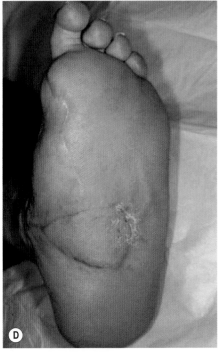

Fig. 8.22 **(A)** Design of a medially-based V-Y advancement flap for closure of a plantar midfoot defect. The direction of the flap is dependent on the mobility of local tissues and the presence of definable perforators. **(B)** The plantar fascia along the edge of the flap is completely incised. Blood supply to the V-Y flap is derived from direct underlying perforators. For that reason, the flap should never be undermined. **(C)** Maximum advancement on the plantar aspect of the foot is approximately 2 cm. **(D)** Completely healed V-Y flap at 6 months follow-up.

infected wounds.[113] In the setting of exposed bone and/or chronic osteomyelitis, muscle flaps can be used to obliterate dead space and aid in the delivery of neutrophils and parenteral antibiotics to the site of infection.[114,115] Furthermore, in their series of 165 lower extremity free flaps, Hollenbeck *et al.* found that plantar flaps containing a cutaneous paddle were more prone to late ulceration along the interval between the flap and the native plantar skin.[100] This suggests that differences in mobility at the flap interface, rather than tissue composition within the flap, may be more predictive of late

breakdown. Levin advocates a modified insetting technique that incorporates a well-approximated, sigmoidal/tangential closure (i.e., "vest-over-pants"), which is more resistant to the effects of shearing than a simple transverse approximation. The long-term durability and excellent functional outcomes observed with muscle flaps and skin grafts for plantar surface reconstruction have been well characterized by May and colleagues as well as others.[116,117]

Commonly utilized muscle flaps for this region include the rectus abdominus, gracilis, and serratus anterior muscle. The

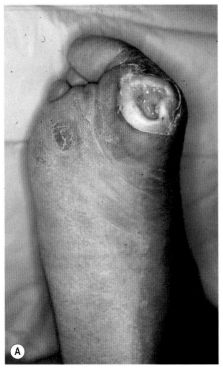
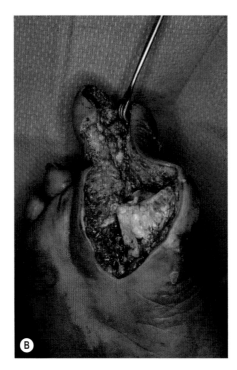
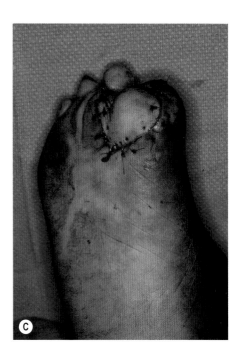
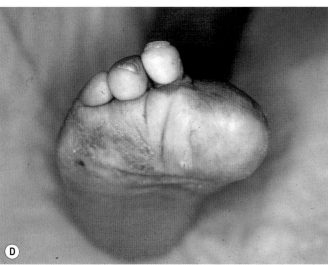

Fig. 8.23 Fillet of toe flap. **(A)** Infected first submetatarsal ulcer with underlying osteomyelitis in a patient with hallux valgus deformity. **(B)** Defect created by excision of the infected ulcer and debridement of the first metatarsal head. A fillet of hallux flap is raised with care taken to preserve the digital neurovascular bundles. **(C)** Rotation and inset of the flap into the distal plantar defect. **(D)** Completely healed fillet of toe flap with excellent contour at 1-year follow-up.

rectus abdominus muscle flap (Fig. 8.24) provides thin and broad coverage, is easy to harvest, and has an excellent pedicle with minimal donor site morbidity.[118] The gracilis muscle (Fig. 8.25) is also an excellent choice for foot and ankle reconstruction.[119,120] It should be harvested from the ipsilateral thigh to limit all incisions to the same extremity. The pedicle is somewhat shorter than that of the rectus abdominus muscle, and thus, depending on the location of the defect and recipient vessels, its utility may be limited. This flap is most useful for heel wounds where micro-anastomoses can be performed to the nearby posterior tibial vessels. Alternatively, using the bottom two or three slips of the serratus anterior muscle (Fig. 8.26) provides adequate soft-tissue coverage with a pedicle length upwards of 18 cm.[121] Therefore wounds on the plantar surface can be reconstructed with anastomoses to the foot's dorsal circulation.

A word of caution regarding the use of the latissimus dorsi flap: while this flap is an attractive option in many other parts of the body, the functional loss of this muscle must be carefully weighed in lower extremity patients who are often crutch- and/or wheelchair-dependent for a prolonged period of time.[122]

Forefoot amputations

Reconstructive surgeons managing patients with foot ulceration should be well-versed in the options available for forefoot amputation, as these procedures often yield the simplest means to provide stable soft-tissue closure and bipedal ambulation. For large ulcers involving the metatarsal head and distal shaft, consideration should be given to partial ray amputation. Resection of the more independent first or fifth

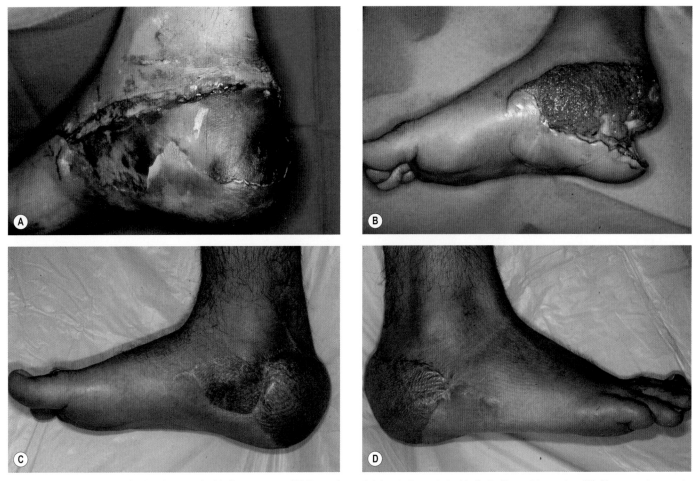

Fig. 8.24 Rectus abdominus free flap for posterior hindfoot coverage. **(A)** Traumatic crush injury to the posterior hindfoot with overlying eschar. **(B)** Clean granular wound and viable heel pad following serial debridement and negative pressure wound therapy. **(C,D)** Medial and lateral views 6 months after definitive coverage with a rectus abdominus free flap and split-thickness skin graft.

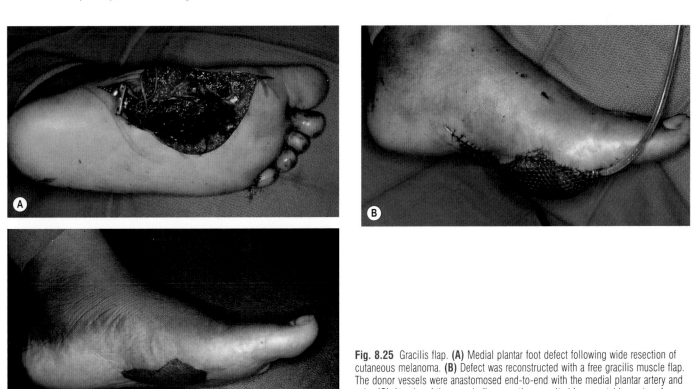

Fig. 8.25 Gracilis flap. **(A)** Medial plantar foot defect following wide resection of cutaneous melanoma. **(B)** Defect was reconstructed with a free gracilis muscle flap. The donor vessels were anastomosed end-to-end with the medial plantar artery and vein. **(C)** Atrophy of the muscle flap over time resulted in acceptable contour for footwear and ambulation.

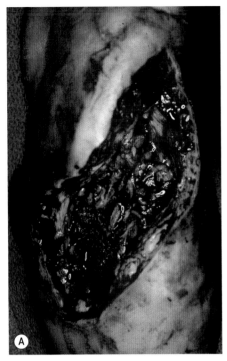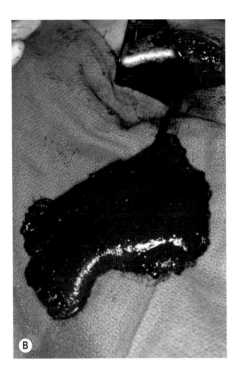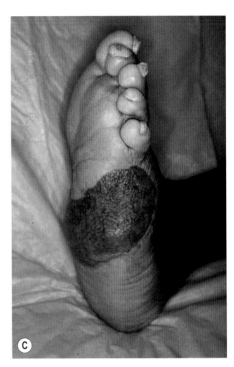

Fig. 8.26 Serratus anterior muscle flap. This diabetic patient sustained a plantar-lateral foot ulceration secondary to Charcot collapse of the midfoot. **(A)** The wound was aggressively debrided resulting in a large soft-tissue defect along the lateral weight-bearing surface of the foot. **(B)** The lower three slips of the serratus anterior muscle were harvested as a free flap to provide soft-tissue coverage. **(C)** The reconstructed foot has remained completely healed after 10 years.

metatarsal will cause less biomechanical disruption than resection of the second, third, or fourth metatarsals, because the central three rays operate as a cohesive unit. Given their importance in ambulation, all efforts should be made to preserve as much metatarsal length as possible.

If ulcers are present under several metatarsal heads, or if resection of one head results in ulceration at an adjacent metatarsal head, a pan-metatarsal head resection should be considered. Additionally, if more than two toes with accompanying metatarsal heads have to be resected, a transmetatarsal amputation is indicated. To maintain biomechanical stability, care should be taken to preserve the normal parabola, with the second metatarsal being the longest. If performed correctly, transmetatarsal amputation provides an excellent functional level for most patients.[123] No formal prosthetic/orthotic is necessary, and the patient may wear normal shoes with a small distal insert. Attention, however, must be paid to avoid equinovarus deformity from loss of the extensors, which often leads to recurrent lateral plantar ulceration. Usually, the Achilles tendon is lengthened to avoid this complication. Alternatively, the extensor and flexor tendons of the fourth and fifth toes can be tenodesed while the ankle is in neutral position so that distal forefoot dorsiflexion is preserved.

Plantar midfoot

The midfoot is defined as the region between the proximal tarsal row and the midshaft of the metatarsals. It comprises the medial non-weight-bearing arch as well as the more lateral weight-bearing soft tissues. Bony prominences associated with midfoot wounds should be resected judiciously. Medial instep wounds result from deformities of the first metatarsal

base, medial cuneiform, and navicular bones. Lateral wounds are often secondary to prominence of the fifth metatarsal base and/or cuboid bones. Limited midfoot fusions should be strongly considered if they will prevent joint subluxation and thereby promote more uniform weight distribution.

More commonly, ulcers on the medial/lateral plantar midfoot are caused by Charcot collapse of the plantar arch. If the underlying shattered bone has healed and is stable, then resection of excess bone can be accomplished via a medial or lateral approach and the ulcer can be left to heal secondarily or covered with a glabrous skin graft and/or local flap. An unstable midfoot skeleton can be excised using a wedge excision and the arch recreated by fusing the proximal metatarsals to the talus and calcaneus via an Ilizarov frame. Shortening of the skeletal midfoot usually permits wound closure either primarily or with a local flap.

Local fasciocutaneous flaps

Small wounds in this region may be closed using any of the options discussed previously for the forefoot (i.e., V-Y advancement, bilobed, rhomboid, transposition, etc.). Local V-Y flaps can be advanced up to 1.5 cm to help close a defect, whereas defects as large as 3 cm in diameter can be closed using double-opposing V-Y flaps. For slightly larger defects, a simple medially-based rotation flap or the pedicled medial plantar fasciocutaneous flap (described in the hindfoot section below) offer effective and versatile options for wound closure.

Neurovascular island flap

The neurovascular island procedures described previously are useful for the coverage of 2–3 cm defects. This repair necessitates a more proximal dissection of the vessels and nerves from the plantar surface of the foot. If the dominant circulation is from the first dorsal metatarsal artery, division of the deep transverse metatarsal ligament will be necessary to permit adequate flap transfer and inset.

Local muscle flaps

If muscle is needed, a pedicled flexor digiti minimi brevis flap (laterally) or a flexor hallucis brevis flap (medially) can be useful. The flexor digiti minimi brevis is a type II muscle that receives its dominant pedicle at the lateral plantar artery take-off of the digital artery to the fifth toe and can be used to cover defects over the proximal fifth metatarsal. The flexor halluces brevis muscle has a similar (type II) vascular anatomy but can be harvested on a much longer pedicle, as an island flap on the medial plantar artery, to reach defects as far as the proximal ankle. Other useful muscle flaps for medial and lateral defects include the pedicled abductor hallucis flap and abductor digiti minimi flap, respectively (both described in the hindfoot section below).

Free tissue transfer

The plantar instep of the foot is of relatively low functional and aesthetic importance. It can be reliably resurfaced using thin, pliable fasciocutaneous or perforator flaps (i.e., radial forearm, parascapular, ALT, etc.). The contralateral sensate free instep flap, based on the medial plantar neurovascular bundle, provides tissue of matching quality for excellent functional and aesthetic results. Larger defects on weight-bearing surfaces should be reconstructed with free muscle flaps and skin grafts for improved long-term stability, as described previously. Great care should be taken to tailor the flap so that it is inset at the same height as the surrounding tissue.

Midfoot amputations

Deformities at the tarsometatarsal junctions (Lisfranc's joint) occur when a shortened gastrocnemius–soleus complex alters normal ankle motion. The inability to dorsiflex the ankle places undue strain across Lisfranc's joint during gait, which leads to increased compensatory motion, joint breakdown, and resultant midfoot deformity. In the absence of protective sensation (i.e., diabetes, peripheral neuropathy), soft-tissue ulceration becomes inevitable.[124] Midfoot amputations may be the preferred "repair" in patients who are not candidates for reconstruction. The procedure is simple and may be performed rapidly without the significant morbidity associated with more complex reconstructions. When executed properly, a functional limb that provides a stable platform for ambulation may be salvaged. The two most common forms of midfoot amputation are the Lisfranc and Chopart amputations.

The Lisfranc amputation involves the removal of all metatarsals with the exception of the very proximal remnant of the second metatarsal, which serves as a keystone area and should be preserved if possible. The direction of blood flow along the dorsalis pedis and lateral plantar artery should be evaluated. Absence of antegrade flow through either mandates preservation of the perforator connecting the two at that level. To prevent a delayed equinovarus deformity, a split anterior tibial tendon transfer to the cuboid with Achilles

tendon lengthening or a simple Achilles tenectomy (removing 1–2 cm of tendon) should be performed at the time of amputation. Closure is most often achieved using the plantar tissue. Postoperatively, the patient's foot is placed in slight dorsiflexion until the wound has healed. Although custom footwear will be required, patients generally return to their previous ambulatory level with little, if any, increase in energy expenditure.[125]

The Chopart amputation involves separating the talus and calcaneus from the navicular and cuboid. A modified version can be performed by splitting the midfoot at the juncture between the navicular/cuboid and the cuneiform bones. With the Chopart procedure, the insertions of both the peroneal tendons and the tibialis anterior tendon will be disrupted, impairing dorsiflexion and foot eversion. A distal Achilles tenectomy (1–2 cm) or a combined Achilles tendon lengthening and tibialis anterior tendon transfer to the lateral talus/calcaneus is, therefore, mandatory to prevent ulceration. When healed, a calcaneal–tibial rod can be used to further stabilize the ankle. Postoperatively, the limb is cast in slight dorsiflexion for 4–6 weeks.[126]

Plantar hindfoot and medial/lateral ankle

Plantar heel defects or ulcers are among the most difficult of all wounds to treat. Reconstruction should provide durable soft-tissue coverage for safe weight-bearing while permitting near normal ankle motion. More than any other region in the foot, the surgeon must consider both form and function when managing wounds in this area. Tendons from muscles of the superficial/deep posterior and lateral compartments of the leg traverse this region as they enter the foot. The posterior tibial artery and tibial nerve lie between the flexor digitorum longus and the flexor halluces longus tendons, posterior to the medial malleolus. These structures, along with the tibialis posterior tendon, travel beneath the laciniate ligament (flexor retinaculum) to enter the foot. The sural nerve and lateral leg compartment musculature also pass posterior to the lateral malleolus on their way to the foot. Loss of tissue in this region can be catastrophic and may permanently cripple the patient or mandate a below-knee amputation. A variety of reconstructive options are available based on the precise location of the defect.

Intrinsic muscle flaps

Three intrinsic foot muscles may be used individually or together to repair small wounds of the hindfoot region: the abductor hallucis brevis (AHB), flexor digitorum brevis (FDB), and abductor digiti minimi (ADM) muscles.[127–130]

Abductor hallucis brevis muscle flap

The AHB is a type II muscle that, despite its limited bulk, provides useful coverage of the medial plantar heel and medial malleolus (Fig. 8.27 ⊙). It is elevated through an incision along the medial glabrous junction. The tendon is divided distally, and the muscle is separated from the medial head of the flexor halluces brevis. Because the dominant blood supply enters the muscle proximally, as branches from the medial plantar artery, the more distal pedicles can be safely ligated. If an increase in the arc of rotation is needed, the medial plantar artery may be ligated distal to the proximal muscle pedicle and dissection continued to its origin off of the posterior tibial artery.

Fig. 8.27 appears online only.

Flexor digitorum brevis muscle flap

The FDB muscle can be useful for heel pad reconstruction, especially if used to fill an existing defect that can be covered by intact glabrous skin from the heel (Fig. 8.28). It is a type II muscle whose blood supply is derived from branches off both the medial and lateral plantar arteries, with the latter usually being dominant. The lateral plantar artery courses deep to the proximal muscle belly where the dominant pedicle enters the muscle. A midline plantar foot incision through the skin and plantar fascia is used to harvest the muscle. The four flexor tendons are divided distally and the muscle is dissected proximally off the underlying quadratus plantae muscle.

Further mobilization is possible by harvesting the flap on the lateral plantar artery and continuing the pedicle dissection to its origin within the tarsal tunnel; however, this approach is not routinely recommended. The muscle is then turned on itself (180°) to fill the posterior/plantar defect.

Abductor digiti minimi muscle flap

Despite its limited size, the ADM is the workhorse flap for lateral heel and distal lateral ankle wounds (Fig. 8.29). It is mobilized via an incision along the lateral glabrous junction. This type II muscle is detached from the lateral fifth metatarsophalangeal joint by dividing the tendinous insertion. It is then elevated off the flexor digiti minimi to the level of the proximal fifth metatarsal. The minor pedicles enter the muscle medially. Its dominant blood supply enters at the medial proximal corner of the muscle and is derived from the lateral

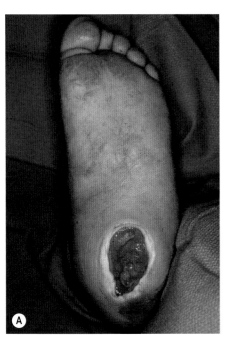

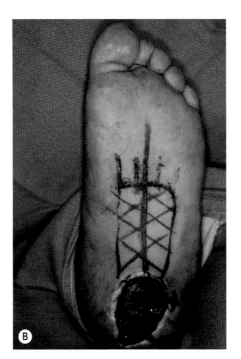

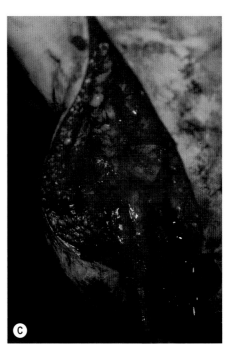

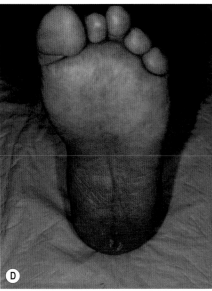

Fig. 8.28 Flexor digitorum brevis flap for heel pad reconstruction. **(A)** Plantar heel ulcer in a diabetic patient with calcaneal gait. **(B)** Outline of the flexor digitorum brevis flap drawn on the plantar surface of the foot. **(C)** A midline plantar foot incision is used to harvest the muscle, and the four flexor tendons are divided distally. The muscle is then dissected proximally and turned on itself (180°) to fill the plantar heel defect. **(D)** Coverage of the flap is provided through skin grafting or advancement of intact glabrous skin from the heel as shown.

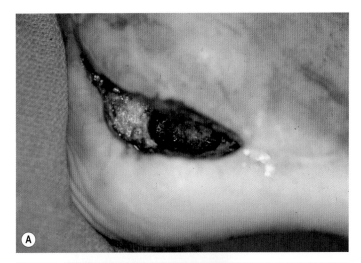

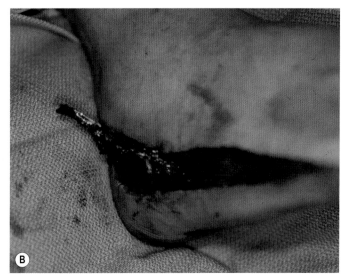

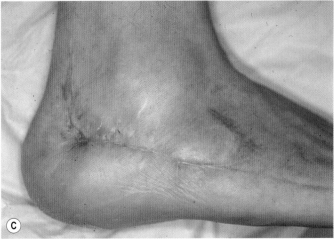

Fig. 8.29 Abductor digiti minimi flap. **(A)** Debrided lateral calcaneal wound with exposed underlying bone. **(B)** The abductor digiti minimi flap is elevated from distal to proximal through a linear incision along the lateral glabrous junction, transposed into the adjacent defect, and resurfaced with a split-thickness skin graft. **(C)** Stable wound coverage is observed after 2 years.

plantar artery. The origin of the muscle can be divided off the lateral calcaneus for improved mobilization and the donor site is typically closed primarily. For larger defects, it can be used in conjunction with either or both of the muscles discussed above.

Medial plantar artery flap

This fasciocutaneous flap provides the most versatile solution for medial or plantar heel reconstruction, providing tissue of similar quality (Fig. 8.30). It was originally described 40 years ago by Taylor and Hopson.[131] Mir had used it over 20 years earlier as a cross-foot flap from the instep of the opposite extremity.[132] A flap as large as 6 x 10 cm can be harvested with ease; however, the donor site must be skin-grafted. Therefore it is important to ensure that the instep is not a primary weight-bearing surface (i.e., Charcot collapse), as this would be a relative contraindication to using this flap.[133,134]

The flap is outlined over the medial instep of the foot and centered on the medial plantar artery using a hand-held Doppler. The distal extent of the flap is incised first through the skin and plantar fascia. The medial plantar neurovascular bundle is readily identified in the cleft between the AHB and the FDB muscles. The vessels are divided distally and elevated with the flap. If the patient is sensate, an intraneural dissection of the medial plantar nerve is performed

to preserve flap sensation and avoid damaging the medial trunk to the hallux. The dissection plane is superficial to the muscles (just deep to the plantar fascia) and includes the deep fascial septa separating the AHB and FDB, which is intimately associated with the vascular pedicle. For most reconstructions, the dissection may stop where the vessels emerge from the lateral border of the AHB muscle. Further mobilization is possible by dividing this muscle and the laciniate ligament and tracing the medial plantar artery to its origin from the posterior tibial artery. If additional pedicle length is needed, the lateral plantar artery can be divided; although, this is not recommended.

Heel pad flaps

Posterior heel wounds often result from prolonged decubitus pressure and usually signify severe vascular disease involving both the posterior tibial and the peroneal arteries. Soft tissue closure can be achieved using a medially- or laterally-based suprafascial flap of the heel pad. The lateral calcaneal flap, in particular, is useful for posterior calcaneal and distal Achilles defects. Its length can be increased (i.e., extended lateral calcaneal flap) by creating an L-shaped design that extends posterior and inferior to the lateral malleolus. The flap is based on the lateral calcaneal artery and is harvested with the lesser saphenous vein and sural nerve to provide

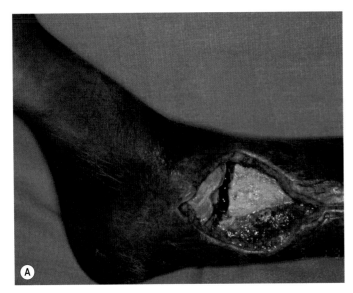

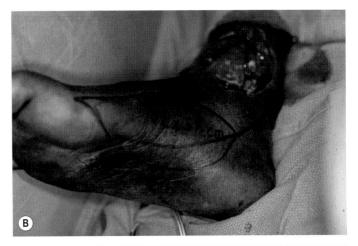

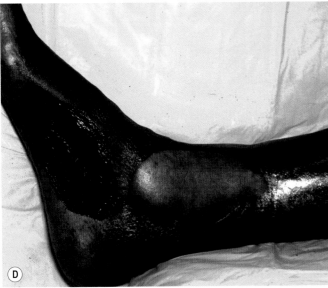

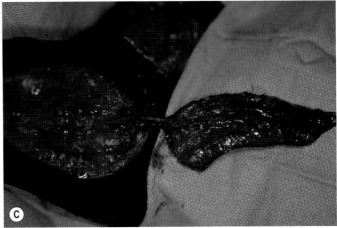

Fig. 8.30 Medial plantar artery flap. **(A)** Open distal tibial fracture. **(B)** Design of a medial plantar artery fasciocutaneous flap along the instep. **(C)** Elevation of the flap on the medial plantar pedicle. **(D)** Viable flap and skin grafted donor site.

cutaneous sensation. Nevertheless, the utility of the lateral calcaneal flap is limited by its difficult harvest, poor donor site, and restricted arc of rotation.

Sural artery flap

The retrograde or reverse sural flap is a versatile neurofasciocutaneous flap that is useful for ankle and posterior heel defects (Fig. 8.31).[135] Occasionally, a median superficial sural artery is seen coursing with the sural nerve; however, in most cases, the flap is supplied by an arterial plexus of vessels that travel along the sural nerve and receive retrograde flow from a peroneal perforator located 5 cm above the lateral malleolus. The artery and sural nerve first course above the fascia and then dive deep to the fascia at the midcalf, while the accompanying lesser saphenous vein remains above the fascia.

The flap is outlined over the raphe between the two heads of the gastrocnemius muscle. A line is drawn from the inferior edge of the flap to the pivot point for the pedicle approximately 5 cm proximal to the lateral malleolus. Flap elevation

begins along its cephalic margin. Through this incision, the lesser saphenous vein and sural nerve are identified superficial and deep to the deep fascia, respectively. Both structures are ligated so that they may be elevated along with the flap and underlying deep fascia. The margins of the flap pedicle should lay 2–3 cm on either side of the Dopplered lesser saphenous vein. Harvesting the overlying skin with the pedicle minimizes torque on the vein as it rotates 180° during inset. The arc of rotation will provide coverage of the lateral/medial ankle and posterior heel/Achilles region. In a well-vascularized extremity, the pedicle can be divided after 3–4 weeks to improve contour of the lower leg. Depending on flap size, the donor site may be closed primarily or covered with a split-thickness skin graft.

While this flap is particularly useful in patients who are not candidates for free tissue transfer, its complication rate is high and primarily related to venous congestion. This can be minimized if the flap is harvested with 3 cm of tissue on either side of the pedicle and with the overlying skin intact.[136] Problems with venous congestion can be further mitigated by

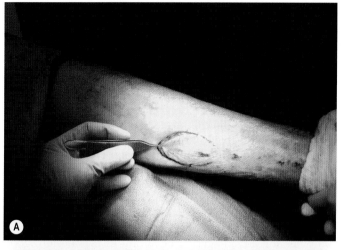

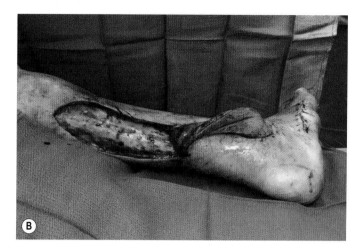

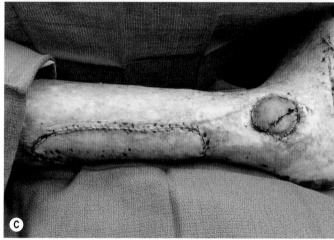

Fig. 8.31 Reverse sural artery perforator flap for coverage of a chronic, unstable wound over the lateral malleolus. **(A)** Initial flap elevation. **(B)** The flap is harvested with 3 cm of tissue on either side of the pedicle keeping the overlying skin intact to minimize torque on the vein as it rotates 180° during inset. **(C)** In a well-vascularized extremity, the pedicle can be divided after 3–4 weeks to improve contour of the lower leg. Depending on flap size, the donor site may be closed primarily or covered with a split-thickness skin graft.

delaying the flap by a few days after ligating the proximal lesser saphenous vein and sural artery.[137,138] The insetting of the flap is critical to avoid kinking of the pedicle. Offloading of the flap and heel during the healing phase may be simplified by using an Ilizarov-type frame. The major donor deficit of this flap is the loss of sensibility along the lateral aspect of the foot, while the skin-grafted depression in the posterior calf may pose a problem should the patient undergo a below-knee amputation in the future.

Free tissue transfer

The hindfoot represents an area of high functional and low aesthetic demand. The same principles apply to the plantar heel as for other weight-bearing regions of the foot. Namely, free muscle flaps surfaced with a skin graft offer a durable and well-contoured reconstruction, capable of withstanding the shear forces of repeated ambulation. Nevertheless, several fasciocutaneous (i.e., radial forearm, lateral arm, parascapular, etc.) and/or perforator flaps (i.e., ALT) have been used successfully as well. With many of these flaps, sensory nerve coaptation to disrupted calcaneal sensory branches may be performed at the time of reconstruction to improve early sensibility.[139–141] However, outcomes and overall benefit of this added procedure remain controversial. Some studies report no differences in flap survival or re-ulceration rates between neurotized and non-neurotized flaps.[142] In the setting of intact

deep sensory pathways, good return of sensibility is often seen in non-innervated flaps by 1 year.[116,140,141] If neurotization of a plantar flap is to be attempted, then proximal dissection of the sensory nerve to a healthier region should be performed to facilitate coaptation without disrupting intact nerve branches.

Hindfoot amputations

The presence of calcaneal osteomyelitis in patients who have limited ambulatory capacity or significant comorbidities may warrant vertical calcanectomy to remove bony prominences/diseased bone and develop soft-tissue envelopes to simplify wound closure. Although patients can still ambulate with a partially resected calcaneus, disinsertion of the Achilles tendon mandates the use of custom orthotics.

Syme first described amputation at the ankle in 1843.[143] The Syme's amputation has a definite role in hindfoot reconstruction and should be considered in the setting of severe osteomyelitis involving the talus and/or calcaneus, in patients who are poor candidates for free tissue transfer, and in diabetic patients with prior contralateral lower extremity amputation. The procedure involves amputation through the distal tibia/fibula, just above the ankle mortise. The talus and calcaneus are carefully removed, leaving behind a vascularly intact heel pad, which is anchored to the anterior surface of the osteotomized distal tibia to provide durable and secure soft-tissue coverage. The procedure can be modified by leaving a 1 cm thick wedge of plantar calcaneal cortex attached to the heel pad and fusing this structure to the distal tibia. Large medial and lateral "dog ears" can be revised during a second operation to minimize tension during initial wound closure. A dorsal flap may be required to facilitate closure if the plantar soft tissues have been compromised by extensive wounds or scars.

For diabetic patients with prior contralateral limb loss, Syme's amputation provides a stable, tailored platform for weight-bearing and ambulation. These patients generally require minimal physical therapy for gait training, and energy expenditure (oxygen uptake, velocity of cadence, and stride length) is consistently better than that measured for both below-knee and above-knee amputees.[144] It is for this specific population that the Syme's amputation is most useful. The key to long-term success with this procedure is having an experienced prosthetist who is skilled at creating well-designed Syme's prostheses.

Achilles region

Wounds involving the posterior hindfoot/Achilles region can be problematic. There are five principles that must be followed in repairing wounds of this unique location: (1) preserve Achilles tendon function, (2) avoid joint/tendon contractures, (3) restore normal anatomy/contour, (4) reconstruct soft-tissue deficiencies, and (5) select donor tissues based upon the specific requirements of the wound. Unfortunately, regional tissue deficits as well as vascular compromise and scarring in this region often preclude attempts at primary wound closure or local tissue rearrangement. Isolated soft-tissue defects with intact paratenon can be managed with a simple skin graft. For defects involving exposed tendon, adequate local wound care and/or NPWT will promote healthy granulation, which can be left to heal secondarily or subsequently skin grafted. The use of a dermal regenerate template (i.e., Integra), with or without NPWT, can provide a healthy dermal layer to facilitate coverage with a thin autograft. Both the VAC and the Ilizarov frame can be used to immobilize and offload wounds around the ankle joint to prevent shear forces from disrupting the healing process.

Local fasciocutaneous flaps

As described above, the extended lateral calcaneal flap and/ or reverse sural flap can be used to provide coverage of small-to-moderate defects in the Achilles region. However, given the inherent difficulties associated with their use (i.e., limited coverage, higher complications, donor site morbidity, etc.), these flaps are typically reserved for patients who have failed previous grafts and are poor candidates for more advanced reconstructive techniques (i.e., free tissue transfer).

Free tissue transfer

Combined defects involving the Achilles tendon and overlying soft tissue pose a significant challenge. Successful reconstruction mandates an accurate evaluation of the patient's preinjury functional status, medical comorbidities, and ambulatory prognosis. For younger, more active patients, functional demands often necessitate a stable gait cycle with normalized range of motion and restoration of power and plantar flexion.

To this end, composite free tissue transfer with a vascularized tendon construct facilitates single-stage reconstruction with contoured, well-vascularized soft-tissue coverage that can withstand a dynamic workload and promote adequate tendon glide with ambulation.[145,146]

At our institution, the composite ALT flap with vascularized fascia lata is the preferred method for reconstructing combined tendocutaneous defects of the Achilles (Fig. 8.32). The fascial sheet of the composite flap is rolled into a tendon-like structure and fixed to the proximal and distal remnants of the Achilles, utilizing multiple non-absorbable, interrupted sutures (Fig. 8.33). If no distal stump is available, the graft is fixed to the calcaneus with a suture anchor. Proximal fixation is accomplished with the ankle joint at 90°. Postoperatively, the ankle is immobilized in the neutral position with an external fixation device for 4 weeks. This construct – which combines the advantages of flexibility in flap design, good skin quality, and minimal donor site morbidity – has been shown in limited series to achieve acceptable ankle power, strength, and range of motion, with improved satisfaction and quality-of-life scores after 1 year.[147,148]

Postoperative care

Patients who have undergone foot reconstruction require a structured, graduated rehabilitation program that is tailored to their functional goals and capabilities. Follow-up should be frequent and involve a multidisciplinary team of specialists (i.e., plastic surgery, vascular surgery, orthopedic surgery, podiatry, infectious disease, primary care, and prosthetist/ orthotist) who are available to participate in the patient's care. Experienced nursing personnel adept at all aspects of wound assessment and care play an integral role as well.

In general, patients are not allowed to bear weight on the operated foot for 4 weeks if the plantar surface was involved. This is of paramount importance to ensure uneventful healing. The use of strict bed rest and/or crutches, walkers, non-mechanized wheelchairs, or rollabouts varies with the nature of the procedure performed and the physical ability and coordination of the patient. Local flaps typically require 1 day of elevation, skin grafts 3–5 days, and free flaps up to 2 weeks. During the bed-rest phase, use of low molecular weight heparin significantly reduces the risk of thromboembolic events. Control of pedal edema is important and may be accomplished through a combination of elevation, NPWT (3–5 days), and/or gentle compression wraps once dependent positioning of the limb is permitted. Sutures are generally removed at 3 weeks in healthy patients, 4 weeks in diabetics, and 6 weeks in patients with renal failure.

With the help of a pedorthotist, appropriate orthotic devices can be prescribed to offload specific parts of the plantar foot. For dorsal wounds, patients are allowed to ambulate far sooner, provided they use a dressing that protects the reconstruction. During healing, a monorail external fixator or Ilizarov frame can be used to immobilize the ankle joint or offload plantar/heel wounds, respectively. The L'Nard splint, or multipodus boot, provides a less invasive option for offloading the heel and immobilizing the ankle joint. For patients who are weight-bearing and ambulatory, the CAM walker boot provides effective immobilization and allows the degree of equinus at the ankle to be adjusted. Following

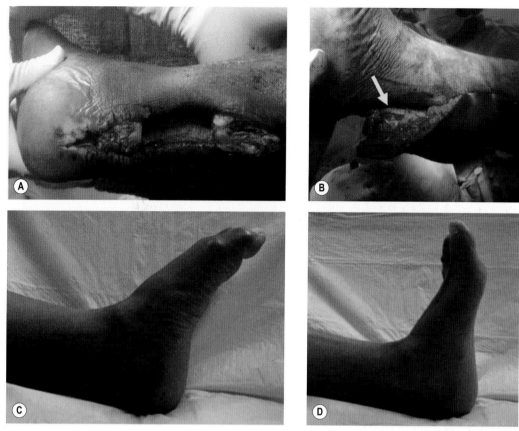

Fig. 8.32 Composite anterolateral thigh/vascularized fascia lata reconstruction of a combined tendocutaneous defect of the Achilles was undergone by a 32-year-old male. **(A)** Segmental loss of the Achilles tendon with large overlying soft-tissue deficit. **(B)** Transfer of the free fasciocutaneous flap and rolled fascia lata to the recipient site. The neo-tendon construct (arrow) is secured to the proximal and distal remnants of the native Achilles using multiple, non-absorbable, interrupted sutures. **(C,D)** Evaluation at 1-year follow-up demonstrating functional range of motion, contour, and aesthetic result of the reconstructed side. *(From: DeFazio MV, Hand KD, Iorio ML, et al. Combined free tissue transfer for the management of composite Achilles defects: functional outcomes and patient satisfaction following thigh based vascularized reconstruction with a neotendon construct. J Reconstr Microsurg. 2014;30(6):431–440.)*

tendon lengthening or transfer, patients should be kept non-weight-bearing for 1 week and in a CAM walker for the next 5 weeks. If compliance is a concern, wrapping the CAM walker in cast material can be helpful. Once healed, the patient will require accommodative shoe wear as well as a course of physical/occupational rehabilitation to regain the strength and mobility needed to live independently at home. If diabetic, vigilant follow-up with a podiatrist for routine preventive foot care is mandatory.

Outcomes

Establishment of a multidisciplinary clinic that provides comprehensive care to patients with diabetic foot ulcers is central to the success of any limb salvage protocol. Such a clinic should be equipped to coordinate diagnosis, offloading, and outpatient preventative care; perform revascularizations, debridements, and reconstructive procedures; aggressively treat infections; and manage medical comorbidities within a multidisciplinary forum.[149] New ulceration, when it occurs, will be detected earlier and lead to management that is more effective at promoting limb preservation. History has demonstrated that routine evaluation and treatment by a comprehensive multidisciplinary team improves the quality and cost-effectiveness of care and can reduce amputation rates by

36–86%.[150–158] These findings mirror the senior author's own 20-year experience managing complex lower extremity wounds in the setting of a multidisciplinary referral center for advanced limb salvage.

Internationally, recurrence rates for healed diabetic foot ulcers range from 60–80%. The importance of offloading and biomechanical stability in the promotion of wound healing and sustained long-term closure has been emphasized previously. However, it is difficult to properly maintain offloading with the use of orthotics alone. In one of the author's own investigations, surgical correction of underlying biomechanical abnormalities (i.e., resection of bony prominences, repair of Charcot midfoot deformities, Achilles tendon lengthening, etc.) at the time of wound closure led to a reduction in ulcer recurrence rates from 25% to 2% over an average follow-up of 5 years.

Summary

Complex lower extremity reconstruction and functional limb salvage is predicated upon the institution of a multidisciplinary collaboration between members of a comprehensive wound care team. Successful healing requires, at a minimum, the presence of adequate local blood flow, a clean wound base, and a biomechanically stable framework to prevent recurrent

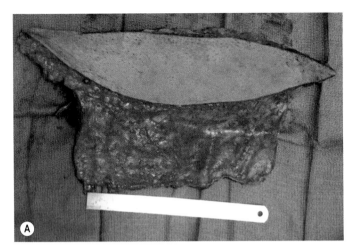

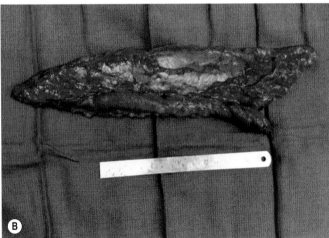

Fig. 8.33 **(A)** Free anterolateral thigh flap with associated strip of vascularized fascia lata following harvest. **(B)** The fascial strip is then rolled to form a neo-tendon construct, which is secured to the proximal and distal remnants of the native Achilles tendon. *(From: DeFazio MV, Hand KD, Iorio ML, et al. Combined free tissue transfer for the management of composite Achilles defects: functional outcomes and patient satisfaction following thigh based vascularized reconstruction with a neotendon construct.* J Reconstr Microsurg. *2014;30(6):431–440.)*

breakdown. Reconstruction of chronic wounds should only be undertaken after the debrided wound manifests signs of healing. The repair is then dictated by the size and location of the wound as well as the patient's goals, functional capacity, vascular status, and medical comorbidities. Most wounds will benefit from simple surgical techniques (i.e., NPWT, delayed primary closure, skin grafting, etc.), while few require more sophisticated modalities (i.e., local, pedicled, or free flaps). Postoperatively, appropriate offloading and rehabilitation, frequent follow-up, and preventative care will minimize complications and promote long-term functional independence. The principles and techniques outlined in this chapter will serve to enhance healing, function, quality-of-life, and survival in patients who face major amputation as the alternative.

 Bonus images for this chapter can be found online at
http://www.expertconsult.com

Fig. 8.2 Effects of elevated serum glucose on blood flow and tissue perfusion.
Fig. 8.4 Blue toe syndrome. **(A,B)** Patient presented with severe pain following sudden appearance of several well-demarcated ischemic lesions involving all 5 digits of the right foot. **(C)** Right lower extremity angiogram demonstrating an ulcerated plaque with organized thrombus in the mid-superficial femoral artery. Percutaneous endovascular intervention was not attempted due to concern over plaque dislodgement and resultant distal embolism. **(D,E)** Open thromboendarterectomy with excision of a 1.5 cm occlusive thrombus.
Fig. 8.6 (A) Preintervention angiogram of the distal right lower extremity in a patient with an ischemic plantar-medial foot wound demonstrating complete occlusion of the posterior tibial artery along with a large mid-level segmental occlusion of the anterior tibial artery (arrow). Additional high-grade stenoses of the proximal anterior tibial and proximal-to-midperoneal arteries are also noted (asterisk). **(B,C)** Postintervention angiograms following percutaneous transluminal angioplasty of the anterior tibial and peroneal arteries revealing widely patent run-off to the foot with no evidence of residual stenosis or occlusion. (From: DeFazio MV, Han KD, Akbari CM, Evans KK. Free tissue transfer after targeted endovascular reperfusion for complex lower extremity reconstruction: setting the stage for success in the presence of multivessel disease. Ann Vasc Surg. 2015;29(6):1316.e7–1316.e15.)
Fig. 8.7 Assessment of Achilles tendon tightness in patients with equinovarus deformity requires that dorsiflexion be tested with **(A)** the leg held in extension (to keep the gastrocnemius muscles at their full resting length) and with **(B)** the knee flexed (which reduces tension on the gastrocnemius). If the ankle only dorsiflexes when the knee is flexed, then tightness of the gastrocnemius muscles is responsible for the equinus posture of the foot and can be released by performing a gastrocnemius recession. If the ankle remains tight during knee extension and flexion, then both gastrocnemius and soleus contributions to the Achilles tendon have to be released, usually percutaneously.
Fig. 8.12 Construction of a closed-system habitat to facilitate free-range maggot debridement therapy for multiple necrotic ulcers involving the dorsal/plantar surfaces of the foot as well as the interstices of the webspaces. Maggots are introduced through the ventilation port, which is sealed with polyester chiffon netting to ensure continuous oxygen penetration. An internal collection chamber is lined with multiple layers of super-absorbent gauze and suspended to prevent pooling of secretions that can irritate the skin and/or lead to barrier disruption.
Fig. 8.13 For larger reconstructions involving mobile and/or weight-bearing surfaces of the foot and ankle, external fixation with an Ilizarov frame is ideal in that it not only provides superior immobilization of the ankle but also suspends the foot and heel, maintains skeletal alignment, and protects the reconstruction from external pressure and potential trauma.
Fig. 8.15 (A) Medial foot defect. **(B)** Lisfranc amputation with rotation of a laterally-based plantar flap for closure. **(C)** Dry gangrenous necrosis of the plantar foot and toes resulting in loss of the majority of the plantar soft tissues. **(D)** Transmetatarsal amputation was performed with preservation of a dorsal soft-tissue flap and use of a skin graft to facilitate closure.
Fig. 8.16 (A) Fibrogranular wound with fibrotic scar tissue overlying the left Achilles tendon and medial malleolus. **(B)** Healthy granulating wound bed following serial debridement and interval negative pressure wound therapy. **(C)** Complete take of a partial-thickness skin graft.
Fig. 8.27 Abductor hallucis brevis flap. Local flaps are particularly useful for coverage of ankle defects with exposed tendon and/or bone. **(A,B)** In this case, the tibiotalar junction could not be completely covered with a local transposition flap. **(C,D)** An abductor hallucis brevis muscle flap was rotated posteriorly into the residual defect and covered with a split-thickness skin graft. **(E)** Follow-up at 1 year demonstrating complete healing without breakdown and acceptable final contour.

5. Taylor GI, Palmer JH. The vascular territories (angiosomes) of the body: experimental study and clinical applications. *Br J Plast Surg.* 1987;40:113–141. *The authors introduce the concept of the "angiosome", which is a 3D unit of tissue fed by a single source artery. The authors evaluated the blood supply to the skin and underlying tissues in fresh cadaver models using ink injection studies, direct dissection, perforator mapping, and radiographic analysis. The blood supply was shown to be a continuous 3D network of vessels supplying all tissue layers through multiple interconnections. The authors plotted an average of 374 major perforators in each subject. This arterial roadmap of the body provides the basis for the logical planning of incisions and flaps, and helps to define the tissues available for composite transfer.*

6. Attinger CE, Evans KK, Bulan E, et al. Angiosomes of the foot and ankle and clinical implications for limb salvage: reconstruction, incisions, and revascularization. *Plast Reconstr Surg.* 2006;117(suppl):S261–S293. *Understanding the angiosomes of the foot and ankle as well as the interaction among their source arteries is clinically useful in reconstructive surgery, especially in the presence of peripheral vascular disease. The authors performed 50 cadaver dissections with methyl methacrylate arterial injections to further define the angiosomes of the lower extremity. They demonstrated six distinct angiosomes of the foot and ankle originating from three main arteries. Blood flow to the foot and ankle is redundant due to multiple arterial–arterial connections between these three major source vessels. Using a Doppler ultrasound probe and selective occlusion, it is possible to determine the patency of these interconnections as well as the direction of blood flow. This step is critical to the planning of vascularly reliable reconstructions, safe exposures, and the most effective revascularization strategy for a given wound.*

8. Neville RF, Attinger CE, Bulan EJ, et al. Revascularization of a specific angiosome for limb salvage: does the target artery matter? *Ann Vasc Surg.* 2009;23:367–373. *The authors conducted a retrospective comparison of outcomes for 52 non-healing lower extremity wounds that required tibial bypass, through either direct revascularization (n=27) to the artery feeding the ischemic angiosome or indirect revascularization (n=25) to an artery unrelated to the ischemic angiosome. Overall, 77% of wounds progressed to healing and 23% failed to heal with resultant amputation. For patients in the direct revascularization cohort, the rates of healing and amputation were 91% and 9%, respectively. In contrast, patients who underwent indirect revascularization experienced a 62% healing rate, with 38% of wounds ending in amputation. The authors concluded that direct revascularization of the angiosome specific to the anatomy of the wound leads to higher rates of healing and limb salvage.*

17. Dellon AL, Mackinnon SE. Chronic nerve compression model for the double crush hypothesis. *Ann Plast Surg.* 1991;26:259–264.

61. Steed DL, Donohoe D, Webster MW, et al. Effect of extensive debridement and treatment on the healing of diabetic foot ulcers. *J Am Coll Surg.* 1996;183:61–64.

69. Mueller MJ, Sinacore DR, Hastings MK, et al. Effect of Achilles tendon lengthening on neuropathic plantar ulcers, a randomized clinical trial. *J Bone Joint Surg Am.* 2003;85:1436–1445. *Limited ankle dorsiflexion has been implicated as a contributing factor to plantar forefoot ulceration and wound chronicity in patients with diabetes mellitus. The authors compared outcomes for 64 patients with diabetes mellitus and a neuropathic plantar ulcer who were treated with total contact casting with and without Achilles tendon lengthening. After two years, the risk for recurrence following Achilles tendon lengthening was 52% less than that for total contact casting alone. The authors concluded that Achilles tendon lengthening should be considered an effective strategy to reduce recurrence of neuropathic plantar forefoot ulceration in patients with diabetes mellitus and limited ankle dorsiflexion.*

74. Argenta LC, Morykwas MJ. Vacuum-assisted closure: a new method for wound control and treatment: clinical experience. *Ann Plast Surg.* 1997;38:563–576.

100. Hollenbeck ST, Woo S, Komatsu I, et al. Longitudinal outcomes and application of the subunit principle to 165 foot and ankle free tissue transfers. *Plast Reconstr Surg.* 2010;125:924–934. *It is known that ill-conceived flap designs may be subject to breakdown, interfere with proper footwear, and/or prevent efficient ambulation. The authors reviewed their experience with 165 lower extremity free tissue transfers and proposed a subunit principle to guide donor site selection based on region-specific functional and aesthetic demands. Flap survival was 92%, and the overall limb salvage rate was approximately 97.6%. In diabetics, the flap survival and limb salvage rates were 80% and 83%, respectively. Although not statistically predictive, the authors found that plantar flaps containing a cutaneous paddle were more prone to late ulceration along the interval between the flap and the native plantar skin when compared to muscle flaps covered with a skin graft.*

148. DeFazio MV, Han KD, Iorio ML, et al. Combined free tissue transfer for the management of composite Achilles defects: functional outcomes and patient satisfaction following thigh-based vascularized reconstruction with a neotendon construct. *J Reconstr Microsurg.* 2014;30:431–440.

156. Driver VR, Madsen J, Goodman RA. Reducing amputation rates in patients with diabetes at a military medical center: the limb preservation service model. *Diabetes Care.* 2005;28:248–253.

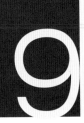

Comprehensive trunk anatomy

Michael A. Howard and Sara R. Dickie

SYNOPSIS

- Many workhorse flaps and reconstructive pursuits involve the trunk.
- Familiarity with the vascular relationships and tissue types within this anatomy is integral to a plastic surgeon.
- What follows is a detailed anatomy of the trunk including the chest, abdomen, back, and perineum.

Access the Historical Perspective section and Fig. 9.1 online at

http://www.expertconsult.com

Basic science and disease process: embryology of the trunk

In the third week of gestation, formation of the axial skeleton begins. The bony skeleton, muscles, fascia, and skin are derived from mesodermal somites bordering the central notochord. Pluripotent mesenchymal cells differentiate into fibroblasts, osteoblasts, and chondroblasts and other progenitor cells that will build the tissues of the fetal body. The axial skeleton consists of skull, vertebral column, ribs, and sternum. The appendicular skeleton includes the pelvic and pectoral girdles. The skeleton begins to chondrify in the 6th week of gestation. The process of ossification can last from a few months gestation until young adulthood. Progenitor skeletal muscle cells divide into dorsal (epaxial) and ventral (hypaxial) divisions along with a corresponding spinal nerve. The extensor muscles of the vertebral column, derived from the epaxial myotomes, are innervated by posterior rami of the spinal nerves. All of the other muscles of the trunk are derived from the hypaxial myotomes and are innervated by the ventral rami. Most skeletal muscles are fully developed by birth.[3]

Angiogenesis begins in the 3rd week of gestation. Primordial blood vessels begin to form in the extraembryonic mesenchyme of the yolk sac. Mesenchymal cells differentiate into angioblasts, forming aggregate blood islands. These begin to coalesce into primitive endothelium. Near the end of the 3rd week, this same process is evident within the embryo itself, and by the beginning of the 4th week, the embryo has a functional circulatory system.[3] At birth, the main vessels and perforators to the skin are present. The entire body is lined by superficial fascia[4] that lies just below the dermis and is surrounded by varying amounts of adipose tissue. It serves to encase, support, and protect the fatty and muscular layers of the body and to support the overlying skin in the dynamic movements of the underlying muscle. In certain areas it is adherent to the deep fascia or periosteum, and at these places the body contour is defined by creases and convexities. Where there are bulges and plateaus the connections between superficial and deep systems are looser. As an individual grows, vessels stretch from their origins, usually in areas near joints or fixed fascial planes of the body. Taylor noted that areas that were mobile had cascades of arterial supply that tended to originate from the fixed areas distant from the tissue supplied by the vessel. He asserted that these perforators were present at birth and grew along the fascial planes and stretched as the individual grew and developed.[2]

Back

The back provides support for the head and shoulders while walking upright. Near the midline, the paraspinous muscles run in a vertical fashion and are mainly responsible for spinal support and protection. Moving laterally and superficially, muscles become broad and are responsible for movement of neck, shoulders, hips, and extremities. Dense adhesions between the superficial fascia and the skin of the back prevent shearing of the tissues. The spine has dense fascia surrounding the spinal processes, which attaches to the dermis. This creates the central midline. There are several notable, bony

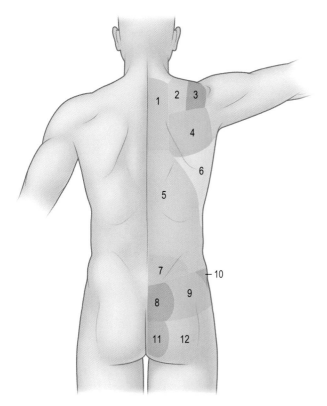

Fig. 9.2 Surface anatomy and vascular angiosomes of back and buttock. (1) Transverse cervical, (2) suprascapular, (3) acromiothoracic, (4) circumflex scapular, (5) posterior intercostals, (6) thoracodorsal, (7) lumbar perforators, (8) lateral sacral perforators, (9) superior gluteal, (10) deep circumflex iliac, (11) internal pudendal, (12) inferior gluteal.

landmarks in the neck and back region: palpable at the base of the neck is the vertebra prominens of the C7 spinous process. The root of the scapular spine is at the level of T3, and the angle of scapula is at T7. Typically, the spinous process of T12 is palpable. The bilateral iliac crest forms the hips at the level of L4. The posterior inferior iliac spine is parallel to S2 (Fig. 9.2).

The *thoracolumbar fascia* is the investing fascia of the back. It encases the paraspinous muscles as well as the quadrates lumborum. It is continuous with the nuchal fascia of the neck, attaches medially to the spinous processes of the thoracic vertebrae, laterally to the angles of the ribs, and inferiorly to the posterior iliac spine. It is supplied by the lumbar and thoracic perforators, as well as the distal end arteries of the superior gluteal artery inferiorly and the thoracodorsal artery superiorly.[5]

The broad, flat latissimus muscle can usually be seen on both sides of the lower midback in thin, muscular individuals. The posterior axillary fold is formed by its tendon as it crosses from the back to insert on the humerus. The *triangular space* of the posterior axilla is defined by the teres minor superiorly, teres major inferiorly, and the long head of the triceps laterally (Fig. 9.3). Through it courses the circumflex scapular artery and two venae comitantes.

There are two spaces referred to as the lumbar triangle. These are areas of the back that do not contain all of the muscular layers. The inferior or *petit triangle* is bound by the latissimus medially, the external oblique laterally, and the iliac crest inferiorly. Its base is comprised of the internal oblique

muscle (see Fig. 9.3). The superior or *Grynfeltt triangle* is created by the 12th rib superiorly, the quadrates lumborum medially, and the internal oblique laterally. The floor is comprised of the transversalis muscle (not shown). No vessels or named nerves travel through these spaces. The *lumbocostoabdominal triangle* is formed by the external oblique, the serratus posterior inferior, the erector spinae, and the internal oblique.

Muscles[6]

The *trapezius* is a large flat muscle that crosses many joints and has multiple actions on the neck, back, and shoulder including elevation, retraction, and rotation of the scapula. Typically it is divided into superior, middle, and inferior portions. Medially it is attached to the spinous processes of C7–T12 vertebrae, the superior nuchal line, and ligamentum nuchae. Laterally, it attaches to the lateral third of the clavicle, the medial acromion process, and the scapular spine. This is the only muscle of the back innervated by a cranial nerve. Upon exiting the skull, the spinal accessory nerve pierces the sternocleidomastoid muscle and passes through the posterior cervical triangle. It enters the trapezius muscle 5 cm above the clavicle, sending a branch to the upper portion of the muscle. The remainder of the nerve runs caudally along the anterior border of the muscle until the fibers desiccate inferiorly. The trapezius receives sensory innervation from cervical nerves C3 and C4. Typically described, the trapezius has Mathes and Nahai type II vascular anatomy receiving blood supply from branches of the transverse cervical artery, which will be described in greater detail later.

The *levator scapulae* originates from transverse processes of C1–C4 and inserts on the superior part of medial border of scapula. It is innervated by dorsal scapular nerve and spinal nerves C3 and C4, and its blood supply is via the dorsal scapular artery. Its main action is elevation of the scapula and depression of the glenoid.

The *Rhomboid* major and minor lay between the medial borders of the scapula to the spinous processes of C7–T5 vertebrae. Their action is to retract the scapula, depress the glenoid, and fix the scapula to the thoracic wall. They are innervated by the dorsal scapular nerve, and blood supply is mainly via the dorsal scapular artery.

The *supra and infraspinatus* muscles originate in their respective scapular fossa and insert into the superior and middle facet of the greater tubercle of the humerus. They are innervated by the suprascapular nerve and receive blood supply from the suprascapular and branches of the circumflex scapular arteries. They act to help abduct the arm and stabilize the humerus in the glenoid cavity.

The *subscapularis* originates in the subscapular fossa and inserts at the lesser tubercle of the humerus. It is innervated by the subscapular nerve. It serves to medially rotate and adduct the arm. Its blood supply is via the subscapular artery.

The *teres minor* originates at the superior lateral border of scapula and inserts into the inferior facet of greater tubercle of humerus. It is innervated by the axillary nerve and receives blood supply via a branch of the circumflex scapular artery. It assists in lateral rotation of the arm.

The *teres major* originates at the dorsal surface of inferior angle of scapula and inserts into the intertubercular groove of humerus. It is innervated by lower subscapular nerve and receives blood supply via branches of the circumflex scapular

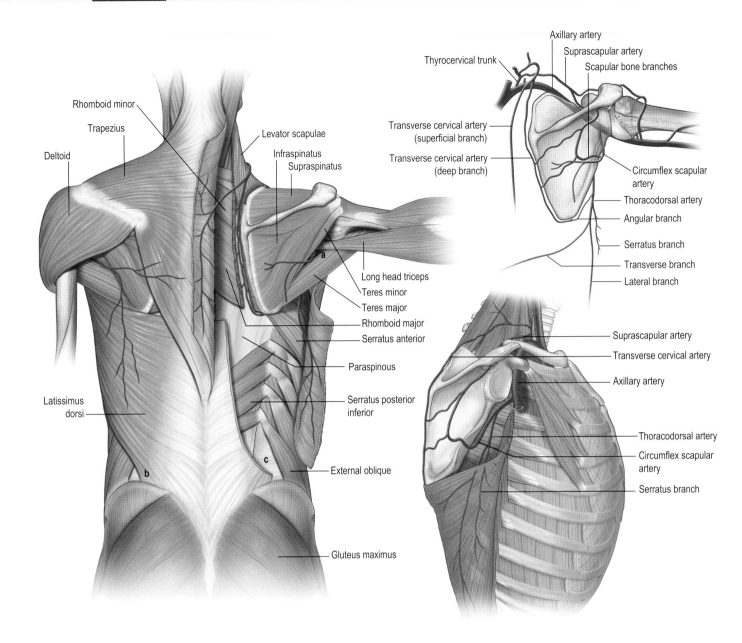

Fig. 9.3 Superficial and deep musculature of the back showing vascular relationships. (a) The triangular space is defined by the teres minor, teres major, and long head of the triceps muscle; (b) lumbar triangle of petit; (c) lumbocostoabdominal triangle.

and thoracodorsal arteries. Its action is to adduct and medially rotate the arm.

The *latissimus* muscle originates at the medial attachment to spinous processes of T7–T12, thoracolumbar fascia, and the iliac crest. It inserts on the intertubercular groove of the humerus. It is innervated by thoracodorsal nerve and functions to extend, adduct, and medially rotate the shoulder. The main vascular pedicle is the thoracodorsal artery, with segmental blood supply arising from intercostals and lumbar perforators medially. The latissimus dorsi is described as Mathes and Nahai type V muscle.

The *serratus posterior* (superior and inferior) are extrinsic muscles of back that lie in an intermediate layer between paraspinous and more superficial latissimus and trapezius muscles. The superior portion of serratus posterior originates at the spinous process of C7–T3 and inserts on the superior border of ribs 2–5. It is innervated by intercostal nerves 2–5

and elevates the ribs during inspiration. The inferior serratus posterior originates at the spinous processes T11–L3 and the thoracolumbar fascia and inserts on the inferior border of ribs 9–12. It is innervated by intercostal nerves 9–11 and the subcostal nerve and serves to depress the ribs on expiration.

The *paraspinous* muscles are referred to as the intrinsic muscles of the back, spanning from occiput to sacrum. They are intricate muscles that interconnect the spinous and transverse processes of the vertebral bones with the ribs and primarily support and protect the spinal column. Their movements include spinal rotation and lateral bending of neck. Innervation is via dorsal primary rami of the spinal nerves. There are three layers of the paraspinous muscles: a deep layer referred to as the transversospinal group (semispinalis, multifidus, rotators); an intermediate layer, the erector spinae group (spinalis, interspinalis, intertransverse, longissimus, and iliocostalis); and a superficial layer, the spinotransverse group (splenius cervicis and capitis). The blood supply to these muscles is segmental stemming from posterior branches of intercostals, lumbar, and sacral arteries, classifying these muscles as Mathes and Nahai type IV.

Vascular anatomy

The *suprascapular* artery is a branch of the thyrocervical trunk. It travels anterior to the trapezius along the shoulder and supplies the upper scapula and the scapular muscles.

The dominant blood supply to the trapezius is via branches of the *transverse cervical artery*. Originating from the thyrocervical trunk, it passes through the posterior triangle of the neck to the anterior border of the levator scapulae muscle.[7] Here, it divides into deep and superficial branches. Upon entering the muscle the superficial branch divides again into an ascending and descending branch. It is the descending branch, sometimes referred to as the *superficial cervical artery* (SCA), which supplies the middle and lateral portions of the trapezius. Once the deep branch separates from the superficial branch, it courses below the levator scapulae to the undersurface of the rhomboids. A perforating branch emerges from between the rhomboid muscles and becomes the main supply to the trapezius inferior to scapular spine (see Fig. 9.3). The deep branch, also referred to as the *dorsal scapular artery* (DSA), supplies the lower middle and inferior portion of the trapezius and the skin paddle above and lateral to it overlying the latissimus. Through the years there have been many anatomic studies attempting to define the blood supply to the trapezius. Some of the confusion arises simply from nomenclature. In 2004, Hass published a large cadaver study, finding, in nearly 45% of specimens, the DSA arose from the subclavian artery or costocervical trunk. In the remaining 55%, the DSA formed a trunk with the SCA and/or the suprascapular artery. The trapezius also receives segmental blood supply medially from the intercostal arteries 3–6, leading some investigators to classify this muscle as Mathes and Nahai type V.[8]

The *subscapular artery* arises from the third portion of the axillary artery and branches into the circumflex scapular and the thoracodorsal arteries. Occasionally the circumflex scapular arises directly from the axillary artery. The *circumflex scapular artery* passes through the triangular space and gives off perforating branches to the superior lateral border of the scapula. There is rarely a defined medullary branch; however, a segment of bone measuring 10–14 cm along the lateral border can usually be harvested reliably on these small perforators.[9] The main artery goes on to divide into a small ascending branch, which is occasionally absent, and more robust transverse and descending branches. These supply the scapular and parascapular flaps, respectively. These arteries run in the subcutaneous plane and are paralleled by two venae comitantes. The venous outflow follows the subscapular system and eventually drains into the axillary vein.[10]

After branching from the subscapular artery, the *thoracodorsal artery* passes along the deep surface of the latissimus and continues caudally 1–4 cm posterior to the lateral border of the muscle. As the artery descends, a branch or branches supply the lower portion of serratus anterior. After this, it divides into a lateral (or descending) branch and a transverse (or horizontal) branch. Angrigiani described three musculocutaneous perforators that reliably left the lateral branch of the

thoracodorsal artery piercing the latissimus muscle and supplying the skin and subcutaneous tissue of the lateral infrascapular back. The proximal perforator exits 8 cm below the posterior axillary fold and 1–4 cm posterior to the lateral border of the muscle. Other smaller perforators were found along a similar trajectory inferiorly and obliquely located along the lateral border of the latissimus (see Fig. 9.3).[11]

Seneviratne *et al.* described the *angular artery* as a branch from the subscapular system that supplied the lower lateral segment and the angle of the scapula. It can arise from the latissimus or serratus branch of the thoracodorsal artery or at a trifurcation with both vessels. From its origin to where it penetrates the bone measures approximately 7 cm and is reliably found between the teres minor and serratus anterior on its way to the dorsal surface of the scapular angle. This artery allows a strip of bone up to 3 cm of the lateral scapular angle and 6 cm of the vertebral surface to be harvested as a composite graft with muscle, fascia, or skin.[12]

The *intercostal* and *lumbar arteries* supply much of the skin and musculature of the midback. Perforators emerging from these vessels pass through the paraspinous muscles in three adjacent columns that parallel the spinous processes laterally at 3, 5, and 8 cm. These segmental perforators have longitudinal anastomotic connections to one another.[13]

The *superior gluteal artery* arises from the internal iliac artery and passes through the greater sciatic foramen. At approximately 6 cm below the PSIS and 4–5 cm lateral to the sacral midline, the artery passes between the gluteus medius and piriformis muscle to enter the gluteus maximus. It sends nutrient branches to the muscle and continues to the overlying skin and soft tissue. The *inferior gluteal artery* also arises from the internal iliac artery. It passes through the lesser sciatic foramen, inferior to the piriformis muscle, to supply the lower gluteal skin and soft tissue (Fig. 9.4).

Chest

The clavicle and manubrium create the cranial border of the chest. The midpoint of the clavicle defines a plumb line drawn down the anterior chest and is referred to as the midclavicular line. The xiphoid and the synchondrosis of ribs 7–10 create the caudal border of the chest. The diaphragm is attached to the posterior surfaces of the xiphoid process and the lower six ribs and costal cartilages. Laterally, the chest is bordered by the anterior axillary fold, which is created by the pectoralis major tendon as it inserts on the humerus (Fig. 9.5). The *deltopectoral triangle* is pierced by the cephalic vein as it joins the axillary vein, bound medially by the clavicle, superiorly by the deltoid, and inferiorly by the pectoralis major muscle. Spanning the triangle and coursing beneath the pectoralis major is the clavipectoral fascia, a thick, dynamic fascial sling. Lateral to the triangular space is the *quadrangular space* of the axilla. Its boundaries include the teres major inferiorly, teres minor and subscapularis superiorly, the long head of triceps medially, and the surgical neck of the humerus laterally. Through it passes the posterior circumflex humeral artery and axillary nerve.[5]

The nipple–areolar complex is located slightly lateral to the midclavicular line and at or near the fourth rib. Innervation of the nipple is by the fourth intercostal nerve, and blood

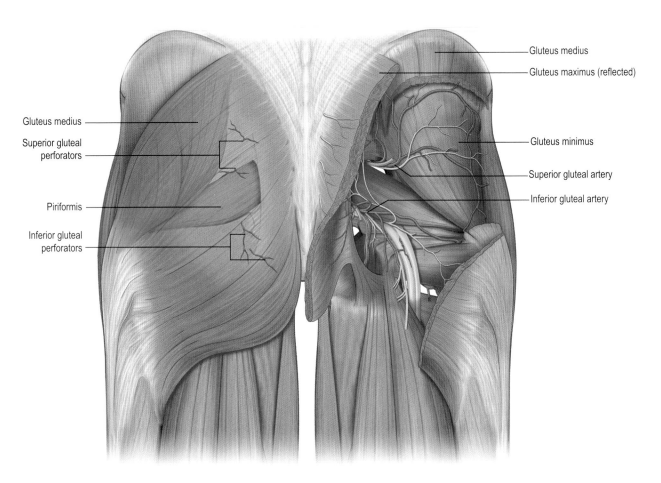

Gluteus medius

Superior gluteal
perforators

Piriformis

Inferior gluteal
perforators

Gluteus medius

Gluteus maximus (reflected)

Gluteus minimus

Superior gluteal artery

Inferior gluteal artery

Fig. 9.4 Superficial and deep musculature of the buttock showing vascular relationships of superior and inferior gluteal artery.

supply is via perforators from the internal mammary artery at the fourth rib as well as the intercostal arteries and the end arteries of the thoracodorsal and thoracoacromial arteries. For females, depending on the size, shape and ptosis of the breast the nipple could be any distance from the fourth rib, but the neurovascular supply remains consistent. The milk ridge refers to a primitive line of ectodermal tissue extending from the axilla to the groin. At any point along this line, breast and nipple tissue can develop. During embryologic development this line appears and subsequently involutes; however, remnants of this tissue can give rise to supernumerary nipples or ectopic breast tissue.[14]

The superficial fascia that lies just below the skin and subcutaneous tissue is present in the chest as it is in the rest of the body. Over the area of the breast this fascia splits into a superficial and a deep layer (Fig. 9.6). These layers support the breast parenchyma and glandular tissue against the chest wall. Running perpendicular between these two layers and into the deep fascia of the chest are *Cooper's ligaments*. These suspensory ligaments support the breast parenchyma yet allow breast mobility. They stretch with growth of the breast during puberty, pregnancy, and weight changes. Loss of elastic fibers in Cooper's ligaments leads to breast ptosis. The superficial fascia of the chest transitions into Scarpa's fascia as it enters the abdomen below the level of the bony thorax.

There are 20–30 axillary lymph nodes draining most of the mammary gland and the anterolateral chest wall as well as the posterior thoracic and scapular regions. The parasternal nodes drain the medial mammary gland and the medial chest wall.

Muscles[6]

The *pectoralis major* is a fan-shaped muscle with a sternal and a clavicular origin. The middle and inferior portion originate at the sternum and costal cartilages of ribs 2–6. The clavicular head originates at the medial clavicle. The muscle inserts into the lateral edge of the intertubercular groove of the humerus (Fig. 9.7). It is innervated by the lateral and medial pectoral nerves. Its action is to adduct and medially rotate the humerus and draw the shoulder anteriorly. The blood supply is Mathes and Nahai type V. The dominant pedicle is the pectoral branch of the thoracoacromial trunk. Secondary blood supply is via the internal mammary artery perforators along its medial border. Laterally, it receives perforators from the thoracic intercostal vessels and some branches from the lateral thoracic artery.

The *pectoralis minor* is a flat fan-shaped muscle that sits below the pectoralis major. It originates lateral to the costal cartilage of ribs 2–5 and inserts as the coracoid process of the scapula. The main innervation is by medial pectoral nerve and occasionally by a small branch of the lateral pectoral nerve.[15] Along with serratus anterior and the rhomboids, the pectoralis minor stabilizes the scapula against the chest wall. The blood supply is variable but has been reported to arise from three sources. The thoracoacromial and lateral thoracic arteries

4–6. The medial chest wall is supplied by branches of the internal mammary artery. The lateral and superior chest wall is supplied by branches of the subclavian and axillary vessels.

The *internal mammary* artery branches from the subclavian artery and runs 1–2 cm lateral to the sternum on the inner surface of the thoracic cavity. Perforating vessels arise at each intercostal space 2–6 and pass superior to the rib margin. These perforators then pass through the pectoralis major at its sternal origin and supply the anterior chest wall and the medial breast parenchyma. Typically the perforator from the 2nd or 3rd interspace is larger than the others and is referred to as the principal perforator.[18]

The *axillary* artery begins as the subclavian artery passes out of the chest past the first rib and ends as it enters the arm passing the teres major, becoming the brachial artery. It is classically divided into three parts having specific branches originating from each. The first part is medial to the pectoralis minor tendon as it inserts onto the acromion, giving rise to the superior thoracic artery. The second part is behind the tendon and gives rise to the thoracoacromial trunk and the lateral thoracic artery. The third part is lateral to the tendon and gives off the subscapular artery and the anterior and posterior humeral circumflex arteries (see Fig. 9.7).

The *superior thoracic* artery is a small vessel that courses medially to the pectoralis minor. It occasionally gives off a muscular branch along the intercostal muscles of the 1st and 2nd rib. It has anastomosis with perforators from these ribs.

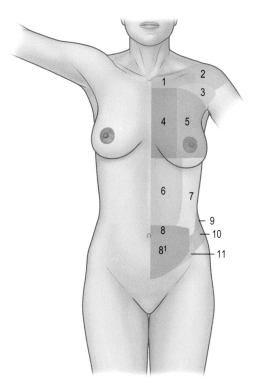

Fig. 9.5 Surface anatomy and vascular angiosomes of the chest and abdomen. (1) Clavicular branch thoracoacromial trunk, (2) acromial branch thoracoacromial trunk, (3) deltoid branch thoracoacromial trunk, (4) internal mammary perforators, (5) pectoral branch thoracoacromial trunk, (6) superior epigastric, (7) intercostal perforators, (8) deep inferior epigastric, (8¹) superficial inferior epigastric (overlying angiosome of DIEP) (9), (10) deep circumflex iliac, (11) superficial circumflex iliac.

provide the main and the most consistent blood supply. The superior thoracic artery, a direct branch of the axillary artery, has also been reported to supply this muscle.[16] Mathes and Nahai originally classified this muscle as class III.

The *serratus anterior* lies below and lateral to the pectoralis major on the anterolateral aspect of the thorax. It originates on ribs 1–9 and inserts on the anterior surface of the medial border of the scapula. Its action is to protract and superiorly rotate the scapula, holding it against the chest wall. Innervation is via the long thoracic nerve, which runs superficial to the muscle along its course.[17] The serratus has a dual blood supply to its upper and lower muscular slips from the lateral thoracic and thoracodorsal system, classifying it as Mathes and Nahai type III.

The *intercostal muscles* include the external, internal, and innermost intercostal muscles, which are layered muscles between each rib. They are layered such that fibers from each pass in opposite directions aiding in expansion and compression of the ribs during respiration. The neurovascular bundles supplying these muscles run on the inferior surface of the rib between the internal and innermost intercostal muscle.

Vascular anatomy

Blood supply to the skin and soft tissues of the anterior chest is derived from a highly interconnected network of named vessels and choke anastomoses. The lateral and inferior pectoralis margins are supplied by perforators from the posterior intercostal arteries and the anterior intercostal arteries of ribs

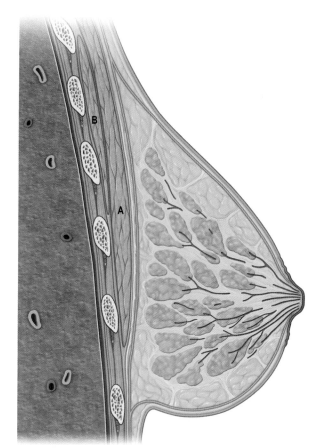

Fig. 9.6 Superficial (green) and deep (gray) fascia of the chest wall and breast. (A) Pectoralis major. (B) Pectoralis minor.

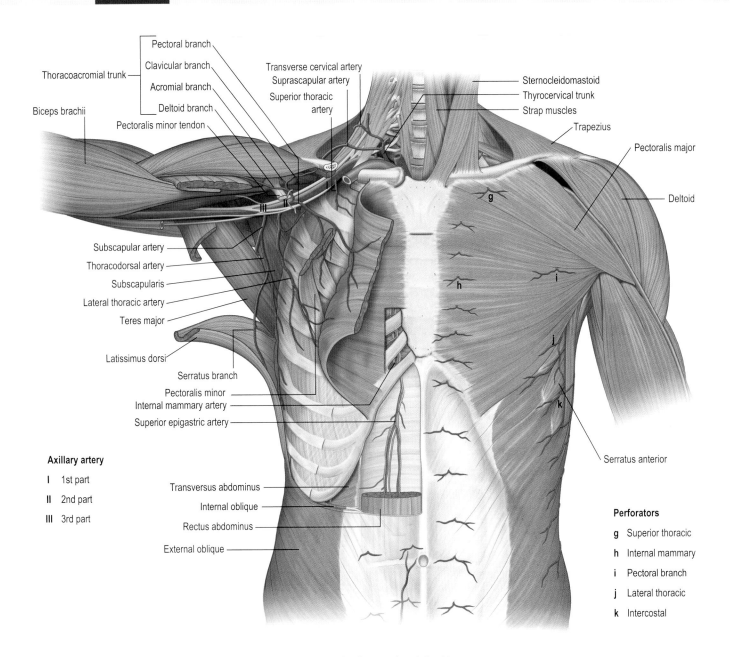

Fig. 9.7 Superficial and deep musculature of the chest and upper abdomen showing vascular relationships.

The *thoracoacromial trunk* gives rise to four branches: the clavicular, acromial, deltoid, and pectoral. The pectoral branch supplies the pectoralis major muscle and the superior portion of pectoralis minor. It originates below the pectoralis minor, passing medially and penetrating the clavipectoral fascia 6–10 cm lateral to the sternoclavicular joint. As it travels along the undersurface of the pectoralis major, small perforating branches pass through the muscle and supply the overlying skin of the superior and lateral chest. The pectoral artery is paralleled by two venae comitantes, which coalesce near the clavicle and enter the axillary or subclavian vein as a single vessel. This is usually within 1–2 cm of where the thoracoacromial trunk arises from the second portion of the axillary artery.[19]

The *lateral thoracic* artery supplies the upper four to five slips of the serratus anterior muscle. Smaller penetrating

vessels enter the underlying rib and periosteum allowing the muscle to be harvested with bone for composite flaps. Variations in blood supply to this muscle have been reported in that the lateral thoracic artery occasionally supplies the lower portion of the muscle.[20] Perforators from the lateral thoracic artery supply the skin and subcutaneous tissue of the superolateral thorax and lateral breast parenchyma.

The *subscapular* artery leaves the third portion of the axillary artery and within 1–4 cm gives rise to circumflex scapular and the thoracodorsal arteries. The prior passes through the triangular space of the back. The thoracodorsal proceeds caudally, providing a branch to the serratus anterior, then passes to the undersurface of the latissimus dorsi muscle. The serratus branch runs superficial to the muscle along with the long thoracic nerve and provides segmental branches to the lower five slips of that muscle.

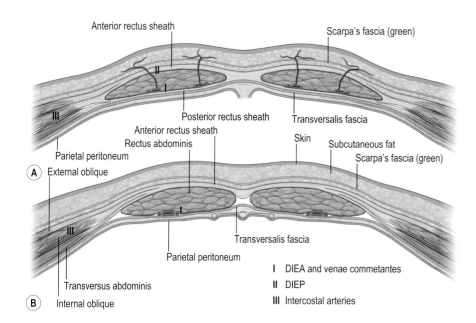

Anterior rectus sheath

Scarpa's fascia (green)

Posterior rectus sheath

Transversalis fascia

Anterior rectus sheath

Skin   Subcutaneous fat

Rectus abdominis

Scarpa's fascia (green)

Parietal peritoneum

(A) External oblique

Transversalis fascia

Parietal peritoneum

I DIEA and venae commetantes

Transversus abdominis

II DIEP

(B) Internal oblique

III Intercostal arteries

Fig. 9.8 (A) The rectus sheath above the arcuate line showing the layers of muscular aponeurosis. **(B)** The rectus sheath below the arcuate line, showing transversalis fascia as the only posterior layer between the rectus and the peritoneum.

The *anterior* and *posterior circumflex humeral* arteries are the last branches to arise from the axillary artery. The posterior circumflex artery passes through the quadrangular space along with the axillary nerve. It supplies the deltoid muscle and the posterior shoulder joint. It has anastomotic connections to the anterior circumflex artery on the lateral side of the humerus.

Abdomen

The abdomen is bound superiorly by the osteocartilaginous framework of the thorax, laterally by the anterior axillary line and the iliac crest, and inferiorly at the level of the inguinal ligament and its insertion to the pubic tubercle. The umbilicus is located in the midline, approximately at the level of the iliac crest. Three tendinous inscriptions traverse the rectus muscle. Zones of adherence where the deep fascia is connected to the deep dermis by vertical fibrous septae gives rise to what is commonly known as the "six pack" abdomen (see Fig. 9.5).

Superficial fascial attachments to the deep fascia create contour differences between the sexes. Men tend to have a zone of adherence along the iliac crest giving rise to a square hip shape. Women tend to have a more curvilinear hip outline due to a zone of adherence several centimeters below the iliac crest.[4] The female abdomen is defined by an hourglass shape. Areas of fat accumulation tend to be inferior to the umbilicus and in the hips. The male abdomen is V-shaped with indentations at the muscular transcriptions and areas of fat accumulation tending to be circumferential in the midabdomen and flank.

Tissue layers of the abdominal wall from superficial to deep are the skin and subcutaneous fatty fascia known as Camper's fascia, deeper superficial fascial layer called Scarpa's fascia, adipose tissue, deep fascia, muscle, and peritoneum surrounding the abdominal contents.[5] The term "Scarpa's fascia" was derived from the first description of this fascial layer in the early 19th century.[21] In modern-day vernacular, Scarpa's fascia has become synonymous with the superficial fascia of the body; however, classically it is only present as the distinct membranous layer in the area of the lower abdomen. Scarpa's fascia is made up of fibrous and adipose tissue with solitary, evenly interspersed elastic fibers. It is contiguous with the linea alba at the midline. Superiorly, it merges with the superficial fascia of the chest and laterally the external oblique fascia. The inferior lateral border includes the *fascia lata* at the thigh and medially the pubis. In males, Scarpa's fascia is contiguous with the *fundiform ligament*, a thickening of the fascia at the pubic bone that surrounds the base of the penis.[22]

The deep fascia of the abdomen consists of the aponeurotic fascia of the paired flat muscles. The convergence of this fascia lateral to the rectus muscle bilaterally is referred to as the *linea semilunaris*. Medial to these lines, the rectus muscle is encased by the *rectus sheath* (Fig. 9.8A). The anterior rectus sheath is composed of the aponeurosis of the external oblique muscle and the anterior aponeurosis of the internal oblique muscle. The posterior rectus sheath is made up of the posterior aponeurosis of the internal oblique and the aponeurosis of the transversus abdominis muscle. In the midline, the anterior rectus sheath fuses with the posterior rectus sheath to form the *linea alba*, which spans from the xiphoid process to the pubic symphysis. Superior to the costal margin, the posterior wall of the rectus sheath is deficient because the transversus abdominis muscle passes internal to the costal cartilages and the internal oblique muscle is attached to the costal margin. Midway between the umbilicus and the pubis is the *arcuate line*. This is the caudalmost edge of the posterior rectus sheath. Caudal to this line, the aponeurosis of the transverses abdominus and the posterior aponeurosis of the internal oblique pass anteriorly to join the anterior rectus fascia, and there is no longer a defined posterior rectus sheath (Fig. 9.8B). Only the very thin transversalis fascia overlying the parietal peritoneum separates the rectus muscle from the peritoneal cavity. Here, between the undersurface of the rectus muscle and transversalis fascia is a layer of adipose tissue that encases the deep inferior epigastric artery and its venae comitantes.

Muscles[6]

The *rectus abdominis* originates at the pubic symphysis and pubic crest. It inserts into the xiphoid process and costal cartilage of ribs 5–7 (Fig. 9.9). It is innervated by the ventral rami of spinal nerves T7–T12. Its main action is to flex the trunk and compress the abdominal viscera. Its blood supply is via the superior epigastric artery and deep inferior epigastric artery, which classifies this muscle as Mathes and Nahai type III.

The *external oblique* originates from the external surface of the lower eight ribs and inserts into the linea alba, pubic tubercle, and iliac crest. The *internal oblique* muscle originates at the thoracolumbar fascia, iliac crest, and lateral half of inguinal ligament. It inserts at the inferior border of ribs 10–12, the linea alba, and the pubis. The *transversus abdominis* muscle originates from the internal surface of costal cartilage ribs 7–12, thoracolumbar fascia, iliac crest, and lateral third inguinal ligament. It inserts at the linea alba, pubic crest, and pectin pubis. These three layered muscles derive innervation from spinal nerves T7–T12 and L1 and act to compress and support the abdominal viscera and to flex and rotate the trunk. Blood supply is segmental via the lower thoracic intercostal vessels, classifying these muscles as type IV.

Vascular anatomy

In 1979, Huger described the cutaneous blood supply to the abdomen, and this theory was supported by anatomic studies of Taylor. Huger's zone I is located medially and supplied by perforators from the deep epigastric system. Zone II includes the lower lateral abdomen, which is supplied by the external iliac system comprising of the superficial inferior epigastric artery and the superficial and deep circumflex iliac arteries. Zone III is lateral; this is supplied by the intercostals and subcostal arteries.[23] These three zones have a rich arcade of anastomosis and choke vessels.

The *deep inferior epigastric artery* (*DIEA*) is a branch of the external iliac artery (Fig. 9.10). It emerges from the medial

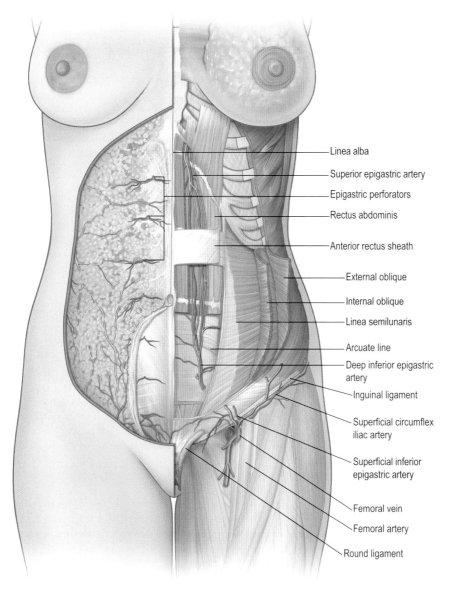

Linea alba
Superior epigastric artery
Epigastric perforators
Rectus abdominis
Anterior rectus sheath
External oblique
Internal oblique
Linea semilunaris
Arcuate line
Deep inferior epigastric artery
Inguinal ligament
Superficial circumflex iliac artery
Superficial inferior epigastric artery
Femoral vein
Femoral artery
Round ligament

Fig. 9.9 Superficial and deep anatomy of the abdomen showing muscular layers and fascial layers with vascular relationships.

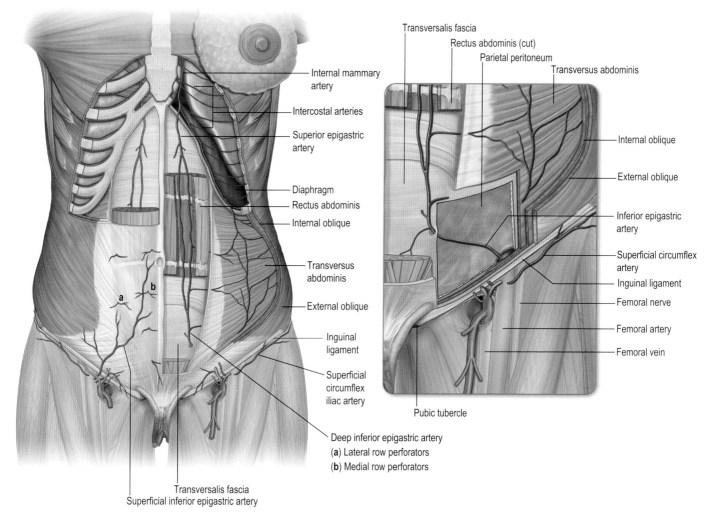

Internal mammary artery

Intercostal arteries

Superior epigastric artery

Diaphragm

Rectus abdominis

Internal oblique

Transversus abdominis

External oblique

Inguinal ligament

Superficial circumflex iliac artery

Deep inferior epigastric artery

(a) Lateral row perforators

(b) Medial row perforators

Transversalis fascia

Superficial inferior epigastric artery

Transversalis fascia

Rectus abdominis (cut)

Parietal peritoneum

Transversus abdominis

Internal oblique

External oblique

Inferior epigastric artery

Superficial circumflex artery

Inguinal ligament

Femoral nerve

Femoral artery

Femoral vein

Pubic tubercle

Fig. 9.10 Superficial and deep muscular layers showing vascular anatomy from iliac and femoral branches. (a) Lateral row perforators from DIEA, (b) medial row perforators from DIEA.

wall of the external iliac artery and pierces the transversalis fascia to course along the posterior surface of the rectus muscle. As the DIEA approaches the arcuate line it divides into a medial and lateral branch and occasionally a third branch providing direct blood supply to the umbilicus. The medial and lateral branches of the DIEA give off perforating vessels to the fasciocutaneous tissue overlying the midabdomen. The dominance of one or the other branch is variable. There are between four and seven perforators in a given individual, usually clustered in the periumbilical region.[24] At the level of the umbilicus there are anastomotic connections to the *superior epigastric artery*, which is a continuation of the internal mammary artery in the chest.

The *deep circumflex iliac artery* (DCIA) originates from the external iliac artery near the origin of the DIEA. The DCIA travels along the iliacus muscle giving off a large ascending branch 1 cm medial to the ASIS. The artery then pierces the transversalis fascia and travels along the internal lip of the iliac crest just lateral to a line of attachment of iliacus to transversalis fascia. Along the medial surface of the iliac crest there are several periosteal branches. Approaching the flank, the transverse branch of the DCIA forms anastomotic connections with the lumbar and iliolumbar arteries. Superficial perforating branches of the DCIA supply an oval-shaped

area of skin along the iliac crest (see Fig. 9.10). Two venae comitantes parallel the DCIA along its course and drain into the external iliac vein as a single vessel.[25,26]

The *superficial inferior epigastric artery* (SIEA) is a branch of the proximal femoral artery arising 2–3 cm below the inguinal ligament. The branching pattern is variable and reported as either an independent branch, from a common trunk with the superficial circumflex iliac artery, or from another branch of the femoral artery such as the external pudendal. The SIEA was originally reported to be present in only 60% of individuals,[27] but current anatomic studies support anecdotal evidence suggesting this artery is more ubiquitous.[28] The vessel travels from its origin superolaterally and pierces Scarpa's fascia 0.5 to 4 cm above the inguinal ligament midway between the ASIS and the pubic tubercle. It travels just superficial to the fascia as it branches medially and laterally to supply the lower hemi-abdominal skin.[29] This vessel and its anastomotic connections do not reliably cross midline. Venous return of the subcutaneous tissue supplied by the SIEA is via two vessels. One vein accompanies the SIEA in its course, and a larger medial vein is almost always present in a more superficial plane. The medial vein often drains into the saphenous bulb but may at times be found to join the smaller vein and drain directly into the femoral vein.[22]

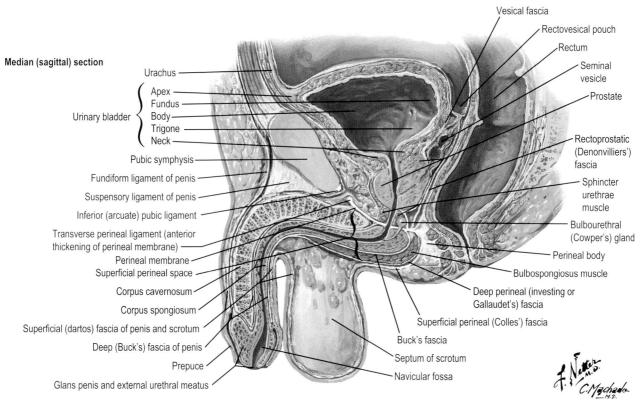

Median (sagittal) section

Urachus

Apex
Fundus
Body — Urinary bladder
Trigone
Neck

Pubic symphysis

Fundiform ligament of penis

Suspensory ligament of penis

Inferior (arcuate) pubic ligament

Transverse perineal ligament (anterior thickening of perineal membrane)

Perineal membrane

Superficial perineal space

Corpus cavernosum

Corpus spongiosum

Superficial (dartos) fascia of penis and scrotum

Deep (Buck's) fascia of penis

Prepuce

Glans penis and external urethral meatus

Vesical fascia
Rectovesical pouch
Rectum
Seminal vesicle
Prostate
Rectoprostatic (Denonvilliers') fascia
Sphincter urethrae muscle
Bulbourethral (Cowper's) gland
Perineal body
Bulbospongiosus muscle
Deep perineal (investing or Gallaudet's) fascia
Superficial perineal (Colles') fascia
Buck's fascia
Septum of scrotum
Navicular fossa

Fig. 9.11 Cross-section anatomy of male pelvis. *(From: Netter; www.netterimages.com. © Elsevier Inc. All rights reserved.)*

The *superficial circumflex iliac* artery is a branch of the femoral artery and usually emerges near the origin of the SIEA or shares a common trunk. This vessel passes over the inguinal ligament superiorly into the abdominal wall running in the superficial fascia along the iliac crest. It supplies the skin and subcutaneous tissue for 10–20 cm in an area of the infero-antero-lateral abdominal wall. It is paralleled by a vein that drains into the greater saphenous vein.

The *intercostal* arteries travel into the abdomen between the internal oblique and the transverses abdominis muscle.

Nerves

Sensory and motor innervation to the anterior abdominal wall is via paired spinal nerves running between the internal oblique and the transversus abdominis muscles and give rise to parallel dermatomes of the abdomen. The ventral rami of T5–T11 and subcostal (T12) provide innervation of the anterior abdominal wall from the periphery of the diaphragm to the superior iliac spine. The *ilioinguinal nerve* passes between the internal oblique and transversus abdominis supplying the hypogastric region and iliac crest. The iliohypogastric nerve innervates skin of the scrotum, labia majora, mons pubis, and medial thigh.

Pelvis

The pelvis consists of a bowl-shaped arrangement of bones connecting the trunk to the legs. It contains the intestines, urinary bladder, and internal sex organs. Paired ilia, ischia, and pubic bones connect anteriorly at the pubic symphysis and posteriorly at the sacrum. The muscles of the pelvic floor

provide the inferiormost border of the peritoneal cavity. Below these are the perineal structures of the male and female anatomy (Figs. 9.11, 9.12).

Female perineum

The external genitalia are derived from ectoderm. The sex-specific genital characteristics start to develop in the 7th week of gestation, appear at the 9th week, and become fully differentiated by the 12th week. Estrogen produced by either the placenta or the fetal ovaries is responsible for female genital differentiation. The genital tubercle arises from mesenchyme at the superior end of the cloacal membrane and becomes the clitoris. The urogenital folds and labial scrotal folds border the cloacal membrane. These become the labia minora, fusing posteriorly to form the frenulum, and labia majora, respectively.[3] The mons pubis and labia majora are covered by stratified squamous epithelium with a thick keratinized layer containing multiple hair follicles. Below the skin of the labia majora is superficial fatty fascial tissue continuous with the Camper's fascia of the abdomen. The deep superficial fascia of the perineum is referred to as Colles fascia and is the perineal extension of Scarpa's fascia. The labia minora, clitoris, urethral, and vaginal opening are covered by stratified squamous epithelium with a thin keratinized layer. There is no adipose tissue below the labia minora, only elastic and fibrous connective tissue and multiple eccrine, apocrine, and sebaceous glands, which serve to lubricate the surface of this delicate tissue (Fig. 9.13).

The perineum is divided into two adjacent triangles (Fig. 9.14). The anterior urogenital triangle is bound by the pubic symphysis, the conjoint ramus of the ischium and pubis, and

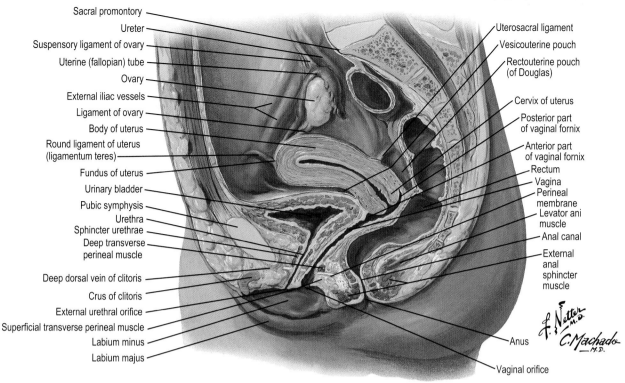

Sacral promontory
Ureter
Suspensory ligament of ovary
Uterine (fallopian) tube
Ovary
External iliac vessels
Ligament of ovary
Body of uterus
Round ligament of uterus (ligamentum teres)
Fundus of uterus
Urinary bladder
Pubic symphysis
Urethra
Sphincter urethrae
Deep transverse perineal muscle
Deep dorsal vein of clitoris
Crus of clitoris
External urethral orifice
Superficial transverse perineal muscle
Labium minus
Labium majus

Uterosacral ligament
Vesicouterine pouch
Rectouterine pouch (of Douglas)
Cervix of uterus
Posterior part of vaginal fornix
Anterior part of vaginal fornix
Rectum
Vagina
Perineal membrane
Levator ani muscle
Anal canal
External anal sphincter muscle
Anus
Vaginal orifice

Fig. 9.12 Cross-section anatomy of female pelvis. *(From: Netter; www.netterimages.com.* © *Elsevier Inc. All rights reserved.)*

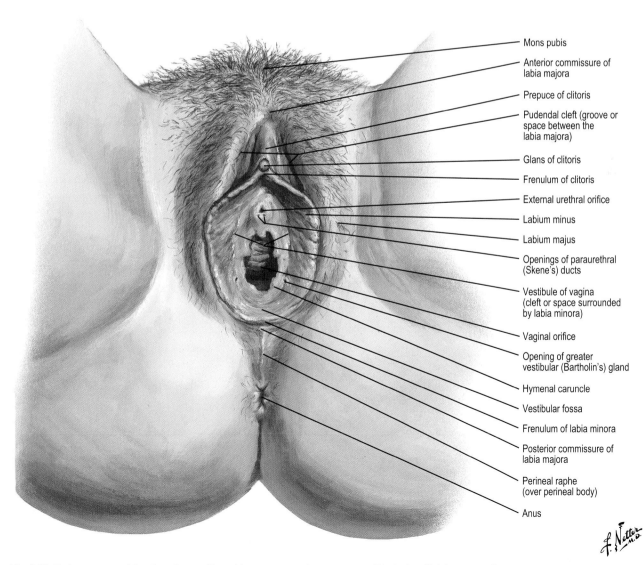

Mons pubis
Anterior commissure of labia majora
Prepuce of clitoris
Pudendal cleft (groove or space between the labia majora)
Glans of clitoris
Frenulum of clitoris
External urethral orifice
Labium minus
Labium majus
Openings of paraurethral (Skene's) ducts
Vestibule of vagina (cleft or space surrounded by labia minora)
Vaginal orifice
Opening of greater vestibular (Bartholin's) gland
Hymenal caruncle
Vestibular fossa
Frenulum of labia minora
Posterior commissure of labia majora
Perineal raphe (over perineal body)
Anus

Fig. 9.13 Surface anatomy of female perineum. *(From: Netter; www.netterimages.com.* © *Elsevier Inc. All rights reserved.)*

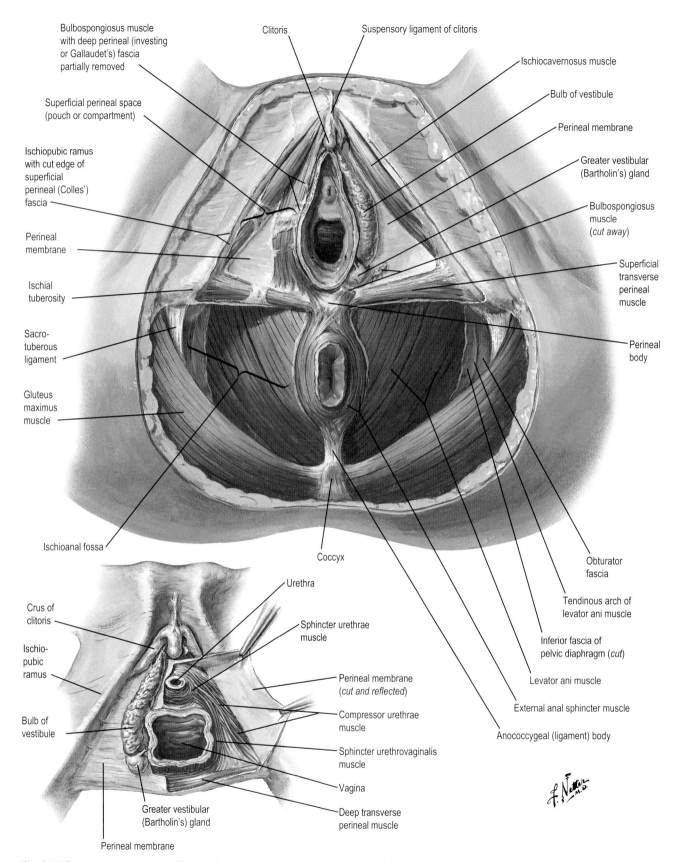

Bulbospongiosus muscle with deep perineal (investing or Gallaudet's) fascia partially removed

Superficial perineal space (pouch or compartment)

Ischiopubic ramus with cut edge of superficial perineal (Colles') fascia

Perineal membrane

Ischial tuberosity

Sacro-tuberous ligament

Gluteus maximus muscle

Ischioanal fossa

Clitoris

Suspensory ligament of clitoris

Ischiocavernosus muscle

Bulb of vestibule

Perineal membrane

Greater vestibular (Bartholin's) gland

Bulbospongiosus muscle (*cut away*)

Superficial transverse perineal muscle

Perineal body

Obturator fascia

Tendinous arch of levator ani muscle

Inferior fascia of pelvic diaphragm (*cut*)

Levator ani muscle

External anal sphincter muscle

Anococcygeal (ligament) body

Coccyx

Crus of clitoris

Ischio-pubic ramus

Bulb of vestibule

Urethra

Sphincter urethrae muscle

Perineal membrane (*cut and reflected*)

Compressor urethrae muscle

Sphincter urethrovaginalis muscle

Vagina

Deep transverse perineal muscle

Greater vestibular (Bartholin's) gland

Perineal membrane

Fig. 9.14 Female urogenital triangle. *(From: Netter; www.netterimages.com. © Elsevier Inc. All rights reserved.)*

the deep transverse perineal muscle spanning the ischial tuberosities. The posterior anal triangle lies behind a line drawn between the ischial tuberosities and contains the anus. The urogenital triangle is divided into a deep and superficial space. Colles fascia forms the roof of the superficial perineal space. Laterally, this fascia is firmly attached to the fascia lata of the thigh at the ischiopubic ramus and defines the perineal thigh crease. Posteriorly, the fascia surrounds the superficial transverse perineal muscle and anchors to the inferior fascia of the urogenital diaphragm.[5]

The superficial perineal space contains the ischiocavernosus muscle that overlies the crus of the clitoris, the bulbospongiosus muscle that overlies the bulb of the vestibule, the superficial transverse perineal muscles, and the greater vestibular glands. The superficial perineal artery and vein travel within this space. The inferior fascia of the urogenital diaphragm, referred to in some texts as the deep perineal or Gallaudet fascia, forms the deep margin of this space. The urethral and vaginal openings pass through here. Posteriorly, the Gallaudet fascia encases the bilateral perineal muscles and fuses in the midline to form the perineal body.

Deep to the Gallaudet fascia is the deep perineal space. This contains the proximal urethra, the external urethral sphincter muscle, and the deep transverse perineal muscles. The terminal branches of the internal pudendal artery travel within this space as they make their way to the clitoris. As they exit the space anteriorly, between the transverse perineal ligament and the arcuate pubic ligament, they become the dorsal artery and the deep dorsal vein of the clitoris. The end branch of the pudendal nerve, the dorsal nerve of the clitoris, travels with these vessels.

Vascular anatomy

The two main vascular pedicles supplying the female perineum are the deep external pudendal artery supplying the anterior labial structures and the internal pudendal artery supplying the clitoris and posterior labial structures (Fig. 9.15). The *deep external pudendal artery* is a branch of the femoral artery. It passes into the subcutaneous plane approximately 8–10 cm from the pubic symphysis and travels along the adductor longus. At 4–6 cm from the pubic symphysis the artery splits into an abdominal branch and a perineal branch. The latter is called the anterior labial artery and supplies the superior third of the labia majora. The second major pedicle arises from the internal pudendal artery supplying the posterior structures and the clitoris. The *superficial perineal artery* is a branch of the internal pudendal artery as it arises from Alcock's canal along the ischium. The superficial perineal artery has two branches, the internal posterior labial artery and the external posterior labial artery. Both supply the posterior two-thirds of the labia minora and majora.[30] The internal pudendal artery continues anteriorly within the deep perineal space to become the *dorsal artery of the clitoris.*

The venous drainage of the perineum patterns the arterial supply. Anteriorly, these vessels drain into the saphenous vein and then the femoral vein. Posteriorly, the superficial perineal veins drain into the internal pudendal vein, which drains to the internal iliac vein.

Innervation to the vulvar structures is via the ilioinguinal nerve, genitofemoral nerve, and the perineal branch of the femoral cutaneous nerve of the thigh. The superficial perineal nerve, a branch of the pudendal nerve, supplies the posterior two-thirds of the labia, and the terminal branch of the pudendal nerve becomes the dorsal nerve to the clitoris.

Male perineum

At the 6–7th week of gestation, testosterone produced by the fetal testes induces the genital tubercle to elongate to form the phallus. An ingrowth of ectoderm along the ventral surface of the penis forms the urethral groove as surface ectoderm fuses in the midline enclosing the spongy urethra within the penile shaft. The corpora cavernosa and corpus spongiosum are developed from mesenchyme within the phallus. The labioscrotal swellings enlarge and fuse to form the scrotum. Circular ectodermal invagination at the glans forms the foreskin. The foreskin is adherent to the glans penis until birth or early infancy.[3]

Descent of the testes into the scrotum begins around the 26th week. Shortly after their descent, the inguinal canal contracts around the spermatic cord. Development of the inguinal canal involves dissention of the gubernaculum, which originates at the inferior pole of the gonad. It passes through the abdominal wall and attaches to the labioscrotal swellings. The processus vaginalis develops ventral to the gubernaculum and travels along the same path carrying extensions of the layers of abdominal wall. These will become the walls of the inguinal canal. The place where the processus passes through the transversalis fascia becomes the deep inguinal ring.

Superficial structures of the male perineum include the penis and scrotum (Fig. 9.16). The penis consists of the root, body, and glans. The paired corpora cavernosa and ventral corpus spongiosum are specialized erectile tissue surrounded by a fibrous outer layer, the tunica albuginea. At the base of the penis the corpora cavernosa split to become the crura of the penis and the corpus spongiosum thickens to become the bulb of the penis. The crura and the bulb, which are surrounded by the ischiocavernosus and bulbospongiosus muscles, respectively, form the root of the penis and lie in the superficial perineal space (Fig. 9.17). Also contained in this space is the proximal spongy urethra, superficial transverse perineal muscles, superficial perineal vessels, and branches of the pudendal nerve. The deep perineal space contains the transverse perineal muscles, the external urethral sphincter, the bulbourethral glands, and the terminal branches of the internal pudendal vessels as they travel to become the deep artery of the penis, the dorsal artery, and the deep dorsal vein of the penis.[5]

In men, Colles' fascia is continuous with the spermatic cord and dartos fascia encasing the penis and scrotum. The suspensory apparatus of the penis consists of the fundiform ligament, the suspensory ligament proper, and the arcuate subpubic ligament. The fundiform ligament is superficial and is an extension of Scarpa's fascia running from the level of the pubic bone around the base of the penis and attaching to the septum of the scrotum. The suspensory ligament proper is deep to the fundiform ligament and bridges between the symphysis pubis and the tunica albuginea of the corpus cavernosum. The arcuate subpubic ligament runs a similar course to the suspensory ligament proper. The suspensory ligaments maintain the base of the penis in front of the pubis and act as a major point of support for the erect penis during intercourse.[31]

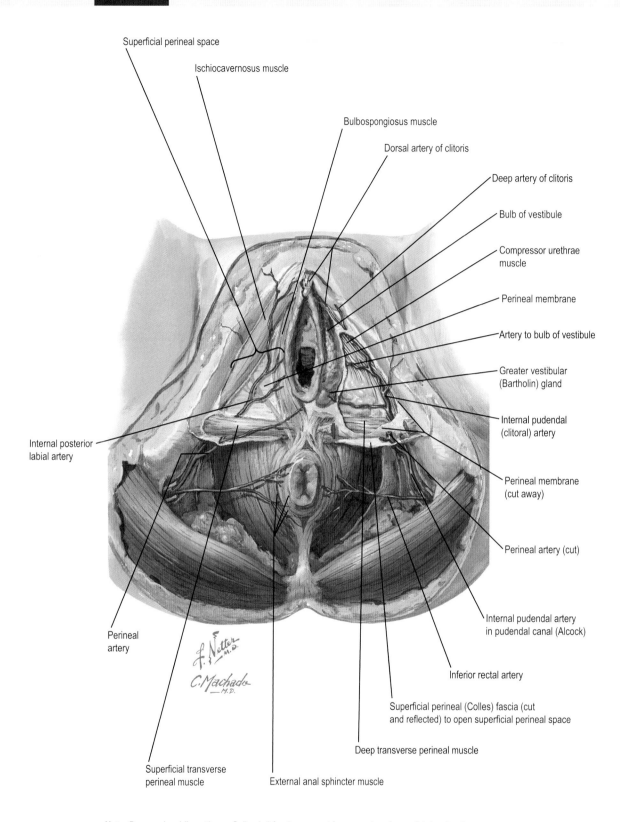

Superficial perineal space

Ischiocavernosus muscle

Bulbospongiosus muscle

Dorsal artery of clitoris

Deep artery of clitoris

Bulb of vestibule

Compressor urethrae muscle

Perineal membrane

Artery to bulb of vestibule

Greater vestibular (Bartholin) gland

Internal pudendal (clitoral) artery

Perineal membrane (cut away)

Perineal artery (cut)

Internal pudendal artery in pudendal canal (Alcock)

Inferior rectal artery

Superficial perineal (Colles) fascia (cut and reflected) to open superficial perineal space

Deep transverse perineal muscle

External anal sphincter muscle

Superficial transverse perineal muscle

Perineal artery

Internal posterior labial artery

Note: Deep perineal (investing or Gallaudet) fascia removed from muscles of superficial perineal space.

Fig. 9.15 Vascular anatomy of the female perineum. *(From: Netter; www.netterimages.com. © Elsevier Inc. All rights reserved.)*

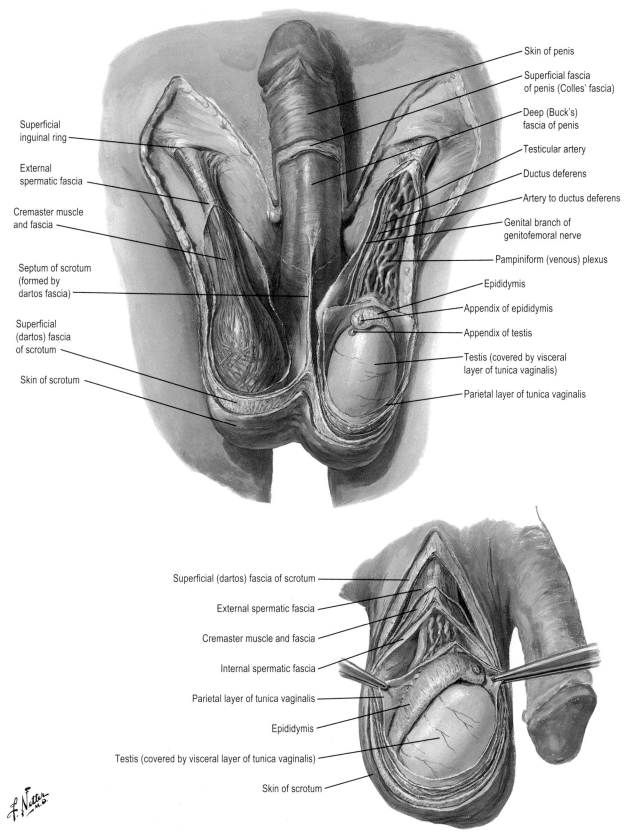

Skin of penis

Superficial fascia
of penis (Colles' fascia)

Deep (Buck's)
fascia of penis

Testicular artery

Ductus deferens

Artery to ductus deferens

Genital branch of
genitofemoral nerve

Pampiniform (venous) plexus

Epididymis

Appendix of epididymis

Appendix of testis

Testis (covered by visceral
layer of tunica vaginalis)

Parietal layer of tunica vaginalis

Superficial
inguinal ring

External
spermatic fascia

Cremaster muscle
and fascia

Septum of scrotum
(formed by
dartos fascia)

Superficial
(dartos) fascia
of scrotum

Skin of scrotum

Superficial (dartos) fascia of scrotum

External spermatic fascia

Cremaster muscle and fascia

Internal spermatic fascia

Parietal layer of tunica vaginalis

Epididymis

Testis (covered by visceral layer of tunica vaginalis)

Skin of scrotum

Fig. 9.16 Superficial structures of male perineum and their fascial layers. *(From: Netter; www.netterimages.com.*

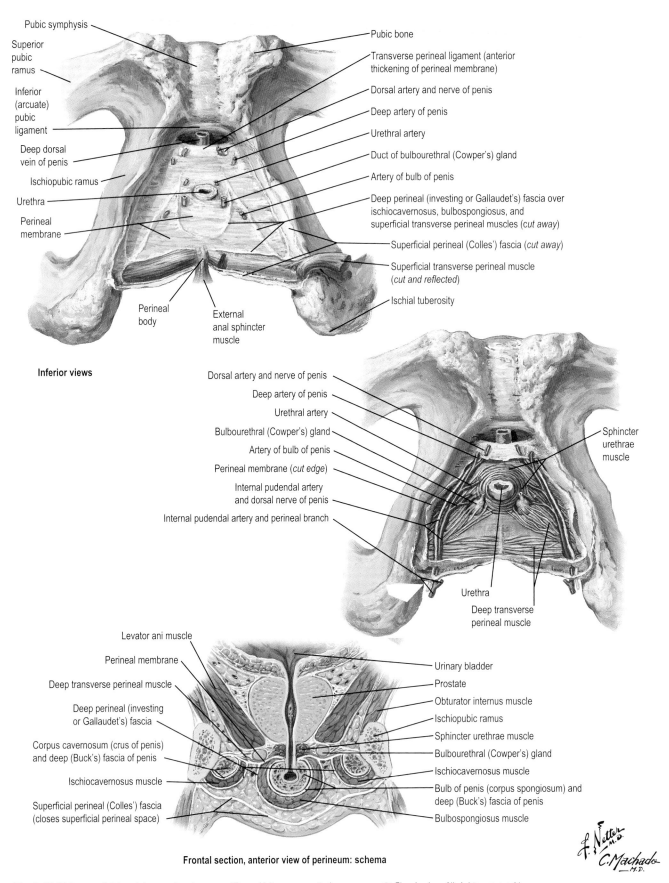

Pubic symphysis

Superior pubic ramus

Inferior (arcuate) pubic ligament

Deep dorsal vein of penis

Ischiopubic ramus

Urethra

Perineal membrane

Perineal body

External anal sphincter muscle

Pubic bone

Transverse perineal ligament (anterior thickening of perineal membrane)

Dorsal artery and nerve of penis

Deep artery of penis

Urethral artery

Duct of bulbourethral (Cowper's) gland

Artery of bulb of penis

Deep perineal (investing or Gallaudet's) fascia over ischiocavernosus, bulbospongiosus, and superficial transverse perineal muscles (cut away)

Superficial perineal (Colles') fascia (cut away)

Superficial transverse perineal muscle (cut and reflected)

Ischial tuberosity

Inferior views

Dorsal artery and nerve of penis

Deep artery of penis

Urethral artery

Bulbourethral (Cowper's) gland

Artery of bulb of penis

Perineal membrane (cut edge)

Internal pudendal artery and dorsal nerve of penis

Internal pudendal artery and perineal branch

Sphincter urethrae muscle

Urethra

Deep transverse perineal muscle

Levator ani muscle

Perineal membrane

Deep transverse perineal muscle

Deep perineal (investing or Gallaudet's) fascia

Corpus cavernosum (crus of penis) and deep (Buck's) fascia of penis

Ischiocavernosus muscle

Superficial perineal (Colles') fascia (closes superficial perineal space)

Urinary bladder

Prostate

Obturator internus muscle

Ischiopubic ramus

Sphincter urethrae muscle

Bulbourethral (Cowper's) gland

Ischiocavernosus muscle

Bulb of penis (corpus spongiosum) and deep (Buck's) fascia of penis

Bulbospongiosus muscle

Frontal section, anterior view of perineum: schema

Fig. 9.17 Male superficial and deep perineal spaces. (From: Netter; www.netterimages.com. © Elsevier Inc. All rights reserved.)

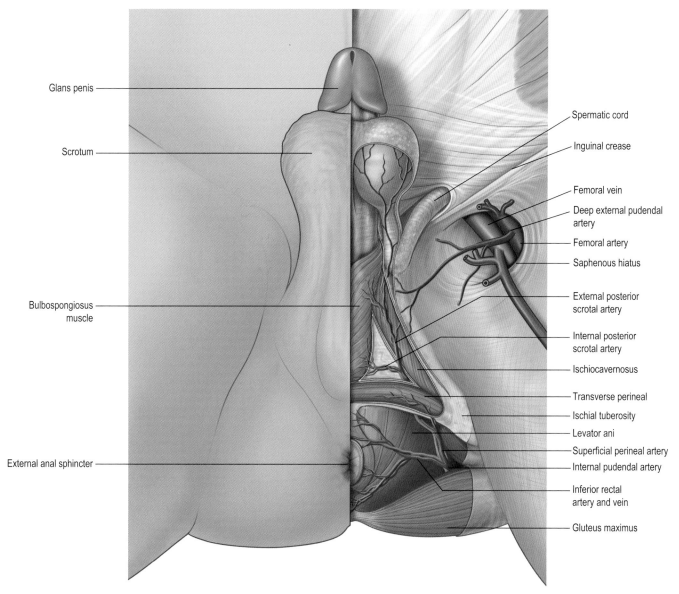

Glans penis

Scrotum

Bulbospongiosus
muscle

External anal sphincter

Spermatic cord

Inguinal crease

Femoral vein

Deep external pudendal
artery

Femoral artery

Saphenous hiatus

External posterior
scrotal artery

Internal posterior
scrotal artery

Ischiocavernosus

Transverse perineal

Ischial tuberosity

Levator ani

Superficial perineal artery

Internal pudendal artery

Inferior rectal
artery and vein

Gluteus maximus

Fig. 9.18 Vascular anatomy of the male perineum.

The scrotum supports and encases the testicles (see Fig. 9.17). The *dartos* fascia, which lies just under the skin, is a thin musculofascial layer that regulates the temperature of the testicles by contracting and relaxing, bringing the scrotum closer or further from the ambient heat of the body. The *cremaster* muscle originates at the inferior internal oblique muscle, inguinal ligament, pubic tubercle, and pubic crest. It inserts into the investing fascia of the spermatic cord and testes. Its function is to retract the testicles. It is innervated by the genital branch of the genitofemoral nerve.[5]

Vascular anatomy

There are three main arterial pedicles to the male perineum (Fig. 9.18). The *deep external pudendal artery* is a branch of the femoral artery and supplies the anterior perineum. It courses from the saphenous hiatus and provides supply to anterior structures. It divides into two branches at the level of the spermatic cord to become the *internal anterior scrotal artery* supplying the base and dorsum of the penis, ventral scrotum, perineal fat, and anteromedial spermatic–scrotal fascia. The *external anterior scrotal artery* supplies the lateral scrotum. The *superficial perineal artery* is a terminal branch of the internal pudendal artery. Its course takes it superficial to the superficial transverse perineal muscle and lateral to the bulbocavernosus muscle. It has three branches. The *internal posterior scrotal artery* supplies the dorsal scrotum and raphe. The *external posterior scrotal artery* supplies the posterior-lateral spermatic cord fascia. The *transperineal arteries* provide anastomotic connection to the anterior vessels. The third arterial supply is the *funicular artery*, a branch of the deep inferior epigastric artery that crosses just below the inguinal ligament and supplies the anterior perineum, giving off terminal branches to the cord.[32] The deep structures of the penis are supplied by the *dorsal artery* and the *deep artery* of the penis, which are terminal branches of the pudendal artery.

Venous drainage parallels the arterial supply. Venous supply of the penile shaft is variable and can drain via the deep external pudendal system or toward the infraumbilical system of the superficial inferior epigastric or superficial external pudendal veins.[31]

 Bonus images for this chapter can be found online at **http://www.expertconsult.com**

Fig. 9.1 Mathes and Nahai Classification of the vascular anatomy of muscle. Type I, single vascular pedicle; type II, dominant pedicle(s) plus minor pedicles; type III, two dominant pedicles; type IV, segmental pedicles; type V, dominant pedicle plus secondary segmental pedicles. (From: Mathes SJ, Nahai F. Classification of the vascular anatomy of muscles: experimental and clinical correlation. Plast Reconstr Surg. 1981; 67(2):177–187.)

 Access the complete reference list online at   **http://www.expertconsult.com**

1. Mathes SJ, Nahai F. Classification of the vascular anatomy of muscles: experimental and clinical correlation. *Plast Reconstr Surg.* 1981;67:177–187. *Original article defining variation in muscle perfusion as it relates to reconstructive surgery.*

2. Taylor GI, Palmer JH. The vascular territories (angiosomes) of the body: experimental study and clinical applications. *Br J Plast Surg.* 1987;40:113–141. *Sentinel article laying groundwork for angiosome theory.*

3. Moore KL, Persaud TVN. *Before We Are Born: Essentials of Embryology and Birth Defects.* 5th ed. Philadelphia: WB Saunders; 1998. *Used as cardinal reference for embryologic origins of trunk and perineum.*

4. Lockwood TE. Superficial fascial system (SFS) of the trunk and extremities: a new concept. *Plast Reconstr Surg.* 1991;87: 1009–1018.

5. Moore KL, Agur AM. *Essential Clinical Anatomy.* 2nd ed. Baltimore: Lippincott Williams & Wilkins; 2002. *Textbook of anatomy for general structure and surface anatomy.*

6. Olson TR, Pawlina W. *ADAM Student Atlas of Anatomy.* Baltimore: Williams & Wilkins; 1996. *Atlas of anatomy for general structure and muscular anatomy.*

10

Reconstruction of the chest

David H. Song and Michelle C. Roughton

Access video content for this chapter online at expertconsult.com

SYNOPSIS

- Chest wall reconstruction frequently requires both bony and soft-tissue support.
- Skeletal support is accomplished with mesh, acellular dermal matrix, or autogenous material.
- Soft-tissue coverage can be achieved with local muscle flaps, omentum, or local tissue rearrangement.
- Proper treatment of mediastinitis includes debridement, rigid sternal fixation when possible, and soft-tissue coverage.
- Intrathoracic reconstruction is indicated for difficult empyemas and bronchopleural fistulas. Commonly latissimus is used for space filling and reinforcement of ischemia-prone areas.

 Access the Historical Perspective section online at
http://www.expertconsult.com

Introduction

Chest wall reconstruction can be generalized to include skeletal support and soft-tissue cover. Skeletal support to prevent open pneumothorax and prevent or reduce paradoxic chest wall motion is usually required when the defect exceeds 5 cm in diameter. Generally, this corresponds to those defects exceeding a two rib resection. This rule of thumb, however, is somewhat region dependent (Table 10.1). Posterior chest wall defects may tolerate up to twice the size of those in the anterior and lateral chest due to scapular coverage and support.[1,2] Furthermore, without truly rigid chest wall reconstruction, i.e., methyl methacrylate, titanium, or rib graft, some paradoxic chest wall motion is expected and is usually well tolerated in patients without underlying pulmonary disease.[3]

Options for skeletal support include various mesh products including polytetrafluoroethylene (PTFE, Gor-Tex), polypropylene, Mersilene (polyethylene terephthalate)/methyl methacrylate,[4] titanium, and acellular dermal matrix

(Fig. 10.1). Furthermore, use of tensor fascia lata (TFL) and thoracolumbar fascia as both graft and flap reconstruction has been described. Little data exists as to outcome comparisons between these options. However, in a retrospective review of 197 patients, PTFE and polypropylene appear to be equivalent in complications and outcomes.[1] Another smaller retrospective review of 59 patients prefers Mersilene-methyl-methacrylate sandwich (MMM) to PTFE due of decreased paradoxic chest wall motion.[5] Yet another group retrospectively evaluated 262 patients and, despite an increased risk of wound complications, prefers rigid to pliable mesh (MMM), especially for larger resections.[6] As alloplastic implants tend towards an increased infection rate when compared to autogenous material or acellular dermal matrix, the authors prefer to avoid all alloplastic mesh when possible.

Chest wall reconstruction frequently requires some form of soft-tissue coverage as many of these defects result from full-thickness resections. Reconstructive goals include wound closure with maintenance of intrathoracic integrity, restoration of aesthetic contours, as well as minimization of donor site deformity.

Recruitment of local muscles with or without overlying skin is often the first line of reconstructive treatment. These muscles include pectoralis major, latissimus dorsi, serratus anterior, rectus abdominus, and external oblique. The omentum may also be used. Commonly, the ipsilateral latissimus muscle is divided during thoracotomy incisions, and the authors encourage early communication between surgeons if there are multiple teams.

Pectoralis major

Pectoralis major, a muscle overlying the superior portion of the anterior chest wall, is the workhorse for chest wall reconstruction, especially for defects of the sternum and anterior chest. Its main function is to internally rotate and adduct the arm. Additionally, this muscle serves as the foundation for the female breast, and when absent, such as in Poland syndrome, reconstruction may be indicated for aesthetic reasons

Table 10.1 Chest wall regions	
Anterior	Between anterior axillary lines
Lateral	Between anterior and posterior axillary lines
Posterior	Between posterior axillary lines and the spine

(Fig. 10.2). It originates from the sternum and clavicle and inserts along the superomedial humerus in the bicipital groove. Its dominant pedicle is the thoracoacromial trunk, which enters the undersurface of the muscle below the clavicle at the junction of its lateral and middle third. Segmental blood supply is derived from internal mammary artery (IMA)

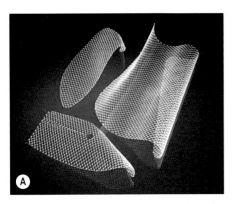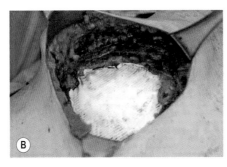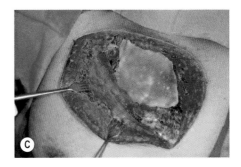

Fig. 10.1 Implantable mesh products including polypropylene, polytetrafluorethylene (PTFE, Gore-Tex), and acellular dermal matrix.

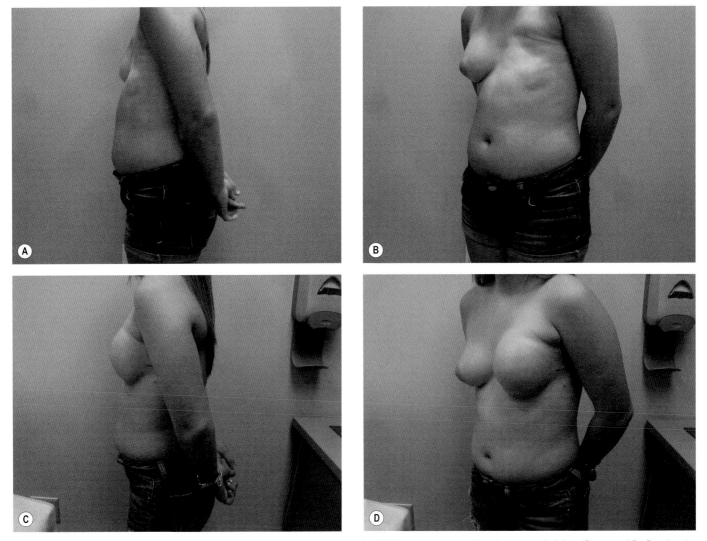

Fig. 10.2 Left sided Poland's syndrome. With tissue expander and acellular dermal matrix (ADM), placed through a lateral transverse incision. *(Courtesy of Dr. Roughton.)*

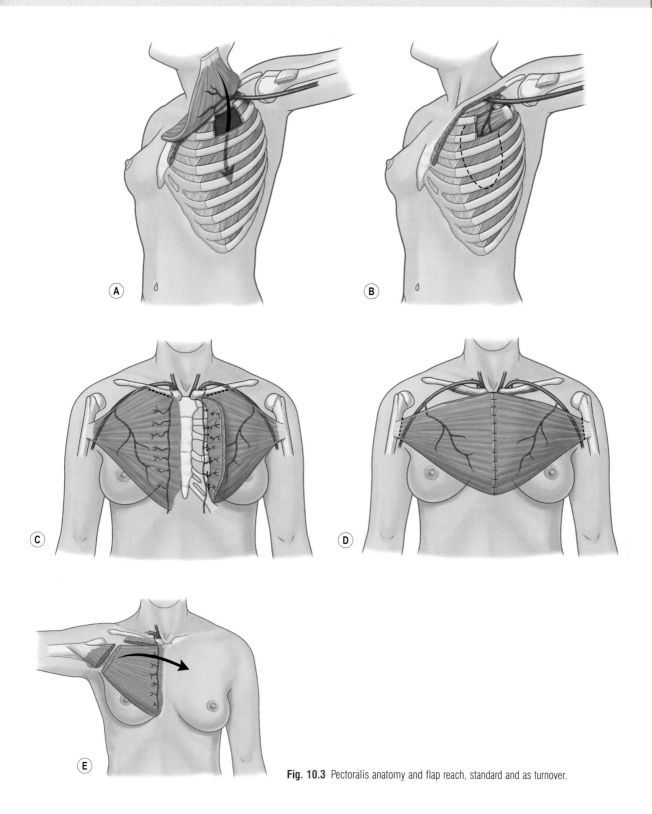

Fig. 10.3 Pectoralis anatomy and flap reach, standard and as turnover.

perforators. It will easily cover sternal and anterior chest wall defects as an island or advancement flap. It can also be turned over, based on the IMA perforators, and, with release of its insertion, cover sternal, mediastinal, and anterior chest wall defects. As a turnover flap, the anterior axillary fold may be preserved. In order to place the muscle intrathoracically, a portion of the second, third, or fourth rib will be resected (Fig. 10.3). The muscle may be harvested with or without a skin paddle. Donor site deformity including scar placement and loss of anterior axillary fold may be aesthetically displeasing.[7]

Latissimus dorsi

Latissimus dorsi, a large, flat muscle covering the mid and lower back is often recruited for chest wall reconstruction especially when significant bulk and mobility is required. It is easily placed into the chest for intrathoracic space-filling. It is known as the climbing muscle and adducts, extends, and internally rotates the arm. It originates from the thoracolumbar fascia and posterior iliac crest and inserts into the superior humerus at the intertubercular groove. Superiorly it is attached to the scapula, and care must be taken to carefully separate this muscle from the serratus at this point to avoid harvesting both muscles. Its dominant blood supply is the thoracodorsal artery, which enters the undersurface of the muscle 5 cm from the posterior axillary fold.[8] Segmental blood supply is derived from the posterior intercostal arteries as well as the lumbar artery. Based upon its thoracodorsal pedicle, the muscle can easily reach the ipsilateral posterior and lateral chest wall including those defects involving anterior chest wall, sternum, or mediastinum. It can also be turned over and based upon the lumbar perforators. In this fashion, it can reach across the midline and back again. Again, it can be moved intrathoracically with rib resection. Donor site morbidity can include shoulder dysfunction as well as unattractive scarring.[9] However, our experience suggests these concerns are minimal. Also, transposition of this muscle can blunt or obliterate the posterior axillary fold resulting in some asymmetry.[7] We advise caution in patients who have undergone previous thoracotomy and modified radical mastectomy as the muscle or blood supply may have been divided. Muscle sparing thoracotomy incisions may be helpful in preoperative planning. (See Figs. 10.4 & 10.5.)

Serratus anterior

Serratus anterior is a thin broad multi-pennate muscle lying deep along the anterolateral chest wall. It originates from the upper eight or nine ribs and inserts on the ventral-medial scapula. It functions to stabilize the scapula and move it forward on the chest wall such as when throwing a punch. It has two dominant pedicles including the lateral thoracic and the thoracodorsal arteries. Division of the lateral thoracic pedicle will increase the arc posteriorly, and similarly division of the thoracodorsal will increase the arc anteriorly. The muscle will reach the midline of the anterior or posterior chest. More commonly, however, it is used for intrathoracic coverage, again requiring rib resection. An osteomyocutaneous flap may be harvested by preservation of the muscular connections with the underlying ribs. Donor site morbidity is related to winging of the scapula and can be avoided if the muscle is harvested segmentally and the inferior three or four slips are harvested.[7] (See Fig. 10.6.)

Rectus abdominus

Rectus abdominus is a long, flat muscle that constitutes the medial abdominal wall. It originates from the pubis and inserts onto the costal margin. It can easily cover sternal and anterior chest wall defects and can also fill space within the mediastinum. It has two dominant pedicles, the superior and inferior epigastric arteries and functions to flex the trunk. With division of the inferior pedicle, the muscle will cover the mediastinum and the anterior chest wall. It can be harvested with an overlying skin paddle, and usually the resulting cutaneous defect can be closed primarily. When taken with overlying fascia, there is a risk for resultant

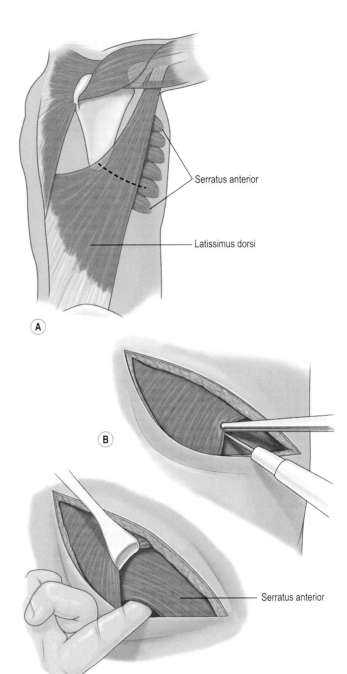

Fig. 10.4 Muscle sparing thoracotomy. *(From: Ferguson MK. Thoracic Surgery Atlas. Edinburgh: Elsevier©; 2007.)*

hernia, and at times, mesh reinforcement of the abdominal wall is necessary. Caution is also advised for patients with prior abdominal incisions as the skin perforators or intramuscular blood supply may have been previously violated.[7] (See Fig. 10.7.)

External oblique

External oblique is a broad, flat muscle that originates from the lateral lower eight ribs and inserts onto the iliac crest and linea semilunaris. It easily covers lower anterior chest wall

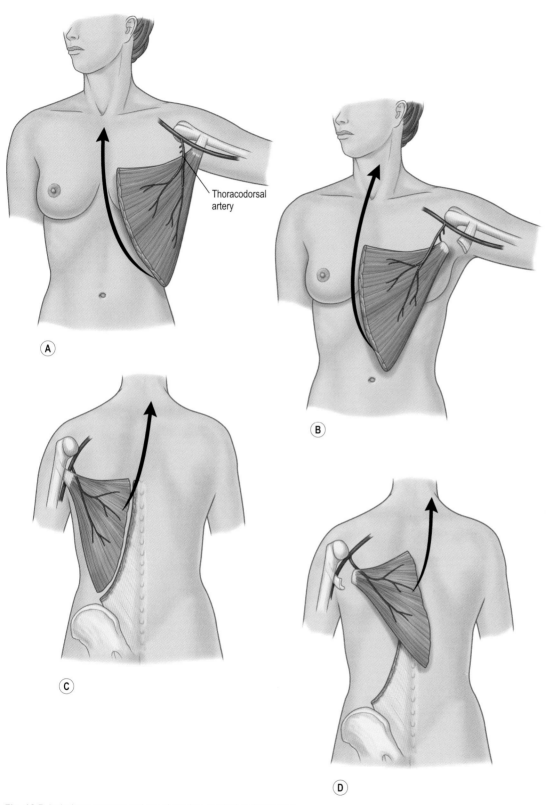

Thoracodorsal
artery

Fig. 10.5 Latissimus anatomy and arc of rotation standard and turn over.

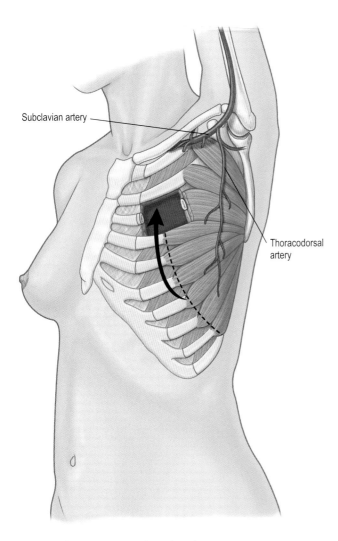

Subclavian artery

Thoracodorsal artery

Fig. 10.6 Serratus anatomy and arc of rotation.

defects as a rotational flap and has a segmental blood supply from the posterior intercostal arteries, which enter the muscle at the midaxillary line. It functions in situ as an important strength layer of the abdominal wall, and thus its harvest tends to be a second-line option when the latissimus is not available. A similar flap can be made with overlying soft tissue leaving the muscle intact as well.[7] (See Fig. 10.8 – external oblique anatomy and arc of rotation.)

Omentum

The omentum comprises visceral fat and blood vessels that arises from the greater curve of the stomach and is also attached to the transverse colon. This flap can easily cover wounds in the mediastinum and anterior, lateral, and posterior chest wall. It has two dominant pedicles, the right and left gastroepiploic arteries. The greatest benefit of this flap is the pedicle length that can be easily elongated with division of internal arcades. The flap is mobilized onto the chest or into the mediastinum from a tunnel through the diaphragm or over the costal margin. Caution is again advised for patients with prior laparotomy incisions as the omentum may have significant intra-abdominal adhesions or have been previously

resected. Furthermore, when transposing the omentum over the costal margin, by necessity a portion of the abdominal fascia must be left open to allow egress. This area is prone to hernia.[7] (See Figs. 10.9–11.)

Key points

- Skeletal chest wall support may be achieved with mesh, acellular dermal matrix, or autogenous material such as tensor fascia lata. The former is more prone to infection. Rigid skeletal support prevents paradoxic chest wall motion although this is usually well tolerated.
- Pectoralis muscle is the workhorse for sternal and anterior chest wall defects.
- Latissimus muscle is known for its bulk and ability to reach intrathoracic defects. Caution is advised for patients with previous thoracotomy incisions as it may have been divided. Less commonly the thoracodorsal vessels will have been clipped during modified radical mastectomy.
- Serratus muscle is less bulky than the latissimus but will function to cover lateral chest wall defects and some intrathoracic needs.
- Rectus abdominus is an excellent choice for sternal and anterior chest wall defects, especially the lower two-thirds. Furthermore, it can be used to fill space within the mediastinum.
- External oblique is well positioned for a rotational flap and easily covers lower anterior defects.
- The omentum can reach almost any chest wall defect. Its greatest advantage is its pedicle length, which can be extended by dividing the arcades.

Patient selection/approach to patient

The importance of a multidisciplinary approach to chest wall reconstruction cannot be underestimated. These patients, whether suffering from malignancy, infection, or trauma, are often also plagued with cardiac or respiratory insufficiency, diabetes, obesity, malnutrition, tobacco use, and generalized deconditioning. Thorough workup including pulmonary function testing, physical therapy and nutritional assessment, smoking cessation, and preoperative control of blood sugar, outcomes may be optimized. Furthermore, communication between referring surgeon and reconstructive plastic surgeon is crucial to properly define preoperative reconstructive expectations as well as incision planning with caution to spare chest wall musculature if required. Occasionally preoperative imaging may be used to confirm suspected vascular injury to commonly used muscle pedicles, e.g., thoracodorsal vessels during mastectomy.

Acquired chest wall deformities are commonly the result of iatrogenic injury. Chest wall wound infections, mediastinitis, osteoradionecrosis (ORN), refractory empyemas, and bronchopleural fistulae can all necessitate a reconstructive surgeon. The surgeon is generally well prepared to reconstruct any defect with utilization of the workhorse flaps described above, combined with general principles of thorough debridement and skeletal stabilization. Common chest wall reconstructive problems are described below.

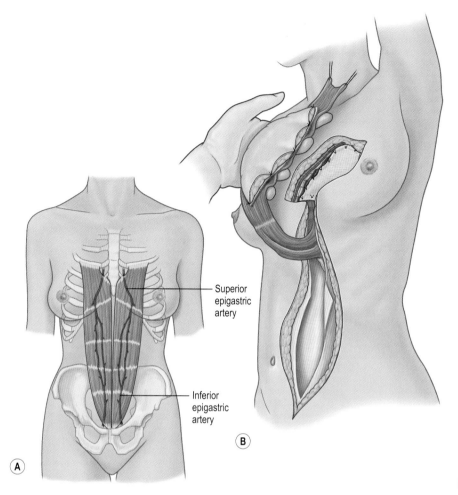

Superior epigastric artery

Inferior epigastric artery

Fig. 10.7 Rectus anatomy and arc of rotation.

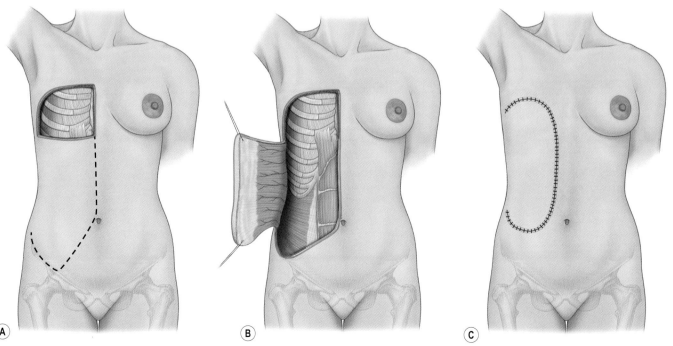

Fig. 10.8 External oblique anatomy and arc of rotation.

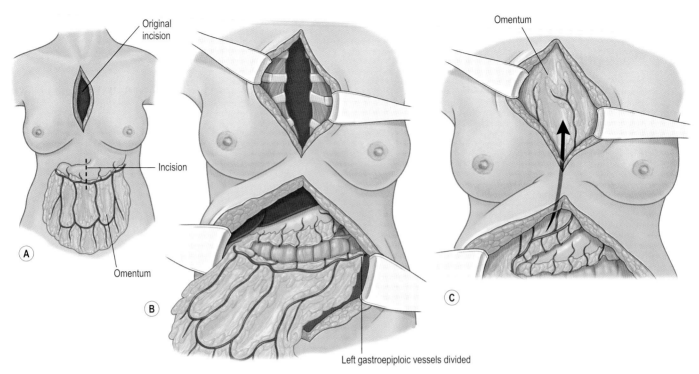

Fig. 10.9 Omentum anatomy.

Chest wall tumors

Basic science/disease process

Primary tumors of the chest wall comprise only 5% of thoracic neoplasms.[14] Half of these are considered benign.[15] The most common benign tumor is osteochondroma and is resected only when symptomatic. The most common primary malignant tumors are sarcomas, chondrosarcoma from the bony structures, and desmoid tumors from the soft tissue. Sarcoma resection is recommended to include a 4 cm margin of normal tissue and thus will almost always necessitate significant chest wall reconstruction[16] (Figs. 10.12 & 10.13). Over half of

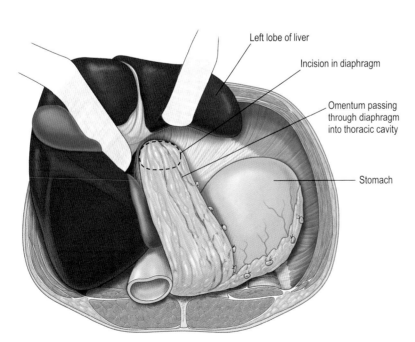

Fig. 10.10 Omentum is passed through cruciate incision in diaphragm under the left lobe of the liver.

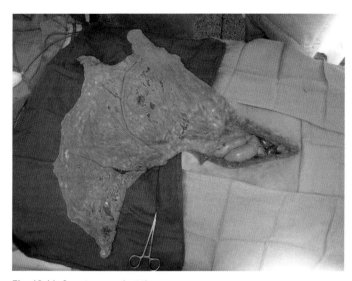

Fig. 10.11 Omentum arc of rotation.

malignant chest wall lesions represent metastatic disease, with breast and lung cancers being the most common.[17]

Diagnosis/presentation/patient selection

For relief of symptoms including pain, ulceration, and foul odor, and occasionally for disease control, even metastatic lesions may necessitate resection. (See Fig. 10.14.)

Treatment/surgical technique

Like other neoplasms, metastatic tumors are resected with a margin of normal tissue, and thus they too will frequently require skeletal support as well as recruitment of soft tissue in the form of pedicled or free flaps.

Outcomes

Not all metastatic resections are palliative. The 5-year survival rate following resection of chest wall recurrence of breast cancer is reported to be as high as 58%.[18]

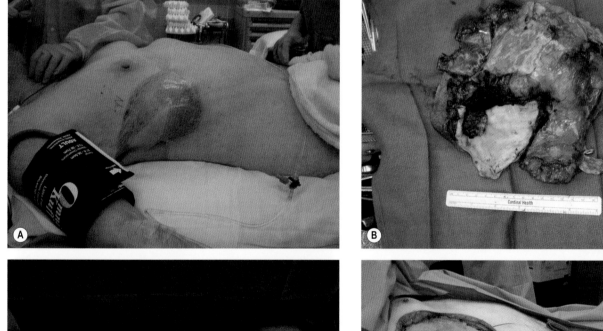
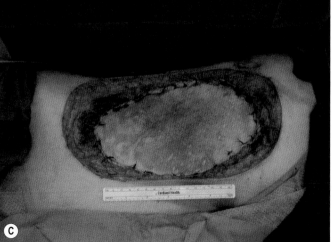
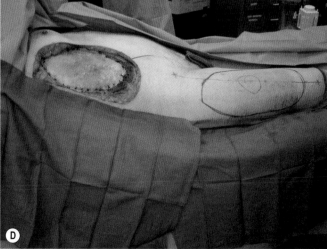

Fig. 10.12 Multipe recurrent osteosarcoma. Initial reconstruction included ipsilateral latissimus, free contralateral latissimus. Third recurrence, resection involved 6 ribs and the previously implanted mesh. Reconstructed with free anterolateral thigh (ALT) flap to the deep inferior epigastric artery/deep inferior epigastric vein (DIEA/DIEV). *(Courtesy of Dr. Song.)*

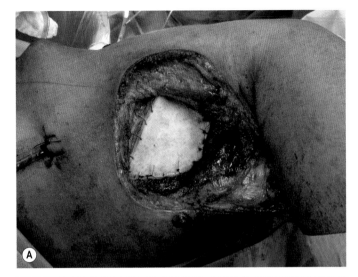

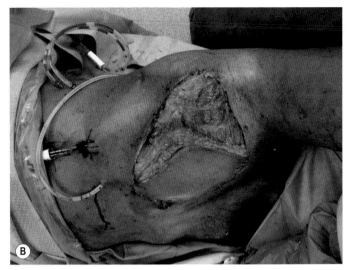

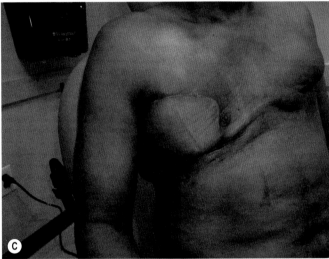

Fig. 10.13 Radiation-induced rhabdomyosarcoma of anterolateral chest wall, resection of ribs 3–5, and adherent right middle lobe (RML). Reconstruction with porcine acellular dermal matrix (ADM) and latissimus myocutaneous flap and skin graft. *(Courtesy of Dr. Roughton.)*

Mediastinitis

Basic science/disease process

Mediastinitis occurs in 0.25–5% of patients undergoing median sternotomy.[19–21] Historically, mortality approached 50% in these patients.[9] Sternal wound infections may be classified into three distinct types as described by Pairolero (Table 10.2).[22] Type I wounds occur in the first several postoperative days and are usually sterile. This is consistent with early bony nonunion and may represent the earliest stage of infection and perhaps even the portal of entry for skin flora. Type II infections, occurring in the first several weeks postoperatively, are consistent with acute deep sternal wound infection including sternal dehiscence, positive wound cultures, and cellulitis. Type III infections, presenting months to years later, represent chronic wound infection and uncommonly represent true mediastinitis. They are usually confined to the sternum and overlying skin and may be related to osteonecrosis or persistent foreign body.

Speculation exists that dehiscence of the sternum precedes infection of the deeper soft tissues within the mediastinum.

Table 10.2 **Classification of infected sternotomy wounds**

Type I	Type II	Type III
Occurs within first few days	Occurs within first few weeks	Occurs months to years later
Serosanguineous drainage	Purulent drainage	Chronic draining sinus tract
Cellulitis absent	Cellulitis present	Cellulitis localized
Mediastinum soft and pliable	Mediastinal suppuration	Mediastinitis rare
Osteomyelitis and costochondritis absent	Osteomyelitis frequent, costochondritis rare	Osteomyelitis, costochondritis, or retained foreign body always present
Cultures usually negative	Cultures positive	Cultures positive

(Adapted from Pairolero and Arnold. Chest wall tumors. Experience with 100 consecutive patients. *J Thorac Cardiovasc Surg*. 1985;90:367–372.)

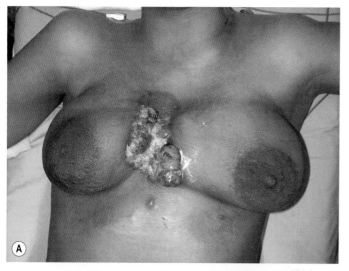

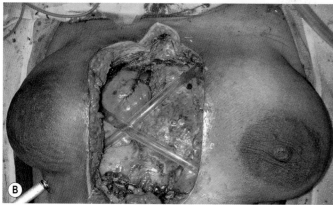

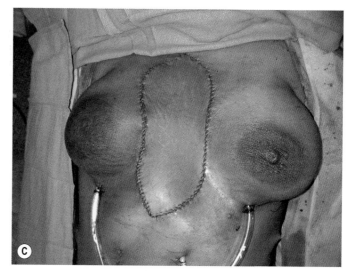

Fig. 10.14 Sternal metastases from breast cancer, resection, and vertical rectus abdominus myocutaneous [FLAP] (VRAM) flap coverage. *(Courtesy of Dr. Song.)*

Like other fractures in the body, such as the lower extremity and the mandible, sternal instability may perhaps encourage infection rather than result from it.[23]

Diagnosis/patient presentation

Preoperative risk factors for the development of mediastinitis include older patients, chronic obstructive pulmonary disease (COPD), smoking, end stage renal disease (ESRD), diabetes mellitus (DM), chronic steroid or immunosuppressive use, morbid obesity including large, heavy breasts, prolonged ventilator support (>24 h), concurrent infection, and reoperative surgery. Other variables include off midline sternotomies, osteoporosis, use of left internal mammary artery (LIMA) or right internal mammary artery (RIMA), long cardio-pulmonary bypass runs (>2 h), and transverse sternal fractures.[24,25] A high index of suspicion is encouraged for any patient with sternal instability or "click". However, firm diagnosis of mediastinitis or deep sternal wound infection is made by isolation of an organism from mediastinal fluid or tissue and observing chest pain or fever associated with bony instability.[26]

Treatment/surgical technique (Video 10.1 ▶)

Consistent with fundamental plastic surgery principles, treatment of infection, including that of the mediastinum (Fig.

10.15),[27] will require adequate drainage and debridement. Quantitative tissue culture facilitates this debridement.

If tissue culture is positive, >10 organisms per cm³ of tissue, indicating deep sternal wound infection rather than early sternal dehiscence, early debridement is encouraged and should be performed urgently. A thorough debridement includes the removal of sternal wires and extraneous foreign bodies including any unnecessary pacing wires and chest tubes (Fig. 10.16). Sharp debridement of necrotic and/or purulent tissue is performed until remaining tissue appears healthy and bleeding.[28,29] Radical sternectomy is not indicated, and sternal salvage should be attempted if the bone is viable. This may be determined by bleeding from the marrow and the presence of hard, crunchy cortical bone. Topical antimicrobials such as silver sulfadiazine and mafenide creams are employed to gain and maintain bacteriologic control of the wound. Subatmospheric pressure wound therapy may be utilized to increase wound blood flow and expedite granulation tissue, thereby decreasing dead space.[30,31] This has been shown to decrease the number of days between operative debridement and definitive closure of sternal wounds.[20]

Fixation of the sternum or residual sternal bone is crucial for bony healing. Furthermore, this fixation prevents paradoxic motion of the anterior chest wall and may improve many complications seen with sternal nonunion such as chronic chest wall pain and abnormal rubbing or

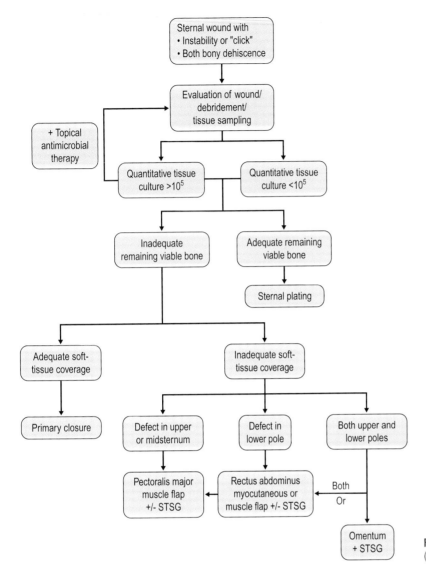

Fig. 10.15 Management of sternal wounds. Split thickness skin graft (STSG).

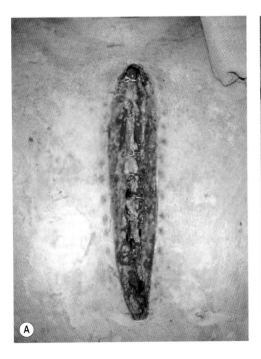

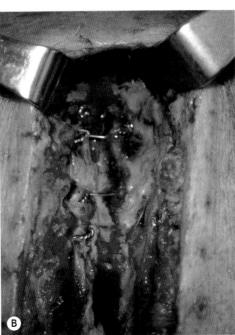

Fig. 10.16 Thorough debridement requires removal of necrotic tissue and foreign bodies. (Courtesy of Dr. Song.)

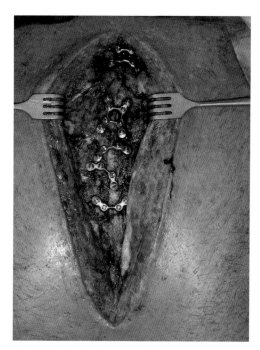

Fig. 10.17 Rigid fixation is crucial for sternal union.

clicking sensations.[32] For adults, titanium plates are used (Fig. 10.17).

Occasionally, sternal dehiscence occurs early in the postoperative course, consistent with type I sternal wound infections. This is secondary to mechanical failure of wire closure rather than infection. The wounds are sterile and should proceed to rigid sternal fixation. More commonly, however, patients will present with sternal nonunion in a delayed fashion. In the absence of infection, the residual viable bone can be plated directly. Importantly, a paradigm shift has occurred in the authors' institution such that patients who are deemed high risk for mediastinitis and sternal dehiscence are plated prophylactically.[33,34] Several plating systems exist all designed to facilitate ease of application as well as emergent chest re-entry.

Once rigid fixation is achieved, soft-tissue closure must be addressed. As very limited soft tissue exists over a normal sternum, residual local tissue following debridement of mediastinitis will often prove inadequate for plate coverage. Thus muscle flap coverage is indicated. When the wound involves the upper two-thirds of the sternum, pectoralis major muscle advancement or turnover flaps are easily harvested and are the first line therapy for wound closure (Fig. 10.18). Caution is advised for turnover flaps when the ipsilateral IMA has been harvested for coronary artery bypass graft (CABG). Furthermore, emergent chest re-entry will, by definition, devascularize this turnover flap. Additionally, when the lower sternal pole lacks coverage, the pectoralis may be inadequate based on its limited arc of rotation. For these cases, the rectus abdominus muscle flap is a better choice (Fig. 10.19). It may be used despite LIMA or RIMA harvest based upon the eighth intercostal artery, its minor pedicle. If the rectus is unavailable secondary to previous surgery, a pedicled omental flap should be considered for soft-tissue sternal coverage. Finally, if the omentum has been previously resected or the patient has had multiple prior abdominal operations, the latissimus dorsi flap

can be used. This may be harvested with a skin island and allow chest wound closure.[35] Skin grafting, if required, may be employed for closure of either the sternal wound or flap donor site.[18]

Empyema and bronchopleural fistula

Basic science/disease process

Empyema is defined as a deep space infection between the layers of visceral and the parietal pleura. Empyema and bronchopleural fistulas often are found in concert and plague pneumonectomy and partial pneumonectomy defects. The chest cavity, unlike most other regions in the body, is rigid and non-collapsible. Thus deep space infections, such as empyemas, are unlikely to heal without collapse of dead space or filling of the cavity. Older techniques, such as open chest drainage and the use of Eloesser flaps, designed to decrease intrathoracic dead space, (Fig. 10.20) have fallen out of favor.

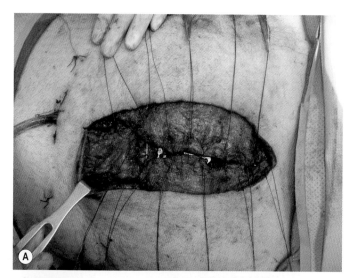
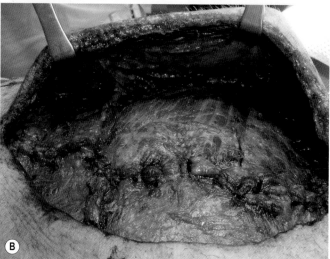

Fig. 10.18 Bilateral pectoralis advancement flaps. Muscle sutured together in midline. *(Courtesy of Dr. Roughton.)*

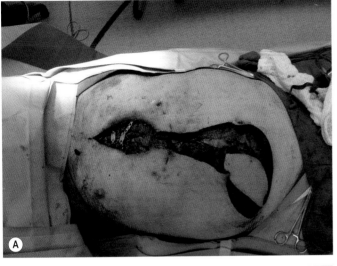

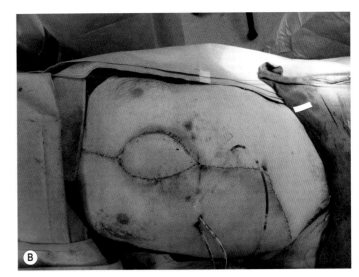

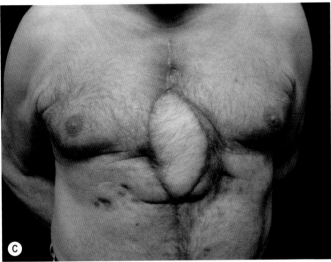

Fig. 10.19 Oblique rectus abdominus myocutaneous flap for inferior pole sternal coverage. *(Courtesy of Dr. Roughton.)*

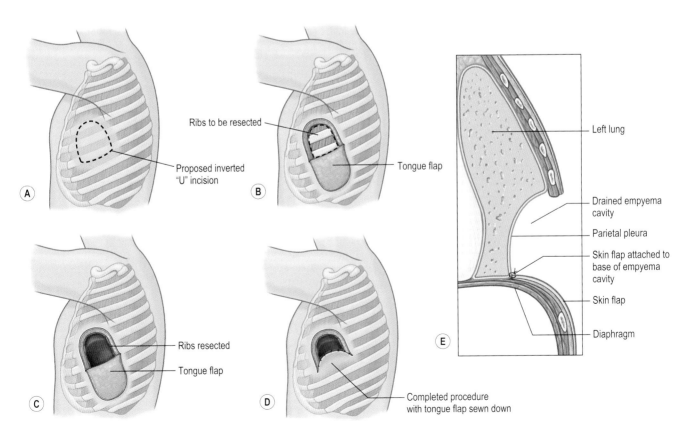

Ribs to be resected

Proposed inverted "U" incision

Tongue flap

Ribs resected

Tongue flap

Completed procedure with tongue flap sewn down

Left lung

Drained empyema cavity

Parietal pleura

Skin flap attached to base of empyema cavity

Skin flap

Diaphragm

Fig. 10.20 Eloesser flap. Skin flap sewn to parietal pleura.

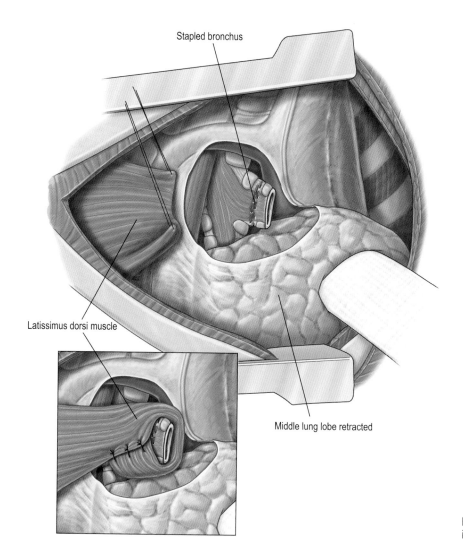

Stapled bronchus

Latissimus dorsi muscle

Middle lung lobe retracted

Fig. 10.21 Bronchopleural fistula with latissimus muscle introduced intrathoracically for reinforcement.

The bronchial stump, created after pneumonectomy, can also become a reconstructive challenge. If it dehisces, by definition, a bronchopleural fistula is created. This phenomenon, a massive air leak between the large airways and the chest cavity, is unlikely to resolve without the interposition of healthy tissue in the form of flap coverage.[36] (See Fig. 10.21.)

Surgical technique

The omentum, latissimus dorsi, serratus anterior, pectoralis major, and rectus abdominus muscles have all been described for space filling and reinforcement of the bronchial stump.[37,38] An often encountered problem with intrathoracic space filling is the sheer volume required to totally obliterate the thoracic cage. This can be overcome with thoracoplasty (meaning partial rib/cage collapse) or with the use of multiple flaps.[39] As a single flap, however, the latissimus muscle is often the preferred choice given its volume.

Outcomes

Outcomes following muscle flap transposition are reported as quite successful with 73% resolution or prevention of infection in Arnold and Pairolero's retrospective review of 100 patients with severe intrathoracic infections.[28] Several smaller and more recent studies report even higher rates of success.[26,40,41] In fact, prophylactic use of the latissimus muscle for reinforcement of the bronchial stump in high-risk patients is the standard of care in some centers.[42]

Osteoradionecrosis

Basic science/disease process

The use of adjuvant radiation therapy is becoming increasingly common in the treatment of both breast and lung cancer. As such, osteoradionecrosis (ORN) of the ribs is becoming an increasing problem for reconstructive surgeons. Radiation injury and tissue damage may not become clinically apparent for months to years after exposure, especially in tissues with slow cell turnover such as bone. Although the mechanism is poorly understood, radiation leads to an increased production of cytokines, collagen deposition, and scarring within affected tissues, as well as vascular damage leading to relative hypoxia (Figs. 10.22 & 10.23). The severity of radiation-induced necrosis is related to several factors including total dose, dose per

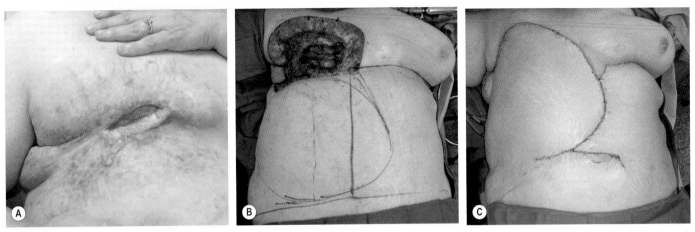

Fig. 10.22 **(A)** Osteoradionecrosis of ribs following chest wall radiation for breast cancer. **(B,C)** Following radical resection, serratus thoracoabdominal flap is planned and inset. Note all incisions kept supraumbilical to preserve lower abdominal donor site for future autologous breast reconstruction. *(Courtesy of Dr. Gottlieb.)*

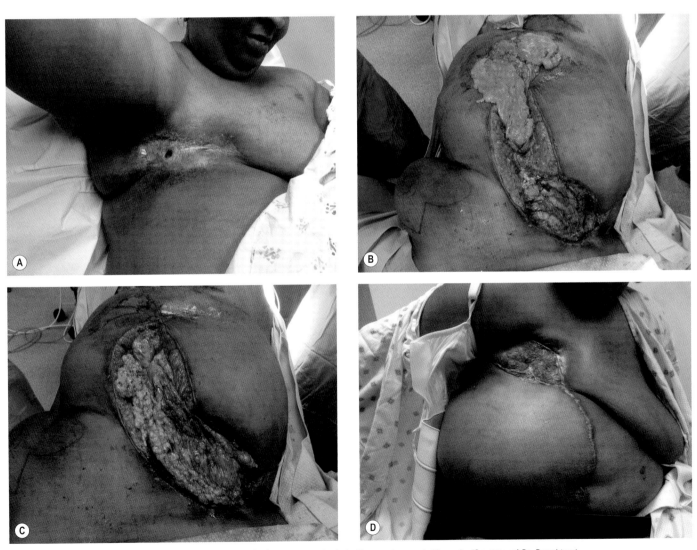

Fig. 10.23 Osteoradionecrosis following chest wall radiation for breast cancer treated with omentum and skin graft. *(Courtesy of Dr. Roughton.)*

fraction, frequency of administration, and whether it is combined with chemotherapy. Smaller doses per fraction appear to be better tolerated.[43] Note that this entity may be difficult to diagnose radiographically and demands a high level of clinical suspicion.

Treatment/surgical technique

Some advocate hyperbaric oxygen (HBO) therapy for ORN. However, for ORN of the mandible, a prospective, randomized, placebo-controlled trial showed the HBO group actually fared worse than their counterparts.[44] Anecdotally, the authors have not found this therapy to be essential or especially helpful and do not routinely pursue it. Management of ORN of the chest wall consists of wide local excision and reconstruction. In addition to osteonecrosis, radiation damage also affects overlying soft tissues creating hyperpigmentation, decreased pliability, and even ulceration. However, note that this decrease in chest wall pliability may make skeletal reinforcement unnecessary for borderline sized defects. Recruitment of healthy tissue in the form of local myocutaneous flaps is recommended for coverage of resultant chest wall defects and any skeletal reinforcement as indicated.

Osteomyelitis

Basic science/disease process

Chest wall osteomyelitis most commonly results from contiguous spread of infection, either from pneumonia or empyema. Hematogenous spread is also possible. Infectious etiology tends to be bacterial, with mycobacterial and fungal sources less likely. It frequently coexists with ORN as well.

Diagnosis/patient presentation

Osteomyelitis produces symptoms including fever, chest pain, and localized swelling of the chest wall.[45]

Treatment/surgical technique

Similar to osteomyelitis of other areas of the body, antibiotics and surgical excision are recommended. Chest wall reconstruction should proceed similarly to other areas of resection with rigid support when indicated and soft-tissue coverage in the form of local muscle flaps. In an infected field, however, the authors strongly discourage use of prosthetic material. When skeletal stabilization is indicated, autogenous material or acellular dermal matrix is preferred.

Traumatic chest wall deformities

Basic science/disease process

Chest trauma results from both penetrating and blunt injuries, which damage underlying bony and soft tissues. This may occur with or without further injury to vital organs or great vessels within the thoracic cage.

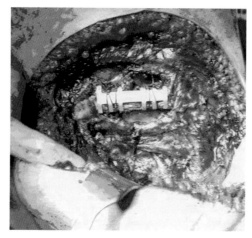

Fig. 10.24 Judet struts. *(From: Surgical Stabilization of Severe Flail Chest, Fig. 7, reproduced with permission from CTSNet, Inc. © 2010. All rights reserved.)*

Diagnosis/patient presentations

Severe paradoxic chest wall motion, in the form of flail chest, may be seen following significant chest trauma. This results from multiple adjacent rib fractures, broken in two or more places, creating a flail segment.

Patient selection/treatment/surgical technique

Patients with traumatic chest wall deformities should initially be stabilized according to Advanced Trauma Life Support (ATLS) protocol. Chest tubes and positive pressure ventilation should be initiated as indicated. For patients with respiratory compromise, rigid fixation of the flail segment may be indicated. This is accomplished traditionally with the use of mini-plates, thicker titanium recon bars, or Judet struts (Fig. 10.24). Significant loss of chest wall, seen in massive crush injuries, should be managed again with rigid support to the remaining viable chest wall and concomitant soft-tissue coverage.

Outcomes

Traditionally patients were treated with expectant management; however, rib plating has been shown to reduce ventilator dependence and ICU stay as well as incidence of pneumonia in patients with flail chest.

Secondary procedures

Chest wall reconstruction has been, over the last three decades, very successful. Cases of failure commonly result from inadequate control of infection or residual tumor burden. In either case, an aggressive resection is often indicated and the use of a second flap. Another unfortunate complication of skeletal chest wall reconstruction is infection of alloplastic mesh products. In these cases, removal of the infected prosthesis and use of acellular dermal matrix, autologous fascia, or even contralateral ribs may be indicated.

Access the complete references list online at   **http://www.expertconsult.com**

1. Deschamps C, Tirnaksiz BM, Darbandi R, et al. Early and long-term results of prosthetic chest wall reconstruction. *J Thorac Cardiovasc Surg.* 1999;117(3):588–592. *The authors review their experience with nearly 200 patients requiring chest wall reconstruction over 15 years. Mesh is utilized (polypropylene and polytetrafluoroethylene) for skeletal support, and over half of the patients required muscle transposition for soft-tissue coverage. Wound healing was complete for 95% of patients, although 24% experienced local cancer recurrence.*

6. Weyant MJ, Bains MS, Venkatraman E, et al. Results of chest wall resection and reconstruction with and without rigid prosthesis. *Ann Thorac Surg.* 2006;81(1):279–285.

7. Zenn MR, Jones G. *Reconstructive Surgery: Anatomy, Technique, and Clinical Applications.* St Louis (MO): Quality Medical Publishing; 2012. *This textbook detailing nearly all commonly used flaps in plastic surgery continues to be an excellent reference for relevant anatomy, flap selection, and arc of rotation.*

13. Pairolero PC, Arnold PG. Thoracic wall defects: surgical management of 205 consecutive patients. *Mayo Clin Proc.* 1986;61(7):557–563.

19. Jurkiewicz MJ, Bostwick TJ, Bishop JP, et al. Infected median sternotomy wound: successful treatment with muscle flaps. *Ann Surg.* 1980;191(6):738–743.

20. Sarr MG, Gott VL, Townsend TR. Mediastinal infection after cardiac surgery. *Ann Thorac Surg.* 1984;38:415–423.

23. Gottlieb LJ, Pielet RW, Karp RB, et al. Rigid internal fixation of the sternum in postoperative mediastinitis. *Arch Surg.* 1994;129(5):489–493.

28. Dickie SR, Dorafshar AH, Song DH. Definitive closure of the infected median sternotomy wound: a treatment algorithm utilizing vacuum-assisted closure followed by rigid plate fixation. *Ann Plast Surg.* 2006;56(6):680–685. *This paper contains a treatment algorithm for mediastinitis, emphasizing debridement, the use of sub-atmospheric pressure, rigid fixation, and soft-tissue coverage.*

33. Song DH, Lohman RF, Renucci JD, et al. Primary sternal plating in high-risk patients prevents mediastinitis. *Eur J Cardio-Thor Surg.* 2004;26:367–372. *This is a case-controlled study of prophylactic sternal plating in high-risk patients. The group who was plated experienced no mediastinitis while 14.8% of the control group, closed with wire, developed mediastinitis.*

38. Arnold PG, Pairolero PC. Intrathoracic muscle flaps. An account of their use in the management of 100 consecutive patients. *Ann Surg.* 1990;211(6):656–660. *The authors detail a 73% success rate with treatment and prevention of intrathoracic infection following muscle transposition into the chest of high-risk patients.*

11

Reconstruction of the soft tissues of the back

Gregory A. Dumanian and Vinay Rawlani

SYNOPSIS

- Reconstruction of the soft tissues of the back at first may seem to be a daunting task compounded by large wounds, unfamiliar and segmental anatomy, radiation, hardware, and difficulties with postoperative positioning.
- Many of the conditions treated require significant coordination with surgical colleagues. The conditions may be unfamiliar to the plastic surgeon and without parallels elsewhere in the body, an example being pseudomeningoceles filled with cerebrospinal fluid (CSF).
- The goal of this chapter is to provide the reader with real-life solutions to difficult problems involving back wounds.

Introduction

The back is 18% of the total body surface area; however, until recently, reconstruction of the back was neglected in plastic surgery texts. From the nape of the neck, to the anterior axillary lines, to the inferior gluteal crease, the only area well known to the plastic surgeon is the buttocks for the treatment of pressure sores. What changed the equation were the advances made in spine surgery and instrumentation. In decades past, spinal fusions were often performed by removing discs and scraping the endplates of vertebral bodies. These procedures were not limited by the surrounding soft tissues. This changed with improvements in surgical hardware that allowed for longer constructs for spinal stability. Simultaneous anterior and posterior spine exposures for rigid fixation greatly stripped and elevated the surrounding soft tissues, and correspondingly pushed the soft tissues past the point where wound healing would be automatic. In response to the need created by our surgical colleagues, surgical procedures to reliably close the back were developed.

Patient presentation

Midline back wounds

When a spine surgeon calls to discuss new drainage from a midline spine wound, the thought process for treatment should be methodical and thorough. When was the last procedure performed, and did the procedure involve the placement of hardware? What type of hardware is present, and is it locally prominent or is it low profile? Did the spine surgeons place hardware on the anterior or lateral aspect of the vertebral bodies, or rather was it only posterior? Have there been any dural tears that were repaired, and do the spine surgeons have any evidence of a CSF leak? After obtaining an understanding of what was done, an evaluation of wound healing issues is necessary. Is the patient markedly malnourished and catabolic? Is obesity and dead space management the problem? Has the patient been radiated for a spinal cord metastasis with the associated stiff and edematous soft tissues? Next, an examination of the patient is often telling of what needs to be done. Continued soiling of dressings with fluid and dieback of wound edges often point to deep fluid collections emerging from around the spinal hardware. Further understanding of the time course of the drainage also points to the underlying pathology. Early postoperative episodes of drainage less than 4–6 weeks after the spine surgery are typically successfully treated with repeat surgery and soft-tissue reconstruction with hardware preservation. However, drainage that has been only partially treated with a small debridement or treated solely with IV antibiotics only to resurface months later is more difficult to treat. In fact, a chronic hardware infection defined as bacteria in association with hardware greater than 6 months after placement is typically not a situation that plastic surgery can definitively treat without hardware removal.

Much can be learned with the simple examination of a patient's spine X-ray in terms of the existence and location of hardware. Do the plain films demonstrate hardware immediately deep to the wound or drainage areas? Plain films of the spine are also obtained to reveal the length of the construct when present, degenerative spine disease, and the presence or absence of fusion. CT and MRI scans are helpful when looking for fluid collections, pseudomeningoceles, and inflammation of the soft tissues. A key issue is if fluid collections are above or below the standard back muscle closure or fascial plane. If fluid or a hematoma is seen deep to the musculature, a deep hardware infection is more likely. Unfortunately, the spinal hardware causes artifacts in both CT and MRI scans, lowering their ability to demonstrate fluid collections with high accuracy.

Non-midline back wounds

While midline wounds are either due to pressure sores or spine procedures, non-midline wounds represent a much more heterogeneous collection of etiologies and therefore require a wide range of solutions. Much like acquired wounds elsewhere in the body, wounds of the non-midline back are due to poor wound healing after access incisions of the chest cavity or retroperitoneum, necrotizing infections, or tumor excision. Traumatic injuries are uncommon. A working knowledge of the conditions facing the thoracic surgeon is important in these instances. Thoracotomy incisions sometimes break down in the face of an empyema, persistent air leaks, radiation, and malnutrition. Desmoid tumors, soft-tissue sarcomas, and even neglected skin cancers can leave large defects of the back. For these patients, a more standard thought process and wound management often suffices. The wounds are typically flat and often allow skin grafting. When flaps are needed to cover bone or prosthetic material, the same muscles that are used to cover the midline spine are often available and easier to mobilize to the lateral back due to the lateral placement of their pedicles. The lateral tissues, being more mobile than the midline tissues, are easier to transpose for adjacent tissue transfers. Free flaps are facilitated as they have larger inflow vessels available nearby, such as the axillary artery, than exist for midline reconstructions.

Patient treatment

Local wound care

For superficial relatively painless wounds without exposed hardware, local wound care with dressings is a relatively risk-free way to achieve wound closure. Draining midline incisions tend to have wide areas of undermining along the length of the closure. These tunnels can typically be opened in the office with a local injection of anesthesia and finger fracturing of the incision. A long wound without tunnels with a saucer shape typically heals faster than small wounds with a fishbowl shaped internal wound, due to the improved ability to cleanse the surface of the internal wound. Therefore tunnels should be opened along old incision lines. All necrotic tissue should be debrided. All non-absorbable sutures, such as braided polyester, should be removed. Obtaining local wound control with wide exposure of the wound is a tried and tested method for the first step in healing. Patients are often unaware of the real size of the wound and must be

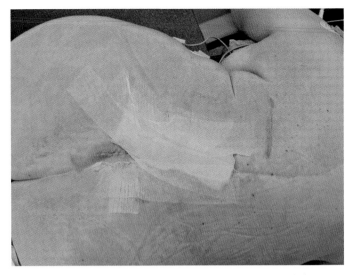

Fig. 11.1 Lumbar incision draining serous fluid 2 weeks after lumbar fusion.

prepared for the resulting appearance of the surgical site after opening of the tunnels.

Much depends on the patient's home situation. Dressings can be simple wet-to-wet saline dressings, with showering twice a day to cleanse the surface of the wound. Subatmospheric pressure dressings can be employed, but the tubing is sometimes difficult to place under back bracing devices (Figs. 11.1–11.3). This does well for obese patients with thick subcutaneous tissues, who otherwise tend to dehisce suture lines due excessive weight and suture pull-through. After a wound has granulated, if it is painful, then delayed primary closure or skin grafts can be performed if the wound is sizeable. However, the risks of these secondary closure procedures often outweigh the benefits. The subcutaneous tissue stiffens during the time of obtaining local wound control, and it is difficult to re-elevate and close without a fairly sizeable procedure.

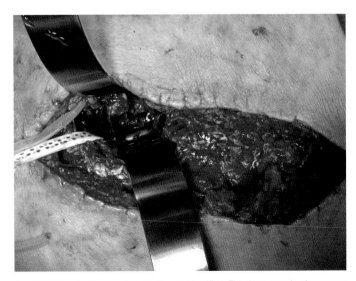

Fig. 11.2 A subcutaneous hematoma was identified. The deep muscle closure was opened, and there was no purulence or fluid present. The muscles were reclosed, and a subatmospheric pressure dressing applied.

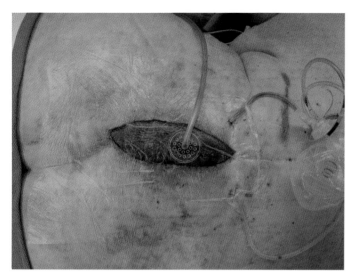

Fig. 11.3 Subatmospheric pressure dressing used to aid in delayed primary closure of the skin flaps.

Operative debridement

Patients with persistently draining wounds after spine surgery associated with hardware should be evaluated critically for an operating room debridement. Secondary indications for a debridement include unexplained fevers and fluid collections seen on imaging scans. The patient should be readied for surgery with large intravenous lines and in a warm operating room. The large exposed surface areas can allow the patient to rapidly cool, with the associated coagulopathies and increased blood loss that occurs. Blood should be available for a transfusion. Due to the segmental nature of the vascularity, surgery does not typically expose large blood vessels, but rather many small ones, and the blood loss is rather constant throughout the case.

The maneuvers in the operating room are a critical step in the treatment of patients with postsurgical back wounds. A thorough incision and drainage should be performed for patients with unexplained or purulent drainage through their incision. The entire length of the incision should be opened as wide as necessary to explore for purulence and drain fluid collections. The erector spinae muscle closure should be reopened for cultures and to evaluate for liquefying hematomas. In addition, the surgeon should know at the beginning of the debridement whether a laminectomy was performed at the original spine surgery, in order to prevent injury to the spinal cord and dura during the incision and drainage. If this is the case, the spine team should be available to assist in opening the wound.

At this point, the surgeon will need to make a decision as to the quality of the tissues. Non-purulent benign fluid collections in the subcutaneous tissues with no purulence deep to the musculature can be reclosed over drains, or else closed secondarily with a subatmospheric pressure dressing (see above, local wound care). Purulent and deep collections require additional decisions. If the local wound is so purulent as so preclude an immediate re-closure, then all non-viable tissue should be debrided and the wound irrigated and left open for local wound care. This can be done with dressing changes over several days until the second trip to the operating room. Alternatively, a subatmospheric pressure dressing may be applied.

For those deep wounds judged amenable to re-closure, a radical incision and drainage is performed. This should involve the surgical excision of scarred tissues where possible to reveal supple soft tissues with pulsatile bleeding. Scar tissue, though it bleeds, does not bleed in a pulsatile fashion due to the small size of the vessels that developed during prior wounding. Pulsatile bleeding at wound margins has been shown to correlate with wound healing in problematic incisions, such as distal foot amputations. Tissues with a pseudobursa should be excised, as this too represents scar tissue. Tissue that is stiff is unyielding and does not conform well, and so the tissues should be removed until they are soft to palpation. Pulsatile irrigation with saline is gentle to tissues that cannot be removed and cleanses surface bacteria.

An interesting issue is the removal of non-viable elements such as hardware and bone graft. While plastic surgery teaching emphasizes the removal of all non-vascularized surfaces, in this case the hardware acts to stabilize the wound. An orthopedic principle is that the most effective way to fight infections is to have rigid bone fixation. Therefore hardware that is well fixed should remain in place in early hardware infections. This is done both to stabilize the wound for improved healing, as well as to avoid the surgery involved with removing and replacing hardware. Long-term maintenance of the hardware as well as clinical and radiographic evidence of fusion is well documented in patients that were returned to the operating room for washouts within 6–8 weeks after placement. As stated previously, hardware colonized after 6 months is defined as a chronically infected foreign body, and salvage of this hardware is much less likely in the long-term. Another issue is the endogenous and exogenous bone graft placed to achieve a fusion. In the absence of definitive studies, it seems reasonable to remove a non-incorporated and easy to remove graft, but to leave in place a graft that has, in any way, begun to stick to the local tissues due to inosculation. Loose hardware should be removed and replaced in a secure fashion if deemed necessary.

Wound "shape" is an important concept for reconstruction of the soft tissues of the back and is especially true for the depth of the wound. The back has lordotic and kyphotic regions in the normal condition, and these contours can be dramatically changed with pathology. These curves make postoperative positioning difficult when the surgical incision involves the most prominent portion of the back. The depth of the procedure performed by spine surgeons is also important. For example, a patient with a laminectomy has a deeper wound than when the spinous processes are intact. Also, spinal hardware serves to create a local prominence in contradistinction to the depth of the surgical dissection. A prime reason for persistent fluid collections is the 3D space between a laminectomy and the adjacent vertically oriented bars. Crosslinks between the bars further prevent soft tissues from collapsing into the space immediately over the midline. Finally, laterally placed hardware can be poorly covered by soft tissue and be the originators of pressure sores. This is especially common when hardware inserts into the posterior superior iliac spines for pelvic fusions. Therefore in the treatment of wounds of the spine, the 3D shape should be evaluated and converted as much as possible to a 2D wound. Prominent hardware should be exchanged for something with

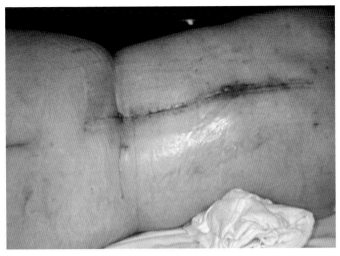

Fig. 11.4 Purulent drainage from a back wound 2 weeks after posterior spinal fusion.

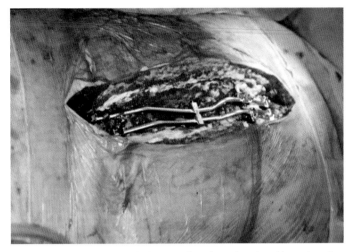

Fig. 11.6 Hardware revised to be less prominent in conjunction with erector spinae muscle flaps.

a lower profile (Figs. 11.4–11.7). Incomplete corrections of spine deformities should be revised in patients to better re-create the natural contours. The deeper the hole, the more a flap should be "dropped into" the defect, rather than tissue simply slid towards the midline. Teamwork between the spine and the soft-tissue surgeons is often necessary to appropriately treat problems of wound shape and contour.

The status of the CSF and dura is also critical for treatment of certain back wounds. The dura is opened and closed in a planned fashion in numerous instances, including the treatment of spinal cord malignancies, untethering of the spine for patients with a history of cord lipomas and spina bifida, and treatment of pseudomeningoceles. Unplanned tears of the dura also occur in laminectomy procedures. The low-pressure CSF leaks and the continuing fluid build up push the soft tissue away from the leakage site and thereby prevent soft-tissue collapse of the space. The CSF fluid in fresh postoperative cases can also become infected, and exists in association with surgical wounds of the back. Treatment of patients with CSF leaks will be discussed later in this chapter.

Flap closure

Principles

The first step in reconstruction is a timely debridement, as has been emphasized already. The second step is local wound control with a radical debridement of all stiff and scarred tissue. For the reconstruction, the surgeon should never rely on scar tissue as a positive factor for wound healing. The more completely the old scar can be excised and replaced with non-scarred new soft tissues, the better the reconstruction. Finally, the procedure with the highest chance for success and with the lowest morbidity should be selected for the patient.

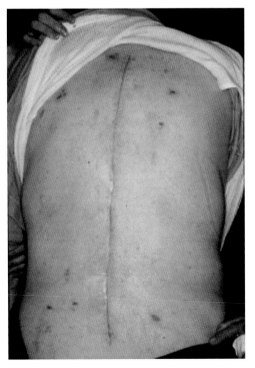

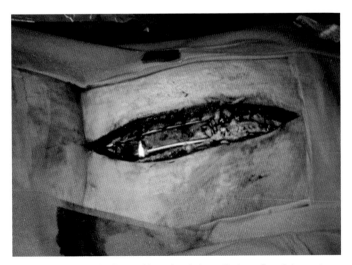

Fig. 11.5 Prominent hardware with exudate between the bars. Crosslinks create a hardware "cage" to prevent soft tissue from collapsing to the depth of the surgical dissection.

Fig. 11.7 Healed wound in this patient after optimizing both the hardware architecture and the soft tissues.

Central questions to be answered relate to the presence or absence of a fusion, and the vertebral levels involved.[1] When an instrumented fusion has been performed, the erector spinae musculature function is no longer necessary, and the muscles are completely expendable in terms of a reconstruction. The fusion rods prevent postoperative motion and, when the erector spinae muscles are re-approximated in the midline, they tend to stay in place. Spine patients without fusions still require the function of the erector spinae musculature when healing is completed for flexion and extension of the spine. These patients do better with flaps that are "dropped into" the defect, rather than with erector spinae muscles that are closed side to side and that would dehisce with back flexion.

Possible flap choices for spine closure

Erector spinae muscle flaps

The erector spinae muscles, also called the paraspinous muscles,[2] are expendable after a previous spine fusion and no longer functional for spine extension and flexion. The dissection of these muscles proceeds in a stepwise fashion in order to move them towards the midline. This flap is appropriate from the high cervical area to the low lumbar area, but it will not adequately cover an occipito-spinal fusion, and nor will it be sufficient for low lumbosacral lumbosacral soft-tissue coverage. One must be careful in its use when a lateral approach to the spine has been made, because the muscle can be transected for access.

First, skin flaps are elevated superficial to the thoracolumbar fascia (Fig. 11.8). With a retractor putting tension on the soft tissues, the granulation tissue is entered using a cautery and a blunt plane is elevated with finger dissection. The latissimus muscle and trapezius muscle should stay attached to the skin. The dissection is easiest inferior in the lumbar area where the muscle is round and large, and most confusing superiorly where the muscle is thinnest and becomes attached to the undersurface of the trapezius. The erector spinae muscles have a convex shape, and there is a rounded aspect

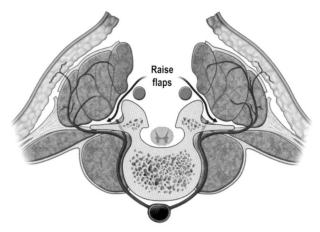

Fig. 11.9 A dissection is then performed to release the medial and deep attachments of the erector spinae muscles to the spine and transverse processes. The lateral blood supply is approached from the deep aspect of the muscle.

of the muscle that then descends laterally towards the more lateral neck, thoracic, and lumbar areas. It is in this groove that segmental blood vessels enter the lateral and deep aspects of the longissimus and iliocostalis muscles. Continuation of these blood vessels is superficial to the skin and the latissimus muscle in the thoracolumbar area. While the surgeon is elevating the skin flaps, the perforators and dorsal sensory nerves going up to the skin can often be identified and preserved to maintain skin vascularity. To lessen the chance of marginal skin perfusion and to limit a future potential seroma cavity, undermining should not be overdone.

The thoracolumbar fascia is incised, much like the development of any standard bipedicled flap, in order to mobilize the erector spinae muscle and/or overlying skin to the midline. When the original dissection is superficial to the fascia and the fascia remains attached to the muscle, this facilitates the later closure and the fascial release is critical to the movement of the muscle. Occasionally the fascia remains attached to the skin during the initial elevation. In this case, muscle mobilization is facile, but the skin is more difficult to close in the midline. Therefore an incision of the fascia along its length allows the skin to move medially and to provide the excess for debridement and re-closure. The dissection up until this point is rather easy and bloodless, but only moves the muscle an estimated 30% of its potential. Complete mobilization of the muscle requires a dissection along the deep aspect of the erector spinae (Fig. 11.9). Again with tension applied to the tissue with retractors, cautery dissection of the deep and medial attachments of the erector spinae will mobilize the muscle and detach it from the lateral aspects of the transverse processes of the spine. It will by necessity divide the medial row of blood vessels entering the paraspinous muscles, but the prior dissection to identify the lateral vessels entering the muscle will suffice to preserve vascularity. One technique is to have the fingers of the non-dominant hand in the lateral groove at the site of the lateral perforators while bluntly elevating the medial aspect of the muscle with the thumb and index finger. The medial muscle elevation is a powerful means to allow the paraspinous muscles to "unfold" like an accordion to be advanced towards the midline (Figs. 11.10 & 11.11). The muscle changes shape from being a round muscle mass to being more elliptical. Advancement of the muscle is a

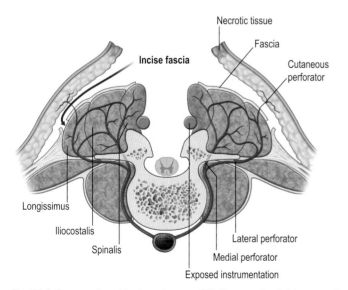

Fig. 11.8 Cross-section of lumbar spine area. Skin flaps are elevated to expose the thoracolumbar fascia and to reach the region of the lateral pedicle entering the erector spinae muscles. The thoracolumbar fascia is incised to allow a medial movement of the muscles.

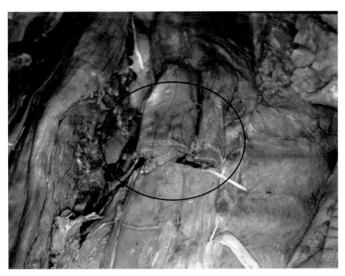

Fig. 11.10 Cadaver dissection of the erector spinae muscles at the lumbar level.

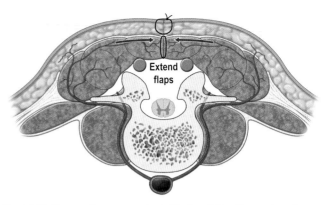

Fig. 11.12 The muscles are approximated in the midline. The erector spinae muscles unfurl, changing shape from circular to elliptical.

different process from simply releasing the thoracolumbar fascia and "rolling" the dorsal aspect of the muscle towards the midline.

With the skin and muscle flaps so created, it is now quite easy to distinguish stiff and inflamed tissue from more normal soft tissue. The medial aspect of the skin, subcutaneous tissue, and paraspinous muscles is sharply debrided. The muscles are brought together in the midline (Fig. 11.12), and any extra tissue can be imbricated to help fold the soft tissue into crevices between vertically oriented hardware bars (Fig. 11.13A–F). Drains are left both deep and superficial to the erector spinae closure and are kept until the drainage is minimal. When the closure of the erector spinae muscles is of good quality, there is no need for a second overlying muscle flap using the trapezius or the latissimus muscles.

Latissimus muscle or myocutaneous flap

The latissimus muscle is a well-known and understood flap.[3] Based on the thoracodorsal pedicle, the muscle can be moved superiorly up to the level of the top of the scapula. Based on its minor perforators that also supply the paraspinous muscles,

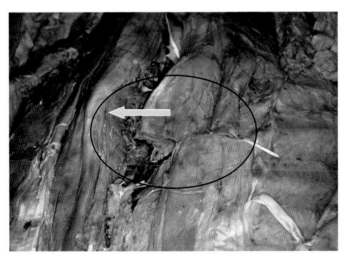

Fig. 11.11 Release and medial movement of the muscles.

the latissimus can reach the lower lumbar area. An advantage of the latissimus is being able to be "dropped in" to a hole, and so it is useful for patients that have not been fused, or for more lateral defects. The muscle can reliably carry a skin paddle, and this often helps in the inset of the flap. Caution should be made for patients that have had thoracotomy incisions, as the muscle is often divided. The latissimus muscle is a good but second-line flap for the coverage of midline back wounds. In comparison to the paraspinous flaps, the latissimus flap can only cover a spine wound 10–12 cm in length, while the erector spinae flaps can cover practically the entire length of the spine. The dissection required to elevate the latissimus muscle takes more time and effort than for the erector spinae. While the morbidity of flap elevation is low, there is a long-term potential functional loss, especially for those patients who may need to utilize crutches or wheelchairs. The latissimus muscle is a good choice for a radiated wound of the midback, where the patient has not been fused, and the erector spinae musculature is in the field of radiation (Fig. 11.14A–C).

Patients undergoing latissimus flaps should have a thorough debridement of their wounds. The flap dissection is best begun in an area where the anatomy has not been distorted by prior incisions. For instance, flaps based on paraspinous perforators should begin in the axilla with the identification of the muscle and division of the thoracodorsal pedicle. It is easier than one would expect to be in the wrong plane and to divide these small paraspinous perforators when the dissection is begun in the midline wound.

The orientation and design of the skin paddle should be done carefully. For flaps based on the thoracodorsal pedicle, a skin paddle oriented with its long axis perpendicular to the midline will result with the skin paddle vertically oriented. Closure of the donor site initially oriented perpendicular to the spine does not make the midline spine any more difficult to close due to added tension. Another helpful skin paddle is a V-Y design (Fig. 11.15A–D) with the latissimus muscle and overlying skin advanced medially along the submuscular loose areolar plane. This flap can be re-elevated and moved a second time if necessary.

Trapezius muscle flap

The trapezius flap is useful for high cervical wounds because the paraspinous musculature is of limited mobility and size

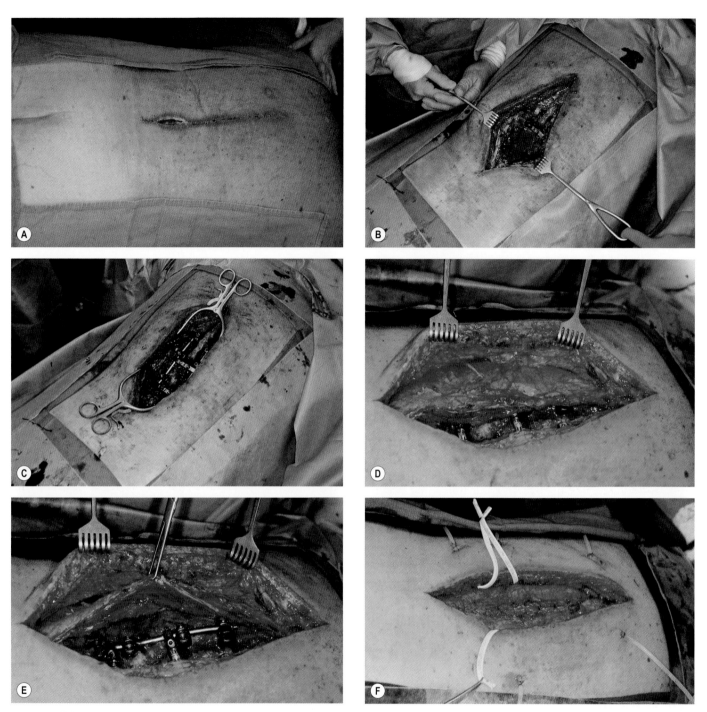

Fig. 11.13 (A) Patient with a long thoracolumbar fusion with drainage 3 weeks after a posterior spinal fusion. Note the erythema of the staple line. **(B)** Complete opening of the superficial and deep tissues reveals an infected fluid collection surrounding the hardware. A crossbar is visible. **(C)** The wound is radically debrided to reveal the entire spinal hardware construct. The hardware seems solidly fixed to the bone. **(D)** Dissection deep to the thoracolumbar fascia to the lateral border of the erector spinae muscles. A large nerve traveling through the muscle to the overlying skin is spared. **(E)** Dissection on the deep aspect of the erector spinae muscles to the level of the lateral perforators. **(F)** Erector spinae muscles closed in the midline.

at that level. In addition, the trapezius flap may have a variable blood supply. The superficial branch of the transverse cervical artery (superficial cervical artery (SCA)) and/or the deep branch of the transverse cervical artery (dorsal scapular artery (DSA)) are the main pain pedicles. Segmental thoracic perforators can supply a "turnover" trapezius flap, analogous to what is more routinely done for the pectoralis muscle;

however, these are morbid in terms of shoulder stabilization. The occipital artery supplies the superior aspect of the flap and can be use to cover small cervical wounds.

The most common trapezius flap elevation is based upon the main pedicle supplied by the branches of the transverse cervical artery. The dissection begins with identification of the distal and inferior triangular aspect of the trapezius where it

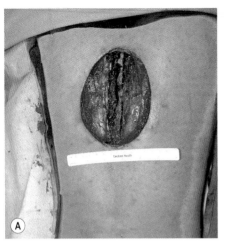
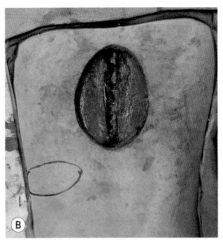
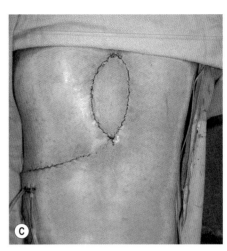

Fig. 11.14 **(A)** A 26-year-old man had a recurrent desmoid tumor removed from his thoracic spine area. There is exposure of the spinous processes. There is no hardware present. **(B)** A skin paddle slightly less wide than the defect and oriented at a right angle to the long axis of the wound is drawn out. **(C)** Final inset of the Latissimus Myocutaneous Flap. The flap donor site is oriented perpendicular to the long axis of the defect so that closure of the donor site will not make the recipient site more difficult to close.

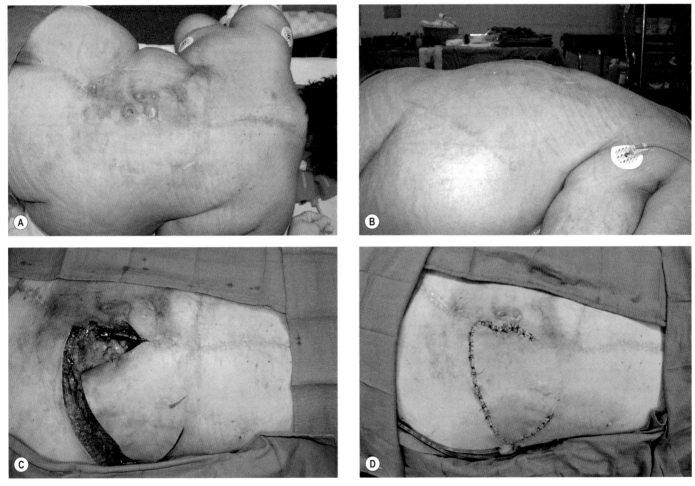

Fig. 11.15 **(A)** A 57-year-old female with a complex history of back surgery, revisions, and flaps. She has already had erector spinae flaps and a left latissimus flap for closure. She presents with a new area of exposed hardware due to a pressure sore. She is not yet fused, and removal of the hardware is not possible. **(B)** The area of the pressure sore is at a kyphotic area of the lumbosacral spine. The optimal way to treat this condition is to correct the spinal deformity at the same time as improving the soft tissues. **(C)** A myocutaneous latissimus flap with the skin paddle advanced in V-Y fashion is elevated after debridement. **(D)** Closed incisions. As might be anticipated, several months later she presented with a new pressure sore at the same spot. She subsequently underwent successful correction of the spinal deformity and a readvancement of the V-Y flap for coverage.

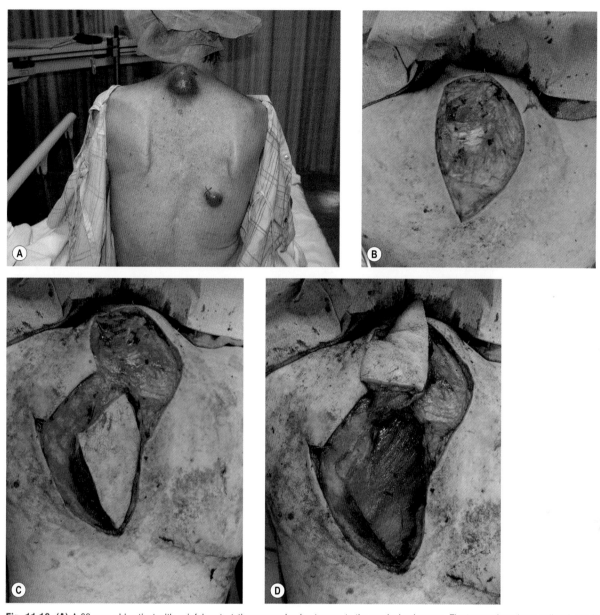

Fig. 11.16 (A) A 60-year-old patient with painful metastatic neuroendocrine tumors to the cervical spine area. The tumors have been radiated, precluding closure with skin grafts. **(B)** Wound after tumor excision. **(C)** Incised myocutaneous trapezius flap. The skin paddle was oriented at the inferior aspect of the muscle. **(D)** Trapezius flap during inset with 180° twist. The superficial dorsal scapular artery was not included with this flap, resulting in mild hypoperfusion of the skin paddle. The donor site was closed in the vertical midline.

just overlaps the latissimus muscle, because the crossing muscle fiber directions of the two muscles are quite distinct in this area. The main branch enters the muscle approximately 7–8 cm lateral to the midline and at the level of the spinous process of C7 on its deep aspect.[4] A skin paddle overlying the muscle can be taken to help with the inset. The more cephalad and larger the skin paddle, the better the reliability (Fig. 11.16A–D), as the skin overlying the caudal trapezius is often supplied by the angular branch of the thoracodorsal system. Further cephalad and lateral to the elevated skin paddle, the upper back skin is elevated off the trapezius. The deep dissection is then performed, with the muscle elevated off the paraspinous musculature and the rhomboids, taking care to elevate the pedicle. The medial attachments are thickest, and then a plane between the two muscle groups is reached where

dissection is easy. The main pedicle is encountered and, with this vessel under direct view, the lateral aspect of the muscle is divided. Movement of the flap is tested, and the lateral muscle division is extended if greater mobility is required for wound coverage. The higher the dissection continues, the higher the morbidity due to shoulder drop but the greater the arc of rotation of the muscle.

Because of its sizeable donor site morbidity for the shoulder, the indication for the trapezius flap is in a non-fused patient with a radiated deep back wound where the erector spinae have been involved in the field of radiation. As the muscle is typically turned 90° for inset, the length of midline coverage by the trapezius is usually short, and either a combination of two trapezius flaps or else the trapezius flap with erector spinae flaps should be planned for long wounds.

Superior gluteal artery

The superior gluteal artery flap technique is the most challenging of all of the reconstructive soft-tissue procedures for the spine, but it is a necessary and useful procedure.[5] The flap should not be attempted unless the surgeon has had significant experience with perforator flaps and the surgical management of sacral pressure sores. A line is drawn between the superior-lateral aspect of the sacrum and the posterior-superior iliac spine. From a point that bisects this line, a second line is drawn toward the greater trochanter. This second line represents the path of the superior gluteal artery and is the long axis of the flap. A skin paddle is designed that encompasses the Doppler signal of the perforator of the superior gluteal artery and is oriented laterally towards the greater trochanter (Fig. 11.17A–F). This will be the lateral most tissue to be captured by the superior gluteal artery perforator.[6] To improve the reliability of the tissue, a strip of gluteus muscle oriented underneath the skin paddle can be taken along with the perforator. This is a different orientation than the skin paddle used for closure of sacral pressure sores, where extra skin is taken medial to the Doppler signal. The superior border of the skin is incised, and the skin flap elevated until the perforator from the superior gluteal artery is seen to be entering the skin paddle. Medial to this, the gluteus muscle is split to aid in the dissection of the pedicle. These patients typically have some motor dysfunction, and their gluteus muscles are thin and atrophic. With the pedicle under full view, the remainder of the skin paddle can be incised and the flap dissection completed. If there is difficulty with identification of the SGA perforator, additional muscle should be elevated with the skin paddle, or a decision made to dissect the other buttock. Medially, any muscle along the pedicle will resist the 180° flip required of the pedicle for the flap to reach the midline. Muscle found around the pedicle that impedes this 180° turn should be excised so that there is no tension on the flap to reach the lumbosacral spine. The skin paddle is de-epithelialized and will be able to cover the dura. The donor and recipient sites are closed over drains. Avoidance of a three-way incision with a small skin bridge and tunneling of the flap under this area also assists in the final closure. Alternatively, the flap may be transferred as a propeller flap with the skin paddle designed lateral to the perforator and rotated 180° medially into the defect. Given the difficulty of this flap and its perforator in general, caution is advised with the propeller design.

The buttocks are an area not typically reached by the spine surgeons. Both buttocks should be prepped into the field, in case there is an injury to the pedicle. In patients with buttock weakness preoperatively, the stronger side should be used. Caution should be observed with regard to patients who are markedly obese, and those with prior pressure sore procedures. A complete pressure relief bed is necessary for 10–14 days after the procedure to prevent pressure on the pedicle as it runs from the lateral sacrum towards the midline. Drains are often required for several weeks in the donor site. The procedure does not cause much pain or dysfunction long-term.

Closed suction drainage between the base of the wound and the flap should be maintained until less than 30 cc a day emerges in the bulbs. The more drains, the better, and for large procedures even 4–6 bulbs have been required. Furthermore, postoperative placement on a pressure relief air fluidized bed will allow the patient to lie directly on the flap without causing a pressure injury to the tissues. It is suspected that compression of the flap directly onto the wound bed has beneficial effects in helping the wound to seal.

Omentum

The primary criterion for using a pedicled omental flap includes scarred, irradiated, divided, and otherwise unusable back musculature suitable for local flap transfer in a patient in need of soft-tissue coverage of thoracolumbar spinal instrumentation (Fig. 11.18A–C).[7] The second criterion includes extremely deep wounds, such as those of patients with coverage needs of both anterior and posterior instrumentation, and for patients in whom the abdominal cavity is already entered for exposure. Absolute contraindications to the use of a pedicled omental flap include a history of intra-abdominal malignancy and a previously resected omentum. Relative contraindications include morbid obesity and the potential for intra-abdominal adhesions from previous laparotomies. The zone of coverage for an omental flap is from the lumbosacral recess inferiorly up to the level of the midscapula superiorly.

Close coordination is required between the spine and the plastic surgery teams. Typically, a posterior spinal instrumentation for stabilization is performed before the omental flap is harvested. The abdomen is entered either through an upper midline incision, a Kocher, or a right paramedian incision. After entering the peritoneal cavity and identifying the omentum, dissection begins by liberating the omentum and transverse colon such that they can be lifted out of the abdominal cavity. Traction on the tissues will aid in demonstrating the fusion plane between the omentum and the transverse mesocolon. The omentum can be dissected from its attachments to the transverse colon with a minimum of sharp dissection; blunt dissection is adequate. The dissection, if performed in the correct planes, should be avascular and not require the ligation of vessels. It is critical to not confuse the transverse colon blood supply with an omental vessel. Inclusion of the middle colic vessels with the flap may potentially devascularize the colon. Performed correctly, the entire colon from the hepatic flexure to the splenic flexure can be mobilized away from the omentum and stomach. Attention to detail should be made when putting traction on the left side of the omentum. Adhesions to the spleen can cause bleeding from the splenic capsule, and in the worst case require a splenectomy.

Next, a decision is made regarding whether to base the flap on the right or left gastroepiploic artery. The right-sided vessel is usually larger; the left is used when the spine exposure includes a left flank incision. The omentum is mobilized off the stomach by taking down the short gastric vessels. One should not attempt to travel great distances for each tie, as this tends to shorten the reach of the flap. The gastroepiploic vessel courses 1–2 cm from the edge of the stomach and should not be encroached by the ties. The stomach should be decompressed with a nasogastric tube, and this tube should remain in place for several days so that gastric distension will not cause any of the vessel ligatures on the greater curve to pull off. After compete mobilization of the gastroepiploic vessel off the stomach, it can be followed to the area where it emerges as the gastroduodenal artery (a branch off the hepatic

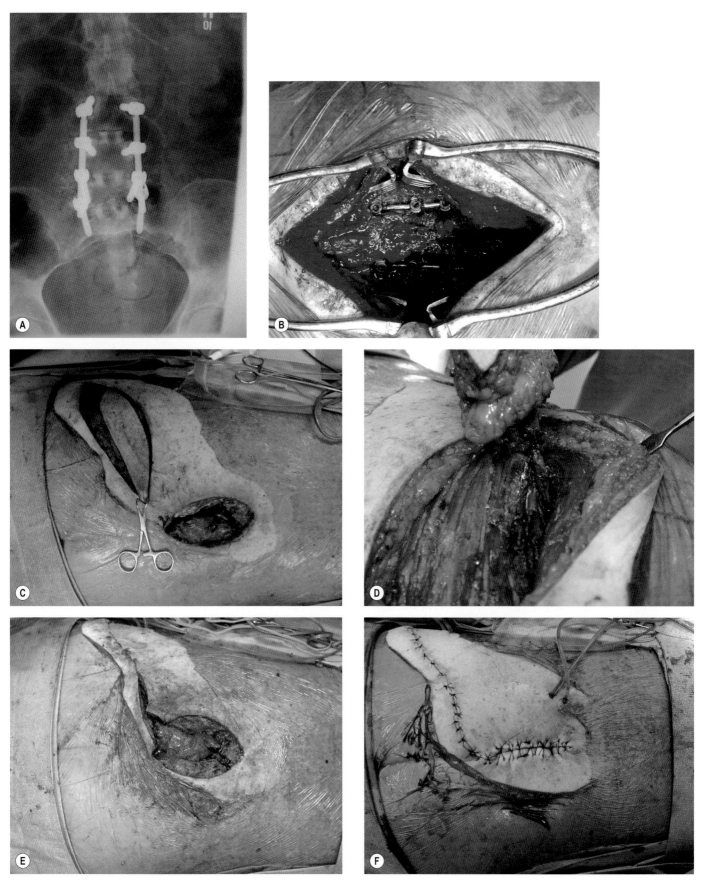

Fig. 11.17 (A) Radiograph of low lumbar fusion of a patient with drainage 3 weeks after spinal fusion. **(B)** Intraoperative view after debridement fusion site. **(C)** Incised skin paddle for left superior gluteal artery perforator (SGAP) flap. The staple marks the audible Doppler signal of the SGAP perforator to the skin. **(D)** Vascular pedicle to the superior gluteal artery perforator flap. Muscle around the pedicle must be minimized to allow for a facile flip of the flap to the midline. **(E)** The skin paddle is de-epithelialized and placed to fill the lumbosacral recess. **(F)** Closed incisions.

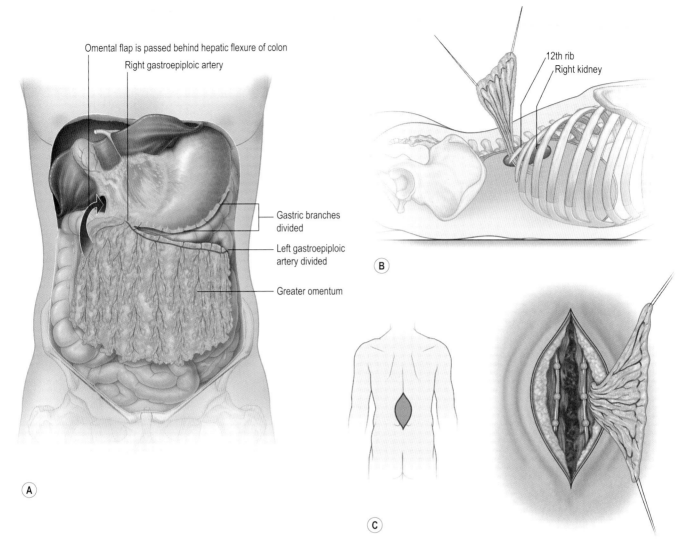

Fig. 11.18 Diagram of a pedicled omental flap for coverage of the spine.

artery/celiac plexus just inferior to the pylorus and still superior to the transverse colon mesentery). The artery and vein should not be skeletonized, so that the surrounding soft tissue can help prevent unexpected tension on the vessels during the tunneling process. Sutures can also be used in this area to prevent tension and thrombosis of the pedicle.

The passage of the omentum toward the spinal column requires creativity and knowledge of anatomy of the gastro-duodenal artery and its relationship to the attachments of the colon to the retroperitoneum. The most straightforward means to tunnel the omentum to the spine is to mobilize the hepatic flexure and right colon toward the midline. This is an avascular plane, and the mobilization of the colon is greatly simplified by the prior elevation of the omentum off the colon. The line of lateral peritoneal reflection (the white line of Toldt) is incised, exposing the retroperitoneum. The omental flap is then positioned behind the colon in the right paracolic gutter. The right kidney and Gerota's fascia is mobilized medially, and the omentum is "parked" on top of the 12th rib, which is confirmed by palpation. The abdomen is then closed in standard fashion and the patient re-prepped in the prone position.

The 12th rib is identified by palpation after elevating the latissimus muscle and skin off the rib cage. Lateral to the paraspinous muscles, the 12th rib is excised, the periosteum opened, and the omental flap will be immediately identifiable (Fig. 11.19A & B). The only confusion would be if Gerota's fascia were entered and the perirenal fat mistaken for the omental flap. The integrity of blood flow through the pedicle is assessed with a Doppler probe. Multiple drains are used in the closure in order to avoid seroma formation and problematic fluid collections. When skin is not available for coverage of the omentum, a negative pressure suction dressing is applied immediately onto the flap and a delayed skin graft performed.

Adjacent tissue transfers/perforator flaps

Adjacent tissue transfers without a defined blood supply and perforator flaps are two ends of a spectrum of possible reconstructions of the soft tissues of the back. In adjacent tissue transfers such as V-Y, transposition, and rotation flaps, the thick soft tissues of the back will create large dog ears, and

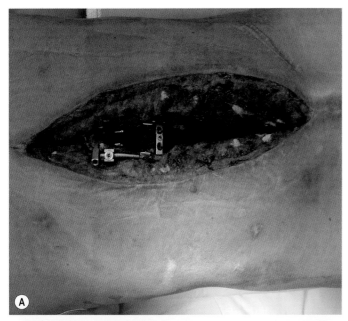

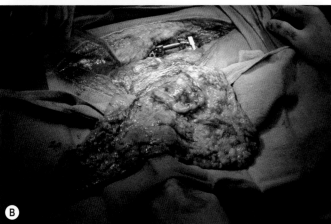

Fig. 11.19 (A) A paraplegic patient had an anterior and posterior fusion, all from the posterior approach. The spinal cord was tied off for access anteriorly. A deep infected fluid collection resulted, with the anterior and posterior hardware acting as a solid "cage". It was anticipated that flaps from the back would not be able to fill this deep hole. **(B)** The omentum has been harvested from an anterior approach and parked under the 12th rib. From the back, the 12th rib was excised and the omentum pulled posteriorly. The flap successfully filled the 3D space created by the hardware "cage".

donor sites will typically need to be covered with skin grafts. Keystone-style flaps are particularly useful advancement flaps of the back. A broad base to a keystone ensures incorporation of perforators; however, mobility requires release of the deep fascia. Perforator flaps, on the other hand, will allow transposition and insets in a more facile manner, and are especially useful in the iliolumbar and scapular areas.[8–10] Typically perforators of the thoracic and lumbar areas are located within 10 cm of the midline and will often exist lateral to the spinal erector muscles. However, the stresses on the soft tissues of the back with movement in and out of bed and with position changes will make the delicate nature of perforator flaps difficult to protect. In addition, these rearrangements of skin will do better with flat lateral wounds, rather than potential 3D wounds of the midline spine.

External oblique flap

Patients with huge lower lateral thoracic and lumbar wounds can be closed with pedicled external oblique turnover flaps.[11] These patients will have large radiated wounds where the remaining soft tissues could not be expected to accept a skin graft, or where there was a prosthetic material used for reconstruction of the posterior abdominal wall. These large, flat flaps can be thought of as an interface to help with healing of skin grafts to the wound bed. Done either unilaterally or bilaterally, the muscle is exposed with wide elevation of the abdominal skin, done through an oblique incision paralleling the dermatomes. Then, the insertion of the muscle is divided, just as it fuses with the anterior rectus fascia. Much like a components separation procedure, the external oblique is bluntly elevated towards the posterior axillary line off the internal oblique, to the point where segmental vessels enter the muscle. The muscle is flipped on itself 180° to cover the defect and to subsequently be skin grafted. When the flap is done unilaterally, the corresponding muscle imbalance of the anterior abdomen may cause an unusual contour of the abdominal wall.

Tissue expansion

Tissue expansion can be preferable to other solutions for reconstruction of the soft tissues of the back in certain instances. Those situations are more for pediatric cases than for adults and include the closure of wounds for giant congenital nevi excisions. Rarely, the soft-tissue defects in children before spine surgery will be amenable to a planned prior tissue expansion. The indications for tissue expansion are scarred local tissues, laterally displaced muscles, and a need for spinal instrumentation (Fig. 11.20A–D). The largest expanders possible should be placed immediately adjacent to the area that will require coverage, and the long axis of the expander should be oriented in a superior-inferior direction to allow for a medial sliding of the expanded tissue with a minimum of back-cuts and transposition flaps. Incisions for placement should be made radially to the closest edge of the expander to decrease the chance of extrusion of the implant through this newly placed scar. Ports should be placed over bony prominences to facilitate their palpability.

Free flap coverage of the back

Soft tissues

The erector spinae muscles are able to cover practically the length of the spine. However, patients exist that are not candidates for this procedure. Scarred erector spinae muscles from previous advancements or neuromuscular conditions such as polio cannot be moved to the midline. Eector spinae flaps are also not possible in patients who have received wide field radiation. One can feel on preoperative examination of these patients a woody non-yielding of the soft tissues even 6 cm from the midline. These situations are best treated with free flaps, especially when the defect is longer than 12 cm, preventing the use of a transposition of the latissimus or trapezius muscle (and when the omental flap is not possible). The difficulty with free flap coverage of the spine is finding a suitable donor vessel.[12] Possibilities include the superior gluteal artery pedicle and intercostal vessels. A long saphenous vein graft anastomosed to the common femoral artery

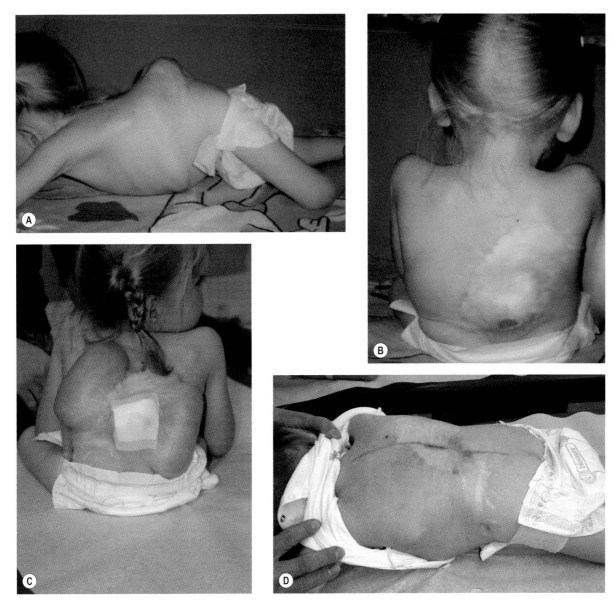

Fig. 11.20 **(A)** Lateral photo of a young child with a significant congenital spine defect. **(B)** Previous attempts at correction have produced numerous scars. A well-cared-for pressure sore is at the apex of the deformity. **(C)** Bilateral subcutaneous tissue expanders placed on the posterior trunk. **(D)** Healed incision after spine correction and advancement flap closure with expanded skin flaps.

can provide both inflow and outflow when divided for a lower trunk defect, and a long cephalic vein graft tied to the external carotid can bring inflow for an upper trunk flap. A latissimus dorsi flap can be harvested in the prone position with proper prepping and draping (Fig. 11.21A–C).[13] Free flaps are for defects that are both long and wide. Multiple position changes of the patient are required, and the long vein grafts when used are prone to twists and spasm. Some allow the vein graft loop to "mature" for a period of time to ensure that spasm will not cause a flap loss. While possible, this makes the final anastomosis to the arterial pedicle more difficult due to size mismatches, adds a separate operative procedure, and is generally not necessary.

Bone

The vertebral bodies of the spine are typically reconstructed with cages and bone grafts when corpectomies are performed,

and with good results. Certain patient subpopulations exist where vascularized bone is preferable. In these patients, more rapid incorporation of the bone graft due to its viable osteocytes reduces the chance for construct failure and infection. It is difficult to define exactly who should receive vascularized bone flaps, as the success rates of non-vascularized autograft and allograft are high. Fusions longer than three vertebral bodies in length, previous failed reconstructions, a history of radiation, esophagocutaneous fistula onto the fusion site, and active osteomyelitis may all be indications for a free fibula flap to the anterior spinal column.[14,15] In the cervical esophagus, after stabilization of the posterior spine, the anterior construct is readied using a bone template of extra fibula taken from the flap. The flap is made ischemic after being preshaped on the leg according to the template and then placed into a trough created within the anterior vertebral bodies to accept the fibula flap. The trough must be slightly wider than the bone flap so that there will be no shear force or compression of the

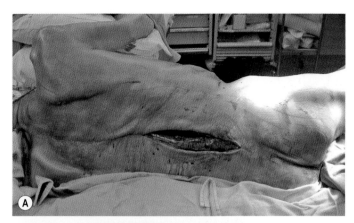

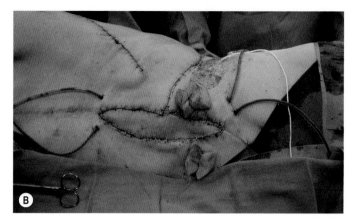

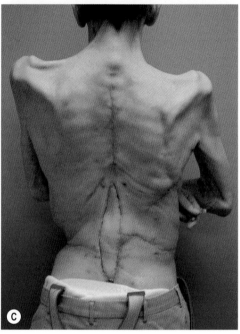

Fig. 11.21 (A) A 73-year-old man with a history of polio who has had a hardware instrumentation and prophylactic closure of his spinal fusion with erector spinae flaps. Due to the fibrotic nature of his muscles, an infected fluid collection developed. This situation was remedied with a free flap to the back. He is in the lateral decubitus position at the time of his first debridement. **(B)** A myocutaneous latissimus flap is elevated and anastomosed to a long saphenous vein graft loop with inflow from the right common femoral artery and outflow through the saphenous vein to the common femoral vein. The skin paddle facilitates a solid inset of the flap. **(C)** Long-term result.

pedicle running along the side of the bone. Narrowing of the diameter of the fibula is often necessary. The bone is stabilized with kick plates superiorly and inferiorly, and vascular anastomosis is then performed to the external carotid or the transverse cervical vessels. The prior spine stabilization makes the neck, by definition, less mobile, and therefore the vascular repairs may be best done with loop magnification. In the thoracic area, vascular inflow is either end to end from a segmental lumbar vessel or off a saphenous vein patch of the aorta fashioned by vascular surgery.

Vascularized bone reconstruction of the spine

A straightforward means of bringing vascularized bone to the anterior aspect of the thoracic spine is with a pedicled rib flap. For patients undergoing both anterior and posterior fusion of the spine with an associated thoracotomy for access, a pedicled rib based on its intercostal neurovascular bundle can be harvested. Unlike vascularized fibula flaps, the vascularized rib brings viable osteocytes but no structural support to the spine. The rib graft can either be placed next to or within the metal cage that is used for structural replacement of the

vertebral body.[16] The rib area near the costal cartilage is the actual bone that is used for the flap. The curved rib along the axillary line is excised, creating the neurovascular pedicle that is necessary for the rib flap to be positioned without tension.

Flap selection by region

Cervical region

The cervical spine area is more often instrumented from the anterior rather than the posterior approach. Wounds of the anterior cervical spine are uncommon, and when they occur can be in association with esophageal injuries. Wounds of the posterior cervical spine are more common. Etiologies of these wounds include pure soft-tissue defects without involvement of the spine, pressure sores, complications after laminectomy for radiated cancer excisions, and complications after placement of hardware for fusions. Soft-tissue defects without spine involvement are treated depending on the size and location of the defect either with skin grafts or adjacent tissue transfers. Pressure sores tend to be treated conservatively with pressure relief. Laminectomies are performed for spinal cord pressure from metastases, and the wound beds are typically radiated.

Trapezius pedicled flaps are the preferred treatment for these patients, as the erector spinae muscles are stiff and immobile from the cancer treatment. The more laterally placed trapezius muscles are typically pliable and non-radiated, allowing them to be mobilized and "dropped in" to the defect. The erector spinae muscles also tend to dehisce in the midline from neck flexion in the absence of spinal hardware. Complications after placement of hardware have been discussed earlier. In most cases, the erector spinae muscles can be mobilized to the midline with both superficial and deep releases. The cervical muscles are thin, located underneath the trapezius muscle, and become smaller as they insert on the occiput. In the cervical region, the trapezius and skin should be elevated as one unit to then identify the paraspinous muscles, and these planes can be confusing. Beginning inferiorly where the trapezius has a unique triangular shape and then proceeding superiorly is a technique for being in the correct plane.

Thoracic region

Like the cervical region, defects of the thoracic area include pure soft-tissue defects without involvement of the spine, pressure sores, complications after laminectomy for radiated cancer excisions, and complications after placement of hardware for fusions. Soft-tissue defects without spine involvement are treated depending on the size and location of the defect either with skin grafts or adjacent tissue transfers. The scapular and parascapular flaps can be helpful in closing some of these soft-tissue defects without spine involvement. In these cases, the donor site should be oriented perpendicular to the long axis of the wound to facilitate closure.[17] Alternatively, when closure of the donor site aids in the closure of the wound, the flap can be half the width of the wound and a pure 180° flip of the flap based on an underlying perforator will allow closure of both the wound and the donor site. Pressure sores tend to be treated conservatively with pressure relief. However, in some instances, a true spine correction for deformity is what is required to definitely treat the wound. Laminectomies are performed for spinal cord pressure from metastases, and the wound beds are typically radiated. Latissimus flaps based on the paraspinous perforators are ideal for allowing the muscle to be "dropped in" these defects, and thereby not manipulating the radiated and stiff erector spinae muscles. Myocutaneous latissimus flaps have easier insets with the overlying skin paddle sewn to the adjacent midline skin of the back.

Wounds of the thoracic back after spine surgery and placement of hardware are best treated with erector spinae flaps. There is no need for a "double muscle" closure with further mobilization of a latissimus flap if the erector spinae muscles come together normally. Rarely, the 3D shape of the wound is sizeable and requires modification of the spinal hardware. Even more rarely, after transection of the spine or corpectomy, the wound will be extremely deep. In these circumstances, the pedicled omental flap is ideal for filling the defect and helping achieve closure. These unusual circumstances often require either erector spinae flaps or latissimus flaps to aid in the closure.

Lumbar region

The high lumbar area is the optimal area for re-closure with erector spinae flaps. The muscles are largest in this area and

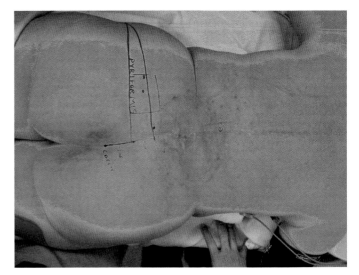

Fig. 11.22 This 50-year-old female has a recurrent fluid collection in the low lumbar spine after fusion. The initial plan is to perform a superior gluteal artery flap.

exist in a lordotic area of the back that is protected from pressure. The lateral perforators are easy to visualize as they enter the muscle. The only difficulty in this area is management of the often-thick subcutaneous tissue. Seromas can be problematic after elevation of the skin in order to mobilize the underlying muscle. Allowing the drains to stay for a prolonged period of time, as well as quilting sutures from the subcutaneous tissue down to the muscle bed, is helpful in preventing this postoperative aggravation. Other flaps are also possible for the lumbar area. Turnover latissimus flaps can reach this area, but only with some difficulty (Figs. 11.22 & 11.23). Sliding of myocutaneous latissimus flaps elevated from the lower lumbar area and transposed medially provides thick coverage of the spine, but only at the expense of a skin grafted donor site.[18] The omentum will also reach this area with some ease.

The inferior region of the lumbar spine is best covered with superior gluteal artery based flaps as described below. Often,

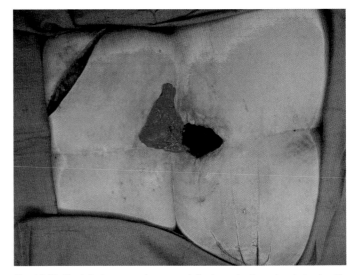

Fig. 11.23 The latissimus muscle can reach the lower lumbar spine, but only with extensive dissection, and the muscle that reaches the area is small and unable to fill the space well.

a gluteal flap will be combined with erector spinae flaps for coverage of a longer lumbar and lumbosacral defect. Another problem area is the posterior superior iliac spine, which is a site where bone grafts are harvested. Fluid collections, hematomas, and scar tissues develop from procedures on this area. Lateral dissection of the erector spinae muscles can be made confusing and difficult in this area that has had prior surgical exploration for bone grafts.

Lumbosacral region

The recess between the sacrum and the inferior aspect of the spine is best filled with a superior gluteal artery based flap. The erector spinae muscles are thin and laterally displaced in this area, precluding their use. Omental flaps require position changes in the operating room and bowel dissection. Random pattern skin flaps of the lumbar tissue or perforator based flaps are possible but are difficult to inset and control in an area that is subjected to high shear forces with position changes. Finally, while latissimus flaps can be mobilized to reach this area, there are many wounds that are simply too big for the latissimus muscle to reach and fill the entire cavity (Fig. 11.24).

Patients undergoing a full sacrectomy for tumors can undergo bilateral gluteus myocutaneous flaps if the superior and/or inferior gluteal arteries are preserved during the sacrectomy. For these patients, the plastic surgery team can mobilize the gluteus maximus off the sacrum, exposing the pedicles to the muscle and the sacrotuberous ligaments. The spine surgeon can then perform the tumor excision. Closure of the gluteus muscles in the midline, as in the case of a pressure sore, can be done with V-Y advancement of the skin paddles if necessary. Finally, for low rectal tumors with invasion into the sacrum, a transabdominal flap based on the inferior epigastric artery is feasible. The oblique rectus abdominis musculocutaneous (ORAM) flap, using a skin paddle based in an oblique direction off the periumbilical perforators and using only the lower aspect of the rectus muscle, can easily bring non-radiated skin to the lumbosacral

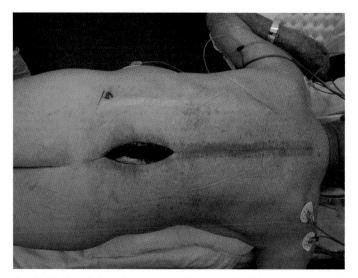

Fig. 11.24 The latissimus flap can be mobilized to reach this wound. However, the wound is large and it would be difficult for the latissimus flap to reach and fill this wound. This wound is better treated with a superior gluteal artery perforator flap for the lumbosacral recess, and bilateral erector spinae flaps for the lumbar area.

area.[19] The vertical rectus abdominis myocutaneous (VRAM) is another common design to achieve wound closure, but requires the harvest of more muscle.[20] These abdominal flaps need to be harvested in the supine position and parked adjacent to the sacrum. After sacrectomy, the flap can be retrieved from the posterior approach and inset.

For the majority of patients with lumbosacral defects, the tissue near the trochanter can be elevated with the blood vessels in continuity with the superior gluteal artery for soft-tissue coverage (Fig. 11.25A–D). This can be done as a pure perforator flap, or else with a strip of gluteus muscle under the skin paddle (which is de-epithelialized). As the flap is typically flipped 180°, the skin paddle will rest over the dura. To re-emphasize, this is a different design from the superior gluteal artery perforator (SGAP) flaps that are for sacral pressure sores. The proximal aspect of the pedicle must be dissected free of any muscle, as the muscle will obstruct the pedicle from being flipped towards the midline. Patients with longer wounds extending to the midlumbar area may need additional mobilization of the erector spinae muscles to the midline.

Patients undergoing this procedure do not complain of significant buttock morbidity after flap harvesting. Most of these patients have chronic lower spine dysfunction and buttock weakness before surgery, and so they are not used to robust gluteus maximus muscles for ambulation. In fact, the muscle atrophy typically present facilitates dissection. If the patients have any elements of motor strength imbalance, then the "stronger" side should be used for the flap elevation as that side has more to give if additional weakness were to develop.

Wounds of the lateral back

Soft-tissue reconstruction of the lateral back has certain special characteristics. In the thoracic area, if the rib cage is intact, most wounds are closeable with local wound care, latissimus flaps, parascapular/scapular flaps, serratus flaps, or posterior movement of a perforator flap from tissues in the anterior axillary line area. If the ribs are involved, then a decision about possible reconstitution of the pleural line needs to be made. Most authorities recommend that three or more ribs are reconstructed with a prosthetic patch, and this patch then needs to be covered with soft tissues. However, when the rib defect is located under the scapula, then the scapula serves to protect and camouflage any defect and larger rib resections are tolerated.

The lateral lumbar area in adults is protected typically by its lordotic shape, and the only structure that needs to be reconstructed is the posterior aspect of the abdominal wall. All other wounds can be closed with local wound care, skin grafts, or transfer of the latissimus muscle. In rare instances, which are radiated and require vascularized soft tissue for closure, an external oblique pedicled flap is possible.

Special clinical situations

Prophylactic closure of back incisions

Spine teams have noted the efficacy of muscle flap closure for open spine wounds, and this has led to the introduction of

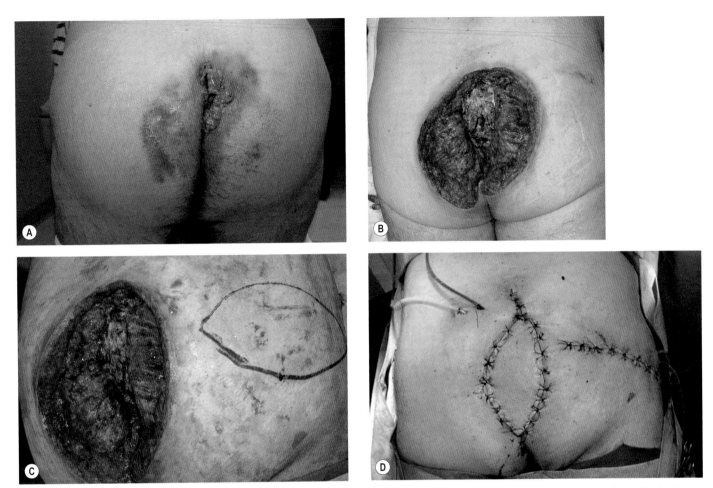

Fig. 11.25 (A) Large Marjolin's ulcer found in a chronic pilonidal cyst in an ambulatory patient. **(B)** Tumor excision. **(C)** A superior gluteal artery perforator flap is drawn out. The long axis of the skin paddle is perpendicular to the long axis of the defect to facilitate closure. The tumor excision and the final closure were staged to allow for definitive pathologic clearance of the margins. **(D)** Flap inset into the defect.

prophylactic use of muscle flaps at the time of spine surgery.[1,21] The same algorithms described earlier in this chapter are used, but they are applied at the time of the back procedure rather than only when there is a complication. It is difficult if not impossible to define exactly who needs a prophylactic soft-tissue reconstruction of the back. Patients with previous hardware infections, a woody feel to the soft tissues at the time of surgery, prior back surgery, long reconstructions greater than six vertebral bodies, CSF leaks, and a history of radiation to the area all seem to be appropriate candidates for soft-tissue reconstruction. However, should one prior surgery of the back require flap dissection and muscle mobilization? What about a reconstruction that is seven vertebral bodies in length in a patient who has not previously undergone a procedure? Should a remote history of a CSF leak require a prophylactic flap? Each muscle mobilization can only be performed once, and subsequently a different reconstruction would be required if there was an additional complication. At tertiary medical centers, if one includes long reconstructions in patients with prior surgeries or radiation, then practically every closure would involve plastic surgery.

Studies making the case for plastic surgery closures have compared historical wound complication rates to wound rates after muscle flaps. The entire field of spine surgery has evolved over the last decade, and historical comparisons are in all likelihood not accurate. Front and back stabilizations of the spine are more infrequent than, in the past, with shorter surgeries and less stress on the patient. Better instrumentation and the use of bone morphogenetic protein have improved the bone fusion rates, allowing subtle alterations in spine technique. The skill of the plastic surgeon in performing a standard soft-tissue closure is also not factored into the equation when considering the expected wound rate of a subpopulation of problematic patients are closed in standard fashion by spine surgeons. In an ideal world, every patient should have a closure by plastic surgery to potentially decrease complication rates. In the real world, with schedules and desires for simplicity and cost containment, a more limited number of patients should receive a prophylactic closure. In our center we limit prophylactic closures to patients with prior infections, muscles that will not close in the midline due to tissue loss or prior surgery, a history of radiation and a woody feel to the tissues, and CSF leaks (Figs. 11.26–11.28). Spine surgeons and plastic surgeons that work together frequently as a team will find a "comfort zone" to consult for possible closures neither too often, nor too late.

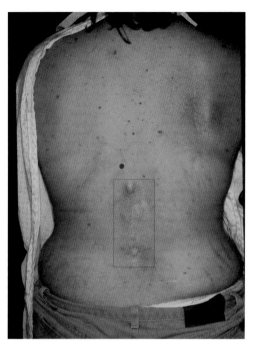

Fig. 11.26 This patient, with previous back surgery, radiation, a long planned fusion length, and a wide woody feel to the soft tissues, should have a planned prophylactic flap closure. She underwent closure with a pedicled omental flap.

Chronic hardware exposures

Chronic hardware exposures act differently from acute exposures and are arbitrarily defined as an exposure occurring more than 6 months after placement. From experience, long-term coverage of chronically exposed hardware is not successful. A hardware infection is likely to be present in patients

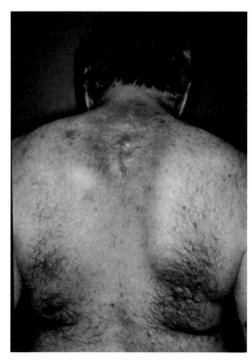

Fig. 11.27 This man has a wide radiated defect and a prior laminectomy. A long fusion is planned.

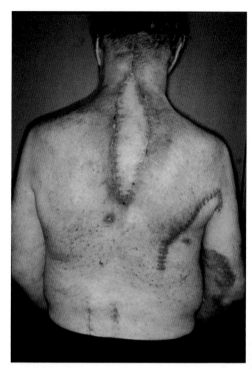

Fig. 11.28 The midline tissue was completely replaced with a free myocutaneous latissimus flap. A long cephalic vein graft loop was fashioned with inflow taken off the external carotid artery. Prophylactic flaps require a high level of coordination between spine and plastic surgery teams.

presenting with small areas of drainage where on palpation a piece of hardware can be reached. Similarly, patients with fluid collections or "fluid cysts" in association with hardware have chronic infections. These infections can be present for months or years without suppurating or making the patient overly ill, which is undoubtedly due to the low virulence of the organism, such as *Staphylococcus epidermidis*.

Debridement, irrigation, and soft-tissue coverage of these chronic exposures may be initially successful, but eventually fail. Perhaps these procedures can buy enough time for the spine to achieve clinical and radiographic evidence of fusion. However, for most patients the involved hardware should be removed. The question is: should all of the hardware be removed, or just a local portion (such as a large bolt) and the soft tissues closed (Fig. 11.29A–D)? These are decisions made in the operating room. All hardware in association with exudative fluid should be removed, and well-incorporated hardware encased in bone should be allowed to remain. No flaps are typically required for closure when all of the hardware is removed as outcomes depend more on the structural stability of the spine than on any soft-tissue work. The soft tissues are simply approximated over drains, and complete healing is the rule rather than the exception. Antibiotics are not needed for prolonged periods in these situations.

Esophageal fistula after spine procedures

A brief mention of this spine related soft-tissue complication is made, despite the wound being on the anterior surface of the torso rather than the posterior surface. A small number of patients undergoing cervical spine fusion will suffer a traumatic injury to the esophagus, causing drainage and

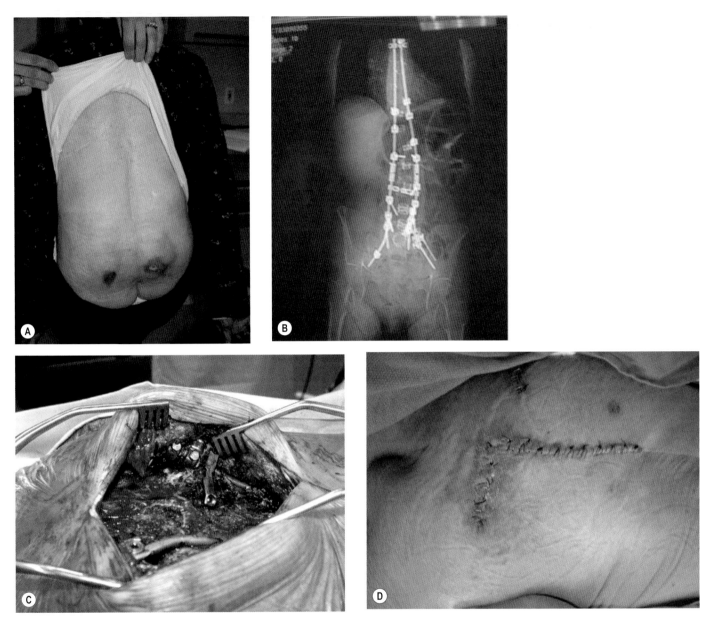

Fig. 11.29 (A) Patient over 1 year after thoracosacral fusion with bilateral lower back wounds. Large pelvic rim bolts are palpable from within the wound. The patient has not achieved clinical and radiographic evidence of fusion. **(B)** Radiograph of construct. **(C)** Large bolts from the hardware to the posterior iliac crest are visible with minimal soft-tissue cover. No purulence is noted around more superior hardware. **(D)** The bolts were excised and the superior hardware was allowed to remain in place with a good long-term result.

contamination of the fusion site.[22] Another group of patients will develop a pressure sore of the cervical spine hardware into the esophagus, and so the hardware can be seen during an esophagoscopy. Everything depends on the timing of the esophageal leak with the placement of the hardware. If the esophageal injury occurred at the time of hardware placement, then the spinal fusion is not solid, and the hardware is still needed. Simple repair of the esophageal defect is problematic even without the spine issues, as the standard treatment by otolaryngology is to drain fluid collections and let the wounds heal by secondary intention. Improvement of the soft tissues between the spinal hardware and the cervical esophageal repair is important. Local flaps from the neck, the pectoralis flap, and omental free flaps are all thin flaps that

can be interposed into this space. The omentum is perhaps best able to deal with the contaminated drainage, and it easily conforms to the space crevices. Incisions on both sides of the neck facilitate bringing of the flap completely across the anterior body of the cervical spine. However, this would simultaneously put both recurrent laryngeal nerves at risk. Pectoralis flaps are perhaps best avoided in spinal cord patients that use their accessory chest muscles to breathe. Gastrostomy tubes obviate the need to eat in the postoperative period and are extremely helpful. Even more rarely, the esophageal leak requires removal of the previously placed construct used to fuse the anterior vertebral bodies. A short fibular free flap "press-fit" into the defect can be used in this situation to achieve fusion, but to stay completely autogenous in the reconstruction. A longer fusion of the posterior spine is required for these cases so that neck movement will not cause the free fibula flap to extrude anteriorly. The microvascular surgeon used to head and neck reconstructions for cancer will be frustrated in these cases by the lack of neck movement for positioning and the soft tissues of the neck (that did not have a lymphadenectomy) that limit exposure.

Patients that develop pressure sores of the hardware into the cervical esophagus are often found months after the cervical fusion, and the hardware can often be removed. Repair of the esophagus if possible and interposition of the soft-tissue flap is much easier in the absence of hardware and when the bone is fused.

Bonus content for this chapter can be found online at
http://www.expertconsult.com

Special Clinical Considerations
"Tethered cord surgery" or "lipomas of the spine".
Pseudomeningocele repair and cerebrospinal fluid leaks.
Fig. 11.30 (A) This 45-year-old female had a lipoma resected from her spinal cord in infancy. Now, she has a recurrent "lipoma" and symptoms of a tethered spinal cord. **(B)** The dura is entered and the spinal cord dissected from scar tissue, holding it inferiorly. A dural patch is constructed. A temporary lumbar drain is visible and is used to keep cerebrospinal fluid pressure low in the immediate postoperative period. **(C)** A superior gluteal artery perforator flap is placed over the dural repair. The tissue of the flap is taken from the right buttock in this case, and near the trochanter.

Access the complete reference list online at **http://www.expertconsult.com**

1. Dumanian GA, Ondra SL, Liu J, et al. Muscle flap salvage of spine wounds with soft tissue defects or infection. *Spine.* 2003;28:1203–1211. *Long-term results of successful salvage of posterior hardware with soft-tissue reconstruction of the back is presented.*

2. Wilhelmi BJ, Snyder N, Colquhoun T, et al. Bipedicle paraspinous muscle flaps for spinal wound closure: an anatomic and clinical study. *Plast Reconstr Surg.* 2000;106:1305–1311. *This is an early description of paraspinous muscle flaps for repair of soft-tissue defects after spine surgery.*

6. Nojima K, Brown SA, Acikel C, et al. Defining vascular supply and territory of thinned perforator flaps: part II. Superior gluteal artery perforator flap. *Plast Reconstr Surg.* 2006;118:1338–1348. *This paper illustrates the performance of superior gluteal artery flaps that can then be used for spine reconstruction.*

7. O'Shaughnessy BA, Dumanian GA, Liu JC, et al. Pedicled omental flaps as an adjunct in complex spine surgery. *Spine.* 2007;32:3074–3080. *Small series illustrating the use of pedicled omental flaps in spine reconstruction surgery.*

14. Lee MJ, Ondra SL, Mindea SA, et al. Indications and rationale for use of vascularized fibula bone flaps in cervical spine arthrodeses. *Plast Reconstr Surg.* 2005;116:1–7.

15. Erdmann D, Meade RA, Lins RE, et al. Use of the microvascular free fibula transfer as a salvage reconstruction for failed anterior spine surgery due to chronic osteomyelitis. *Plast Reconstr Surg.* 2006;117:2438.

16. Said HK, O'Shaughnessy BA, Ondra SL, et al. Integrated titanium and vascular bone: a new approach for high risk thoracic spine reconstruction: P34. *Plast Reconstr Surg.* 2005;116:160–162.

17. Mathes DW, Thornton JF, Rohrich RJ. Management of posterior trunk defects. *Plast Reconstr Surg.* 2006;118:73e–83e.

18. Mitra A, Mitra A, Harlin S. Treatment of massive thoracolumbar wounds and vertebral osteomyelitis following scoliosis surgery. *Plast Reconstr Surg.* 2004;113:206–213.

20. Glass BS, Disa JJ, Mehrara BJ, et al. Reconstruction of extensive partial or total sacrectomy defects with a transabdominal vertical rectus abdominis myocutaneous flap. *Ann Plast Surg.* 2006;56:526–530.

21. Garvey PB, Rhines LD, Dong W, Chang DW. Immediate soft-tissue reconstruction for complex defects of the spine following surgery for spinal neoplasms. *Plast Reconstr Surg.* 2010;125:1460–1466. *Large series of prophylactic flaps from the MD Anderson group demonstrates improved outcomes.*

23. Duffy FJ, Weprin BE, Swift DM. A new approach to closure of large lumbosacral myelomeningoceles: the superior gluteal artery perforator flap. *Plast Reconstr Surg.* 2004;114:1864–1868.

12

Abdominal wall reconstruction

Mark W. Clemens II and Charles E. Butler

 Access video content for this chapter online at expertconsult.com

SYNOPSIS

- Defects due to failed laparotomy closures, tumor ablation, congenital anomalies, and trauma are the most common indications for abdominal wall reconstruction (AWR).

- Ventral hernias can be the result of a genetic predisposition in impaired collagen formation or due to acquired structural collagen abnormalities from mechanical strain and predisposing risk factors, such as tobacco use, diabetes, and obesity.

- Direct suture repair of ventral hernia defects results in an extremely high rate of recurrence compared with mesh reinforcement of similar hernia defects.

- Tissue-based bioprosthetic mesh has gained popularity for its use in complex AWRs due to the lower rates of mesh infection, fistula formation, and mesh explantation than the rates reported with synthetic mesh.

- Successful surgical techniques require complete fascial coaptation, inset of mesh under physiologic tension, judicious use of drainage catheters, and reduction of subcutaneous dead space with quilting sutures.

- Adjunctive reconstructive techniques such as components separation with musculofascial advancement flaps, pedicled muscle flaps, and free flaps are important for assisting in fascial closure and soft-tissue coverage of large abdominal wall defects.

 Access the Historical Perspective section online at
http://www.expertconsult.com

Introduction

The principle goal of reconstructive surgery is to restore form and function, and ideally to restore "like with like". For the abdominal wall, this maxim dictates that reconstructive surgeons must anatomically repair abdominal defects by re-establishing the integrity of the myofascial layer, protecting abdominal viscera, providing durable cutaneous coverage, and minimizing the risk of hernia recurrence (i.e., restoring form and function). In the United States, there are an estimated four million laparotomies performed annually carrying a 2–30% incidence of incisional hernia, which produces roughly 150 000–250 000 ventral hernias.[1] This equates to a cost of approximately $2 billion dollars, which is at a time when healthcare is transitioning toward value-based reimbursement and pay for performance concepts, and where efficiency and cost containment are prioritized with little tolerance for complications.[2] There have been three quantum advances in abdominal wall reconstruction over the past year 25 years that define the field. The first development was the surgical technique of components separation as described by Ramirez *et al.* in 1990.[3] Creation of musculofascial flaps with medialization of the rectus complexes allowed for complete midline fascial coaptation by releasing the external oblique aponeuroses and posterior rectus sheath bilaterally. The second major advancement was the observation in prospective randomized controlled trials that direct suture repair of ventral hernia defects results in an unacceptably high rate of recurrence compared with mesh reinforcement of repairs.[4] This important concept indicates that restoration of integrity to the abdominal wall is a slow process that requires recuperation and fascial support through a critical remodeling period, and that this is affected by mechanical strain, genetic predisposition in collagen formation, and predisposing risk factors, such as tobacco use, diabetes, nutritional status, and obesity. The third development was the introduction of bioprosthetic mesh to act as a tissue scaffold for collagen deposition as an alternative to synthetic meshes in selected indications. Each of these surgical advances work synergistically to improve durability and resilience, while mitigating complications. This chapter will focus on patient diagnosis, pertinent anatomy, basic aspects of these techniques, postoperative care, and outcomes, as well as adjunctive procedures, such as workhorse flaps, that are essential for reconstructive surgeons.

Basic science/disease process

Indications for abdominal wall reconstruction are multifactorial and include tumor ablation, congenital anomalies, trauma, and iatrogenic complications second to laparotomies. Each indication has an underlying distinct pathophysiology, which must be specifically addressed for successful surgical correction. Hernias of the abdominal wall can result from genetically impaired collagen formation, deposition, organization, or degradation; from wound-healing deficiencies; and from injury, failed laparotomy closures, or failed hernia repairs.[12–14] Decades ago, it was suggested that both primary and recurrent hernias resulted from abnormal collagen metabolism.[15,16] Original proposed risk factors for the development of hernias included tobacco use and a strong family history of hernia, which suggests a genetic predisposition. Subsequently, ratios of type I and type III collagen and tissue metalloprotease expression in patients with inguinal and incisional hernias were studied in an attempt to isolate an etiology.[17] Further studies suggested that mechanical strain on load-bearing tissues can induce secondary changes in tissue fibroblast function that in turn can result in failure of abdominal wall repairs.[18] Although more studies are needed, it is evident that some primary hernias are the result of a genetic predisposition, whereas the rest may be due to acquired structural collagen abnormalities from mechanical strain, with or without associated predisposing risk factors, such as tobacco use, diabetes, advanced age, male sex, sleep apnea, prostatism, and obesity.[19] Factors associated with destruction of the collagen in the lung in chronic obstructive pulmonary disease and emphysema likely result in poor wound healing and increased hernia formation in patients with these diseases.[2] Wound infection is also associated with hernia formation.[20] It has been suggested that the type of suture used during a primary operation affects incisional hernia formation, but there is no conclusive evidence to support this notion.[14] Whether the type of abdominal incision used in the primary surgery influences the occurrence of incisional hernias also remains controversial. A 1995 analysis of 11 publications examining the incidence of ventral hernia formation after various types of abdominal incisions concluded that the risk was 10.5% for midline, 7.5% for transverse, and 2.5% for paramedian incisions.[12] A more recent prospective, randomized trial reported no difference in hernia formation after 1 year when comparing midline and transverse incisions, but did note a higher wound infection rate with transverse incisions.[16]

Given the likely similar rates of incisional hernia formation after transverse and midline incisions, surgeons should plan incisions based solely on the operative exposure desired to safely complete procedures. A factor known to be linked to incisional hernia formation is the manner in which the initial midline myofascial incision is closed. Specifically, animal and human trials have shown that a 4:1 suture to wound length ratio is optimal to reduce wound-related morbidity and incisional hernia formation.[15,17] This suture strategy is often misunderstood; for clarification, it typically involves 5–7 mm fascia bites and 3–4 mm of travel. This "small-stitch" approach results in improved healing and reduced rates of wound infections.

Abdominal wall anatomy

The lateral abdominal wall musculature is composed of three layers, with the fascicles of each muscle directed obliquely at different angles to create a strong envelope for the abdominal contents. Each of the muscles forms an aponeurosis that inserts into the linea alba, a midline structure joining the two sides of the abdominal wall. The external oblique muscle is the most superficial muscle of the lateral abdominal wall. Deep to the external oblique muscle lies the internal oblique muscle. The fibers of the external oblique muscle course from superolateral to inferomedial (as hands in pockets), and those of the internal oblique muscle run perpendicular to the external oblique muscle's fibers. The deepest muscular layer of the abdominal wall is the transversus abdominis muscle; its fibers course horizontally. These three lateral muscles give rise to aponeurotic layers lateral to the rectus abdominis muscle, which contribute to the anterior and posterior layers of the rectus sheath. It is noteworthy that in contradistinction to what is stated in most anatomy books, the transversus abdominis muscle does not insert into the linea semilunaris medially, but instead the transversus abdominis aponeurosis actually forms the posterior rectus sheath and continues as a muscular component laterally in the upper abdomen. This feature is important when considering the technical aspects of a posterior components separation.

The medial extension of the external oblique aponeurosis forms the anterior layer of the rectus sheath. At the midline, the two anterior rectus sheaths form the tendinous linea alba. On either side of the linea alba is a rectus abdominis muscle, the fibers of which course vertically and run the length of the anterior abdominal wall. The width of these muscles averages 5–7 cm in men. Below each rectus muscle lies the posterior layer of the rectus sheath, which also contributes to the linea alba.

Another import anatomic structure of the anterior abdominal wall is the arcuate line, located 3–6 cm below the umbilicus and delineates the point below which the posterior rectus sheath is absent. The arcuate line is composed of the transversalis fascia and peritoneum. Above the arcuate line, the aponeurosis of the internal oblique muscle contributes to both the anterior and posterior rectus sheaths, and the aponeurosis of the transversus abdominis muscle passes posterior to the rectus abdominis muscle to form the posterior rectus sheath as described previously. Below the arcuate line, the internal oblique and transversus abdominis aponeuroses pass completely anterior to the rectus muscle.

The abdominal wall receives the majority of its innervation from the 7th to 12th intercostal nerves and the 1st and 3rd lumbar nerves. These rami provide innervation to the lateral abdominal muscles, the rectus abdominis muscles, and the overlying skin. The nerves traverse the lateral abdominal wall between the transversus abdominis and internal oblique muscles and penetrate the posterior rectus sheath just medial to the linea semilunaris.

The lateral abdominal muscles receive their blood supply from the lower three to four intercostal arteries, the deep circumflex iliac artery, and the lumbar arteries. The rectus abdominis muscles have a more complex blood supply derived from the superior epigastric artery (a terminal branch of the internal mammary artery), the inferior epigastric artery (a branch of the external iliac artery), and the lower intercostal arteries. The superior and inferior epigastric arteries anastomose near the umbilicus. The periumbilical area provides critical myocutaneous perforator vessels that, if preserved, can decrease skin flap necrosis from skin undermining.[21]

Diagnosis/patient presentation

Abdominal wall reconstruction patients have numerous and varied presentations. The most common presentation to reconstructive surgeons is an incisional hernia as sequelae to a previous laparotomy. There are three general indications to repair an incisional hernia: the hernia is symptomatic, causing pain or alterations in the bowel habits; the hernia results in a significant protrusion that affects the patient's quality of life; and the hernia poses a significant risk of bowel obstruction (such as a large hernia with a narrow neck). However, the likely slow continued growth of incisional hernias due to intra-abdominal pressure should also be taken into consideration. In a young patient with a moderate-sized hernia, an initial non-operative approach can result in the need for a more complex reconstruction in the future if the hernia becomes larger and symptomatic. Therefore most surgeons recommend that these hernias be repaired electively when discovered.

Correct diagnosis of abdominal wall defects is critical to proper management. Following appropriate clinical evaluation, imaging studies are a helpful adjunct for detection and diagnosis of abdominal defects and defining the abdominal wall anatomy. Different imaging modalities are available to evaluate abdominal wall defects.[22,23] Computed tomography (CT) allows for visualization of intra-abdominal organs and the abdominal wall, 3D data sets, and multiplanar reformation capabilities. CT scans may assist in detecting bowel obstruction, incarceration, strangulation, and traumatic wall hernias. Magnetic resonance (MR) imaging also permits the detection of abdominal wall hernias though this modality does not usually offer further sensitivity and therefore may be cost prohibitive.[24]

Several classification systems exist that categorize ventral hernias based on complexity, whether they are spontaneous or acquired, or by their location on the abdominal wall (Fig. 12.1). Acquired hernias typically occur after surgical incisions and thus are commonly referred to as incisional hernias. Epigastric hernias occur from the xiphoid process to the umbilicus, umbilical hernias occur at the umbilicus, and hypogastric hernias occur below the umbilicus in the midline. Although not a true hernia, diastasis recti can present clinically as a bulge in the midline. In this condition, the linea alba is stretched, resulting in bulging at the medial margins of the rectus abdominis muscles. There is no fascial ring or true hernia sac. Unless significantly symptomatic, diastasis recti does not generally require surgical reconstruction. In the repair of abdominal wall defects, the surgeon must consider a multitude of factors to identify the appropriate surgical technique to accomplish the reconstructive goals. An individualized approach is required and must take into account the patient's age, comorbidities, physiologic status, defect size, available local tissue, and presence of contamination.

Operative considerations

The goals of ventral hernia repair, regardless of the etiology of the defect, are to re-establish the integrity of the myofascial layer and provide durable cutaneous coverage while minimizing the risk of hernia recurrence. Although it is impossible to restore the abdominal wall to its native state after surgical wounding or to cure patients with hernia of their intrinsic collagenopathies, strategies can be employed to maximize the possibility of a successful outcome in abdominal wall reconstruction. Restoring the layered nature of the abdominal myofascia, the native location of key muscle groups, and the tone and contour of the abdominal wall is often achievable with contemporary surgical maneuvers. The importance of a meticulous dual-layered repair, centralizing the rectus abdominis muscle complexes, and reinforcing the repair with mesh, especially for hernias larger than 4 cm in greatest dimension, cannot be overemphasized.[25]

The description by Ramirez et al. of the surgical technique of component separation (CS) facilitates medicalization of the rectus musculofascia, and thus midline abdominal closure by releasing the external oblique aponeuroses and posterior rectus sheath bilaterally. Although CS will often allow for midline fascial re-approximation, which is the optimal situation, occasionally this will not be possible, particularly for larger hernias, and the myofascial edges will need to be bridged with mesh. Data have shown that defect size reduction, especially if less than 150 cm², will lead to the lowest recurrence rates.[26] All attempts should be made to avoid a bridged mesh repair because there is a clear trend toward higher recurrence rates compared with when the fascia can be re-approximated over a mesh repair.[27] There are several other theoretic advantages to re-approximating the linea alba. If one considers the linea alba as the tendinous insertion of the rectus and oblique muscles and borrows from the concepts of tendon repair, then it seems logical that the physiologic

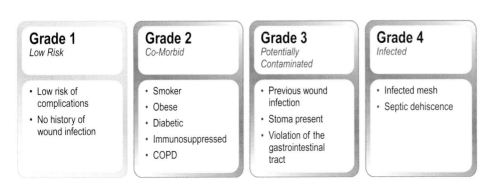

Grade 1 *Low Risk*
- Low risk of complications
- No history of wound infection

Grade 2 *Co-Morbid*
- Smoker
- Obese
- Diabetic
- Immunosuppressed
- COPD

Grade 3 *Potentially Contaminated*
- Previous wound infection
- Stoma present
- Violation of the gastrointestinal tract

Grade 4 *Infected*
- Infected mesh
- Septic dehiscence

Fig. 12.1 Ventral Hernia Working Group's ventral hernia grading scale. COPD, chronic obstructive pulmonary disease. *(From: Ventral Hernia Working Group, Breuing K, Butler CE, Ferzoco S, et al. Incisional ventral hernias: review of the literature and recommendations regarding the grading and technique of repair. Surgery. 2010;148(3):544–558, © Elsevier, 2010.)*

tension of the abdominal wall should be restored during ventral incisional hernia repair. Some authors have evaluated the functional improvement in patients in whom the midline fascia was restored and noted a 40% improvement in the abdominal wall function after repair.[28] Although every attempt to re-establish the midline is advisable, accomplishing that goal is not always feasible, and not all patients can tolerate the intraperitoneal compression required (which can result in intraperitoneal hypertension, pulmonary compromise, or abdominal compartment syndrome). Understanding all of the approaches for abdominal wall reconstruction, and particularly myofascial advancement flaps, is critically important to determining the least invasive procedure to provide a long-lasting repair with an excellent functional outcome for the patient. An understanding of the available reconstructive techniques and an honest assessment of his or her ability to perform each of these techniques should also guide the surgeon in establishing the most appropriate repair for the patient.

Mesh reinforcement of fascial closure is advised for hernia defects larger than 74 cm², even when the myofascia can be closed without tension. Randomized prospective studies have shown significantly lower early and late hernia recurrence rates when mesh is used.[4,29] Mesh materials can be placed in several different configurations: interpositional (mesh edge to the fascial edge), inlay [or sublay] (dorsal to the rectus muscles), or onlay (ventral to the rectus muscles). The interpositional technique has been largely abandoned by most surgeons owing to an unacceptably high hernia recurrence rate. Options for inlay mesh placement include retrorectus (between the rectus abdominis muscles and posterior rectus sheath), preperitoneal (between the posterior rectus sheath and preperitoneal fat), or intraperitoneal. The location of mesh placement plays a critical role in optimizing outcomes. Bridging inlay repairs, in which the mesh edges are sutured to the medial fascial edges of the defect without midline re-approximation, give the poorest outcomes.[27] The location on the abdominal wall to which the mesh is sutured varies between surgeons. Fig. 12.2 depicts the mesh being anchored to the lateral aspect of the released external oblique, internal oblique, and transversus muscles. Many surgeons prefer to anchor the mesh to the lateral aspect of the rectus abdominis musculofascial sheath at the semilunar line. The theoretical advantage is that the semilunar line or lateral rectus sheath is a strong aponeurotic buttress and may reduce the risk of suture pull-through. An advantage of suturing the mesh

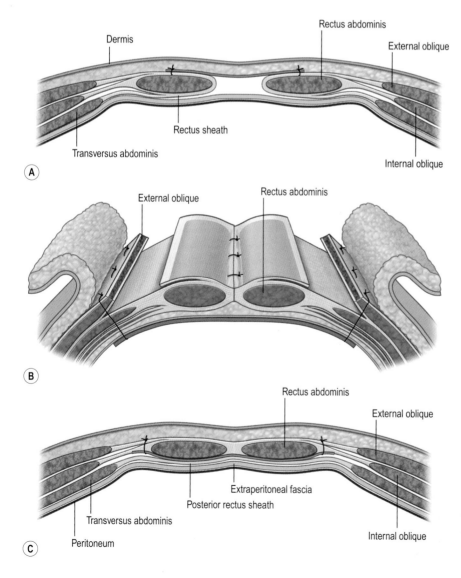

Fig. 12.2 Plane of mesh placement. **(A)** Onlay mesh placement. The mesh is placed superficial to the anterior rectus sheath and the external oblique aponeurosis. **(B)** Intraperitoneal inlay mesh placement. The mesh is placed within the peritoneal cavity deep to the posterior rectus sheath and transversalis fascia laterally. The mesh is anchored laterally, and the anterior rectus sheaths are closed in the midline. **(C)** Above the arcuate line. Retrorectus inlay mesh placement (Rives–Stoppa technique). The mesh is placed within the posterior rectus sheath deep to the rectus abdominis muscle. The mesh is anchored to the linea semilunaris, and the anterior rectus sheaths are closed in the midline.

through the lateral musculature is that there is a greater amount of mesh surface area peripheral to the defect often referred to as a "wide mesh underlay". However, no studies have directly compared these techniques.

Onlay repairs (Fig. 12.2) place the mesh superficial to the anterior rectus sheath and external oblique aponeurosis and re-approximate the fascia over the mesh. The major advantage of this approach is that the mesh is placed outside the abdominal cavity, avoiding direct contact with the abdominal viscera. However, the technique has several disadvantages: a large subcutaneous dissection is required to inset the mesh, which transects skin perforators; there is an increased potential likelihood of seroma formation; the superficial location of the mesh places it in jeopardy of contamination if the incision becomes infected; and a skin wound dehiscence can result in direct external exposure of the mesh. Onlay mesh is usually placed after the fascia is closed in the midline and therefore has little ability to "offload" the fascial tension. In contrast, an inlay mesh inset can be placed with the appropriate physiologic tension to facilitate midline fascial re-approximation as a reinforced, rather than a bridged, repair. In addition, if the midline fascia separates in the early postoperative period, the mesh is often exposed to abdominal viscera. No prospective studies of this technique are available, but a retrospective review reported hernia recurrence rates of 28% with mesh onlay.[30]

Inlay mesh repairs are favorable to overlay repairs because intra-abdominal pressure is distributed against the mesh itself so that tension is spread across the abdominal wall. Inlay mesh placement can be performed in any of three tissue planes: intraperitoneal, retrorectus, and preperitoneal (Fig. 12.2). Mesh should be sutured to the lateral rectus sheath and semilunar line. This location of suture placement can also be used for onlay and inlay techniques. The advantage of the intraperitoneal approach is the avoidance of injury to the posterior sheath and rectus muscle, as well as the fact that concomitant procedures are often performed in the same space (e.g., ostomy takedown or fistula resection). The retrorectus approach has the advantages of being relatively easy to develop (assuming no prior disruptions of this plane) and insulating mesh from the intestines where adhesions may form; this approach also has the theoretical advantage of providing a broad muscle interface with the mesh to facilitate vascularization.[31,32] The preperitoneal approach is a sound option for patients who have a well-developed preperitoneal fat pad, which puts the mesh in direct contact with the posterior sheath.

Regardless of the plane of mesh placement, appropriate tension must be established across the mesh repair. The key is to re-create the physiologic tension across the repair that correlates with the tone of the abdominal wall in a resting state while standing. If excessive tension is placed on the mesh–myofascia suture line, this interface will attenuate and lead to peripheral failure of the mesh repair.

When selecting the appropriate mesh for a patient, the surgeon must consider whether the mesh will be in direct contact with the viscera and whether infection is present or likely. A variety of synthetic mesh products are available for ventral hernia repair. The ideal mesh has not yet been developed but would cause minimal or no inflammatory reaction and be chemically inert, resistant to mechanical stress, sterilizable, non-carcinogenic, hypoallergenic, and reasonably priced.

Each of the commercially available synthetic meshes has some but not all of these properties.

Synthetic mesh materials are classified based on the weight of the material (weight per surface area), pore size, and water angle (hydrophobic or hydrophilic), and whether they include an antiadhesive barrier. When mesh is placed extraperitoneally and there is negligible risk of bowel erosion, a macroporous mesh without an antiadhesive barrier layer is appropriate. Both polypropylene and polyester mesh have been placed successfully in the extraperitoneal position.

Polypropylene mesh is a semirigid, hydrophobic, macroporous mesh that allows for ingrowth of native fibroblasts and incorporation into the surrounding fascia. Placing polypropylene mesh in an intraperitoneal position directly against the bowel is often avoided because of the risk of bowel adhesions to mesh and enterocutaneous fistula formation.[33] Recently, lighter-weight polypropylene mesh has been introduced to address some of the long-term complications of heavyweight polypropylene mesh, particularly adhesions to the bowel. The definition of lightweight polypropylene mesh was arbitrarily set at less than 50 g/m^2, with heavyweight mesh weighing greater than 80 g/m^2. Lightweight mesh products often have an absorbable component that provides initial handling stability; this material is typically composed of polyglactin or poliglecaprone mesh. Whether lightweight rather than heavyweight mesh results in improved patient outcomes is controversial. In a randomized controlled trial evaluating lightweight vs. heavyweight polypropylene mesh for ventral hernia repair, the recurrence rate was more than two times greater in the lightweight mesh group (17% vs. 7% for heavyweight mesh; P=0.05).[34] The use of lightweight polypropylene mesh in the setting of contamination has received renewed interest as a more cost-effective approach than bioprosthetic mesh. Several authors have demonstrated that lightweight polypropylene mesh is relatively resistant to bacterial colonization in experimental models, and small case series have demonstrated safety when utilized in clean-contaminated colorectal cases.[35] Polyester mesh is composed of polyethylene terephthalate and is a heavyweight, hydrophilic, macroporous mesh. Polyester mesh has several different configurations: a 2D flat screen-like mesh, a 3D multifilament weave, and, more recently, a monofilamentous mesh. Uncoated polyester mesh placed directly on the viscera is generally avoided because unacceptable rates of erosion and bowel obstruction have been reported.[36]

For intraperitoneal mesh placement, several options are available. A laminar sheet of mesh with different porosities at different sites and a composite mesh with one side designed to promote tissue ingrowth and the other to resist adhesion formation are available. Laminar mesh is often composed of expanded polytetrafluoroethylene (ePTFE). It has a visceral side that is microporous (3 μm) to resist adhesion formation and an abdominal wall side that is macroporous (17–22 μm) to promote tissue ingrowth. This product differs from other synthetic meshes in that it is flexible and smooth. Some fibroblast proliferation occurs through the pores, but ePTFE has limited fluid permeability. Unlike polypropylene, ePTFE is not incorporated into the native tissue. Encapsulation occurs slowly, and infection can occur during the encapsulation process. When infected, ePTFE mesh almost always requires removal. Polypropylene mesh may be used intra-abdominally so long as the surgeon can ideally separate it from bowel with a tissue interposition such as omentum, hernia sack, or properitoneal tissue. To promote better tissue integration, composite meshes were developed. These products combine the attributes of both polypropylene and ePTFE by layering the two substances. The ePTFE surface serves as a permanent protective interface against the bowel, and the polypropylene side faces the abdominal wall and is macroporous to promote incorporation into the native fascial tissue. Recently, other composite meshes have been developed that combine a macroporous mesh with a temporary absorbable antiadhesive barrier. These mesh materials are made of heavyweight or lightweight polypropylene or polyester and an absorbable barrier typically composed of oxidized regenerated cellulose, hyaluronic acid, omega-3 fatty acids, or collagen hydrogels. Studies in small animals have validated the antiadhesive properties of these barriers, but currently no human trials exist evaluating the ability of these composite materials to resist adhesion formation. When used intra-abdominally, polypropylene mesh can be separated from bowel by interposing soft tissues such as omentum, hernia sac, or properitoneal tissue.

Bioprosthetic meshes are reported to have certain advantages over synthetic meshes because of their potential ability to resist infection and remodel over time, leaving behind host cells and native regenerated collagen. Animal studies have demonstrated a marked reduction in the strength and surface area of adhesions with the use of acellular dermal matrices (ADMs) compared with polypropylene mesh.[37–39] Animal studies have demonstrated rapid host cell and vascular infiltration into ADMs used for hernia repair. These properties are believed to reduce the risk of bacterial infection and potentially allow ADMs to be used in contaminated hernia repairs with a lower risk of infection.[40] Several bioprosthetic meshes are commercially available for abdominal wall reconstruction and are categorized based on the source material (porcine or bovine), processing technique (cross-linked or non-cross-linked), and sterilization technique (gamma radiation, ethylene oxide gas sterilization, or non-sterilized). These products are composed mostly of acellular collagen and theoretically provide a matrix for neovascularization and native collagen deposition. The use of human ADMs has largely been abandoned within abdominal wall reconstruction due to unacceptable long-term elasticity particularly when used in a bridging technique.[41] Bioprosthetic meshes function best when utilized as a fascial reinforcement rather than a bridge or interposition graft.[42] A recent meta-analysis evaluated outcomes with mesh positions in abdominal wall repair.[43] The investigators noted hernia recurrence rates were highest for onlay (17%) placement compared to either underlay (7%) or retrorectus (5%). Seroma rates were lowest following a retrorectus repair (4%). They postulated that this advantage might be due to the improved local blood supply afforded by the retrorectus position; however, larger prospective randomized studies are necessary to confirm these findings. Few data are currently available to assess the long-term durability of bioprosthetic meshes, and no randomized trials have been performed to compare the performance of different bioprosthetic meshes. Furthermore, no data exist directly comparing the outcomes of bioprosthetic mesh vs. synthetic mesh in a clean or clean-contaminated field. Currently, these grafts appear to tolerate placement in a clean-contaminated field, but their long-term durability and role in hernia recurrence are largely unknown. Although bioprosthetic meshes are much more expensive than synthetic meshes, the long-term cost-effectiveness of these materials, particularly in contaminated cases, may be better. More recently, newer bioabsorbable protein meshes that do not biodegrade for several months (unlike polylactic acid-based mesh) have been introduced and proposed as less costly alternatives to bioprosthetic meshes.[44] However, further studies are required before the exact place of these new materials in the armamentarium of the abdominal wall hernia surgeon can be determined.

Surgical technique

Ventral hernia repair proceeds through a previously established midline incision and occurs following adequate adhesiolysis when fascial edges are clearly defined. Mesh is sized to extend at least 4 cm peripheral to the myofascial defect edge and is secured to the musculofascia with permanent interrupted mattress sutures. Intraperitoneal mesh placement may be in direct contact with the abdominal contents if insufficient greater omentum is available to interpose between the mesh and the viscera. It is therefore important to place the sutures close together and tie sutures under direct visualization to prevent entrapment of a loop of intestines. Another technical challenge with this approach is to avoid buckling of the mesh once the midline fascia is approximated. If the midline is going to be approximated, the surgeon can measure the amount of fascial overlap on both sides and inset the mesh appropriately. Ideally, once the mesh is inserted peripherally the midline fascia will be re-approximated, and the mesh and its inset will bear the majority of the tension.

The laparoscopic approach for intraperitoneal mesh placement relies on the same principles as the open technique. Trocars are placed as far laterally as feasible based on the size and location of the hernia. Once the hernia contents are reduced and adhesions are lysed, the defect is measured intraperitoneally and an appropriately sized piece of barrier-coated mesh is fashioned with at least 4 cm of overlap around the defect. The mesh is rolled, placed into the abdomen, and deployed. It is secured to the anterior abdominal wall with preplaced mattress sutures that are passed through separate incisions, and tacking staples are placed between these sutures to secure the mesh 4 cm beyond the defect. The laparoscopic approach offers a significant reduction in postoperative wound morbidity by avoiding subcutaneous tissue dissection. Postoperative pain, however, is often similar to that with an open procedure, and in thin patients a perceptible postoperative bulge may be present.

Mesh can be placed extraperitoneally in either the preperitoneal space or retrorectus position (Fig. 12.2). This technique was initially described by Rives and Stoppa.[31,32] A large piece of mesh is placed ventral to the posterior rectus sheath or peritoneum. This space must first be dissected laterally on both sides of the linea alba to the linea semilunaris. The linea semilunaris is identified by the presence of the intercostal nerves perforating the lateral border of the rectus muscle, as well as the lateral reflection of the posterior sheath as it transitions to the anterior sheath. These neurovascular bundles must be maintained as they provide segmental innervation to the rectus complex. The mesh extends 5–6 cm beyond the superior and inferior borders of the defect. Sutures should be placed under physiologic tension to help medialize the rectus abdominis muscles and prevent buckling of the mesh during midline fascial re-approximation. This approach avoids contact between the mesh and the abdominal viscera. A retrospective review from the Mayo Clinic with a median follow-up of 5 years documented a 5% overall hernia recurrence rate in 254 patients undergoing complex ventral hernia repair over a 13-year period.[45]

Myofascial advancement flaps (Video 12.1 ⏵)

For defects that are too wide to close without undue tension, myofascial release and advancement can be performed. These concepts were originally described by Stoppa and Ramirez, and several modifications have been reported.[46] Myofascial advancement techniques, or components separation, take advantage of the laminar nature of the abdominal wall and the ability to release one muscular or fascial layer to enable medial advancement of another. There are few comparative data to suggest the superiority of one myofascial advancement approach over another, and likely each has a role in abdominal wall reconstruction. If the lateral abdominal compartment must be released, then this can be achieved by open or minimally invasive CS. A minimally invasive CS can be performed various ways, but all of the techniques (to a certain degree) maintain the blood supply to the skin from the underlying rectus abdominis muscles. In contrast, an open CS is performed by raising large subcutaneous flaps to expose the external oblique fascia. The cutaneous perforators emerging from the anterior rectus sheath are ligated and divided to facilitate exposure of the linea semilunaris in its entirety. These flaps are carried laterally past the linea semilunaris. This subcutaneous dissection itself can provide some medial advancement of the abdominal wall skin (Fig. 12.3).

An anatomically precise external oblique aponeurotomy is made 1–2 cm lateral to the linea semilunaris on the lateral aspect of the external oblique aponeurosis from several centimeters above the costal margin to the pubis. It is important to confirm that the incision is not carried through the linea semilunaris, as this would result in a full-thickness defect of the lateral abdominal wall, which is very challenging to repair. The external oblique aponeurosis is then bluntly separated in the avascular plane away from the internal oblique aponeurosis to the midaxillary line, allowing the internal oblique and transversus abdominis muscles with the rectus abdominis muscle or fascia to advance medially as a unit. These techniques, when performed bilaterally, can yield up to 20 cm of mobilization in the midabdomen.

Once the mesh inset and fascial closure are performed, the subcutaneous skin flaps are advanced and closed at the midline. To reduce subcutaneous dead space, interrupted quilting sutures should be placed between the Scarpa fascia and musculofascial repair.[47] This technique also decreases

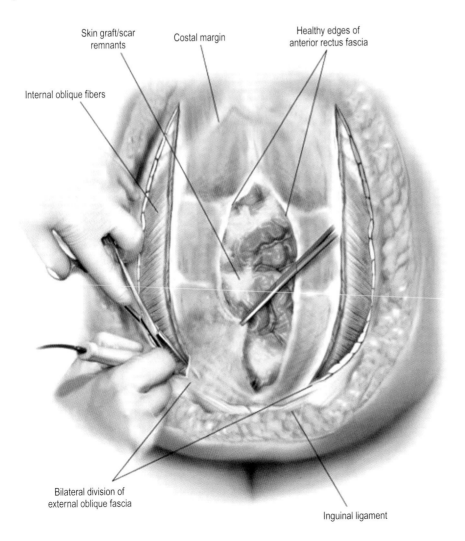

Skin graft/scar remnants

Costal margin

Healthy edges of anterior rectus fascia

Internal oblique fibers

Bilateral division of external oblique fascia

Inguinal ligament

Fig. 12.3 Open component separation. Subcutaneous flaps are elevated off the anterior rectus sheath to expose the external oblique aponeurosis. The external oblique aponeurosis is released from the inguinal ligament inferiorly to above the costal margin superiorly. This allows exposure of the internal oblique muscle fibers once the external aponeurosis is incised. *(From: Rosen M. Atlas of Abdominal Wall Reconstruction, pp. 15–195. © Elsevier, 2012.)*

shear stress, which is thought to contribute to postoperative seroma formation, and decrease the total drain output, allowing the surgeon to place fewer drains and leave them in for a shorter period. After paramedian skin perfusion is critically assessed, a vertical panniculectomy is performed so that the skin is re-approximated in the midline without redundancy.

Open CS often allows tension-free closure of large defects, and recurrence rates as low as 20% have been reported with the use of open CS and mesh reinforcement in large hernias.[48] Recognizing the high recurrence rates with CS alone, several authors have reported series of bioprosthetic or synthetic mesh reinforcement of these repairs; although to date, no randomized controlled trials have demonstrated lower hernia recurrence rates with a specific mesh type. If bioprosthetic mesh is placed, it can be secured in either an underlay or onlay technique; no comparative data exist demonstrating the superiority of either technique. A major limitation of open CS is the wound morbidity associated with the large skin flaps necessary to access the lateral abdominal wall. To avoid this morbidity, several manuscripts have described innovative minimally invasive approaches to CS.[49,50] These approaches are designed to gain direct access to the lateral abdominal wall without creating large skin flaps, creating dead space, or interrupting the primary blood supply to the central abdominal skin by ligation of the rectus abdominis perforator vessels. Laparoscopically, CS is performed through a 1 cm incision below the tip of the 11th rib overlying the external oblique muscle (Fig. 12.4).[51] The external oblique muscle is split in the direction of its fibers, and a standard bilateral inguinal hernia balloon dissector is placed between the external and internal oblique muscles and directed toward the pubis. Three laparoscopic trocars are placed in the space created, and the dissection is carried from the pubis to several centimeters above the costal margin. The linea semilunaris is carefully identified, and the external oblique aponeurosis is incised from beneath the external oblique muscle at least 2 cm lateral to the linea semilunaris. The muscle is released from the pubis to several centimeters above the costal margin. This procedure is performed bilaterally. Comparative data have shown laparoscopic CS to result in a lower rate of wound morbidity than open CS.[49]

A periumbilical perforator-sparing technique of CS may be performed to preserve the blood supply to the anterior abdominal wall skin near the midline and is based primarily on perforator vessels from the deep inferior epigastric vessels. Cadaver dissections and radiographic studies have confirmed that the majority of these vessels are located within 3 cm of the umbilicus.[38] With preservation of these vessels, ischemic complications involving the subcutaneous flaps are significantly reduced.[52] To avoid injury to the periumbilical perforator vessels, a line is marked no less than 3 cm cephalad and 3 cm caudal to the umbilicus. The periumbilical perforator tunnels are begun at the epigastric and suprapubic regions. Subcutaneous tunnels are created using lighted retractors to identify the external oblique fascia. The superior and inferior tunnels are connected using cautery and retractors while maintaining the subcutaneous attachments of the periumbilical region. The linea semilunaris is identified by palpation, and the external oblique is incised 2 cm lateral to this junction. The aponeurotomy is extended several centimeters above the costal margin and to the pubic tubercle. The external oblique muscle is separated from the internal oblique muscle in an avascular plane toward the posterior axillary line. One series reported a significant reduction in wound morbidity with the periumbilical perforator-sparing technique compared with the standard open CS technique (2% vs. 20%; P<0.05).[53] The periumbilical perforator-sparing approach has several limitations. One of the benefits of minimally invasive CS is to reduce subcutaneous dead space. The periumbilical perforator-sparing technique creates considerable dead space and sacrifices more perforator vessels to the skin than other minimally invasive techniques. When skin mobilization is necessary, adequate advancement occasionally can be difficult to achieve because the midline skin is still invested in the periumbilical region. Additionally, the placement of a wide piece of mesh as an underlay can be difficult given the large subcutaneous paddle that is still attached.

Butler and colleagues modified the standard open Ramirez-style procedure that further reduces the subcutaneous dead space and maximizes the blood supply to the abdominal skin with rectus perforator preservation.[47] The minimally invasive components separation (MICS) technique is designed to avoid division of the musculocutaneous perforators overlying the rectus sheath and thus maintain perfusion to the paramedian skin. After lysis of adhesions and identification of the fascial edges, bilateral, 3 cm wide, subcutaneous access tunnels are created over the anterior rectus sheath from the midline to the linea semilunaris at the level of the costal margin (Fig. 12.5). Through these access tunnels, the external oblique aponeurosis is vertically incised 1.5 cm lateral to the linea semilunaris. The tip of a metal Yankauer suction handle (Cardinal Health, Dublin, OH), without suction, is inserted through the opening in the avascular plane between the internal and the external oblique aponeuroses, separating them at their junction with the rectus sheath. The suction tip is advanced inferiorly to the pubis and superiorly to above the costal margin. A narrow incision of 2.5 cm is made inferiorly. Next, lateral dissection between the internal and the external oblique muscles is performed to the midaxillary line. Minimal subcutaneous skin flaps are then elevated over the anterior rectus sheath circumferentially to the medial row of rectus abdominis perforator vessels, and a retrorectus or preperitoneal mesh inlay is generally used. If a preperitoneal inset is used, the preperitoneal fat is dissected from the posterior sheath circumferentially to allow the mesh to be inlaid directly against the posterior sheath or rectus abdominis muscle (below the arcuate line). Mesh is inserted to the semilunar line with #1 polypropylene sutures via the horizontal access tunnels and the cranial and caudal aspect of the defect. Next, the myofascial edges are advanced and re-approximated over the mesh with sutures placed through the myofascia and mesh. Interrupted resorbable 3-0 sutures are placed to affix the posterior sheath to the mesh, thereby obliterating dead space and reducing the potential for fluid collection. Closed-suction drainage catheters are placed in each CS donor site area, in the space between the rectus complex closure and mesh, and in the subcutaneous space. The remaining undermined skin flaps are sutured to the myofascia with vertical rows of interrupted resorbable 3-0 quilting sutures to reduce dead space and potential shear between the subcutaneous tissue and myofascia. A controlled study demonstrated that patients had significantly fewer wound-healing complications (32% vs. 14%, P=0.026) and skin dehiscences (28% vs. 11%, P=0.01) with MICS than with traditional open CS.[47] These improved wound-healing outcomes are likely due

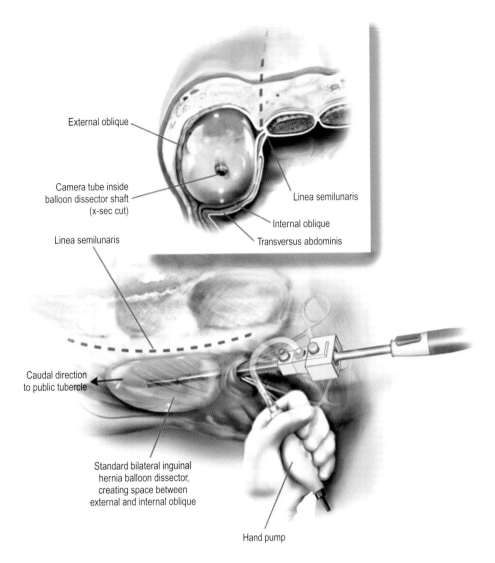

External oblique

Camera tube inside
balloon dissector shaft
(x-sec cut)

Linea semilunaris

Linea semilunaris

Internal oblique

Transversus abdominis

Caudal direction
to public tubercle

Standard bilateral inguinal
hernia balloon dissector,
creating space between
external and internal oblique

Hand pump

Fig. 12.4 Endoscopic component separation.
Access to the external oblique aponeurosis is
achieved through a small incision at the costal
margin through which a balloon dissector is
placed. The external oblique aponeurosis is then
divided from the pubis to above the costal margin.
This minimally invasive approach preserves the
attachments of the subcutaneous tissue (including
myocutaneous perforators) to the anterior rectus
sheath throughout its course. *(From: Rosen M.
Atlas of Abdominal Wall Reconstruction,
pp. 15–195. © Elsevier, 2012.)*

to the preservation of the vascularity of the overlying skin
flaps and reduction of paramedian dead space – the surgical
principles underlying the MICS procedure.

A posterior CS is based on the retromuscular Rives–Stoppa
approach to ventral hernia repair. Unlike the Ramirez CS
focusing on external oblique aponeurosis release, the posterior
CS focuses on transversus abdominis aponeurosis release. As
previously mentioned, the transversus abdominis aponeurosis
actually forms the posterior rectus sheath in the upper two-
thirds of the abdomen. By incising this myofascial aponeurosis,
the surgeon accesses the preperitoneal space. This provides
substantial advancement of both the posterior fascial flap and
the anterior myofascial compartment. The initial release is
completed by incising the posterior rectus sheath approximately 1 cm lateral to the linea alba, and the posterior rectus
sheath is separated from the overlying rectus muscle (Fig.
12.6). The transversus abdominis muscle is incised just medial
to the intercostal nerves, and the underlying transversalis
fascia and peritoneum are identified. This myofascial release
is extended the entire length of the posterior rectus sheath
(Fig. 12.6B). The potential space between the transversus

abdominis muscle and the peritoneum is developed as far
laterally as necessary, even to the psoas muscle if needed. This
plane can be extended superiorly to the costal margin,
retrosternally above the xiphoid, and inferiorly into the space
of Retzius. The posterior sheath is then closed, to completely
exclude any mesh from the viscera. An adequately sized piece
of mesh is then secured, similar to a standard retromuscular
repair, but with greater overlap. The midline is then
re-approximated. In a recent comparative review of open
anterior CS with posterior CS for complex abdominal wall
reconstruction, Krpata *et al.* reported similar fascial advancement but a 50% reduction in wound morbidity with the
posterior approach when compared to an anterior CS.[54]

Postoperative care

In general, abdominal wall reconstruction patients have prolonged postoperative healing periods due to the dynamic
function and mobility of the abdominal musculature. Based
upon specific unique indications, each patient's postoperative

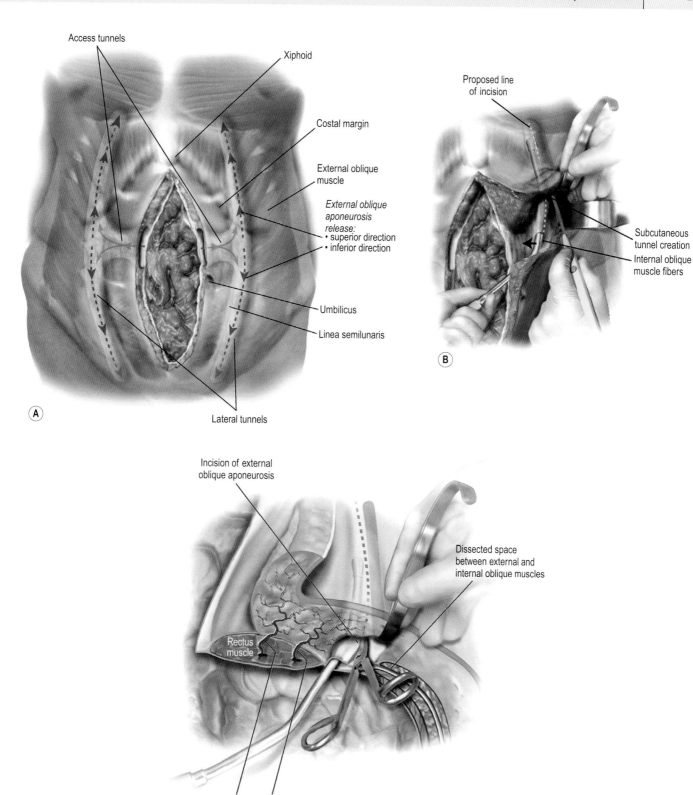

Access tunnels

Xiphoid

Costal margin

External oblique muscle

External oblique aponeurosis release:
• superior direction
• inferior direction

Umbilicus

Linea semilunaris

(A)

Lateral tunnels

Proposed line of incision

Subcutaneous tunnel creation

Internal oblique muscle fibers

(B)

Incision of external oblique aponeurosis

Dissected space between external and internal oblique muscles

Rectus muscle

(C) Intact medial and lateral row musculocutaneous perforators

Fig. 12.5 Minimally invasive component separation (MICS) technique. **(A)** Access to the external oblique aponeurosis is achieved through a small tunnel from the midline to the supraumbilical external oblique aponeurosis. Vertical tunnels are created dorsal and ventral to the planned release site of the external oblique aponeurosis. Periumbilical perforators and the subcutaneous tissue overlying the anterior rectus sheath are left undisturbed. **(B)** The external oblique aponeurosis is then divided from the pubis to above the costal margin. The external oblique aponeurosis in the upper abdomen is released with electrocautery as muscle is transected at, and superior to, the costal margin. **(C)** Scissors are generally used to release the external oblique aponeurosis inferiorly. This MICS approach preserves the attachments of the subcutaneous tissue (including myocutaneous perforators) to the anterior rectus sheath throughout its course. *(From Rosen M. Atlas of Abdominal Wall Reconstruction, pp. 15–195.* © *Elsevier, 2012.)*

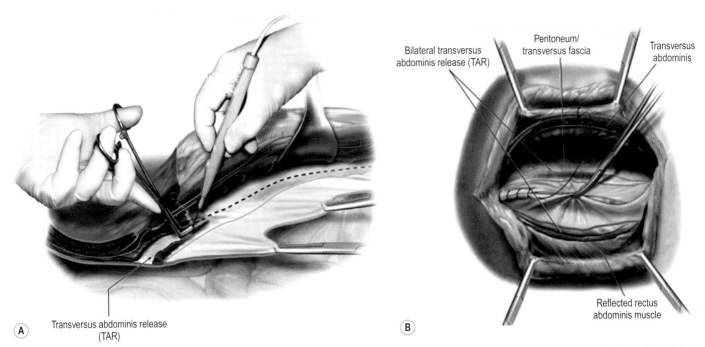

Fig. 12.6 Posterior component separation. **(A)** The initial release is completed by incising the posterior rectus sheath approximately 1 cm lateral to the linea alba, and the posterior rectus sheath is separated from the overlying rectus abdominis muscle. Dissection is carried to the lateral border of the rectus muscle, and the perforating intercostal nerves are identified, marking the linea semilunaris. **(B)** Next, the transversus abdominis muscle is incised just medial to the intercostal nerves, and the underlying transversalis fascia and peritoneum are identified. This myofascial release is extended the entire length of the posterior rectus sheath. The potential space between the transversus abdominis muscle and the peritoneum is developed as far laterally as necessary. *(From Rosen M. Atlas of Abdominal Wall Reconstruction, pp. 15–195.* © *Elsevier, 2012.)*

care regimen should be individually tailored to allow for sufficient healing of the surgical site. Perioperative management of high-risk patients should include appropriate deep venous thrombosis (DVT) chemoprophylaxis according to the Caprini risk score.[55,56] Sequential compression devices and early ambulation should be utilized with low molecular weight fractionated heparins administered postoperatively. Perioperative antibiotics are indicated, and cases with violation of the gastrointestinal tract should be offered broader coverage for anaerobic as well as Gram-negative bacteria. For ventral hernia, closed suction drains are used liberally and are kept in place for an average of 1–2 weeks until there is less than 30 cc per day. Abdominal wall reconstruction patients should refrain from strenuous activities and exercises that isolate the abdominal core for at least 6–12 weeks. Patients may gain comfort from the use on an abdominal binder for 3 months, and then with any expected heavy physical activity thereafter. Routine follow-up includes a physical examination in an outpatient clinic: often performed weekly for 1 month after discharge, then every 3 months for 1 year, and then annually thereafter.

Outcomes/prognosis

Given the wide spectrum of patient characteristics and defect complexities, no single approach to abdominal wall reconstruction and in particular ventral hernia repair will be the best choice for all patients, and comparing different approaches is difficult. Estimated incidences of hernia recurrence have a wide range from 2% to 54%, depending on the type of repair

(mesh 2–36% vs. suture repair alone 25–54%), patient comorbidities, and surgical technique.[1,2,4,25,29] The number of prior attempts of hernia repair is predictive of the relative risk of recurrence. In a study of approximately 10000 patients, 5-year re-operative rate was 23.8% after a primary repair, 35.3% following a secondary repair, and 38.7% after a tertiary repair.[57]

There is no standard nomenclature system to accurately stratify ventral or incisional hernias. This has led to the use of poorly defined, confusing terms such as "complex ventral hernia repair", "large defects", and "loss of abdominal domain". Recently, a group of ventral hernia surgeons (the Ventral Hernia Working Group, VHWG) attempted to develop a classification system for ventral or incisional hernias.[25] The resulting grading system takes into account underlying patient comorbidities and the presence of wound contamination during the repair (Fig. 12.1). In the VHWG system, grade 1 includes hernias in patients with a low risk of complications and no history of wound infection. Grade 2 includes hernias in patients who smoke or have chronic obstructive pulmonary disease, and are obese, diabetic, or immunosuppressed. Grade 3 includes hernias in patients with a previous wound infection, a stoma, or violation of the gastrointestinal tract (i.e., hernias in potentially contaminated surgical fields). Finally, grade 4 includes hernias in patients with infected mesh or septic dehiscence of their wound. Based on this classification system, the VHWG recommended the use of synthetic mesh for grade 1 hernias and bioprosthetic mesh for grades 3 and 4. No consensus recommendations were made for grade 2 hernias. This grading system represents an important first step in developing a classification system to improve reporting and allow appropriate comparative studies to be performed. However, this grading system has not yet been validated in a large patient cohort, and further studies are necessary to validate these results.

Two recent systematic reviews of the use of ADMs in abdominal wall reconstruction have echoed the difficulty of direct comparisons between study results because of differences in patient variables, techniques, nomenclature, and definitions of outcomes.[58,59] The conclusions of these reviews were that there is no consensus on risk factors predicting recurrence or wound morbidity, there is limited consensus on terminology for defect characteristics, and there is no consensus on terminology for outcomes. Clearly, grading systems, such as those described earlier, and the need to accurately assess and report outcomes will be drivers for future studies from multiple institutions and authors that will help define the role of ADMs in AWR.

Several small series with short follow-up have compared the results of laparoscopic ventral hernia repair to those of open ventral hernia repair. A randomized trial by the Veterans Administration compared laparoscopic and open ventral hernia repairs in 146 patients.[60] This series had several important methodologic issues that deserve mention when interpreting the results. First, the authors focused on relatively small defects, with the mean defect size in both groups averaging 46 cm^2. Second, the open technique involved an onlay approach in which subcutaneous flaps are created, and the polypropylene mesh is placed above the fascia. Finally, the mesh placement included only 3 cm of fascial overlap. The authors reported a significantly higher wound morbidity rate with the open approach (23%) than with the laparoscopic technique (6%, odds ratio [OR], 0.2; 95%, confidence interval [CI], 0.1–0.6). Overall recurrence rates were similar in the two groups (8.2% open vs. 12.5% laparoscopic; P=0.44). Although the overall complication rate was lower in the laparoscopic group, the incidence of severe or major complications was higher in the laparoscopic group. Most notably, the rate of enterotomy was higher in the laparoscopic group (4.1%) than in the open group (0%). In general, the laparoscopic approach to ventral hernia repair is a good technique for obese patients or elderly patients with small to medium defects (up to 10 cm wide) in which the morbidity of extensive skin flaps and soft-tissue dissection can be avoided. However, in patients who have severe adhesions or have undergone multiple abdominal surgeries or both, the surgeon should exercise caution when performing adhesiolysis laparoscopically and have a low threshold for conversion to an open approach to avoid bowel injury.

Complications

Infections

Surgical site infections are common after open ventral hernia repair, although the exact incidence is difficult to determine as most series poorly define this outcome variable. Categorization of the intraoperative level of wound contamination, based on the US Centers for Disease Control and Prevention (CDC) criteria, into clean, clean-contaminated, contaminated, and dirty wounds is important to appropriately stratify patients by risk of surgical site infection. Mesh infections are one of the most serious complications that can occur after

ventral hernia repair. Mesh infections are reported to occur in 0–3.6% of laparoscopic ventral hernia repairs and 6–10% of open repairs employing mesh.[61] The most common organism infecting mesh is *Staphylococcus aureus*, seen in up to 81% of cases and suggesting skin flora contamination during mesh implantation. However, Gram-negative organisms, such as *Klebsiella* and *Proteus* spp., have been implicated in up to 17% of mesh infections.[59] In some cases, macroporous polypropylene meshes that become infected can be salvaged with local wound measures and antibiotics and do not require removal. Several reports suggest that lighter-weight polypropylene mesh might be safe in clean-contaminated environments.[62] However, microporous ePTFE mesh does not tolerate infection and almost always requires excision.[63,64]

Seroma

Seroma formation can occur after laparoscopic or open ventral hernia repair. During routine laparoscopic ventral hernia repair, the hernia sac is often not excised; in such cases, a seroma is frequently present postoperatively. It is important to counsel patients so that they are not surprised. In most cases, the seroma will be reabsorbed over time. If symptomatic, the seroma can be aspirated percutaneously. In open ventral hernia repair, drains are often placed in an attempt to obliterate the dead space caused by the hernia and tissue dissection. These drains can cause retrograde bacterial contamination, and seromas can form after drain removal. Long subcutaneous tunnels, meticulous securing of drain exit sites with drain sutures that prevent intussusception of the drain, and meticulous drain exit site wound management using antibiotic impregnated dressings should be utilized to reduce the risk of retrograde bacterial infection. Seroma formation is common after open CS owing to the extensive tissue dissection, and drains may be necessary for up to 4–6 weeks. Intraoperative techniques, such as quilting sutures, fibrin sealant, and postoperative abdominal binders, may help to prevent or reduce seroma formation.[65]

Enterotomy and enterocutaneous fistulas

Unintentional intestinal injury during adhesiolysis can be catastrophic. Appropriate management of an enterotomy during a hernia repair is controversial and depends on the segment of intestine injured (small vs. large bowel) and amount of spillage. Options include aborting the hernia repair, continuing the hernia repair and repairing the enterotomy with local tissue or bioprosthetic mesh using a primary tissue or bioprosthetic mesh repair, or performing a delayed repair using mesh in 3–4 days. When there is gross contamination, the use of synthetic mesh is generally contraindicated. Regardless of the approach taken, it is important that patients understand preoperatively the risk of this complication and how it might alter intraoperative decisions.

The unexpected postoperative appearance of intestinal contents draining through an abdominal surgical incision is a devastating event for the patient and the surgical team. The treatment of patients with enterocutaneous fistulas (ECFs) is complex, and most recommendations are based on expert opinions or single-center retrospective case series.[66] The underlying cause of an ECF has significant implications as to the prognosis for spontaneous closure or need for operative intervention. By definition, an ECF is an abnormal communication between the bowel lumen and the skin. ECFs can be classified based on their anatomy, output, or etiology. The anatomic classification is based on the segment of the intestines that is involved in the fistula: gastrocutaneous, biliocutaneous, enterocutaneous, or colocutaneous. The output classification system is based on the volume of effluent from the fistula: low output (less than 200 mL/day); moderate output (200–500 mL/day); or high output (greater than 500 mL/day). Causes of ECFs include trauma, foreign body, infectious disease, malignancy, and up to 20% of ECFs are related to bowel resection in patients with Crohn's disease.[64] Approximately one-third of ECFs will close spontaneously with appropriate wound care, nutritional support, and medical therapy.[67] Several prognostic factors have been linked to non-healing fistulas. A common mnemonic to describe these factors is FRIENDS of a fistula: foreign body, radiation enteritis, inflammatory bowel disease, epithelialization of the fistula tract, neoplasm, distal obstruction, and ongoing sepsis. With improvements in parenteral nutrition, surgical techniques, and medical care, mortality rates range from 5–25%.[64,65]

There are three phases of ECF management: (1) recognition and stabilization, (2) anatomic definition and decision, and (3) definitive operation. Published guidelines refer to the SOWATS management algorithm: control of sepsis, optimization of nutritional status, wound care, assessment of fistula anatomy, timing of surgery, and surgical strategy.[64] Once a fistula is identified, four factors must be addressed simultaneously: (1) fluid and electrolyte repletion, (2) control of fistula effluent and protection of the surrounding skin, (3) control of infection and drainage of abscesses, and (4) nutritional support. Depending on the location of the fistula along the gastrointestinal tract and the volume of output, significant electrolyte disturbances can occur. In particular, proximal high-output fistulas can result in substantial losses of bicarbonate, which must be adequately replaced. Diligent protection of the surrounding skin is one of the most important and difficult aspects of ECF management. A dedicated enterostomal nurse is essential to the success of wound management as destruction of local skin can seriously affect eventual reconstructive options. In cases in which a fistula is already present, a negative pressure wound therapy (NPWT) device can be helpful to isolate a fistula from the surrounding wound and to allow a skin graft to heal. In cases of uncontrolled intestinal leakage, a proximal diverting stoma can be lifesaving. When a proximal diversion cannot be achieved owing to a foreshortened mesentery or extremely dilated or hostile bowel, appropriate tube drainage can be helpful. Nutritional supplementation is one of the most important aspects of reducing deaths related to ECFs. Nutritional requirements should be adjusted accordingly for patients with proximal high-output fistulas. During initial management of an ECF, parenteral nutritional support is preferred. However, once the sepsis is controlled and the patient is stabilized, enteral feedings are initiated. Enteral feedings preserve the intestinal mucosal barrier, improve immunologic function, and avoid central-line sepsis.

Initially, an abdominopelvic CT study with oral and intravenous contrast is performed. This provides valuable information about undrained collections, bowel length, and the integrity of the anterior abdominal wall. An appropriately performed small bowel X-ray series is also helpful. In conjunction with our radiology team, we perform an initial upper gastrointestinal tract X-ray series with small bowel follow-through using water-soluble contrast material. Next, the fistula is cannulated, and the exact anatomy of the fistula and the remaining small bowel is documented. If necessary, a barium enema is performed to delineate the distal anatomy. In difficult cases, these procedures are performed under endoscopic guidance. Once the entire gastrointestinal tract anatomy is established, a general repair plan for the number of anastomoses, the amount of bowel requiring resection, and the amount of remaining bowel is made. If the fistula output is steadily decreasing and the wound is healing, surgery should be avoided as the fistula might heal spontaneously.[64] The goals of surgical correction of ECFs are to resect the segment of bowel involved in the fistula, re-establish gastrointestinal tract continuity, cover the anastomosis with well-vascularized soft tissue, and provide a stable abdominal wall closure. As the operation is long and difficult, we advocate a two-team approach. The first team is responsible for re-establishing gastrointestinal tract continuity, and the second team performs the abdominal wall reconstruction. An autologous tissue graft or bioprosthetic mesh is preferable to synthetic mesh in this population given the heavy contamination often present as a result of the fistula. Bioprosthetic mesh has been used to bridge the fascial defect in ECF cases with limited success. Although bioprosthetic meshes are very expensive and likely may not prevent a ventral hernia for a long term in these patients, as mentioned, that is not the primary goal of ECF repair. When planning reconstruction of an abdominal wall in the setting of a large hernia defect and a concomitant fistula, it is important to have all of the reconstructive options available and utilize the option that provides the best soft-tissue coverage with the least morbidity for the individual case. In a series of 135 patients with ECFs, Visschers et al.[66] reported successful restoration of gastrointestinal tract continuity in 91% of patients, with a 9.6% mortality rate, despite fairly early surgical repair (mean of 53 days from ECF development). Among 53 patients with concomitant abdominal wall defects, 77% required surgical intervention for closure, and the mortality rate was 15%. Among the 82 patients without an abdominal wall defect, the mortality rate was only 6%. Malnutrition was correlated with failure of surgical closure and increased mortality rates.

Secondary procedures

Composite reconstructions

The goals of abdominal wall reconstruction after full-thickness composite resection are to re-establish the integrity of the myofascial layer and provide external cutaneous coverage. Surgical planning in abdominal wall reconstruction must include accommodating for the loss of both skin and myofascial tissue. Full-thickness loss of the abdominal wall musculofascia and overlying soft tissue – a composite defect – can result from tumor resection, necrotizing soft-tissue infection, or traumatic injury. These clinical scenarios represent the most complicated abdominal wall reconstructions, sometimes requiring multiple staged procedures. Composite defects due to en bloc tumor resection can be repaired at the time of tumor extirpation, provided clear margin status is confirmed. However, composite defects due to necrotizing soft tissue loss or trauma may require serial debridements to control the infectious process, establish the zone of injury, or stabilize the patient before definitive reconstruction of the abdominal wall.

Skin coverage is generally accomplished with local skin advancement and occasionally requires a regional pedicled or free flap with the most common donor site being the thigh or back (Table 12.1). Options for pedicled flaps in the upper abdomen include vertical rectus abdominis muscle flap (VRAM), latissimus dorsi, and omental flaps. Thigh-based flaps, such as anterolateral thigh, vastus lateralis, and tensor fascia lata flaps, are able to reach the lower abdomen and flank as pedicled flaps. If a pedicled flap is not available or feasible, a thoracoepigastric bipedicled fasciocutaneous flap may provide a local tissue alternative and avoid a free tissue transfer. However, when the volume of tissue loss or the arc of rotation needed precludes a pedicled flap transfer, a free flap is required for soft-tissue coverage. The thigh can serve as a source of fasciocutaneous flaps and myocutaneous flaps that provide large skin paddles and significant muscle volume.[68] Recipient vessels in the lateral abdominal wall include the deep inferior epigastric vessels, superior epigastric vessels, internal mammary vessels, intercostal artery perforators, and thoracolumbar perforators. When no local recipient vessels are available, vein grafts to the internal mammary or femoral vessels may be required.

Posterolateral abdominal defects

The anatomic boundaries of the posterior abdominal wall that abut the posterior retroperitoneum include the paraspinous, quadratus lumborum, and iliopsoas muscles. When these muscular layers have been resected, divided, or denervated, their integrity must be restored to prevent a lumbar hernia or bulge.[69] The goal is to support the retroperitoneal viscera and redefine the retroperitoneal reflection to prevent solid organ migration and adrenal or kidney and colon herniation. A true mesh inlay repair may not be feasible owing to the proximity of important neurovascular structures (posteromedial insertion of diaphragm, spine, aorta, and vena cava) to the retroperitoneal defect. In this situation, mesh can be placed in an onlay fashion. When significant dead space exists after reinforcement of the retroperitoneal boundary, a soft-tissue flap can be included to obliterate the dead space and buttress the mesh repair externally. In cases of prior radiation, prior surgery, or excessive skin resection, a pedicled regional or free flap may be required to provide adequate soft-tissue coverage.

Parastomal hernia repair

A parastomal hernia is an incisional hernia defect at the site where the intestine traverses the abdominal wall to create a stoma.[70] Parastomal hernias are a common early complication

Table 12.1 Thigh-based and torso-based pedicled flaps used in abdominal wall reconstruction	
Flap	**Characteristics**
Anterolateral thigh flap	• Large surface area • Minimal donor site morbidity • Generally will reach the periumbilical area but has been reported to reach up to the costal margin • Can reach the ipsilateral posterior superior iliac spine posteriorly and the contralateral fossa laterally • Associated fascia may not be reliable for fascial reconstruction
Tensor fascia lata flap	• Large skin paddle (15×40 cm) • Skin can reach the periumbilical area, but distal skin necrosis is the main shortcoming when TFL is used in abdominal wall reconstruction[48,49] • Adding rectus femoris muscle to TFL with their surrounding fascia allows coverage of larger defects but is still associated with skin necrosis[50]
Rectus femoris flap	• Can be transferred as a muscle flap, musculocutaneous flap, or part of a combined thigh flap based on the lateral circumflex femoral vessel • Provides a long cylindrical muscle, approximately 6 cm wide, and can support a 12×20 cm skin island
Combined thigh flaps	• "Subtotal thigh" flap takes advantage of the versatile lateral circumflex femoral vessel system and can include rectus femoris, TFL, vastus lateralis, and/or ALT flap tissue • Nearly the entire abdominal wall skin can be reconstructed with bilateral pedicled subtotal thigh flaps • Fascial portion of these flaps can be used to repair fascial defects, but mesh is often preferred for reconstruction of the musculofascia, with soft-tissue flaps used for coverage; thigh fascia may be less reliable and can tear along its fibers
Rectus abdominis flap	• Skin paddle can be oriented vertically, horizontally, as an extended deep inferior epigastric artery flap (musculocutaneous flap with lateral skin extension based on the periumbilical perforators), or as a flag flap (skin from the upper abdomen with extensions to the inframammary fold and the anterior axillary line)[51–54] • Useful for defects located at the periphery of the abdominal wall • Generally should be avoided for large abdominal wall defects when the donor site would add to the primary defect
Latissimus dorsi flap	• Arc of rotation of the flap allows coverage of superolateral abdominal wall defects • Can be used as muscle or musculocutaneous flap

ALT, anterolateral thigh; TFL, tensor fascia lata.
(Adapted from Althubaiti G, Butler CE. Abdominal wall and chest wall reconstruction. *Plast Reconstr Surg*. 2014;133(5):688e–701e.)

of stoma formation, with the majority forming 1–2 years after ostomy.[71] The incidence of parastomal hernia varies from 0–39%; the smallest incidence is after loop ileostomy and the greatest after end colostomy. The majority of parastomal hernias are asymptomatic, causing only a cosmetic contour deformity, and therefore can be treated conservatively. Given the challenges in repairing parastomal hernias and the high recurrence rates, surgical intervention should be reserved for hernias that disrupt the ostomy appliance and cause chronic pain, skin breakdown, or intestinal obstruction, incarceration, or strangulation. Reinforcement (either prophylactically or in the treatment of parastomal hernias) with inlay mesh placement in a preperitoneal or intraperitoneal plane has been adopted to further reduce the risk of parastomal hernia. Randomized controlled trials comparing the benefits and risks of mesh reinforcement of stomas with conventional methods of stoma formation have shown that mesh reinforcement reduces parastomal herniation (relative risk [RR] 0.23, 95% CI 0.06–0.81; P=0.02) and the percentage of parastomal hernias requiring surgical intervention (RR 0.13, 95% CI 0.02–1.02; P=0.05) compared with conventional stoma formation.[69] Surgical treatment options for parastomal hernias may include relocation of the stoma or in situ repair of the hernia with or without mesh reinforcement. Repair of the original parastomal defect site with fascial closure and inlay mesh reinforcement, as well as prophylactic reinforcement of a newly created stomal site with mesh, are key to minimizing the risk of parastomal rehernation. Two techniques of intraperitoneal mesh placement are most often used to repair parastomal hernia defects: the keyhole technique and the Sugarbaker technique. The keyhole technique, described in 1977 by Rosin and Bonardi,[72] is performed by placing the bowel through a circular opening in the mesh. The benefit of the technique is that the non-yielding mesh reinforces the attenuated myofascia. The downside of this technique is that the bowel passes perpendicular to the mesh plane, and there is a small area between the bowel serosa and the mesh ring through which the intra-abdominal contents can migrate. In 1985, Sugarbaker[73] described placing a single uncut piece of mesh as an intraperitoneal patch over the parastomal defect and then lateralizing the bowel so as to allow the stoma site to be covered by the mesh (Fig. 12.7). Thus the stoma did not traverse the plane of the mesh repair in a perpendicular fashion but traveled parallel to the mesh before traversing the

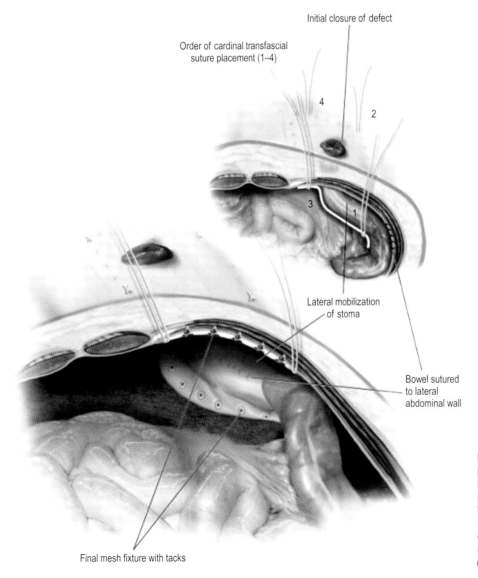

Initial closure of defect

Order of cardinal transfascial suture placement (1–4)

4

2

3

1

Lateral mobilization of stoma

Bowel sutured to lateral abdominal wall

Final mesh fixture with tacks

Fig. 12.7 Sugarbaker parastomal hernia repair. The parastomal hernia annulus is closed and supported by a mesh inlay, directing the bowel laterally and parallel with the abdominal wall. This redirection of the end ostomy reduces the risk of other bowel loops disrupting the plane between the end ostomy and the posterior rectus sheath. *(From Rosen M. Atlas of Abdominal Wall Reconstruction, pp. 15–195. © Elsevier, 2012.)*

abdominal wall. Avoiding direct passage of the bowel through the mesh led to a reduction in rates of both asymptomatic recurrences and those requiring reoperation. The Sugarbaker repair can be performed by open or laparoscopic approaches. An extensive meta-analysis of more than 30 studies, both retrospective and prospective, showed that direct suture repair results in a significantly increased recurrence rate when compared with the keyhole or Sugarbaker mesh repair techniques (OR 8.9, 95% CI 5.2–15.1; P=0.0001).[74] Recurrence rates for keyhole and Sugarbaker mesh repairs have ranged from 6.9% to 17% and do not differ significantly. These findings support the use of a mesh-reinforced parastomal hernia repair technique individualized to the patient's defect and comorbidities and the surgeon's preference.

Conclusion

Given the ever-growing problem of obesity and the increasing complexity of hernia defects, abdominal wall reconstruction remains a challenging and evolving discipline for reconstructive surgeons. The development of national hernia registries and multispecialty collaborative groups is helping to standardize outcome reporting for ventral hernias. Proper surgical technique and patient selection are essential to the successful and durable treatment of the abdominal wall. Further refinements and prospective comparative trials of these procedures is needed to reduce wound morbidity, minimize complications, and define optimal long-term durable repairs.

Access the complete reference list online at   **http://www.expertconsult.com**

3. Ramirez OM, Ruas E, Dellon AL. "Components separation" method for closure of abdominal-wall defects: an anatomic and clinical study. *Plast Reconstr Surg.* 1990;86(3):519–526. *Ramirez and colleagues introduce the concept of musculofascial advancement flaps based upon an anatomic understanding of the fascial planes of the abdominal wall. Cadaver dissections of the abdominal wall were performed to determine the amount of mobilization possible by dissecting layers vs. the entire rectus complex as a block. Mobilization of the rectus complex allowed for the ability to achieve complete fascial coaptation even with wide fascial defects that previously would have been bridged or required distant muscle flaps. This novel concept is now the standard of care and an indispensable technique in hernia repair.*

4. Luijendijk RW, Hop WC, van den Tol MP, et al. A comparison of suture repair with mesh repair for incisional hernia. *N Engl J Med.* 2000;343(6):392–398. *Luijendijk and colleagues performed a prospective multi-institutional European study evaluating 200 cases of primary hernia repair vs. repairs reinforced with mesh. Retrofascial preperitoneal repair with polypropylene mesh was found to be significantly superior to suture repair alone with regard to the recurrence of hernia, even in patients with small defects, at both early and late follow-up. Mesh reinforcement of fascial closure is now the standard for care in hernia repair based upon this landmark article.*

25. Breuing K, Butler CE, Ferzoco S, et al. Incisional ventral hernias: review of the literature and recommendations regarding the grading and technique of repair. *Surgery.* 2010;148(3):544–558. *Breuing and colleagues proposed a grading system of ventral hernias based upon complexity as a surrogate for likelihood of recurrence. The Ventral Hernia Working Group (VHWG) developed a grading system that takes into account underlying patient comorbidities and the presence of wound contamination during the repair. In the VHWG system, grade 1 includes hernias in patients with a low risk of complications and no history of wound infection. Grade 2 includes hernias in patients who smoke or have chronic obstructive pulmonary disease, and are obese, diabetic, or immunosuppressed. Grade 3 includes hernias in patients with a previous wound infection, stoma, or violation of the gastrointestinal tract (i.e., hernias in potentially contaminated surgical fields). Finally, grade 4 includes hernias in patients with infected mesh or septic dehiscence of their wound. Based on this classification system, the VHWG recommended the use of synthetic mesh for grade 1 and bioprosthetic mesh for grades 3 and 4 hernias. The grading system has yet to be formally validated.*

26. Itani KM, Hur K, Kim LT, et al. Comparison of laparoscopic and open repair with mesh for the treatment of ventral incisional hernia: a randomized trial. *Arch Surg.* 2010;145(4):322–328, discussion 328.

40. Itani KM, Rosen M, Vargo D, et al. Prospective study of single-stage repair of contaminated hernias using a biologic porcine tissue matrix: the RICH Study. *Surgery.* 2012;152(3):498–505. *Itani and colleagues performed a prospective multi-institutional study to describe the outcomes of ventral hernia repair in high-risk contaminated patients. Out of 80 patients undergoing open ventral hernia repair with a porcine bioprosthetic mesh reinforcement, defects were classified as "clean-contaminated" (n = 39), "contaminated" (n=39), or "dirty" (n=2). At 24 months, 53 patients (66%) experienced 95 wound events. There were 28 unique, infection-related events in 24 patients. Twenty-two patients experienced seromas, all but 5 of which were transient and required no intervention. No unanticipated adverse events occurred, and no tissue matrix required complete excision. There were 22 hernia (28%) recurrences by month 24. The study advocated the use of non-cross-linked, porcine, acellular dermal matrix in the repair of contaminated ventral hernia in high-risk patients.*

43. Albino FP, Patel KM, Nahabedian MY, et al. Does mesh location matter in abdominal wall reconstruction? A systematic review of the literature and a summary of recommendations. *Plast Reconstr Surg.* 2013;132(5):1295–1304.

45. Iqbal CW, Pham TH, Joseph A, et al. Long-term outcome of 254 complex incisional hernia repairs using the modified Rives–Stoppa technique. *World J Surg.* 2007;31(12):2398–2404.

47. Butler CE, Campbell KT. Minimally invasive component separation with inlay bioprosthetic mesh (MICSIB) for complex abdominal wall reconstruction. *Plast Reconstr Surg.* 2011;128(3):698–709.

66. Visschers RG, Olde Damink SW, Winkens B, et al. Treatment strategies in 135 consecutive patients with enterocutaneous fistulas. *World J Surg.* 2008;32(3):445–453. *In a series of 135 patients with ECFs, Visschers and colleagues[64] reported successful restoration of gastrointestinal tract continuity in 91% of patients, with a 9.6% mortality rate, despite fairly early surgical repair (mean of 53 days from ECF development). Among 53 patients with concomitant abdominal wall defects, 77% required surgical intervention for closure, and the mortality rate was 15%. Among the 82 patients without an abdominal wall defect, the mortality rate was only 6%. Malnutrition was correlated with failure of surgical closure and increased mortality rates. The manuscript highlights the essential management of ECFs including control of sepsis, optimization of nutritional status, wound care, assessment of fistula anatomy, timing of surgery, and surgical strategy.*

13

Reconstruction of male genital defects

Stan Monstrey, Salvatore D'Arpa, Karel Claes, Nicolas Lumen, and Piet Hoebeke

 Access video content for this chapter online at expertconsult.com

SYNOPSIS

This chapter deals with the following topics:
- Genital embryology and anatomy.
- Congenital genital defects:
  - exstrophy and epispadias
  - disorders of sex development (DSD)
  - buried penis and micropenis
  - reconstructive options for penile insufficiency.
- Post-traumatic genital defects:
  - general reconstructive options: skin grafts, pedicled flaps, microsurgical genital reconstruction
  - specific indications: Fournier's gangrene and penile cancer.
- Reconstruction of male genitalia in the female-to-male (FTM) transsexual:
  - vaginectomy, reconstruction of the fixed urethra, and scrotoplasty
  - metoidioplasty
  - complete phallic reconstruction: radial forearm phalloplasty and alternative phalloplasty techniques such as perforator flaps, fibula flap, and muscle flaps.

Introduction

Reconstructive surgery of the male genitalia is performed within a genitourinary reconstructive team: plastic surgeons, urologists, colorectal surgeons, gynecologists, and orthopedic surgeons. The essence of a reconstructive team is reflected in this chapter, which is the collaborative work of plastic surgeons and urologists. Plastic surgery techniques and traditions continue to play an important role in the reconstructive armamentarium of all who intend to repair genital defects.

In this chapter, we first discuss the relevant (genital) embryology and anatomy, then provide a complete overview of congenital and acquired genital deformities, and finally present the scope of past and current surgical techniques that may be used to accomplish the reconstructive goals.

Basic science: genital embryology and anatomy

Genital embryology

Genetic sex

Genetic sex of the embryo is established at conception. The ovum, containing 22 autosomes and an X chromosome, is penetrated by one of the surrounding spermatozoa, half of which have an X chromosome and the other half have a Y chromosome, and receives an X or Y chromosome, thereby establishing genetic sexual assignment.

The embryos of both sexes develop identically for approximately 6 weeks' gestation, the indifferent stage. During this time, the embryo becomes tubularized as the primitive gut is formed to terminate in the cloacal membrane. At the 6th week, the urorectal septum begins to grow downward and inward from the sides into the cloacal cavity, separating the cloaca into the bladder and rectum.

Externally, a mound of mesoderm with a midline groove, known as the indifferent genital tubercle, develops cephalocaudal to the cloacal membrane. As the midline mesenchyme progressively fuses in a caudal direction from the umbilicus, the genital primordials fuse to form a genital eminence.

Gonadal sex

Gonadal sex (differentiated stage) begins at the 7th week of intrauterine life. Evidence suggests that a locus on the Y chromosome (H-Y antigen) induces testicular development by causing differentiation of the seminiferous tubules. Today, many genes are described that play a role in male gonadal development, such as SRY, SOX9, AMH, SF1, DHH, ATRX, and DMRT.

Triiodothyronine (T3) endocrine hormones explain male differentiation. The first is Müllerian-inhibiting factor produced transiently by the Sertoli cells in the seminiferous tubules, which causes regression of the Müllerian duct system (9–11 weeks). The second is a testosterone homologue, produced at the same time by Leydig cells in the seminiferous tubules, that plays two roles: (1) completion of maturation of the seminiferous tubules, epididymides, vasa deferentia, and seminal vesicles, and (2) extratesticular male development by irreversible reduction to dihydrotestosterone by 5a-reductase. The third is dihydrotestosterone, responsible for virilization of the external genitalia and the anterior urethra.

Phenotypic sex

Phenotypic sex is determined by whether the genital tubercle develops into a male or female pattern. In males, urogenital swellings migrate ventrally and anteriorly to form the scrotum. The genital tubercle develops by elongation and cylindrical growth. The urethral folds close over the urethral groove, thereby establishing a urethra and a midline raphe. Mesenchymal tissue coalesces to surround the urethra and form the corpus spongiosum. This development is entirely under the influence (or absence) of testosterone, testosterone derivatives (i.e., dihydrotestosterone), and 5a-reductase and occurs between 6 and 13 weeks' gestation (Fig. 13.1). The prepuce grows to cover the penile glans but is not influenced by dihydrotestosterone.

In females, the lack of testosterone-influenced virilization holds the urogenital sinus and the genital tubercle in a fixed perineal position. The urethral groove remains open (folds develop into labia minora), and the genital tubercle remains stable in size and bends ventrally. The labia majora enlarge, migrate caudally, and fuse to form the posterior fourchette. This lack of closure of the ventral urethra (a nonevent) causes the female perineum to be shorter and the introitus to be more caudally positioned.

Genital anatomy

Male genital anatomy is unique in the human body and has evolved phylogenetically for protection from trauma and disease and to warrant procreation.

Genital fascia

The most obvious protective mechanism is testicular (and penile) withdrawal on exposure to physical stress (like hypothermia or blunt trauma), which causes the unique cremasteric muscles to contract, withdrawing the testicles and shrinking the scrotum as close to the body as possible. Otherwise, the testicles hang free, ostensibly to provide the best environment for sperm development. At the same time, the penile corporal bodies and the urethra also retract and shrink in size, although the penile skin does not have the same retraction properties as the scrotal skin. The penis and the scrotum have redundant skin coverage with their own separate blood supply and underlying supportive superficial fascial system.

The penis contains specially designed tunical tissues that surround the corporal bodies and can expand and, along with venous valve mechanisms, prevent blood outflow during

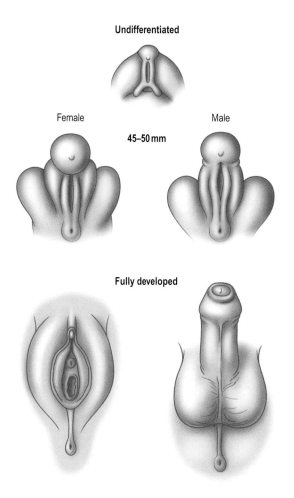

Fig. 13.1 The definitive phenotypic external genital growth that occurs *in utero* under the influence (or absence) of testosterone, dihydrotestosterone, and 5a-reductase. The influence of these virilizing hormones causes the genital tubercle to enlarge, the urethral folds to meet and close ventrally, and the scrotum to migrate medially and posteriorly. Any hormone deficit or receptor site inadequacy leads to an external female genitalia tendency ("phenotype by default").

erections. The tunica albuginea envelops the corporal bodies tightly but is perforated by an intercavernosal membranous septum that allows blood flow between the corpora. The tunical tissues are thick over the dorsal and lateral aspects of each corporal body but thin out in the ventral sulcus – where the urethra and corpus spongiosum are located – and also beneath the glans penis cap so as to have direct vascular contact with the glans.

Overlying the tunica is the deep penile fascia (Buck's fascia), a strong laminar structure that tightly surrounds and binds the corpora cavernosa together and the corpus spongiosum into a single-functioning entity. The urethra and its overlying corpus spongiosum are also protected proximally by surrounding muscles and distally by their location within the intercorporal groove. Buck's fascia carries important neurovascular structures to the glans penis, including the deep dorsal vein and arteries, the deep dorsal nerves of the penis, the circumflex arteries and veins, and the penile lymphatics (Fig. 13.2).[1]

The penile glans itself is a vascular spongiosa containing unique erogenous and tactile sensory endings. The glans epithelium is a unique uroepithelium that contains sensory

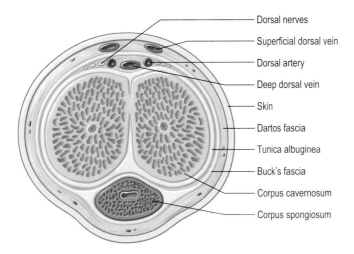

Fig. 13.2 A cross-section of the penile shaft illustrates the superficial and deep fascial layers and their relationships to the corporal bodies and neurovascular structures. *(From: Quartey JK. Microcirculation of penile and scrotal skin. Atlas Urol Clin North Am. 1997;5:1–9.)*

cells, particularly around the corona. The glans is naturally covered and protected by a prepuce made of inner and outer laminae. The inner lamina consists of uroepithelium similar to that of the glans and, in fact, it developmentally separates from the glans in the last trimester and after birth. The outer lamina consists of the same epithelium as the glabrous skin of the penile shaft. Superficial to Buck's fascia, but beneath the penile shaft skin and prepuce, is the superficial fascial system, defined by Dartos fascia. This fascial layer is a continuation of Scarpa's fascia superiorly and Colles' fascia inferiorly and surrounds the penis from the penoscrotal and peno-pubic angles to the prepuce.

The Dartos contains its own vascular plexus that allows overlying skin islands to be elevated on its independent blood supply.

Colles' fascia is a deep, tight, triangular fascial system that arises laterally from the inferior pelvic rami and posteriorly from the perineal membrane to protect the genitalia from toxins, trauma, and infections (and envelops both testicles circumferentially, as the Dartos). Colles' fascia is analogous to the Dartos on the penis, and thus skin island flaps can be elevated on its vascular plexus (see Fig. 9.11).[2]

Overlying both testicles, the epididymides, and the cord structures is a loose, well-vascularized superficial fascial layer: the tunica vaginalis that wraps the testicles. The parietal tunica vaginalis acts as the "vaginal space", which can be likened to the peritoneal cavity. Although the testicles are anchored within the scrotum, they move separately and independently on their cremasteric systems. The neurovascular supply to the testicles is dedicated to the viability of the testicles, epididymides, and cord structures (vasa deferentia) as well as to continued sperm production.

Genital blood supply

The genitalia have two separate arterial systems. The deep system originates from the deep internal pudendal artery. The paired pudendal arteries originate from the internal iliac arteries, pass along the borders of the inferior pelvic rami, and then give off the perineal and scrotal branches before

continuing as common penile arteries. After exiting from Alcock's canal (a split in the obturator fascia that runs from the lesser sciatic foramen to the ischial tuberosity along the sidewall of the ischiorectal fossa), each common penile artery gives off three branches (bulbar, urethral, and cavernosal) and terminates in the dorsal artery of the penis, which runs within Buck's fascia distally to terminate in the balanic arteries. Within Buck's fascia, the dorsal penile arteries are coiled and tortuous compared with the deep dorsal vein, which is linear and straight. This anatomy may be related to erectile function (Fig. 13.3).[3]

The perineal branch of the pudendal artery is just superficial to Colles' fascia and has an unpredictable length, but its central location and strong collateral supply make it a mainstay of genitourinary flap reconstruction. The scrotal branch of the perineal artery passes along the fold between the lateral scrotum and the medial thigh and arborizes within the tunica dartos (Fig. 13.4).

The superficial system originates from the superficial external pudendal arteries – branches of the femoral arteries. The femoral artery typically gives off a superficial external pudendal artery and a deep external pudendal artery. The superficial external pudendal artery supplies vascularity to the dartos fascia and genital skin. The deep external pudendal artery arises as a separate branch and passes into the genital skin as the lateral inferior pudendal artery, which separates into a dorsolateral branch supplying the dorsal and lateral penile shaft skin and an inferior branch supplying the ventral penile skin and the anterior plane of the scrotum (the anterior scrotal artery) (Fig. 13.5). This arrangement allows surgeons to elevate long axial and transverse flaps with relative safety and still cover the shaft donor site with the adjacent skin.

The penile venous system also has a dual blood supply. The superficial system arises from the distal penile shaft and passes

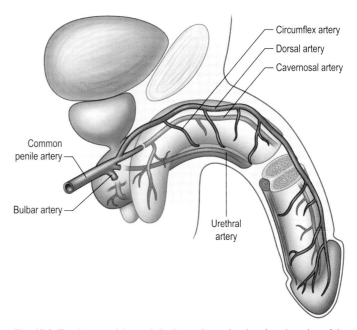

Fig. 13.3 The deep arterial vascularization to the penis arises from branches of the common penile arteries. *(From: Quartey JK. Microcirculation of penile and scrotal skin. Atlas Urol Clin North Am. 1997;5:1–9.)*

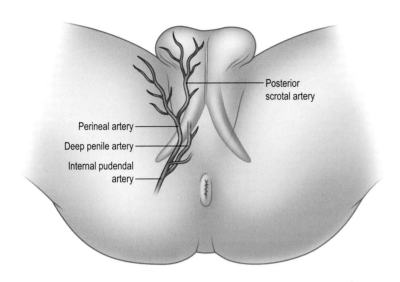

Fig. 13.4 The internal pudendal artery exits Alcock's canal and then divides into the posterior scrotal and perineal arteries. The perineal artery closely follows the crural reflection of Colles' fascia. This anatomy is favorable to dissection, elevation, and transposition of fasciocutaneous flaps that can be rotated into the perineum. *(From: Jordan GH, Stack RS. General concepts concerning the use of genital skin islands for anterior urethral reconstruction. Atlas Urol Clin North Am. 1997;5:23–44.)*

to the superficial dorsal vein within the dartos to drain the penile shaft skin. In approximately 70% of anatomic studies, the superficial dorsal vein empties into the left saphenous vein. Other vascular patterns include connections into the right saphenous vein (10%), left femoral vein (7%), and inferior epigastric vein (3%); in 10%, the superficial dorsal veins empty into the saphenous veins bilaterally. The deep venous system drains the circumflex veins, the deep dorsal vein into the prosthetic plexus and the crural and cavernosal veins into the internal pudendal veins (Fig. 13.6).

The vasa deferentia, epididymides, and testes are vascularized from the retroperitoneal blood supply, primarily the spermatic artery, which originates from the aorta, and the deferential artery, which supplies the vas deferens. In addition, collateral blood supply from the retroperitoneal cremasteric artery follows the vas to become the vasal artery. As the spermatic artery approaches the testis, it divides into the internal testicular artery (which supplies the testis and the adjacent epididymal head and body) and the inferior testicular artery, which passes within the testis. The epididymal tail is supplied by branches of the epididymal, vasal, and testicular arteries.[4]

The veins form the pampiniform plexus, which coalesces around the testis and epididymis to flow into the testicular

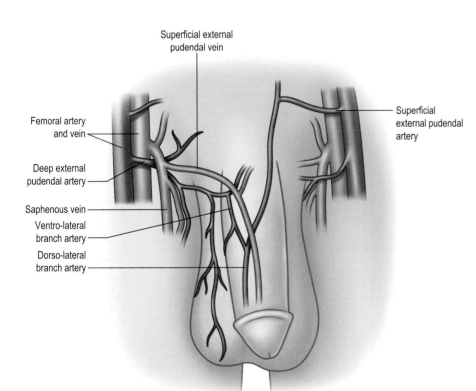

Fig. 13.5 The deep external pudendal vascular system arises from the femoral artery and empties into the saphenous vein. The vessel passes onto the penile shaft and anterior scrotum to vascularize the skin and dartos fascia. *(From: Jordan GH, Stack RS. General concepts concerning the use of genital skin islands for anterior urethral reconstruction. Atlas Urol Clin North Am. 1997;5:23–44.)*

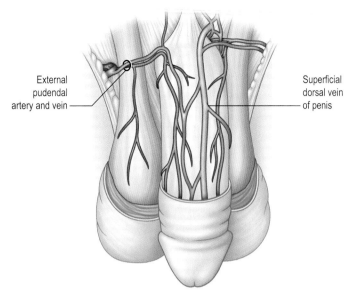

External pudendal artery and vein

Superficial dorsal vein of penis

Fig. 13.6 The superficial dorsal vein of the penis usually empties into the left saphenous system – an anatomic fact that must be taken into account when planning fasciocutaneous flaps. *(From: Jordan GH, Stack RS. General concepts concerning the use of genital skin islands for anterior urethral reconstruction.* Atlas Urol Clin North Am. *1997;5:23–44.)*

veins. The testicular veins then pass in a retroperitoneal plane to empty into the inferior vena cava on the right side and the left renal vein on the left side.

Genital nerve supply

Genital nerves also arise from a dual source and run with the arteries. The pudendal nerve is a mixed motor, sensory, and autonomic nerve that originates from the sacral roots (S2–4), and is the main penile sensory nerve: it passes through the greater sciatic foramen and crosses the pelvic floor to enter the pudendal canal anteriorly, after giving off the inferior rectal nerve, supplying the rectal sphincter and anal skin and conducting the cavernosal reflex before entering Alcock's (pudendal) canal. As the nerve exits Alcock's canal and passes close to the crural tips of the corporal bodies, it divides into the perineal nerve and the dorsal nerve of the penis. The perineal nerve supplies the perineal muscles, the deep structures of the urogenital region, and the posterior scrotal skin. The dorsal nerve of the penis gives off a proximal nerve to the urethra before arborizing into its penile branches. Branches of the nerve pass around the penile shaft within Buck's fascia to innervate the distal shaft and inner lamina of the prepuce and the glans as the major tactile and erogenous source of the penis.

The dorsal nerve of the penis does not provide sensation to the penile shaft. Only the internal preputial plate contains branches of the dorsal nerve of the penis.

The shaft is innervated by ancillary erogenous nerves, including the ilioinguinal nerves, which exit through the external inguinal rings and then innervate the anterior scrotum and the penile shaft skin circumferentially to the level of the prepuce, and branches of the genitofemoral nerves. The scrotum has multiple nerve supplies: the anterior scrotal branches of the ilioinguinal nerve, the genital branches of the genitofemoral nerve (anterior scrotum), and the posterior scrotal branch of the pudendal nerve (posterior scrotum).

Genital lymphatics

Lymphatics of the glans and urethra form a plexus on the ventral side before draining in the deep vein, passing proximally to the superficial inguinal nodes with the distal urethral lymphatics. Some lymphatics also drain in the deep inguinal nodes. The proximal spongy and membranous urethra drains into the external iliac nodes. The lymphatics of the testicles are contained in the spermatic cord and drain in the aortocaval nodes.

Congenital genital defects

Exstrophy and epispadias

Exstrophy of the bladder is an uncommon condition (1/30 000 live births, boys/girls=3:1). The defining features are an open and protruding bladder, an open urethra, and a foreshortened epispadiac penis (Fig. 13.7). The associated spectrum of anomalies may extend to involve the musculoskeletal structures and the gastrointestinal tract. Classic exstrophy – defined by bladder exstrophy, epispadias, diastasis recti, absence of fusion of the pubic symphysis, and deformed pubic escutcheon – occurs in 60% of cases; epispadias alone occurs in 30% of cases, and 10% of cases are more extensive dysmorphias including cloacal exstrophy.

The etiology of exstrophy–epispadias is controversial. It occurs in early gestation between the 3rd and 9th week, but

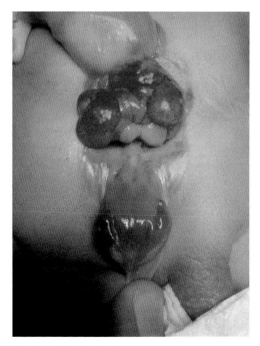

Fig. 13.7 Exstrophy in a boy.

it does not represent an arrest of a normal fetal developmental stage. It is associated with the normal formation and retraction of the cloacal membrane. In the normal fetus, a mesodermal layer of tissue spreads medially to replace the thin cloacal membrane by the 9th week *in utero*. According to Muecke's theory,[5] the cloacal membrane persists and resists any medial migration of mesoderm. The membrane then ruptures, producing a lack of mesodermal tissue to form the anterior abdominal wall and endodermal tissue to form the anterior wall of the bladder. This lack of mesodermal migration also affects the musculoskeletal system: the pubic rami are widely separated, and the inferior pubic rami are consequently laterally rotated. This defect produces a widened and foreshortened urethra and bladder neck, an incompletely formed penis that remains rudimentary and, by definition, is a phallus. According to Mitchell and Bägli,[6] the anomaly is that of a fetal abdominal wall hernia and can be recreated in the laboratory in chickens because they have a persistent cloaca by induction of a localized vascular accident (J. Sumfest, pers. comm. 2002).

The crural bodies are attached to the splayed pubic tubercles, producing a penis that is short, wide, and with dorsal chordee. The corpora are shorter than in a normally developed penis and, unlike in the normal anatomy, independent of each other with no communication through the intercorporal septum. The neurovascular structures to the glans are laterally displaced but move medially at the distal end of the foreshortened penis; the glans is spade shaped and incomplete, and each side is totally dependent on the respective dorsal neurovascular supply. Little circulation passes through the corporal bodies into the glans. The separated pelvic ring also produces a widened scrotum and incompetent pelvic musculature. Therefore the perineum is short, and there is a patulous anus that is anteriorly displaced. The rectus muscles are widely separated, and inguinal hernias are the rule.

Although initial postnatal diagnosis and treatment of bladder exstrophy and epispadias remain in the realm of the pediatric urologist and pediatric orthopedic surgeon, it is important that the plastic surgeon is prepared, if consulted, to help reconstruct such a child. The goals of initial closure are to reconstruct a functional genitourinary system, reduce the risk of bladder squamous metaplasia, and close the pelvic ring by direct closure of the bladder and reconstitution of the pelvic ring. After neonatal closure of the exstrophy, there are asymmetric pubic hairlines. This can easily be reconstructed by creating and mobilizing skin flaps and correcting the pubic hairline.

Different techniques have been described for penile reconstruction[6,7] and although the results of urethral closure have drastically improved, the ideal surgical approach is still controversial: neonatal vs. delayed closure and one stage vs. multistage repair. Phallic length depends on antenatal development, and the majority of these patients end up with small and undeveloped penises, despite the best efforts of their treating surgeons. As they pass through their postadolescent period, many of these young men will benefit from further lengthening procedures or even complete penile reconstruction. In some patients, correction of unaesthetic scars and further release of insufficiently released corpora can help to gain length (Fig. 13.8).

Exstrophy patients miss an umbilicus and are often consulting for umbilical reconstruction. Different techniques have been described with good cosmetic outcomes, but umbilical

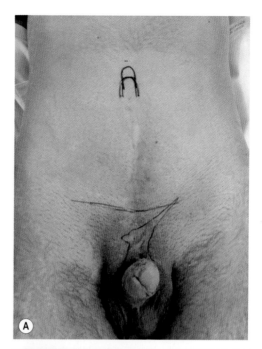
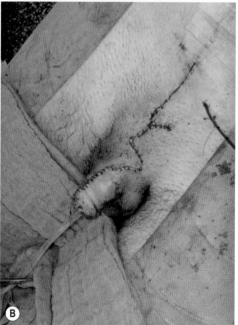

Fig. 13.8 A Z-plasty on the dorsal aspect of the penis extending into the prepubic area can be useful to obtain maximal lengthening.

loss is best prevented by neonatal preservation of the umbilicus and transposition to an abdominal position.[8,9]

In some boys there just is not enough tissue due to underdevelopment or partial or complete loss of penile tissue after primary closure. These patients might be good candidates for phallic reconstruction with free (Fig. 13.9) or pedicled flaps (see below, Fig. 13.12A–C).

Most of these patients have some form of urinary diversion and therefore a non-functional urethra. Although ejaculatory ducts are mostly intact, they are often abnormally positioned as a prepubic fistula. As a consequence sperm production is unpredictable and most of these patients are unable to

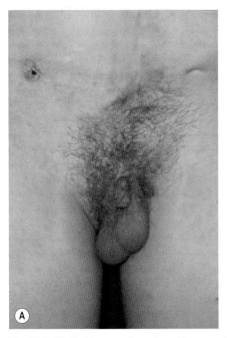
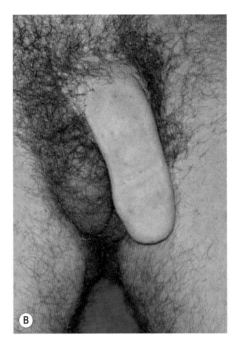
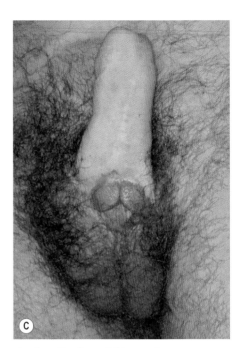

Fig. 13.9 (A) Bladder exstrophy patient with a severely underdeveloped penis who requested a complete penile reconstruction with a free radial forearm flap. **(B,C)** Postoperative result after radial forearm phalloplasty with the small glans incorporated at the base of the reconstructed penis.

procreate naturally. For these reasons, the urethral reconstruction may be a moot point in this group of patients, thus making a phalloplasty, in these "boys without a penis", much easier. The different options and peculiarities for a phalloplasty in an exstrophy patient will be addressed further in this chapter.

Disorders of sex development (formerly "intersex")

Intersex conditions are nowadays defined as disorders of sexual development (DSD).[10] DSDs are beyond the scope of this chapter, and therefore only the conditions in which genital reconstruction is needed will be described: genital ambiguity and absence of Müllerian duct derived structures.

46XX DSD: over-virilized females

The most prevalent condition is congenital adrenal hyperplasia (CAH) where a cortisol synthesis defect causes androgens to be overproduced in a female. This leads to virilization of the female genitalia with urogenital sinus formation (confluence of urogenital tracts), labioscrotal fusion, and clitoromegaly. Surgical correction is needed to separate the urogenital tracts bringing the urethra and the vagina separately to the perineum with a nerve sparing reduction of the clitoris and labial reconstruction. Although optimal timing is controversial, most surgeons agree on early reconstruction.

46XY DSD: under-virilized males

Testosterone synthesis defects and partial androgen receptor insensitivity are among the causes. Patients in this group present genital ambiguity with varying degrees of hypospadia, penoscrotal transposition, and cryptorchidism. Surgical treatment early in life consists of hypospadias repair, correction of penoscrotal transposition, and orchidopexy.

46XY/46XX DSD

This classification refers to varying degrees of genital ambiguity and presence of both male and female or dysgenetic gonads. Reconstruction is done after gender assignment, which is not always obvious. Multidisciplinary teams with expertise in these pathologies are needed to guide diagnosis and treatment in these children.

Genital conditions

This DSD classification includes conditions such as penile agenesis, extreme penoscrotal transposition with rudimentary penis, Mayer–Rokitansky–Kuster–Hauser with absence of Müllerian duct derivates like vagina and uterus, cloacal exstrophy, micropenis, and other genital malformations with normal chromosomes and gonads. All these conditions will eventually require genital reconstruction, although due to their low prevalence, treatment is better centralized.

Buried penis

The buried penis deformity affects pediatric and adult populations. A buried penis is defined as a penis of normal size for age that is hidden within the peripenile fat and subcutaneous tissues (Fig. 13.10 🌐).

Fig. 13.10 appears online only.

In the pediatric population, the fat deposit is often part of the constellation of poor virilization. The abnormal mons fat pad (gynecoid mons) may become associated with generalized obesity in the adolescent patient, and the buried penis must be differentiated from a micropenis in this group. In adults, the problem is almost always associated with obesity and the development of pubic, scrotal, and peripubic ptosis, which must be addressed to correct the hidden penis. Liposuction and lipectomy are part of the treatment in adults,

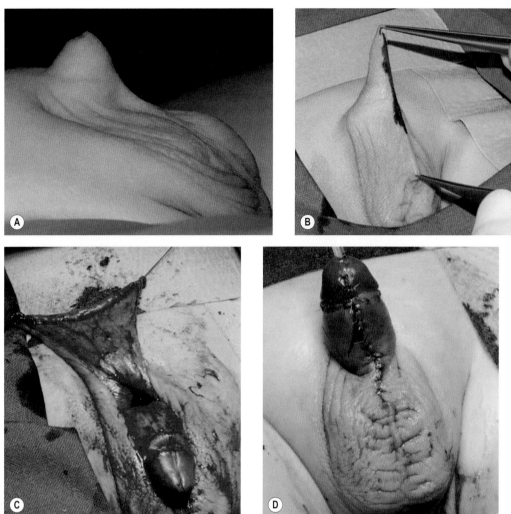

Fig. 13.11 (A) Typical buried penis in an infant. **(B)** Ventral incision of the skin with maximal preservation of skin at the start of the procedure. **(C)** After complete resection of the fibrotic dartos tissue, the penis is released from its buried position and the skin is extendable. **(D)** Coverage of the released corpora with the extended skin creating a penis with normal length.

while in children, with puberty, the prepubic fat deposit often decreases in size and the penis will only be released from the fibrotic dartos tissue.[11,12] Many techniques are described, but the most important steps include keeping all available skin from the start of the procedure, to resect all dartos tissue and to cover the released corpora with the skin (Fig. 13.11).[13]

Reconstructive options for severe penile insufficiency

A clear definition of severe penile inadequacy has not yet been established but can be considered as an insufficient penile length and function to obtain successful sexual intercourse. This implies that puberty must be finished and that the patient must be sexually active. Conditions with penile insufficiency include aphallia or penile agenesis, idiopathic micropenis (stretched penile length in a full-term newborn male <2.5 cm), 46XY DSD, and bladder exstrophy. Reconstructive surgery in these mostly young patients is required because of the devastating effect on psychological and sexual function.

The free vascularized radial forearm flap (RFF) (discussed further below) is considered the gold standard technique in penile reconstruction. The development of perforator flaps has provided new reconstructive options with the advantage of reducing donor site morbidity, increasing the flap's range of motion, and combining different tissue flaps on one single pedicle. The *pedicled anterolateral thigh (ALT) flap* has been shown to provide a valuable phalloplasty alternative specifically in patients with congenital penile insufficiency. This flap is a skin flap based on a perforator from the descending branch of the lateral circumflex femoral artery, a branch from the femoral artery.

There are several reasons why in the "boys without a penis" a pedicled ALT flap can be preferred to the standard RFF (Fig. 13.12):

- A pedicled flap reconstruction (the flap has a sufficiently long pedicle) avoids the technically more complex microsurgical procedure and might also shorten operating time.
- A visible donor site scar on the forearm, often considered as the signature of FTM transsexualism, is avoided and the donor site on the thigh can be more easily concealed.
- Previous reconstructive surgeries at the pelvis, groin area, and lower abdomen (e.g., in the case of bladder exstrophy) might have altered local anatomy and vasculature making a microsurgical anastomosis more difficult.

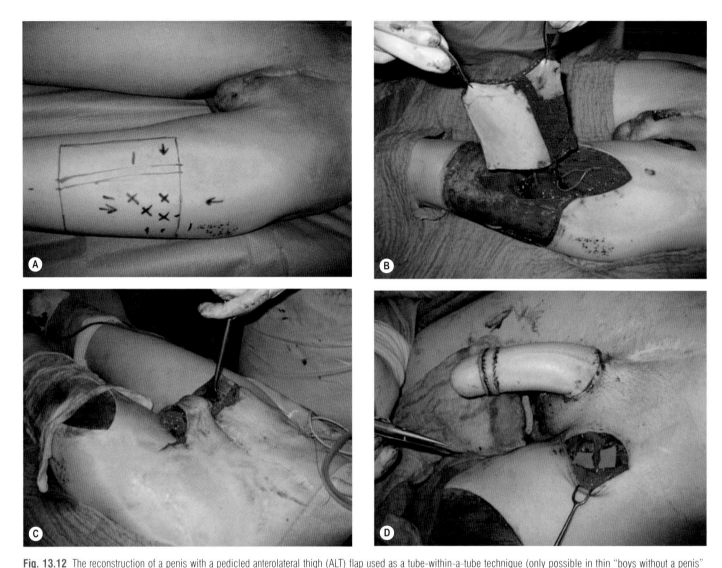

Fig. 13.12 The reconstruction of a penis with a pedicled anterolateral thigh (ALT) flap used as a tube-within-a-tube technique (only possible in thin "boys without a penis" and after defatting). No real urethra was reconstructed here since the patient had a urostomy. **(A)** Preoperative view. **(B)** After flap dissection. **(C)** The flap is tunneled underneath the rectus femoris muscle. **(D)** Suturing and nerve connection (ilioinguinal nerve to lateral femoral cutaneous nerve).

- Though usually thicker than a RFF, the subcutaneous fat layer is thinner than in a (biologically female) transman (the most common phalloplasty patient), facilitating the (urethral)tube-within-a-(penile)tube reconstruction of the penis; moreover, many exstrophy patients have a continent diversion (e.g., appendico-vesicostomy) with a ventral ejaculatory opening left above the scrotum and do not require urethral reconstruction.
- Glandular, penile, and cavernosal tissues are kept at the base of the neophallus to facilitate sexual stimulation and pleasure (Fig. 13.9C). The lateral femoral cutaneous nerve is connected to a dorsal penile nerve, if available, and/or to the ilioinguinal nerve.

A preoperative 3D angio CT-scan provides detailed information on the perforator vessel(s) and the subcutaneous tissue layer.

There is still a lot of controversy as to whether or not to perform a phalloplasty in children. Penile construction in children is similar to that in adults but with one added requirement – growth through puberty to adulthood. Because the phallus is constructed of somatic tissues (showing linear growth) but replaces a penis that is formed by genital tissues (demonstrating a more exponential growth), the growth rates are temporally and quantitatively different during puberty.[14] Care must be taken to accurately predict the anticipated growth rate and to design a phallus that is larger and longer than normal genital size for that age group.[15]

Another issue that we are just now beginning to address is the "correct" age at which to proceed with penile prostheses implantation. Once these boys have reached 18 years and the age of majority, they must be physically and psychologically prepared to manage a phallus that has previously been erectionless.

There is another nagging problem with operating on children – the lack of informed consent. Although the child's best interest and surgery's best intentions are usually served by early reconstruction, there are no long-term studies that have evaluated the results of this surgery over a lifetime or even a generation.

Finally, it comes as no surprise that the large majority of these genitally compromised boys require prolonged psychological therapy to deal with genital loss, surgical trauma, inadequacy, and scarring. These psychological issues are often closely commingled with the need for secondary surgery to complete reconstruction.

Nowhere in surgery is there a stronger need for parental and family support than with these late teenage boys who have essentially undergone years of "surgical abuse".

Post-traumatic genital defects

Post-traumatic genital repair is an uncommon but special chapter in surgical reconstruction. A reconstructive algorithm based on the etiology, an assessment of the extent of injury, and an anatomic inventory includes several goals and observations. First, the anatomically protected position of the genitalia implies that patients who have genital injuries often have large concomitant injuries as well and are in critical conditions. Resuscitation and life support of the patient take precedent over any reconstruction. However, genital reconstruction is of prime relevance, and only hand, eyelid, and lip reconstruction are considered more important in the reconstructive hierarchy. Second, aesthetics are foremost in genital reconstruction. The appearance of the genitalia is important to the self-esteem of a patient who is recovering from trauma. What is frivolous to one person may be a lifelong obsession to another, and genital aesthetics are as valued as other cosmetic areas such as the face, nose, and breasts. Third, the genitalia appear to be a "privileged site" such that the usual postreconstructive sequelae of scarring and contracture are often spared in genital reconstruction. This may be due to the fact that the average adult man has five to eight nocturnal erections every night, thereby inherently stretching scars or skin grafts on the penile shaft. This stretching may counteract and overcome the tendency of myofibroblasts to contract a skin graft or scar.

General reconstructive options

Genital skin grafts

Genital skin loss occurs from burns, avulsion injuries, infections, and gangrene. As a rule, total excision of necrotic genital tissues followed by early skin grafting produces the best results. When the wound is contaminated or infected, adequate debridement of necrotic tissues combined with wound bed preparation prior to skin grafting might be required, and this can be performed with adequate (moist) wound dressings, by temporary coverage with skin allografts, or with the use of topical negative pressure.

The thick split-thickness skin graft is the mainstay of penile reconstruction. The graft should be pliable, placed onto a flat bed, and secured with a tie-over bolus pressure dressing or even better with a special Cavi-Care cylinder type of dressing (Fig. 13.13 ⊕) to reduce the risk of hematoma or seroma formation. Successful skin graft "take" is directly related to a well-vascularized wound bed, meticulous hemostasis, control of erections, an infection-free environment, and adequate immobilization.

Fig. 13.13D–F appears online only.

The donor site should be close to the genitalia, large enough to produce a sheet skin graft, and well hidden. Ideally, the skin graft should be at least 0.018–0.02 inches in thickness and large enough to cover the whole breadth of the penile shaft or scrotum. The skin graft should be sutured circumferentially around the penile shaft with a ventral suture line. As mentioned above, this suture line will not contract, but a Z-plasty is advisable anyway. The graft is then fixed with resorbable sutures to the surrounding skin, the underlying Buck's fascia, and the tunica. Fixation with tissue sealant can improve skin graft fixation and skin graft take in this difficult area.

Extended bed rest is important in the immediate postoperative period to reduce the risk of graft shearing or movement. Amyl nitrate and diazepam (Valium) can be administered to control erections in the early postoperative period. However, erections, massage, and stimulation are recommended for all patients after grafting as soon as there is a full take of the skin graft.

Widely meshed split-thickness skin grafts should never be used on the penile shaft. However, with the so-called "reversed mesh graft" (= non-expanded or 1:1 meshed skin grafts) only puncture-type perforations are made with a V1 carrier (Humeca Ltd, Enschede, the Netherlands; Fig. 13.14), which allow for better fluid evacuation and thus a better skin graft take while still avoiding poor scarring and an unaesthetic mesh pattern long term. These non-expanded meshed split-thickness grafts have also become a mainstay of complicated, staged urethral reconstruction.[16,17] McAninch[18] has described the use of (not too widely) meshed split-thickness skin grafts for scrotal reconstruction. Meshed grafts in this location may produce "good aesthetic results", but they will never measure up to the functional capacity of sheet or 1:1 perforated grafts.

Full-thickness skin grafts also have a place in genital reconstruction, but mostly for smaller skin defects. Full-thickness grafts are particularly useful for coronal sulcus design to prevent "coronal washout" as is usually performed in FTM transsexual patients (see below; Fig. 13.24F).

The same principles apply to scrotal reconstruction. When primary closure is not possible, split-thickness skin grafts are effective if they are placed and immobilized carefully. The testicles must be fixed in an anatomically appropriate position before proceeding with graft coverage. As already mentioned, there is also a place for meshed, non-expanded skin grafts in scrotal and perineal reconstruction because of the uneven and often biconcave contours and, in addition, meshed grafts often emulate scrotal rugae (see below; Fig. 13.18).

Buccal mucosa grafts are often used in urethral reconstruction. They can also be useful in glans reconstruction. After partial penectomy (traumatically or for cancer treatment) the residual corpora are sometimes still long enough to allow for sexual intercourse, but a skin covered penis looks unnatural. Transaction of the suspensory ligament releases the corpora, and the tip of the corpora can be covered by free buccal mucosa grafts that create a mucosa covered glans-like penile tip (Fig. 13.15 ⊕).

Fig. 13.15B & C appears online only.

Genital flaps

For small penile defects, flaps based on the superficial external pudendal system can be used for penile shaft and anterior

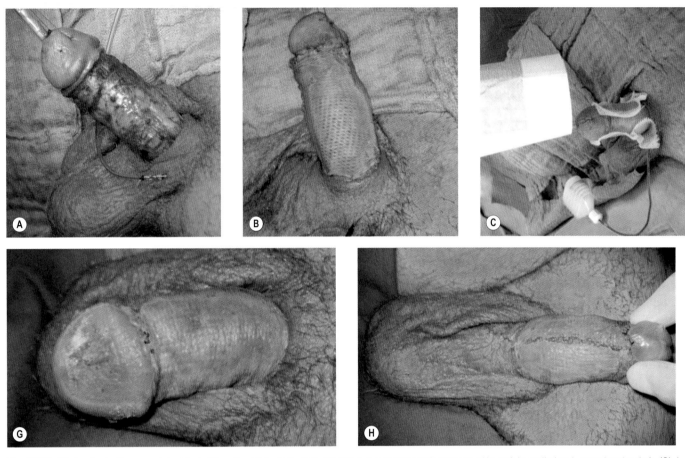

Fig. 13.13 (A) A patient with a complete defect of the skin of the penile shaft. **(B)** The 1 : 1 perforated split-thickness skin graft is applied and sutured to the shaft. **(C)** A Cavi-Care dressing is applied around the skin graft (poured out in a cylinder form around the penis), and this dressing will stay for 1 week. **(G,H)** A complete take of the skin graft is obtained.

urethral reconstruction.[19,20] Proximal penile flaps, vascularized from the lower abdomen and pubis, are less practical for male genitalia reconstruction.

Scrotal flaps have limited applications with the exception of hemiscrotal reconstruction. Although the scrotum has a wealth of well-vascularized skin and subcutaneous tissue, it is ill-suited for genital reconstruction because of its rugous and hairy appearance. A centrally located scrotal flap designed along the medial raphe has been described as a reconstructive flap option for proximal urethral repair,[21] but presurgical depilation is needed. This flap is based on the posterior scrotal artery and can be difficult to mobilize extensively and can cause scrotal tethering. A free oral mucosal graft is a better choice for proximal urethral reconstruction.[22]

In larger defects, there often is a combined penoscrotal defect. Any technique of tissue expansion is risky, especially in the repair of Fournier's gangrene defects due to the bacteriologic environment and the multiple stages needed. Local muscle/myocutaneous flaps, fasciocutaneous flaps, and perforator flaps are among the options for male genitalia reconstruction. Nowadays, the gracilis (purely) muscle flap is no longer considered as "the workhorse of perineal reconstruction" but is useful to cover and vascularize urethral anastomoses and exposed pelvic bones, to reduce the risk of

osteomyelitis, to fill the perineum after exenteration, and to vascularize the perineum in postirradiation injuries.[23]

Fasciocutaneous paragenital flaps that have been used, often with limited application, are the superficial circumflex iliac artery flap,[24] the deep circumflex iliac flap (often combined with an osseous component),[25] the superficial epigastric artery flap,[26] the double-pedicled composite groin flap,[27] the anteromedial thigh flap,[28] the ALT flap,[29] and the pudendal thigh flap.[30,31] The groin flap is based on the superficial circumflex artery, a branch of the femoral artery, and has an unpredictable origin, direction, and size. The flap must often be delayed, attached, or "waltzed" into a central midline position by a secondary procedure to be used as a genital flap. For these reasons, the groin flap has limited primary genital use.

Medial thigh flaps may be based inferiorly on the perineal artery system or superiorly on the external pudendal system and branches of the profunda femoris artery. The inferiorly based flap has been called by several names, including the Singapore flap[30] and the pudendal thigh flap.[32] Originally described to correct vesicovaginal fistulas, the flap is based posteriorly within the crural fold between the scrotum and the medial and extends from the posterior crural fold to the medial groin area anteriorly. Although most flap descriptions have focused on vaginal reconstruction and the correction of

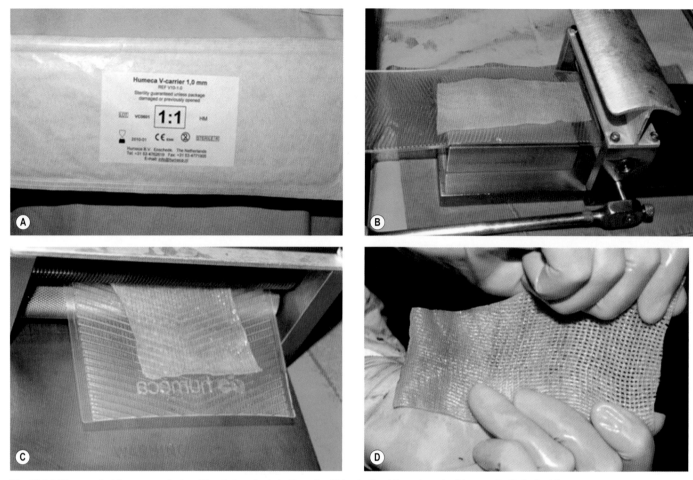

Fig. 13.14 The so-called "reverse-meshed graft" or 1:1 perforated skin graft, obtained with a V1 mesh carrier (Humeca, the Netherlands).

vesicovaginal and rectovaginal fistulas, this flap has been successfully used for male genital or male urethral construction.[31]

To complete the catalogue of fasciocutaneous flaps, the gluteal-posterior thigh flap must also be included.[33, 34] This flap is based on the inferior descending branch of the inferior

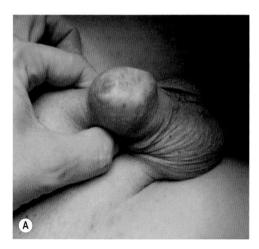

Fig. 13.15 (A) Penis after partial penectomy for spinocellular epithelioma, showing residual corpora, which after release could be sufficient for sexual intercourse.

gluteal artery. Nowadays, this flap has been replaced in most cases by perforator flaps originating from the inferior gluteal artery or IGAP flaps.[35] Additionally, various other new (pedicled) perforator flaps (the so-called "lotus petal flaps") are based on the external pudendal artery and have been described as possible options in the perineal area, although more in female patients.[36]

The formerly more popular musculocutaneous flaps including the vertical and transverse rectus abdominis flap (based on the deep inferior epigastric artery),[37] the gracilis musculocutaneous flap,[38] the rectus femoris musculocutaneous flap,[39] and the tensor fasciae latae musculocutaneous flap[40] have been employed occasionally in genitourinary reconstruction but have only limited use in the reconstruction of male genitalia.

Nevertheless, these flaps can still be an important part of the surgeon's armamentarium in addressing genital injuries after trauma, infection, and cancer and for patients with comorbidities. The trauma, cancer, infection, and comorbid disease that originally contributed to genital tissue loss may also preclude sophisticated microsurgical reconstruction. Thus these flaps are the only hope for functional, albeit suboptimal, genital reconstruction.

In the last decade, myocutaneous flaps have been replaced by their "perforator-type equivalent": the deep inferior epigastric artery perforator or DIEAP flap (with its skin island

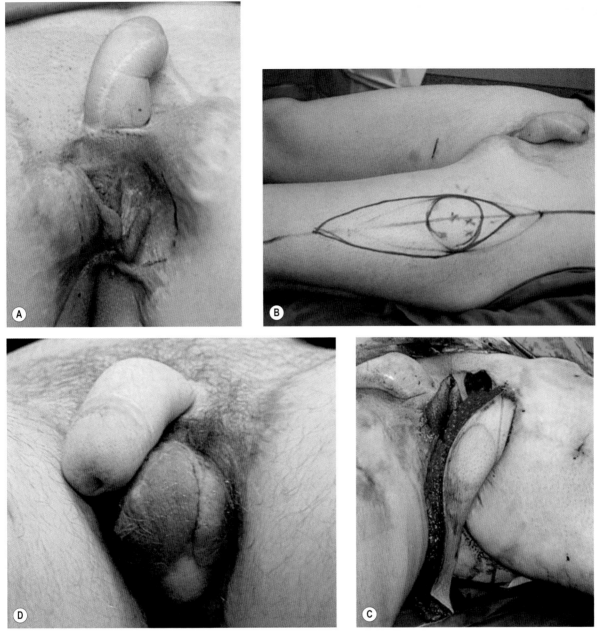

Fig. 13.16 (A) Female-to-male transsexual patient after penile reconstruction with a lack of skin to reconstruct a scrotum. **(B)** Design and dissection of a pedicled anterolateral thigh (ALT) flap. **(C)** Transfer of the ALT flap to the pubic area. **(D)** Postoperative result.

taken either vertically or horizontally) has been reported in a case of penile reconstruction. However, it is mainly the pedicled anterolateral thigh or ALT flap that has become the new "workhorse" nowadays in perineal and male genital reconstruction.[41] For the description of the use of this flap in patients with congenital penile insufficiency we refer to the beginning of this chapter. The pedicled ALT can also be a valuable alternative for the reconstruction of a scrotum (Fig. 13.16).

Microsurgical genital reconstruction

Genital replantation

Microsurgical techniques and free tissue transplantation have become the state-of-the-art treatment for many reconstructive

problems. The first uses of the microscope in genital reconstruction for penile reattachment after amputation were reported independently by Cohen et al.[42] and Tamai et al.[43] in 1977. However, the first account of successful reattachment long predated the introduction of microsurgical techniques. In 1929, Ehrich[44] first reported a successful penile attachment by opposing the lacerated corporal bodies and repairing the overlying tunica. This technique was occasionally successful but usually associated with loss of the overlying skin, glans, sensation, and erectile and voiding function.[45]

Penile replantation often mimics the algorithms of other amputated extremities that are candidates for reattachment. The penis is initially wrapped in saline-soaked gauze and placed into a plastic bag, which in turn is placed in a bag or cooler of ice with water (the so-called "bag-in-a-bag"

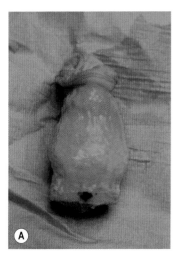
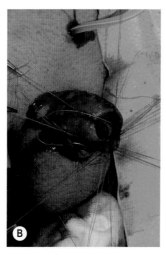
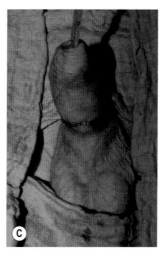
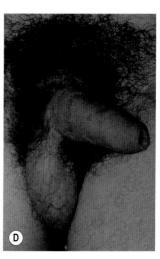

Fig. 13.17 (A) Self-inflicted penile amputation. **(B)** Preparation of microsurgical anastomoses. **(C)** Immediate postoperative result. **(D)** Late postoperative result.

technique). Because genital amputations are often self-inflicted, it is important to involve the psychiatrist even before restorative surgery. After the induction of anesthesia, the proximal and distal ends of the amputated penis are examined microscopically. Minimal debridement is followed by mechanical stabilization of the urethra and re-approximation of the tunica albuginea of the corpora cavernosa.

Revascularization is completed by anastomosis of the deep dorsal arteries, the deep dorsal vein, and the superficial dorsal vein with 9-0 and 10-0 sutures and multiple nerve coaptations with 10-0 and 11-0 nylon sutures. The dartos fascia and skin are then loosely approximated. A suprapubic tube is inserted to divert the urinary flow for 2–3 weeks, and the patient is prescribed bed rest in a warm room.

The ideal candidate for genital replantation is a patient with a clean, sharp cut in which the amputated part has been cooled (Fig. 13.17).

Testicular reattachment has also been reported but requires a sharp amputation etiology for successful anastomosis of the thin-walled arteries and veins that surround and vascularize the testicle, seminiferous tubules, and vasa deferentia.[46,47] Unfortunately, most testicular amputations are of the avulsion or crush type and therefore are not reattachable. Clinically, the only vessel that has adequate caliber is the testicular artery with its venae comitantes.

Two other arteries are also involved in testicular vascularization: the deferens artery, which arises from the inferior vesicular artery and vascularizes the epididymis, and the cremasteric artery, which arises from the inferior epigastric artery and vascularizes the cremasteric muscle and the other cord structures. Both of these arteries are small, flimsy, and often unrecognizable in reattachment circumstances.

There are five factors to be considered before proceeding with testicular reattachment. First: understanding of the three different testicular blood supplies. Second: availability of veins. Third: ischemia time (4–6 h). Fourth: technical feasibility of vasa deferentia anastomosis. A reattached testicle cannot be expected to recover its sperm-producing function, and, even if it does, the sperm count is often too low to be effective. Fifth: maintenance of post-reattachment psychological well-being (particularly in self-mutilation patients). When all of

these points are considered together, the best that can be hoped for with a reattached testicle is maintenance of testosterone secretion. The insertion of a testicular prosthesis combined with hormonal therapy is often a much simpler and equally effective option.

Microsurgical phallic construction

Complete reconstruction of a phallus will be described below.

Penile transplantation

Two attempts at penile transplantation have been reported so far. The first was performed in China and, after initial apparent success, the patient had the transplant removed as he and his wife could not manage to accept somebody else's penis on his body.[48]

The second was performed more recently (December 2014) on a 21-year-old male in South Africa. On March 2015 press reports stated that the patient was doing well and having erections.[49–51]

Penile transplantation has raised some criticism, and to date it is considered as the last option when autogenous reconstruction is not appropriate.[52–54]

Specific reconstructive indications

Fournier's disease

Fournier in 1883 was the first to describe a "fulminant gangrene" of the penis and scrotum that: (1) developed suddenly in previously healthy young men, (2) progressed rapidly, and (3) was idiopathic. Nowadays, every necrotizing fasciitis in the perineum and genitalia is termed Fournier's gangrene.[55]

Fournier's disease is a true genitourinary emergency. Today the etiology is identified in about 95% of cases. Common sources of infection include urogenital disease and trauma (renal abscess), urethral stones, urethral strictures, unrecognized rupture of the urethra when a penile prosthesis is inserted, colorectal causes (ruptured appendicitis), colon cancer, diverticulitis, and perirectal, retroperitoneal, and subdiaphragmatic abscesses and local trauma.[56]

Several systemic conditions have also been associated with Fournier's gangrene and may predispose patients to its development: diabetes mellitus, alcoholism, heavy smoking (more than one pack per day), human immunodeficiency virus infection and acquired immunodeficiency syndrome, and leukemia. Fournier's disease is considered a synergistic necrotizing fasciitis that often includes Gram-positive organisms, Gram-negative organisms, and *Clostridium perfringens* anaerobes in the cultures. The disease often begins as a cellulitis adjacent to an entry wound. The affected area is swollen, erythematous, and tender as the infection begins to include the deep fascia. There is prominent pain as well as fever and systemic toxicity. Scrotal swelling and crepitus quickly increase with the appearance of dark purple areas that become gangrenous. Specific urinary symptoms include dysuria, urethral discharge, and obstruction. A change in mental status, tachypnea, tachycardia, hyperthermia or hypothermia, and the presence of a typical smell indicate a potential Gram-negative sepsis.

A high degree of suspicion is crucial to an early diagnosis. A clinical differentiation between necrotizing fasciitis and simple cellulitis may be difficult initially because the initial signs of pain, edema, and erythema are not distinctive. However, the presence of marked systemic toxicity out of proportion to the local findings should alert the surgeon.

Once the disease is identified, intravenous fluid therapy and broad-spectrum antibiotics should be started in preparation for surgical debridement. Once culture guided antibiotics are begun, anaerobic coverage should be continued regardless of culture results because of the difficulty in culturing these organisms. Immediate surgical debridement is critical, should be aggressive, and continue along fascial planes until all of the devitalized tissues have been removed and viable tissue borders the wound.

Some authors also recommend hyperbaric oxygen therapy in conjunction with debridement and antibiotics to speed up wound healing and minimize gangrenous spread, particularly in patients with *C. perfringens* infections. In addition to hyperbaric oxygen, mechanized wound debridement tools (i.e., topical negative pressure therapy) promote granulation, wound contracture, and reduction of bacterial colonization before reconstruction.

In most cases, reconstruction of the genitalia includes release of the penis and testicles from surrounding granulation tissue; release of scar contracture; split-thickness skin grafts on the penile shaft and peripenile tissues and non-expanded meshed split-thickness grafts of the scrotum, perineum, and crural folds (Fig. 13.18). Flap reconstruction is seldom required.

The mortality rate in Fournier's disease averages approximately 20% but can range from 7% to 75%. Higher mortality rates are found in diabetics, alcoholics, and those with colorectal sources of infection, who often have a greater delay in diagnosis and more widespread extension. To reduce morbidity and mortality, the key is early diagnosis, antibiotic therapy, and surgical debridement.

Penile cancer

In the past, treatment of penile cancer ranged from techniques of local excision to emasculation. Penile cancer involving the redundant preputial and penile skin can be adequately treated

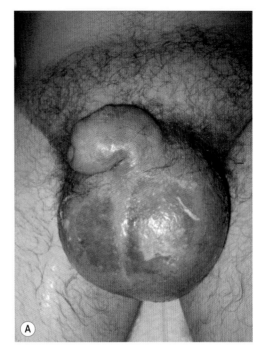

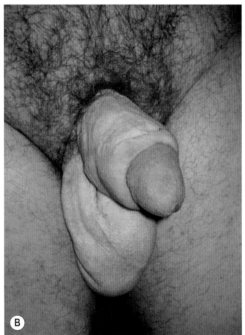

Fig. 13.18 Fournier's gangrene. **(A)** Prior to debridement. **(B)** After skin grafting.

with circumcision. The aggressive treatments used in the past such as partial, subtotal, or total penectomy have lost ground. Since penile cancer involving the spongy erectile tissue of the glans can be treated by "glansectomy", excision can spare the corpora cavernosa and reconstruction is limited to a redefinition procedure or coverage procedure of the distal corporal bodies. Often, just grafting the tips of the corporal bodies provides an excellent functional as well as cosmetic result. Buccal mucosa grafts can be used and create a natural looking glans (Fig. 13.15).

Another surgical method for treating penile cancer involves Mohs surgery. In Mohs surgery, sequential excisions are accomplished until clean margins in all quadrants are achieved. In classic Mohs surgery, the defect is then left to granulate or can be skin grafted.

In patients in whom a true partial penectomy has been performed, either local flaps or microvascular flaps are used to lengthen the penis to incorporate prostheses at a later date. These techniques have poor cosmetic and functional outcomes. It is better to sacrifice the superficial penile tissue saving the remaining corporal bodies to accomplish a true phallic construction. The corporal bodies are incorporated in the base of the microvascular free flap in the case where total penectomy after a total phallic reconstruction is planned (Fig. 13.19). In patients who have had extensive superficial lymph node dissections, angio-CT is performed to identify adequate recipient vessels (deep inferior epigastric vessels and the iliofemoral system). In addition, in cases in which reconstruction is envisioned, if possible, at the time of the extensive exenterative surgery, it is preferable to place intravenous and arterial lines in the dominant forearm, saving the vascularity of the non-dominant forearm for subsequent use in phallic construction.

It is recommended that the surgical oncologist contacts the reconstructive surgeon before exenterative surgery to plan subsequent reconstruction.

Reconstruction of male genitalia in the female-to-male (FTM) transsexual

Reconstruction of the male genitalia in an FTM transsexual individual is more complex than the penile reconstruction in a biologically male patient because of the added difficulties in reconstructing the fixed part of the urethra and the combination with a vaginectomy and a scrotoplasty.

Vaginectomy, reconstruction of the pars fixa of the urethra, and scrotoplasty

This first part of the procedure is usually done by the urologic team, while the team of plastic surgeons harvests the flap. The

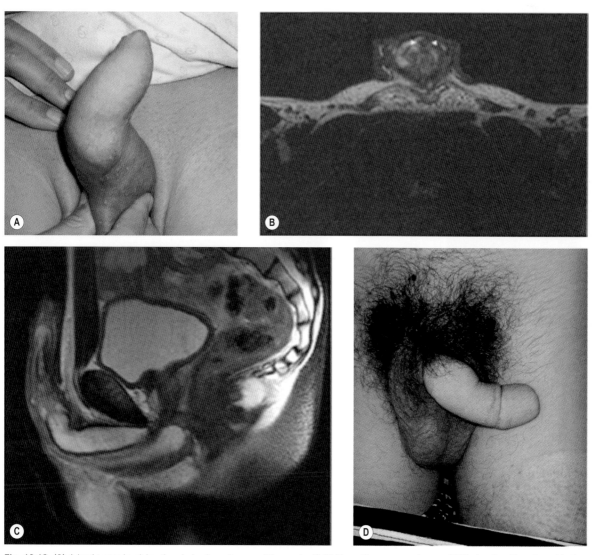

Fig. 13.19 **(A)** A hard tumor involving the whole circumference of the penis. **(B,C)** Magnetic resonance images (MRI) showing disruption of both corpora cavernosa. **(D)** Postoperative result after total penile reconstruction with a free radial forearm flap.

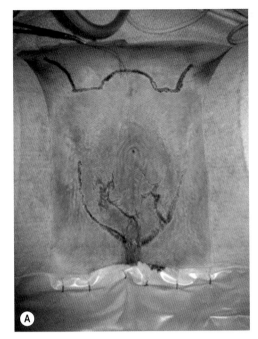

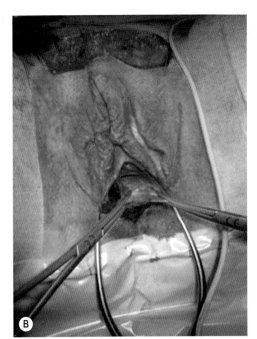

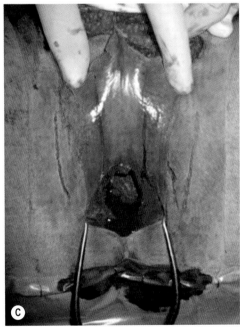

Fig. 13.20 (A) Incision lines of the prepubic area (roman-aqueduct) and of the labia majora for the scrotoplasty. **(B)** Incision of the vaginal introitus starts the vaginectomy. **(C)** Incision lines of the urethral plate between the external urethral orifice and the tip of the clitoris.

patient is positioned in the lithotomy position with supportive boots to avoid compression of the common peroneal nerve and compartment syndrome. A roman-aqueduct-like incision is made in the prepubic area where the phallus will be implanted and the recipient vessels and nerves will be prepared (Fig. 13.20A). Division of the suspensory ligament of the clitoris creates a prepubic space.

First the vesico-vaginal space is infiltrated with diluted xylocaine–adrenaline solution for hydrodissection and hemostasis. The vaginal introitus is incised, and the external urethral sphincter is gently dissected away from the submucosal vaginal tissue. Four mosquito clamps hold the vaginal mucosa (Fig. 13.20B), and the space between the posterior vaginal wall and the rectum is bluntly dissected, and subsequently the space between the anterior vaginal wall

and the bladder is dissected with the electrocautery. Then lateral dissection is started: the levator muscle is released from the lateral vaginal wall using electrocautery for better hemostasis. Dissection is continued until fibrotic tissue of the former hysterectomy is reached. Lateral dissection continues to the midline following this fibrotic plane, and the vagina is removed.

Before urethral reconstruction starts, an 18Fr silicone drain is inserted and a traction suture is placed to hold the enlarged clitoris. The mucosa between the external urethral orifice and the clitoral glans will serve as the urethral plate for the pars fixa of the urethra (Fig. 13.20C). The incision lines are marked (minimum width 2.5 cm), and the urethral plate is dissected away from the inner surface of the labia minora. Now, tubularization of the urethral plate is started at the

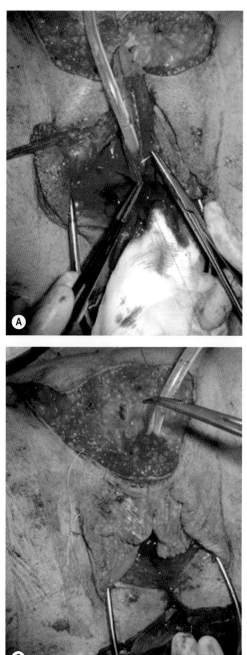

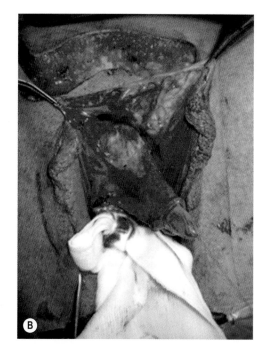

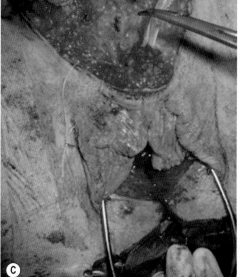

Fig. 13.21 **(A)** Creation of the pars fixa of the urethra by tabularization of the urethral plate. **(B)** Release of the foreskin of the clitoral shaft. **(C)** Tunneling of the clitoris and the distal end of the pars fixa to the prepubic area.

external urethral orifice, with inclusion of the orifices of the paraurethral glands of Skène. Closure of the urethral plate is continued towards the clitoral glans with a running suture in 3-0 Monocryl leaving an oblique distal end for anastomosis with the phallic urethra (Fig. 13.21A). The preputial skin is released from the clitoral shaft, and the clitoral glans is denuded (Fig. 13.21B). One dorsal clitoral nerve (1 or 11 o'clock position) is identified and prepared for later anastomosis. The clitoris and the urethra are tunneled towards the prepubic area and fixed to the pubic symphysis with a Vicryl 2-0 suture (Fig. 13.21C).

Now scrotoplasty is performed: posterior borders of the labia majora are incised (Figs. 13.20A, 13.22B ⬤). The subcutaneous fat is dissected to create two flaps (Fig. 13.22C). The

superficial pelvic floor muscles are now exposed and sutured around the pars fixa of the urethra to close the superficial perineal space (Fig. 13.22A). Abduction and flexion of the hips are reduced in order to facilitate closure with Vicryl 1. The labia majora flaps are now rotated 180° anteriorly towards the base of the foreskin of the clitoris (Fig. 13.22A), and the remains of labia minora are resected as most patients do not want to be reminded to their former female anatomy. The scrotum is placed in front of the patient's legs, and the skin is closed with 3-0 Monocryl (Fig. 13.22).

Fig. 13.22C & F appears online only.

To prepare the pars fixa of the urethra for anastomosis with the phallic pars, 12–16 separate Vicryl 4-0 sutures are placed in its oblique distal end through the prepubic incision. In order to prevent fistula formation, it is advised to catch only submucosa with the suture bite. At the end of the perineal procedure, a suprapubic catheter is inserted.

Metoidioplasty

A metoidioplasty uses the (hypertrophied) clitoris to reconstruct a microphallus in a way comparable with the correction of chordee and lengthening of a urethra in cases of severe hypospadias. Eicher[57] calls it "the clitoris penoid". In metoidioplasty, the clitoral hood is lifted and the suspensory ligament of the clitoris is detached from the pubic bone, allowing the clitoris to extend out further. An embryonic urethral plate is divided from the underside of the clitoris to permit outward extension and a visible erection.[58–61] The urethra is then advanced to the tip of the new penis. The technique is very similar to the reconstruction of the horizontal part of the urethra in a normal phalloplasty procedure. Scrotal reconstruction and vaginectomy are performed during the same procedure.

FTM patients interested in this procedure should be informed preoperatively that voiding while standing cannot be guaranteed, and that sexual intercourse will not be possible (Fig. 13.23).

The major advantages of metoidioplasty are absence of a donor scar, preservation of erectile function even if only in a

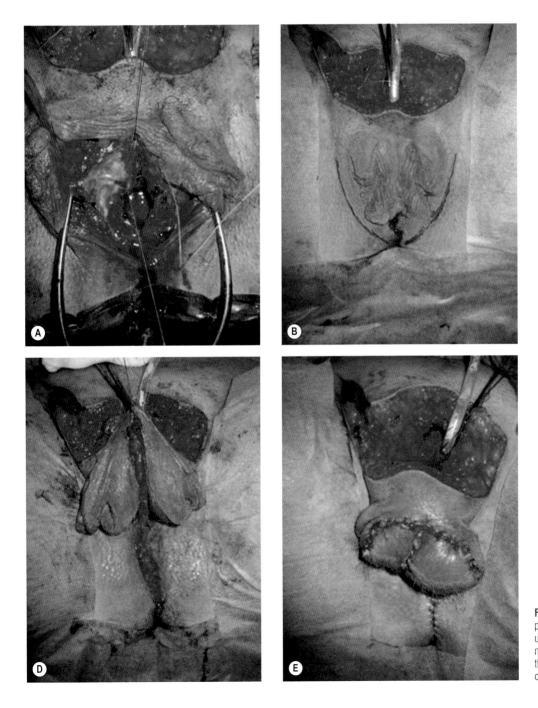

Fig. 13.22 **(A)** Closure of the superficial perineal muscles over the pars fixa of the urethra. **(B)** Incision lines at the labia majora for the scrotoplasty. **(D)** Rotation of the labial flaps 180° anteriorly. **(E)** Closure of the skin and final result.

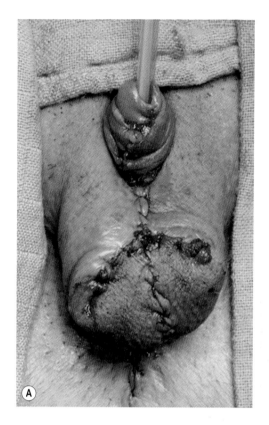
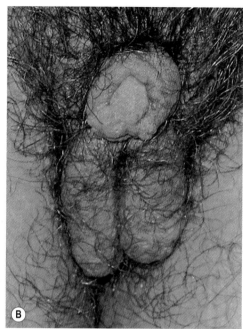

Fig. 13.23 Metoidioplasty. **(A)** Immediate results. **(B)** Late postoperative results.

micropenis, and lower costs compared to a phalloplasty. Complications of this procedure also include urethral obstruction and fistula.

It is always possible to perform a regular phalloplasty (e.g., with a radial forearm flap) at a later stage, and with the likelihood of reduced risk of complications and shorter operating time because vaginectomy, reconstruction of the pars fixa of the urethra, and scrotoplasty have already been performed.

Complete phallic reconstruction

The term "phalloplasty" was first used in 1858 by Sprengler to indicate reconstruction of the integument after decollement (separation of the superficial tissue layers) of the penis.[62] Bogoras, the first to report on the reconstruction of the entire penis, labeled his procedure "penis plastica totalis".[63] He was also the first to use a single abdominal tube, a technique later applied by others. Subsequently, "phalloplasty" was used to describe penile reconstruction.

Following the WWII, some leading plastic surgeons showed an interest in phalloplasty. In 1948, McIndoe[64] improved the abdominal tubed flap by constructing a neo-urethra while raising the tube pedicle with an inlay skin graft. Maltz[65] and Gillies and Millard[66] popularized the technique adding a costal cartilage graft as rigidity prosthesis. Further, Gillies was the first to report the use of this technique in a transsexual patient. The Stanford team[61,67] refined the procedure by tubing an infraumbilical abdominal flap inside out in order to create a skin-lined tunnel as a future urethral conduit. This method reduced the number of stages previously necessary for phalloplasty.

Snyder described phalloplasty with a single pedicled infraumbilical skin flap prelaminated with a superficial

skin-lined conduit.[68,69] In addition, Hester performed phalloplasty in one stage using a vertical, superficial inferior epigastric artery flap with a subcutaneous pedicle in a male born with ambiguous genitalia.[70] After McGregor introduced the groin flap in 1972,[24] Hoopes[71] commented that "the groin flap may prove the method of choice for phallus reconstruction". Orticochea[38] used a gracilis myocutaneous flap in a five-stage phalloplasty procedure and claimed it produced cosmetically and functionally superior results. The Norfolk team also used a unilateral gracilis myocutaneous flap for phalloplasty.[39] Sometimes a combination of flaps was used. Exner[72] implanted rigidity prosthesis in a rectus abdominis muscular flap and used bilateral groin flaps to cover the neophallus.

Once microsurgery established a foothold in genital construction, plastic surgeons began to explore and map out the genital neurovascular supply and to consider expanding the applications of microsurgery to elective reconstruction of the genitalia. Chang and Hwang[73] described an ingenious adaptation of the tube-in-tube concept into a free tissue transfer with the RFF originally described by Song et al.[74]

Since these early reports, a wide variety of other free flaps have also been described for phalloplasty, including the dorsalis pedis flap,[29] the deltoid flap,[75] the lateral arm flap,[76] the fibular flap,[77] the tensor fasciae latae flap,[40] the ALT,[78] and the DIEAP flap.[79] The fact that so many techniques for penile reconstruction exist is evidence that none is considered ideal. Still, most of these articles are only case reports or small series and even nowadays the "old" Chinese flap or RFF is by far (>90%) the most frequently used free flap in the literature[80] and is therefore often considered as the gold standard for penile reconstruction.

Radial forearm flap: technique and long-term results (Video 13.1 ⊙)

Monstrey *et al.* recently published the only large and well-documented, long-term follow-up study on the use of the radial forearm phalloplasty.[79] They described the technique used in 287 consecutive cases and evaluated to what degree this supposed "gold standard" has been able to meet the ideal goals in phallic reconstruction.

Technique

While the urologist is operating in the perineal area in the lithotomy position, the plastic surgeon dissects the free flap of the forearm. The creation of a phallus with a tube-in-a-tube technique is performed with the flap still attached to the forearm by its vascular pedicle. A small skin flap and a skin graft are used to create a corona and simulate the glans of the penis (Fig. 13.24A–F ⊙).

Fig. 13.24D appears online only.

Once urethra lengthening is completed, the patient is put into a supine position to prepare the recipient vessels contralateral to the flap. The free flap can be transferred to the pubic area, and urethral anastomosis is performed first (Fig. 13.24G & H): the radial artery is microsurgically connected to the common femoral artery in an end-to-side fashion, and the venous anastomosis is performed between the cephalic vein and the greater saphenous vein. Alternatively, arterial anastomosis can be done end-to-end to a side branch of the femoral artery. One forearm nerve is connected to the ilioinguinal nerve for protective sensation, and the other nerve of the forearm is connected to one of the dorsal clitoral nerves – that

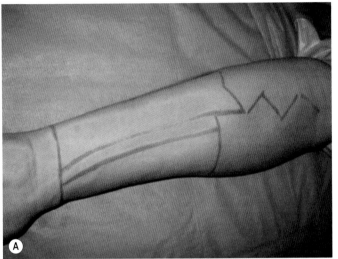

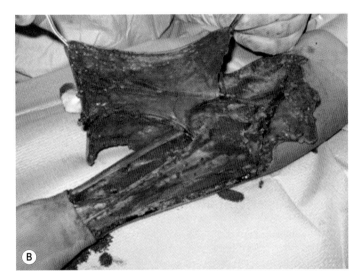

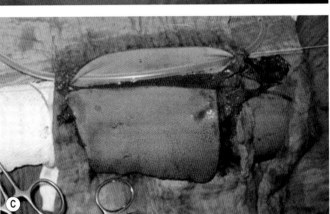

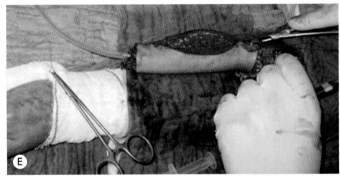

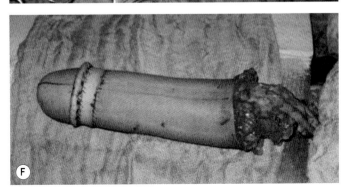

Fig. 13.24 Standard radial forearm technique. **(A)** Design. **(B)** Dissection of the flap. **(C)** Tubing (inner tube) of the urethra. **(E)** Outer tube of the penis itself. **(F)** Creation of the glans of the penis (with penis still attached to the forearm, just prior to transfer to the pubic area).

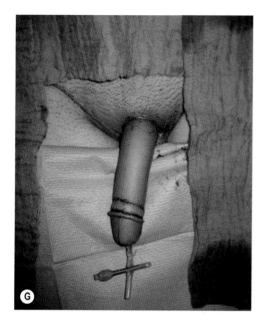

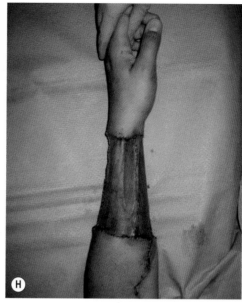

Fig. 13.24, cont'd (G) Immediate postoperative result of the penis. **(H)** The donor site on the arm.

has been previously prepared and marked by the urologist – to restore erogenous sensation. The clitoris is usually denuded and buried underneath the penis, thus keeping the possibility for stimulation during sexual intercourse.

In the first 50 patients of this series, the defect on the forearm was covered with full-thickness skin grafts taken from the groin area. In subsequent patients, the defect was covered with split-thickness skin grafts harvested from the medial and anterior thigh.

All patients receive a suprapubic urinary diversion. They then remain in bed for 1 week, and the transurethral catheter is removed after 10 days if no major local wound healing problems are present. The patient starts voiding at day 12, and the suprapubic catheter is removed at day 14 if no substantial residual urine (>100 mL) is present. The average hospital stay for the phalloplasty procedure is 2.5 weeks.

Tattooing of the glans can be performed after a 2–3 month period, before sensation returns to the penis. Implantation of the testicular prostheses can be performed after 6 months, but it is typically done in combination with the implantation of a penile erection prosthesis, 1 year after the operation, once penile sensitivity is completely restored and has reached the tip of the penis.

Ideal goals

The ideal goals or requirements of a penile reconstruction have been described by Hage and De Graaf[80] and include the following challenges: (1) a one-stage procedure that can be predictably reproduced, (2) an aesthetically acceptable phallus, (3) a phallus that has both tactile and erogenous sensibility, (4) a competent neo-urethra to allow voiding while standing, (5) minimal complications, (6) an acceptable donor site morbidity, (7) a natural-looking scrotum, and (8) enough phallic bulk to tolerate the insertion of a prosthetic stiffener allowing sexual intercourse. What can be achieved with the RFF phalloplasty technique?

A one-stage procedure

It has been accepted that a complete penile reconstruction with erection prosthesis can never be performed in one single operation. Monstrey *et al.* however, early in their series and in order to reduce the number of surgeries, performed a (sort of) all-in-one procedure, which included a subcutaneous mastectomy (SCM) and a complete genito-perineal transformation.[79] However, later in their series they performed the SCM first most often in combination with a total hysterectomy and oophorectomy.

The reason for this change in protocol was that lengthy operations (>8 h) resulted in considerable blood loss and increased operative risk.[81] Moreover, an aesthetic SCM is not to be considered an easy operation and should not be performed "quickly" before the major phalloplasty operation.

An aesthetic phallus

Phallic construction has become predictable enough to refine its aesthetic goals, which include the use of a technique that can be replicated with minimal complications. In this respect, the RFF has several advantages: the flap is thin and pliable allowing the construction of a normal sized, tube-within-a-tube penis; the flap is easy to dissect and is predictably well vascularized making it safe to perform a (aesthetic) glans-plasty at the distal end of the flap. The final cosmetic outcome of a radial forearm phalloplasty is a subjective determination, but the ability for most patients to shower with other men or go to the sauna is the usual cosmetic barometer (Fig. 13.25).

The potential aesthetic drawbacks of the RFF are the need for a rigidity prosthesis, flattening of the reconstructed corona, and possibly some volume loss over time.

Tactile and erogenous sensation

Of the various flaps used for penile reconstruction, the RFF has the best sensitivity.[82,83] Monstrey *et al.*[79] always connect one antebrachial nerve to the ilioinguinal nerve for protective sensation and the other forearm nerve with one dorsal clitoral nerve. The denuded clitoris is always placed directly below the phallic shaft. Later manipulation of the neophallus allows for stimulation of the still-innervated clitoris.

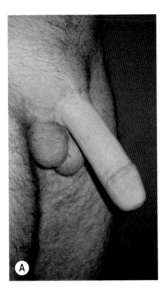

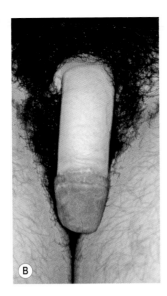

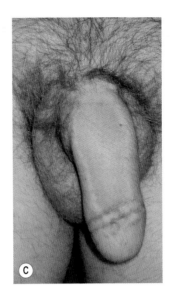

Fig. 13.25 Late postoperative results of radial forearm phalloplasties.

After 1 year, all patients in Monstrey *et al.*'s series[79] had regained tactile sensitivity in their penis, which is an absolute requirement for safe insertion of an erection prosthesis.[82]

In a long-term follow-up study on postoperative sexual and physical health, more than 80% of the patients reported improvement in sexual satisfaction and greater ease in reaching orgasm (100% in practicing postoperative FTM transsexuals).[84]

Voiding while standing

For biologic males as well as for FTM transsexuals undergoing a phalloplasty, the ability to void while standing is a high priority.[85] Unfortunately, the reported incidences of urologic complications, such as urethrocutaneous fistulas, strictures, and hairy urethras, are extremely high in all series of phalloplasties, even up to 80%.[34] For this reason, certain (well-intentioned) surgeons have even stopped reconstructing a complete neo-urethra.[76,78]

Although Monstrey *et al.*[79] reported a 41% (119/287) urologic complication rate, the majority of these early fistulas closed spontaneously and ultimately *all* patients were able to void through the newly reconstructed penis. Since it is unknown how the new urethra – an, on average, 16 cm skin tube – will affect bladder function in the long term, lifelong urologic follow-up was strongly recommended for all these patients.[86]

Minimal morbidity

Complications following phalloplasty include the general complications such as minor wound healing problems in the groin area or (minor) pulmonary embolism despite adequate prevention (interrupting hormonal therapy, fractioned heparin SC, and elastic stockings). A vaginectomy is usually considered a particularly difficult operation with a high risk of postoperative bleeding, but in Monstrey *et al.*'s series no major bleedings were seen.[81] Two early patients displayed symptoms of nerve compression in the lower leg, but after reducing the length of the gynecologic positioning to under 2 h, this complication never occurred again. Apart from the urinary fistulas and/or strictures, most complications of the radial forearm phalloplasty are related to free tissue transfer. The total flap failure in their series was very low (<1%, 2/287)

despite a somewhat higher anastomotic revision rate (12% or 34/287). About 7.3% of the patients demonstrated some degree of skin slough or partial flap necrosis. This was more often the case in smokers, in those who insisted on a large-sized penis requiring a larger flap, and also in patients having undergone anastomotic revision.

With *smoking* being a significant risk factor many microsurgeons and transgender surgeons no longer perform elective microsurgical penile reconstruction on patients who fail to quit smoking 1 year prior to their surgery.

No functional loss and minimal scarring in the donor area

The major drawback of the RFF has always been the unattractive donor site scar on the forearm (Fig. 13.26). Selvaggi *et al.* conducted a long-term follow-up study[87] of 125 radial forearm phalloplasties to assess the degree of functional loss

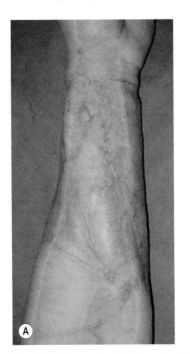

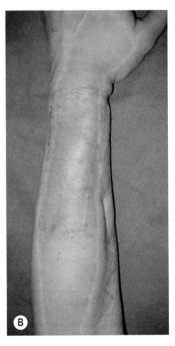

Fig. 13.26 Late result of the donor site at the forearm.

and aesthetic impairment after harvesting such a large forearm flap. An increased donor site morbidity was expected, but the early and late complications did not differ from the rates reported in the literature for smaller flaps as used in head and neck reconstruction. No major or long-term problems (such as functional limitation, nerve injury, chronic pain/edema, or cold intolerance) were identified. Finally, with regard to the aesthetic outcome of the donor site, they found that the patients were very accepting of the donor site scar, viewing it as a worthwhile trade-off for the creation of a phallus. Suprafascial flap dissection, full-thickness skin grafting, and the use of dermal substitutes may improve the forearm scar.

Normal scrotum

For the FTM patient, the goal of creating natural-appearing genitalia also applies to the scrotum. As the labia majora are the embryologic counterpart of the scrotum, many previous scrotoplasty techniques left the hair-bearing labia majora *in situ*, with midline closure and prosthetic implant filling, or brought the scrotum in front of the legs using a V-Y plasty. These techniques were aesthetically unappealing and reminiscent of the female genitalia. Selvaggi in 2009 reported on a novel scrotoplasty technique that combines a V-Y plasty with a 90° turning of the labial flaps resulting in an anterior transposition of labial skin (Fig. 13.27). The excellent aesthetic outcome of this male-looking (anteriorly located) scrotum, the functional advantage of fewer urologic complications, and the easier implantation of testicular prostheses make this the technique of choice.[88]

Sexual intercourse

In a radial forearm phalloplasty, the insertion of an erection prosthesis is required in order to engage in sexual intercourse. In the past, attempts have been made to use bone or cartilage, but no good long-term results are described. The rigid and semirigid prostheses seem to have a high perforation rate and therefore were initially never used in our patients. Hoebeke *et al.*, in the largest series to date on erection prostheses after penile reconstruction, only used the hydraulic systems available for impotent men.[89] A recent long-term follow-up study showed an explantation rate of 44% in 130 patients, mainly due to malpositioning, technical failure, or infection. Still, more than 80% of the patients were able to have normal sexual intercourse with penetration. In another study, it was demonstrated that patients with an erection prosthesis were more able to attain their sexual expectations than those without prosthesis (Fig. 13.28).[90]

A major concern regarding erectile prostheses is long-term follow-up. These devices were developed for impotent (older) men who have a shorter life expectancy and who are sexually less active than the mostly younger FTM patients.

Nowadays some newer semirigid devices are available with less risk of perforation. These therefore have become an option for implantation after phalloplasty.

Conclusion

The authors in this review article conclude that the radial forearm phalloplasty is a very reliable technique for the construction, usually in two stages, of a normal-looking penis that allows the patient to void while standing and also to experience sexual satisfaction.

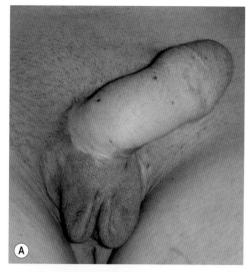

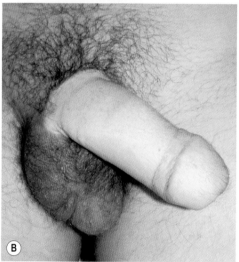

Fig. 13.27 Reconstruction of a lateral looking scrotum with two transposition flaps before and after implantation of prostheses.

The main disadvantages of this technique are the rather high number of initial fistulas, the scar on the forearm, and the potential long-term urologic complications.

Alternative phalloplasty techniques

Perforator flaps

Perforator flaps are considered the ultimate form of tissue transfer. Donor site morbidity is reduced to an absolute minimum, and the usually large vascular pedicles provide an additional range of motion or an easier vascular anastomosis. At present, the most promising perforator flap for penile reconstruction is the ALT flap, which can be used both as a free flap[91] or rather as a pedicled flap (S. Suominen, pers. comm. 1994),[41,92] therefore avoiding the problems related to microsurgical free flap transfer (see above).

The pedicled ALT flap represents the best alternative for penile reconstruction because as a pedicled flap it does not require any microvascular anastomosis, it can be reinnervated like the RFF, and its donor site morbidity is limited to the donor site scar that requires skin grafting and is more easily concealed.

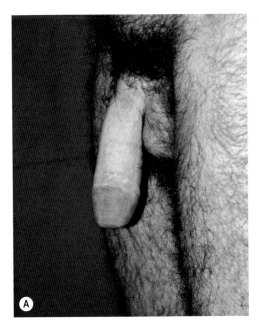

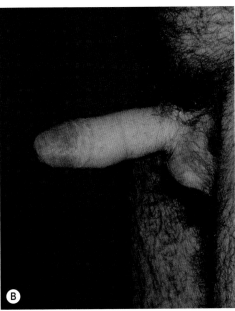

Fig. 13.28 After implantation of an erection prosthesis.

Accurate patient selection is mandatory. Candidates for this technique are patients that:

- Have a pinch test of less than 2 cm in the lateral thigh
- Do not wish to have a forearm scar
- Would accept the scar on the thigh
- Have an insufficient ulnar artery on Allen's test
- Have an adequate, possibly septocutaneous, perforator on angio-CT (or MRI).

We routinely perform a preoperative CT scan to choose the best side for harvest of the ALT flap.[93] The distal most perforator is chosen, and the flap is drawn with the perforator lying close to its proximal margin (Fig. 13.29A) in order to gain pedicle length for tensionless transfer to the pubic area. The proximal incision is performed first, and two sensory branches of the lateral femoral cutaneous nerves are isolated for sensory

coaptation (Fig. 13.29D). Then the medial or lateral incision is performed – according to the surgeon's preferences – and suprafascial dissection is carried out until the perforator is identified. Once perforator dissection is completed, the flap is harvested circumferentially (Fig. 13.29E). In most cases it is sufficient to tunnel the flap underneath the rectus femoris and then under a subcutaneous tunnel to the groin. Both tunnels should be as wide as possible. If additional length is required, the pedicle can be dissected more proximally with sacrifice of the vascular branch to the rectus femoris and also tunneled underneath the sartorius muscle that – in cases of short pedicles – will act as a sling and cause pedicle compression. Once the flap is tunneled and the pedicle is checked (Fig. 13.29F), the flap is wrapped around the reconstructed urethra (see below) and shaped. The coronoplasty is performed 10 days after the operation due to the different vascularization of the ALT compared to the RFF.

The major drawback of the ALT flap is that, unless the patient is extremely thin, the tube-within-a-tube technique cannot be used for urethra reconstruction.

An inner urethral tube can be provided by prefabricating the ALT flap with a split-thickness skin graft. The skin-grafted area should have a width of at least 5 cm to provide an adequate inner tube and prevent future stricture. Still, the quality of the inner urethral tube when lined with skin grafts might be inferior compared to normal skin, resulting in a higher rate of urologic complications (strictures and fistulas) when compared to a RFF tube-within-tube phalloplasty. The shape of a prefabricated ALT phalloplasty is comparable with or even somewhat better than the RFAF phalloplasty if the patient is not too fat and the flap is defatted. This technique can be an excellent backup in redo phalloplasties and in cases when no forearm is available.

To overcome this problem the ALT has either been used alone without urethral reconstruction or combined with a second flap for the inner urethral tube. However, to date, there is no extensive report on this technique apart from one case series and a few case reports.[94–98] We have performed more than 80 phalloplasties with an ALT flap (unpublished data) and – as the ability to void while standing is an essential requirement of a phalloplasty – we have worked on an effective technique of urethral reconstruction. We will go through all the potential alternatives available.

The fabrication of an inner tube for urethral conduit makes the ALT flap procedure in reconstruction of a phallus more complex, especially in the biologically female transman, while in most bladder extrophy patients the inner tube is not necessary as they have a urinary diversion.

As outlined earlier, a tube-within-a-tube, similar to the conventional RFAF phalloplasty procedure, can also be constructed in the case of a pedicled ALT flap, but only in very thin individuals. In most cases, however, the subcutaneous fat is too thick and another technique must be chosen to reconstruct the inner urethral tube.

The use of well-vascularized tissue is necessary. Therefore the inner tube is best made with another flap. A pedicled peritoneal flap, elevated together with the posterior rectus fascia pedicled on a branch of the deep inferior epigastric artery pedicle[99] has been tried in order to reconstruct a urethral conduit, but this was not suitable:[41,100] the inner peritoneal lining easily causes fibrosis resulting in permanent obliteration of the lumen.[100]

Another option could be a pedicled groin flap, turned 180° on its pedicle and transferred to the pubic area, with the proximal part of its pedicle buried subcutaneously. The donor scar can be closed primarily. Because of the thickness of the flap, the same objections can be made as mentioned with the tube-within-a-tube technique and a bulk is left where the pedicle is tunneled.

Eventually, we discovered our current standard technique: a pedicle superficial circumflex iliac (artery) perforator (SCI (A) P) can be harvested as an ultrathin flap but pedicled. This flap

has been described bilaterally for total penile reconstruction, but it carries the major disadvantage of not being sensate, thus making it impossible to safely wear an erectile prosthesis.[101] The SCIAP allows combination of two pedicled perforator flaps (Fig. 13.29A), sensate ALT and SCIAP, without prolonging operative time because the SCIAP flap can be harvested and tubed in the lithotomy position during the urologic part (Fig. 13.29B & C). Then the patient is put back in the supine position, the SCIAP is sutured to the elongated urethra, and

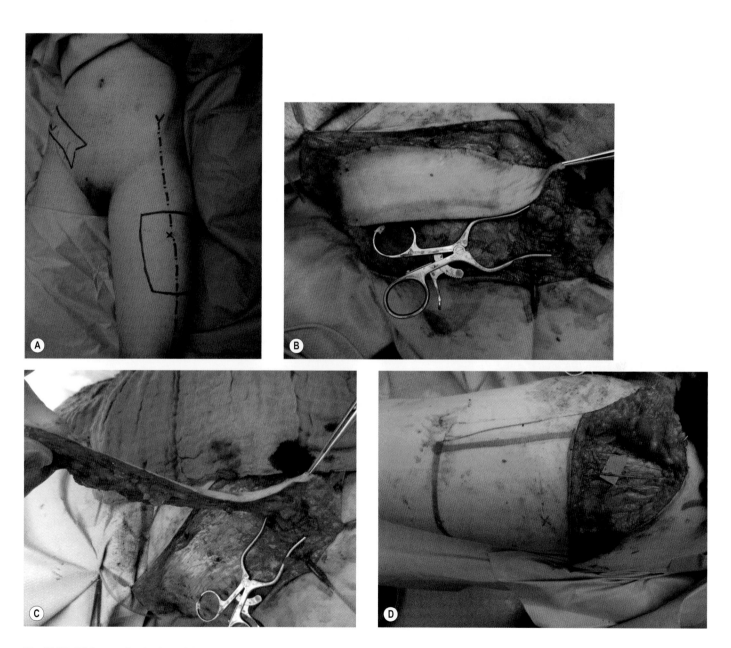

Fig. 13.29 (A) Preoperative drawings of the anterolateral thigh/superficial circumflex iliac artery perforator (ALT/SCIAP) phalloplasty. The ALT is planned based on the angio-CT findings. The SCIAP flap is planned contralaterally to the ALT with a distal "V" shaped tip to compensate for scar retraction at the junction between the pars fixa and the phallic urethra. **(B)** The SCIAP flap at the end of pedicle dissection (left is lateral, the fish hooks are placed caudally). The green backgrounds are placed underneath the SCIAP (lateral) and the superficial vein (medial). There is always a superficial vein draining the skin of the SCIAP, which is only kept when it does not interfere with flap rotation. **(C)** A caudal view of the elevated SCIAP flap shows how thin the flap can be. After elevation the tip and margins of the flap can be further trimmed. Having such a thin flap for urethral reconstruction is very important, especially in the female-to-male (FTM) transgender patient, whose ALTs are usually thicker than in biologic males. **(D)** Once the patient is put back in the supine position, harvesting of the ALT flap is begun. Prior to that, the tubed SCIAP flap is sutured to the pars fixa of the urethra and wrapped in wet gauze while the donor site is closed primarily. The dissection of the ALT flap (right is cranial, top is medial, the knee is on the left side) is begun with proximal incision and identification of two branches of the lateral femoral cutaneous nerve.

Continued

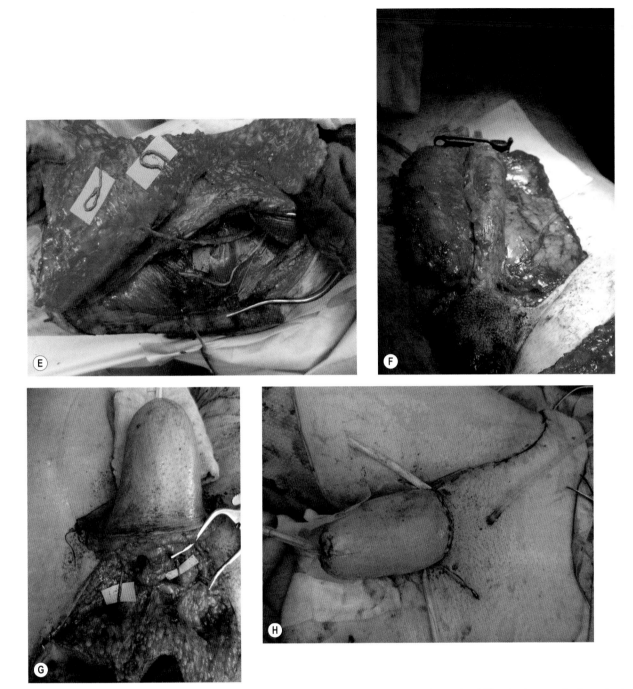

Fig. 13.29, cont'd (E) Same view as Fig. 13.29D. The flap is reflected medially. Pedicle dissection is completed. The retractor separates the rectus femoris and the vastus lateralis muscle. The pedicle between them is evidenced by a green background. The perforator ran for a short distance inside the muscle in this particular case. Between the fishhooks and the retractor a small amount of muscle fiber has been divided to allow for pedicle transfer. Next to it and medially, the intact motor nerve to the vastus lateralis can be seen. Two green backgrounds are placed on the undersurface of the flap with the sensory nerves lying on top of them. **(F)** This caudal view shows the ALT flap after tunneling and before tubing (top is cranial, right is left on the patient's body). The ALT is lying with the skin on the pubic skin; its undersurface is visible with the tubed SCIAP lying on top of it. At this point the ALT will be sutured around the SCIAP. Any undue tension should be avoided and postoperative edema anticipated. Any tension might potentially compromise the flaps. In the case of doubt, a split-thickness skin graft can be placed between the two edges of the ALT in the ventral (less visible) surface of the penis. **(G)** Bird's eye view of the reconstructed penis (left is cranial, top is right) nerve coaptations are the last step to correctly estimate length as the shorter the nerve stump, the faster reinnervation. Two green backgrounds are placed underneath the coapted nerves: the one above is coapted to the right dorsal clitoral nerve, the one below to one of the ilio-inguinal nerves. **(H)** Before and after closure the flap must always be checked because any undue tension or compression on the pedicle must be avoided. A slightly pinker flap with a slightly faster refill like the one shown in this picture is – however – extremely common with pedicled perforator flaps and should not be a cause for concern.

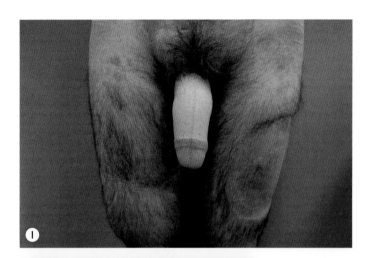

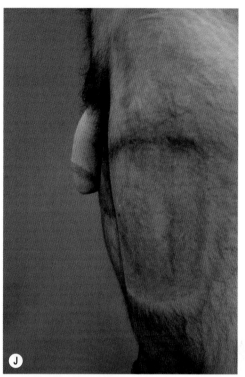

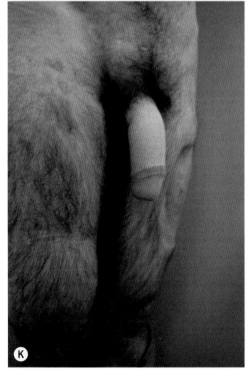

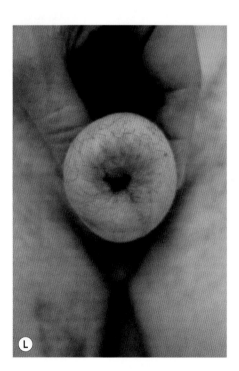

Fig. 13.29, cont'd (I–K) One-year postoperative result before erectile prosthesis implantation. Front, lateral, and three-quarters view. Showing the end result, the flap's donor site on the left thigh, the skin graft donor site on the right thigh, and the barely visible SCIAP flap donor site scar on the right groin. **(L)** Frontal view of the tip of the penis. The external urinary meatus stays patent and allows effective voiding.

the ALT is harvested and transferred (Fig. 13.29D–H). Nowadays, unless there are bilateral groin scars, this is our first choice for urethral reconstruction in combination with an ALT phalloplasty (Fig. 13.29I–L).

A good though demanding alternative is a narrow free RFAF. This flap is thin and very well vascularized (Fig. 13.30). The results of this combined (pedicled ALT+free RFAF) phalloplasty procedure were similar to the results

of the RFAF (only) phalloplasty with regard to the urologic complication rate and were even more pleasing from an aesthetic point of view. The resulting scar on the arm is small and located on the inner side (Fig. 13.30). This scar is easily concealed and acceptable for most FTM transsexuals willing to avoid the circumferential scar. The scar on the leg, although conspicuous, never poses a problem for these patients as it can be more easily hidden than the scar on the arm, which is sometimes considered "the signature" of a phalloplasty procedure. Obviously, this procedure becomes more complex as it combines two flaps, one of which is a free microvascular flap.

Fibular flap and muscle flaps

There have been several reports on penile reconstruction with the fibular flap based on the peroneal artery and the peroneal vein.[102–103] This flap consists of a piece of fibula that is vascularized by its periosteal blood supply and connected through perforating (septal) vessels to an overlying skin island at the lateral site of the lower leg. The advantage of the fibular flap is that it makes sexual intercourse possible without a penile prosthesis. The disadvantages of this technique are the poor quality of flap sensation, a pointed deformity to the distal part of the penis when the extra skin can glide around the end of fibular bone, and that a permanently erected phallus is impractical.

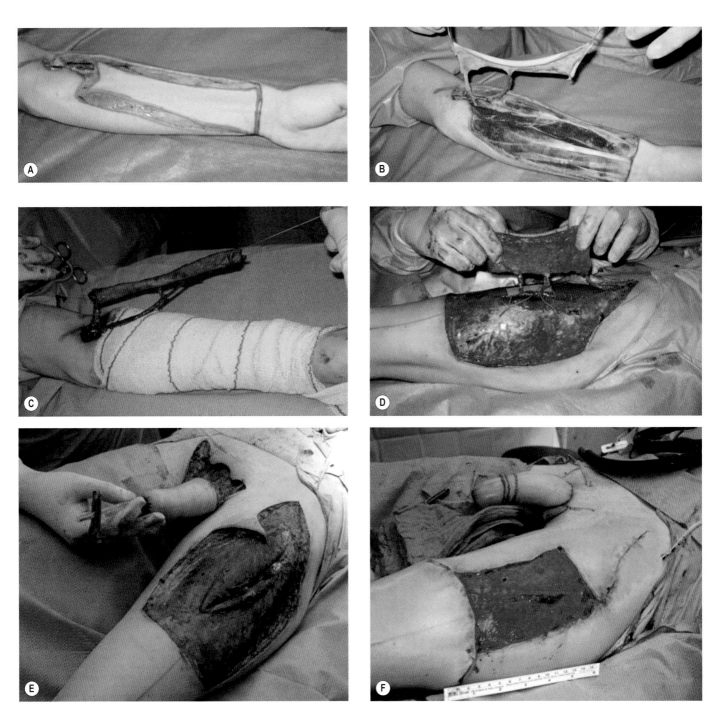

Fig. 13.30 (A,B) Dissection of a narrow free vascularized radial forearm used for the urethra. (C) The radial forearm flap urethra is ready to be transferred to the pubic area. (D) Dissection of the anterolateral thigh (ALT) flap that will be used to wrap around the urethra. (E) Radial forearm flap (RFAF) urethra and ALT wrap-around put into position in the pubic area. (F) After coronoplasty and grafting of the donor area.

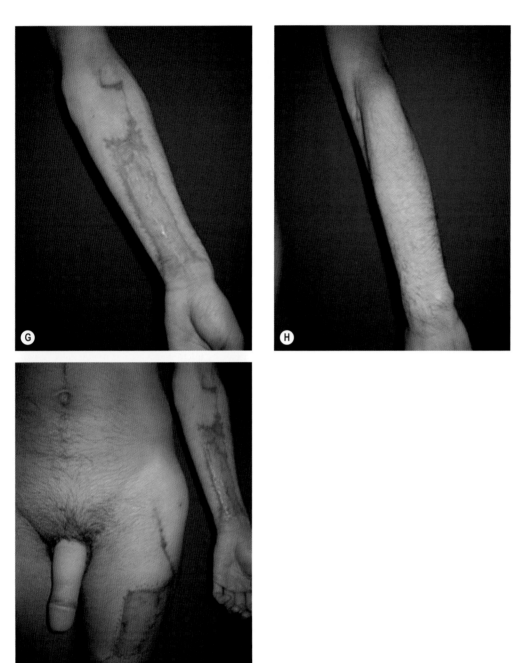

Fig. 13.30, cont'd (G–I) Results after 3 months: the donor site on the inner aspect of the arm is inconspicuous and the donor site on the leg can easily be covered, even with shorts.

Alternative techniques also employ innervated muscle flaps like the free latissimus dorsi[104] and the bilateral pedicled gracilis flap.[105] Both techniques enable contraction of the penis, which is present from the beginning with the gracilis and needs nerve regeneration with the latissimus dorsi. However, no skin sensation is restored, and urethral reconstruction, if attempted, needs multiple stage techniques. These muscle flaps are not reported to have protective skin sensitivity, and subsequently they are not reported to host a penile prosthesis. Vesely[104] reports that 42% of patients have sexual intercourse because muscle contraction allows the penis to stiffen and move during sexual intercourse.

Summary

The importance of a multidisciplinary approach

Gender reassignment, particularly reassignment surgery, requires close cooperation between the different surgical specialties. In phalloplasty, the collaboration between the plastic surgeon, the urologist, and the gynecologist is essential.[106] The actual penile reconstruction is typically performed by the plastic and reconstructive surgeon, but, in the long term, the urologist's role may be the most important for patients who have undergone penile reconstruction, especially because the complication rate is rather high, particularly with regard to the number of urinary fistulas and urinary strictures. The urologist also reconstructs the fixed part of the urethra and is generally the best choice for implantation and follow-up of the penile and/or testicular prostheses. The urologist also addresses later sequelae, including stone formation. More-over, the surgical complexity of adding an elongated conduit (skin-tube urethra) to a biologic female bladder, and the long-term effects of evacuating urine through this skin tube, demand lifelong urologic follow-up.

Therefore professionals who unite for the purpose of creating a gender reassignment program should be aware of the necessity for a strong alliance, mainly between the plastic surgeon and the urologist, which is an absolute requisite for consistently obtaining the best possible results. In turn, the surgeons must commit to the extended care of this unique population that, by definition, will continue well into the future.

Bonus images for this chapter can be found online at
http://www.expertconsult.com

Fig. 13.10 Buried penis: retraction of the peripenile and pubic fat reveals a normal size penis.

Fig. 13.13 (D–F) A Cavi-Care dressing is applied around the skin graft (poured out in a cylinder form around the penis), and this dressing will stay for 1 week.

Fig. 13.15 (B) After penile elongation with release of the suspensory ligament and coverage of the distal part of the penis with buccal mucosa. **(C)** Result of glans reconstruction using buccal mucosa.

Fig. 13.22 (C) Creation of the flaps for the scrotoplasty. **(F)** Closure of the skin and final result.

Fig. 13.24 (D) Tubing (inner tube) of the urethra.

 Access the complete reference list online at   **http://www.expertconsult.com**

6. Mitchell ME, Bägli DJ. Complete penile disassembly for epispadias repair: the Mitchell technique. *J Urol*. 1996;155(1):300–304. *The authors present their technique for epispadias repair in the context of a case series. Phallic disassembly into the urethral plate and bilateral hemicorporeal glandular bodies are the basis for their reconstruction.*

10. Lee PA, Houk CP, Ahmed SF, et al. Consensus statement on management of intersex disorders. International Consensus Conference on Intersex. *Pediatrics*. 2006;118(2):e488–e500. *This paper represents the responses of 50 international experts to a series of literature-based questions. Topics ranging from diagnosis to medical and surgical management, as well as the important role of psychosocial support, are discussed.*

24. McGregor IA, Jackson IT. The groin flap. *Br J Plast Surg*. 1972;25:3.

33. Hurwitz DJ, Swartz WM, Mathes SJ. The gluteal thigh flap: a reliable, sensate flap for the closure of buttock and perineal wounds. *Plast Reconstr Surg*. 1981;68:521. *The authors describe the results of anatomic dissections detailing the gluteal thigh flap's neurovascular morphology. A case series demonstrating the clinical utility of the flap is also presented.*

38. Orticochea M. A new method of total reconstruction of the penis. *Br J Plast Surg*. 1972;25:347–366.

42. Cohen BE, May JW, Daly JS, et al. Successful clinical replantation of an amputated penis by microneurovascular repair. *Plast Reconstr Surg*. 1977;59:276.

55. Eke N. Fournier's gangrene: a review of 1726 cases. *Br J Surg*. 2000;87:718. *This is a meta-analysis of Fournier's gangrene publications from 1950–99. The authors investigate trends in diagnosis and management and conclude that while precise definitions vary, treatment is based on clinical presentation.*

70. Hester TR Jr, Nahain F, Beeglen PE, et al. Blood supply of the abdomen revisited, with emphasis on the superficial inferior epigastric artery. *Plast Reconstr Surg*. 1984;74(5):657–666.

73. Chang TS, Hwang YW. Forearm flap in one-stage reconstruction of the penis. *Plast Reconstr Surg*. 1984;74:251–258. *Single stage free forearm-based penile reconstruction is described in this case series.*

79. Monstrey S, Hoebeke P, Selvaggi G, et al. Penile reconstruction: is the radial forearm flap really the standard technique? *Plast Reconstr Surg*. 2009;124:510–518.

14

Reconstruction of acquired vaginal defects

Leila Jazayeri, Andrea L. Pusic, and Peter G. Cordeiro

SYNOPSIS

- Acquired vaginal defects are most commonly the result of oncologic resections.
- The classification of acquired vaginal defects, based on anatomic location, is defined.
- Current approaches to reconstruction of these defects most commonly involve local or regional flaps.
- Flap selection, based on defect type, is described.
- Surgical technique for commonly indicated flaps is described.
- A cautious approach to postoperative management, as well as careful adjustment of patient expectations, is critical in the care of these patients.

 Access the Historical Perspective section online at **http://www.expertconsult.com**

Introduction

Acquired vaginal defects most commonly result from the resection of pelvic malignant neoplasms. Advanced colorectal carcinomas frequently involve the posterior vaginal wall, and carcinoma of the bladder may extend into the anterior vaginal wall. Primary tumors of the vaginal wall may also result in any number of vaginal defects. Local extension or recurrence of uterine or cervical malignant neoplasms can necessitate pelvic exenteration and total vaginal resection. Trauma or burns to the vaginal area may also result in vaginal distortion; however, the relatively protected position of the vagina makes these deformities much less common.

Irrespective of their etiology, vaginal defects may range from a small mucosal defect to total circumferential loss. In addition, tumor ablation may necessitate the resection of nearby pelvic contents and/or vulvar and perineal tissue. The subsequent pelvic dead space or resulting perineal defects are critical considerations in the final reconstruction.

Anatomic considerations

The close anatomic relationship between bladder, vagina, and rectum needs to be appreciated by the reconstructive surgeon. Ligamentous support of these organs is interrelated, and surgical dissection of any one structure may lead to prolapse and herniation of the remaining components. In addition, pelvic exenteration may disrupt or devascularize the pelvic floor musculature. The pelvic sidewalls define a fixed anatomic space that, once cleared of the pelvic organs, will either delineate a dead space or invite small-bowel prolapse and adhesions.

The vagina is essentially a distensible cylindrical pouch (Fig. 14.1). Normal length is 6–7.5 cm along its anterior wall and 9 cm along the posterior wall.[7] It is constricted at the introitus, dilated in the middle, and narrowed near its uterine extremity. In its normal anatomic position, the vagina tilts posteriorly as it extends up into the pelvis, forming a 90° angle with the uterus. Careful orientation of the neovagina is important to successful reconstruction and ultimate sexual function. The introitus is a frequent site of contracture after reconstruction, and any distortion of its normal position relative to other structures, such as the urethral orifice, perineal body, and anus, should be addressed. If no resection of the external vulva and perineum is required, great care must be taken to avoid their distortion because this may also have an impact on sexual function and body image.

Diagnosis

The classification of acquired vaginal defects is based on their anatomic location (Fig. 14.2). This classification will help to guide reconstructive efforts. There are two basic types of vaginal defect: partial (type I) and circumferential (type II). These basic types can be further subclassified. Type IA defects are partial and involve the anterior or lateral wall. These defects may result from the resection of urinary tract

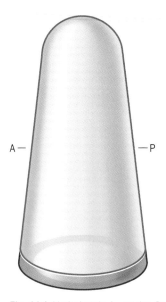

Fig. 14.1 Vaginal vault. A, anterior; P, posterior.

malignant neoplasms or primary malignant neoplasms of the vaginal wall. Type IB defects are partial and involve the posterior wall. These defects, which tend to be the most common type of vaginal defect requiring reconstruction, result primarily from extension of colorectal carcinomas. Type

TYPE I: PARTIAL DEFECT

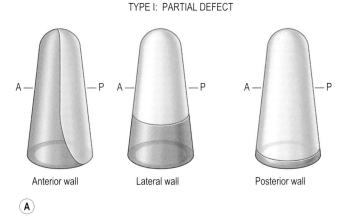

Anterior wall   Lateral wall   Posterior wall

(A)

TYPE II: CIRCUMFERENTIAL DEFECT

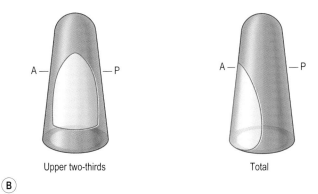

Upper two-thirds   Total

(B)

Fig. 14.2 Classification system of acquired vaginal defects. **(A)** Type I: partial defect. **(B)** Type II: circumferential defect. A, anterior; P, posterior.

IIA defects are circumferential defects involving the upper two-thirds of the vagina. These defects are typically the result of uterine and cervical diseases. Type IIB defects are circumferential, total vaginal defects that are commonly the result of pelvic exenteration. These defects result in considerable soft-tissue loss, dead space, as well as distortion of the introitus.

In addition to the vaginal defect one must consider the extent of the pelvic dead space in ablative surgeries such as APRs and pelvic exenterations. In an APR the entire rectum anal canal and anus are removed and a permanent colostomy is created. When pelvic exenteration is performed, all the organs from the pelvic cavity are removed. The urinary bladder, urethra, rectum, and anus are removed in addition to the vagina, cervix, uterus, fallopian tubes, ovaries, and, in some women, the vulva, and in men, the prostate. In this procedure both a colostomy and urinary diversion are created.

Patient selection/preoperative considerations

Successful management of patients undergoing vaginal reconstruction is dependent upon a multidisciplinary approach. The oncologic and reconstructive surgeons need to communicate well in terms of both the expected defect and the reconstructive options that are available to that specific patient. The anesthesia team needs to be well advised of the nature of the procedure and the hemodynamic stress that can be expected intraoperatively. Also, early involvement of a psychiatrist and a sex therapist may be warranted.

The radiation oncologist is an important participant in the overall treatment plan. Many patients have had previous radiotherapy, and others may be receiving intraoperative radiotherapy or placement of a brachytherapy cannula. The radiotherapy plan has important implications for the choice of flap as both the recipient and donor sites can be affected by radiation injury. In addition, the medical oncologist should be involved with the decision-making as many patients may receive pre- and postoperative chemotherapy. Surgical procedures should be timed to minimize the effects of chemotherapy on wound healing, as well as to avoid unnecessary delays in starting chemotherapy protocols.

Most important to the success of the reconstruction is the full and informed involvement of the patient and her family. It is important to be specific about the goals of vaginal reconstruction with patients, which include effective wound healing and restoration of body image and sexual function[8] (Box 14.1). For those women motivated to preserve sexual function, a comprehensive program of sexual rehabilitation may be

BOX 14.1 **The major goals of vaginal reconstruction**

- To promote effective wound healing, facilitating postoperative radiation therapy and chemotherapy
- To decrease pelvic dead space, thus decreasing fluid loss, metabolic demands, and infection
- To restore the pelvic floor, preventing herniation and small-bowel fistula
- To re-establish body image
- To re-establish sexual function

warranted. Ratliff *et al.* investigated sexual adjustment after vaginal reconstruction with gracilis myocutaneous flaps and found that, although 70% of patients were judged to have a physically adequate vagina, fewer than 50% resumed sexual activity.[9] Absence of pleasure (37%), problems with vaginal dryness (32%), excess secretions (27%), self-consciousness about ostomies (40%), and self-consciousness about nudity in front of their partner (30%) were the most frequent concerns. Preoperative and postoperative counseling, in addition to postoperative rehabilitation strategies (vaginal dilators, lubricants, and topical estrogens) have been suggested as the best way to influence these outcomes positively and give patients the best hope of functional and psychological recovery.[8,10] The psychologist and sex therapist should be an integral part of the ablative–reconstructive team. In addition, at most tertiary care institutions, specialized nursing teams can help the patient and her family prepare for the psychological distress that they may experience.

Treatment/surgical technique

There are five basic goals in vaginal reconstruction (Box 14.1). Selection of the optimal reconstructive method to achieve these goals is based on the type of defect and the characteristics of the patient. Small defects that can be closed without tension will ideally be closed primarily. In the case of the irradiated wound, however, one must proceed cautiously with primary closure. Rarely is skin grafting alone an adequate alternative for oncology patients.

Proceeding along the reconstructive ladder, regional flaps continue to be the most frequently used and effective procedures. Many flaps have been described, none of which are ideal for all defect types (Table 14.1).[11–17] To simplify surgical decision-making, a reconstructive algorithm has been developed on the basis of defect type (Fig. 14.3).[18]

Type IA defects, which involve only the anterior or lateral vaginal walls, usually require little tissue bulk and small to moderate surface coverage. The modified Singapore (vulvoperineal or pudendal thigh) fasciocutaneous flap is ideal in this setting.[15,16] It provides a highly vascularized, reliable, and pliable flap that conforms well to the surface of the vaginal cylinder. This flap is based on the posterior labial arteries and innervated by perineal branches of the posterior cutaneous nerve of the thigh.[19] The flaps are raised in the thigh crease,

Table 14.1 Previously described flap options for vaginal reconstruction

Defect type	Flap option
IA	Singapore (i.e., pudendal fasciocutaneous)
IB	Pedicled rectus myocutaneous Pedicled rectus musculoperitoneal Muscle-sparing rectus myocutaneous
IIA/B	Vertical rectus abdominis myocutaneous Gracilis Singapore Pedicled jejunum Sigmoid colon

lateral to the hair-bearing labia majora, and may be designed to measure 9×4 cm to 15×6 cm.[15,16] The posterior skin margin is marked at the level of the posterior fourchette (Fig. 14.4A). The skin, subcutaneous tissue, deep fascia of the thigh, and epimysium of the adductor muscles are raised (Fig. 14.4B). Posteriorly, the base of the flap is undermined at the subcutaneous level to facilitate rotation and insetting. Depending on the defect, unilateral or bilateral flaps may be developed (Fig. 14.4C). The flaps may be inset by tunneling under the labia majora or by division of the labia at the level of the fourchette. The donor site is closed primarily (Figs. 14.4D & 14.5).

Type IB defects, which encompass the posterior vaginal wall, frequently require greater soft-tissue bulk to fill the dead space made by resection of the rectum. Here, the preferred choice is the pedicled rectus myocutaneous flap. This highly reliable flap provides both large surface area and large volume, and the skin can be used to replace the entire posterior vaginal wall. The healthy muscle and subcutaneous tissue bring well-vascularized tissue to the pelvis, obliterate dead space, and separate the contents of the abdominal cavity from the zone of injury. When used for vaginal reconstruction, the flap is based on the deep inferior epigastric vessels that arise from the external iliac arteries and enter the rectus muscle along its posterolateral surface 6–7 cm above its insertion on the pubis (Fig. 14.6). In planning the flap, one must ensure that these vessels are not divided as part of the cancer resection. One must also ensure that the muscle itself is not violated during placement of the stoma. In addition, good communication between the reconstructive surgeon and the colorectal surgeon

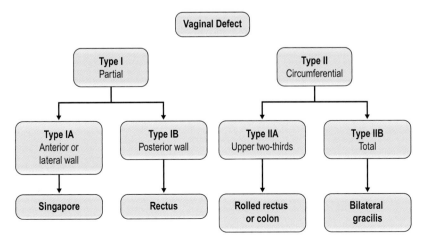

Fig. 14.3 Algorithm for reconstruction of the vagina based on defect type.

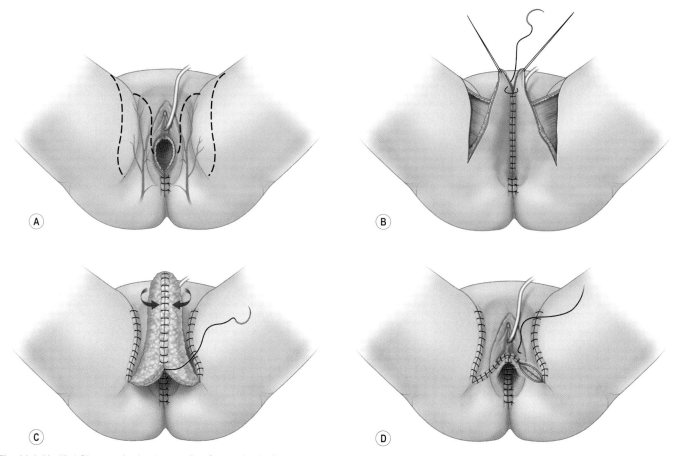

Fig. 14.4 Modified Singapore fasciocutaneous flap. See text for details.

is required when planning the stoma. Usually the stoma is placed on the patient's left side, thus sparing the right rectus for reconstruction. If there is only one available rectus for both stoma placement and the reconstructive donor site, the colorectal surgeon may be able to place the stoma through an empty rectus sheath, or through the external oblique. Communication with the colorectal surgeon is also required for incision

planning. If the right rectus is to be used for reconstruction, ask the colorectal surgeon not to plan the abdominal incision around the left side of the umbilicus, as this will lead to vascular compromise of the umbilicus when harvesting the rectus flap.

Either a vertical or transverse skin island design may be used for the rectus myocutaneous flap, depending on the size

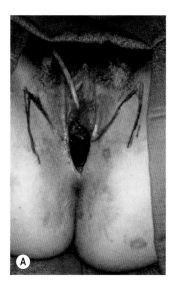
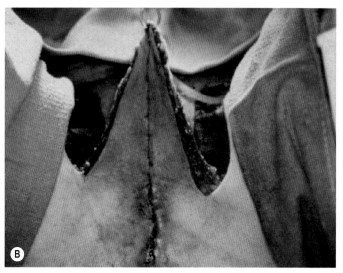
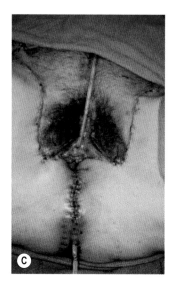

Fig. 14.5 (A) Marking of the modified Singapore fasciocutaneous flap. **(B)** Flap elevation. **(C)** Flap inset.

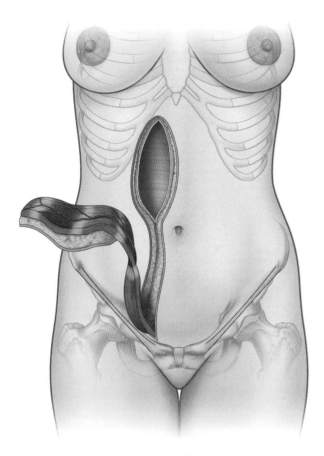

Fig. 14.6 Pedicled rectus myocutaneous flap.

of the defect and the characteristics of the patient's abdominal wall. For posterior wall reconstruction, the vertical rectus abdominis myocutaneous (VRAM) design is usually preferable because it maximizes blood supply by centering the skin island over the medial and lateral rows of perforators, and does not interfere with the contralateral muscle and stoma placement.

Both the vertical and transverse rectus abdominis myocutaneous flaps can be designed up to 10×20 cm in size with easy donor site closure. When the flap is inset into a posterior wall defect, care must be taken to avoid constriction or tension on the vascular pedicle as this is the principal cause of flap failure. Leaving the distal muscle insertion intact to decrease tension on the pedicle is helpful in this regard (Fig. 14.7).

The rectus abdominis musculoperitoneal flap is a modification rectus flap for type I vaginal defects. Here a patch of posterior rectus sheath and peritoneum above the arcuate line is harvested with the rectus to the exact dimensions of the resected vaginal mucosa. The pedicled flap is then transposed into the vaginal canal, and the peritoneal patch is sutured to the edges of the vaginal mucosa. This technique avoids the need for harvesting skin and anterior rectus sheath. The peritoneum has previously been shown to re-epithelialize to squamous epithelium, making it indistinguishable from vaginal mucosa.[17]

Type IIA defects are circumferential defects involving the upper two-thirds of the vagina and, like type IB defects, they are well reconstructed with the pedicled rectus myocutaneous flap due to its skin and soft-tissue bulk. The rectus is preferable to bilateral gracilis flaps because the intervening vulvar

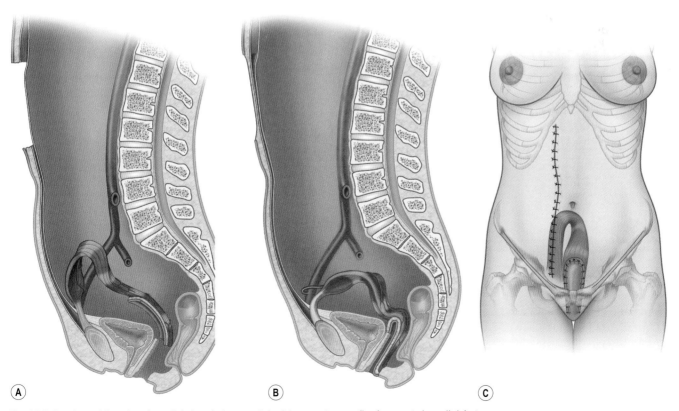

(A)   **(B)**   **(C)**

Fig. 14.7 Rotation and insetting of a pedicled vertical rectus abdominis myocutaneous flap for a posterior wall defect.

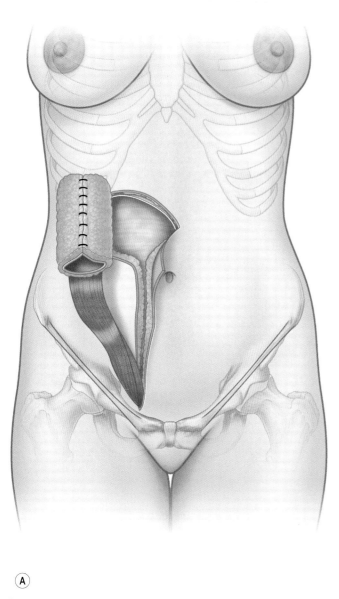

(A)

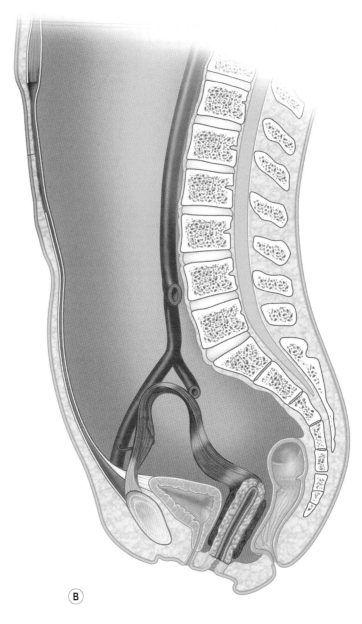

(B)

Fig. 14.8 Tubing and insetting a pedicled rectus flap for a circumferential defect.

and pelvic floor musculature prohibits transfer of the gracili to the defect. When using the rectus myocutaneous flap for these defects, the cutaneous portion of the flap is tubed. A transverse skin island is easier to manipulate and leaves a slightly longer pedicle than the VRAM. A flap width of 12–15 cm will provide a neovagina with a 4 cm diameter.[20] Once tubed, the flap is then sutured to the remaining vaginal cuff from above (Fig. 14.8).

The sigmoid colon or jejunum may also be used to reconstruct type IIA defects for patients in whom the rectus flap cannot be utilized. For the sigmoid colon flap, a segment of colon is isolated and pedicled on a branch of the inferior mesenteric artery.[12] For the jejunum flap, a 15 cm segment of jejunum is isolated and pedicled on the fourth branch of the superior mesenteric artery, approximately 30 cm distal to the ligament of Treitz.[21] For both of these flaps the bowel is stapled

closed superiorly, and sutured inferiorly to the vaginal cuff. Excessive secretions and unpleasant odor, especially for the sigmoid colon, persist as common patient complaints and limit the usefulness of these techniques.[22]

Type IIB defects are circumferential defects involving the entire vagina and frequently the introitus. These are usually total pelvic exenteration defects. Given the need for a large skin island, bilateral gracilis flaps are an excellent reconstructive choice for these defects. The subcutaneous tissue and muscle of the two conjoined flaps will provide a large volume of soft tissue that can obliterate the dead space within the pelvis. The vascular supply of the gracilis flap is the medial femoral circumflex artery, which enters the gracilis muscle 7–10 cm below the pubic tubercle (Fig. 14.9A). An elliptical skin island approximately 6×20 cm can be designed centered over the proximal two-thirds of the muscle, with the anterior border of

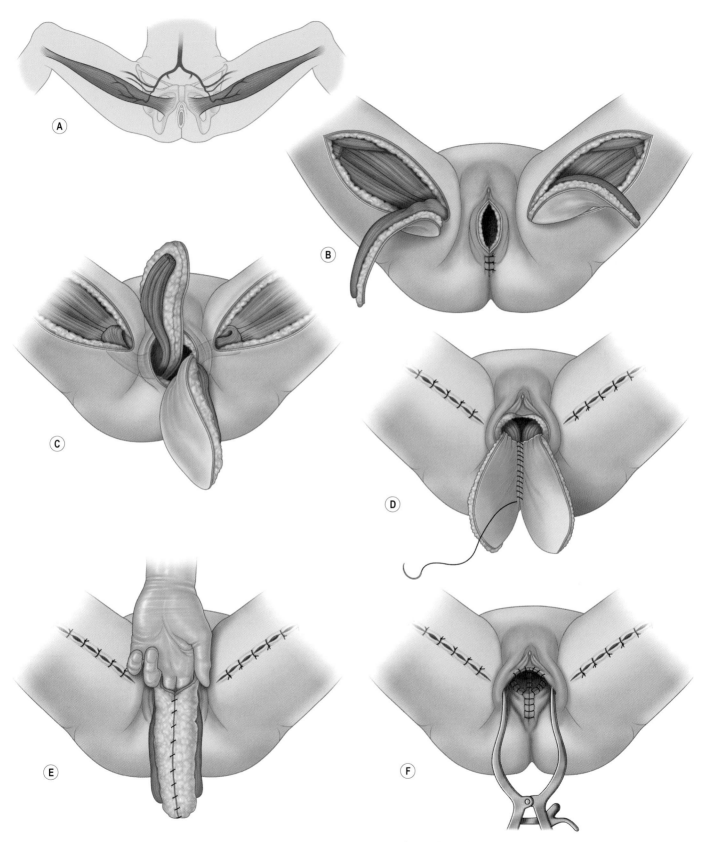

Fig. 14.9 Anatomy, design, elevation, and insetting of bilateral gracilis flaps for a type IIB defect. See text for details.

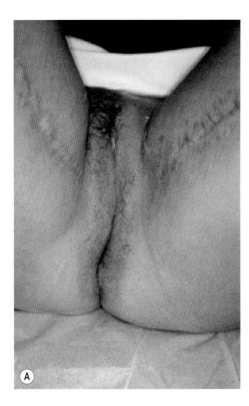

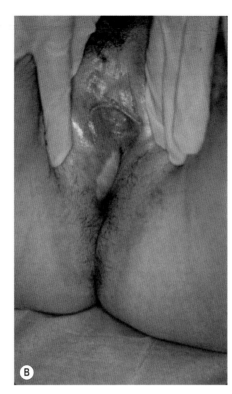

Fig. 14.10 Postoperative results of a vaginal reconstruction using bilateral gracilis flaps.

the incision lying on a line between the pubic tubercle and the semitendinosus tendon. Once elevated, the flaps are tunneled subcutaneously into the vaginal defect (Fig. 14.9B & C). The flaps are then sutured in the midline, and a neovaginal pouch is formed (Fig. 14.9D & E). The neovaginal pouch is then inserted into the defect, and the proximal flap edges are sutured to the introitus (Figs. 14.9F & 14.10). The flap can maintain some sensation for pressure through branches of the obturator nerve.[22]

Additional surgical considerations

While the majority of patients can be reconstructed by using an algorithm based on defect type, a few may require a modified approach. In addition to the type of vaginal defect, consideration should be given to patient specific risk factors, the surrounding surgical defect, and the need for postoperative radiation and/or chemotherapy. Obesity, for example, has been shown to be a significant risk factor for poor wound healing after rectus flap reconstruction.[6] Obese patients with type IIB defects therefore may be better reconstructed with thin, bilateral Singapore flaps. Alternatively, the rectus may be used without its cutaneous portion and a skin graft applied directly to the muscle over a vaginal stent. In elderly patients or patients with significant comorbidities who are unlikely to resume intercourse after reconstruction, a full vaginal reconstruction may be omitted. Using a rectus muscle flap to obliterate dead space within the pelvis may still be of wound-healing benefit to these patients.

In addition to patient specific risk factors, and the vaginal defect, consideration must be given to surrounding surgical defects as well. When the ablative surgeon resects nearby pelvic contents, the resulting non-collapsible dead space may need to be addressed. Such is the case in low rectal tumors requiring APR or more advanced rectal cancers requiring

pelvic exenteration, both of which result in a poorly vascular dead space often requiring chemoradiotherapy. In these cases local flaps can be used to obliterate the non-collapsible dead space with vascularized tissue. Butler compared immediate VRAM flap reconstruction of irradiated APR wounds that could have been closed primarily vs. primary closure.[11] The flap group had significantly lower incidence of perineal abscess (9% vs. 37%, p=0.002), major perineal wound dehiscence (9 vs. 30%, p=0.014), and drainage procedures required for perineal/pelvic fluid collection (3% vs. 25%, p=0.003) than the control group. Although both groups could have been closed primarily, bringing in healthy vascularized tissue reduced major perineal wound complications by filling the dead space, separating the bowel from the underlying perineum, and closing the perineal skin defect with non-irradiated flap skin.

Finally, in patients with previous vaginal reconstruction and recurrent disease, the choice of regional flap might be extremely limited, perhaps warranting free flap reconstruction.[23,24] Several pedicled perforator flaps recently described are good alternative options in these cases. Examples include the muscle-sparing vertical rectus,[25] the deep inferior epigastric perforator (DIEP) flap,[26,27] superior and inferior gluteal artery perforator (SGAP and IGAP) flaps,[28] anterolateral thigh (ALT) flaps,[29] and even free-style perforator flaps.[30]

Postoperative care

Immediate perioperative period

At the end of the reconstructive case, it is imperative to leave a pelvic drain in place in order to drain the fluid that will inevitably collect in any remaining dead space. While these drains typically drain a large amount, the goal should be to keep it in place until the patient is mobile and the drainage begins to decrease, rather than reaching below a certain set point.

Postoperatively, careful attention must also be paid to the patient's hemodynamic and nutritional support. All patients should receive deep-vein thrombosis prophylaxis and be placed on a fluidized mattress and given instructions not to sit for a minimum of 4 weeks. Positioning is difficult due to these restrictions, and patients should be encouraged to lie on either side, stand, or walk. Prophylactic perioperative antibiotics are often used.

Long-term care

The placement of a vaginal stent intraoperatively is not routine for all flap reconstructions. However, once the flap is healed, gradual dilatation with a lubricator may be important in order to increase the size of the orifice. If the patient wishes to use the neovagina for intercourse, she should be told that dilatation must be continued on an ongoing and regular basis for life. Dilatation can begin at approximately 2 months post-reconstruction, as long as everything has healed well. Custom dilators are usually constructed for each patient. Estrogen creams applied to reconstructed type I defects can also be helpful to maintain lubrication.

Complications, prognosis, and outcomes

Complications

The principal early complications after vaginal reconstruction include infection and pelvic abscess, delayed wound healing, and flap loss. While the risk of infection and pelvic abscess is decreased when flap reconstruction is performed after vaginal resection, it still remains significant at approximately 10%.[5,11,14] Perioperative antibiotics, adequate drainage, and patient positioning, as mentioned in the previous section, are all important preventive measures. Once a pelvic infection is established, percutaneous or operative drainage is generally necessary to prevent worsening sepsis. The incidence of delayed wound healing or wound dehiscence varies widely in the literature, ranging up to 46% of patients.[31] Radiotherapy, obesity, and smoking are all risk factors for poor wound healing that should be considered preoperatively. The most common location for wound separation is the posterior perineal closure site, which usually responds to conservative management.

Flap loss, both partial and complete, is a major postoperative problem that will delay adjuvant therapy and increase patient morbidity. The incidence of flap loss depends on the type of flap used, surgical technique, and patient characteristics. When used for vaginal reconstruction, the VRAM flap is highly reliable with less than 5% incidence of total or partial flap loss; gracilis myocutaneous flaps are less reliable with a 10% to greater than 20% incidence of total or partial flap loss.[32–34] The success rate of both of these flaps depends on careful attention to design and surgical technique. The modified Singapore flap is susceptible to apical necrosis, but complete flap loss occurs in up to 15%.[14,19] Partial flap loss may be managed by debridement and local wound care. In the setting of irradiated tissue, full debridement and reconstruction with an alternative flap may be required. In general, the overall complication rate for the VRAM is lower than either the gracilis or Singapore flaps in vaginal reconstruction (32%, 62%, and 47%, respectively).[32]

In addition to complications at the site of the vaginal reconstruction, one must also consider potential donor site complications. For all potential donor sites, hypertrophic scarring, infection, and wound-healing problems must be considered. When harvesting the rectus myocutaneous flap for vaginal reconstruction, an abdominal donor site complication rate of 16–30% has been reported, including such complications as dehiscence, delayed healing, or hernia.[11,35] However, comparing abdominal complications in similar patients without flap reconstruction shows similar abdominal complication rates, thus questioning whether harvesting the rectus muscle adds significant morbidity to these patients.[11] Thigh abscess or hematoma, infection, sensory anomalies, or hypertrophic scarring are the most common complications in patients who have had their gracilis muscles harvested, occurring in up to 40% of patients.[33,35]

Prognosis and outcomes

After pelvic exenteration, there is a 40–60% chance of 5-year survival among patients with gynecologic cancer. Among APR patients, there is a 25–40% chance of 5-year survival.[4] For the patients who do well with their disease and ultimately achieve wound healing, sexual function and body image are fundamental quality-of-life issues. Vaginal reconstruction has been associated with improved body image and sexual function.[36,37] In a pooled analysis of patients undergoing vaginal reconstruction by local flaps, 122 of 246 (50%) patients resumed sexual activity postoperatively.[38] Anatomic reconstruction of the vagina does not equate with restoration of sexual function for a variety of reasons. In a review of 44 patients who underwent bilateral gracilis flap reconstruction, Ratliff et al. found that 33% complained of vaginal dryness, whereas 28% complained of excess vaginal secretions. Twenty percent thought their neovagina was too small, whereas 5% found it to be too large. Eighteen percent had flap prolapse, and a further 18% had pain with intercourse.[9] The most important determinant of postoperative sexual activity, however, is prior sexual activity, and this is not affected by the type of reconstruction.[32,38] Extensive preoperative counseling is essential to ensure realistic patient expectations regarding postoperative sexual function.

Access the complete references list online at **http://www.expertconsult.com**

11. Butler CE, Gundeslioglu AO, Rodriguez-Bigas MA. Outcomes of immediate vertical rectus abdominis myocutaneous flap reconstruction for irradiated abdominoperineal resection defects. *J Am Coll Surg*. 2008;206(4):694–703. *In this retrospective case series, the* *authors assess the impact of immediate closure of irradiated APR defects with VRAM flaps as compared to primary closure. They conclude that VRAM flaps reduce perineal wound complications without increasing early abdominal wall complications.*

13. McCraw J, kemp G, Given F, et al. Correction of high pelvic defects with the inferiorly based rectus abdominis myocutaneous flap. *Clin Plast Surg.* 1988;15(3):449–454.

14. Shibata D, Hyland W, Busse P, et al. Immediate reconstruction of the perineal wound with gracilis muscle flaps following abdominoperineal resection and intraoperative radiation therapy for recurrent carcinoma of the rectum. *Ann Surg Oncol.* 1999;6(1):33–37. *This is a retrospective case review evaluating the efficacy of gracilis flaps for immediate perineal reconstructions. This modality was found to decrease the rate of major wound infections significantly in this population.*

16. Woods JE, Alter G, Meland B, et al. Experience with vaginal reconstruction utilizing the modified Singapore flap. *Plast Reconstr Surg.* 1992;90(2):270–274. *The authors describe a modification of the Singapore flap in which the labia majora are released, yielding good contour and no flap loss. The technique is illustrated and sample cases are described.*

17. Wu LC, Song DH. The rectus abdominis musculoperitoneal flap for the immediate reconstruction of partial vaginal defects. *Plast Reconstr Surg.* 2005;115(2):559–562.

18. Cordeiro PG, Pusic AL, Disa JJ. A classification system and reconstructive algorithm for acquired vaginal defects. *Plast Reconstr Surg.* 2002;110(4):1058–1065. *A classification system for acquired vaginal defects is presented based on a 7-year case review. From this experience, the authors derive a reconstructive algorithm and conduct an outcomes assessment.*

33. Nelson RA, Butler CE. Surgical outcomes of VRAM versus thigh flaps for immediate reconstruction of pelvic and perineal cancer resection defects. *Plast Reconstr Surg.* 2009;123(1):175–183. *The authors compare the efficacy of VRAM flaps to that of thigh flaps in immediate pelvic and perineal reconstruction. VRAM flaps are found to reduce major perineal wound complications without increasing early abdominal wall morbidity.*

15

Surgery for gender dysphoria

Loren S. Schechter

Access video lecture content for this chapter online at expertconsult.com

SYNOPSIS

- The goal of surgery is a successful functional and cosmetic result.
- Surgery is only one factor in the overall therapeutic process.
- Multidisciplinary care is essential for the transgender individual.
- Surgical techniques for transwomen include penile inversion and intestinal transposition.
- Surgical techniques for transmen include metoidioplasty and pedicled/free flap phalloplasty.
- Secondary surgical procedures for the face and breast/chest are available for transgender individuals.

 Access the Historical Perspective section online at
http://www.expertconsult.com

Introduction

Gender dysphoria – definition

The term gender dysphoria describes a heterogeneous group of individuals who express varying degrees of dissatisfaction with their anatomic gender, and the desire to possess the secondary sexual characteristics of the opposite sex.[1] For these individuals, surgical therapy plays a pivotal role in relieving their psychological discomfort.[2] As noted by Dr. Milton Edgerton in 1983, "transsexualism is a severe, and pathologic condition that is undesirable for both the patient and society... and non-surgical treatment continues to be expensive, time-consuming, and enormously disappointing".[3]

While the intent of Dr. Edgerton's statement is accurate, there have been significant advances not only in the understanding, management, and care of transgender individuals but also in the social and political climate over the past 35 years. In fact, in 2010 the World Professional Association for

Transgender Health (WPATH) released a statement recommending the de-psychopathologization of gender nonconformity stating that "the expression of gender characteristics, including identities, that are not stereotypically associated with one's assigned sex at birth is a common and culturally diverse human phenomenon [that] should not be judged as inherently pathological or negative".[4]

Goals of therapy

Congruent genitalia

WPATH developed the *Standards of Care* to help provide "the highest standards" of care for individuals. The *Standards of Care* state that the overarching treatment goal is "...lasting personal comfort with the gendered self, in order to maximize overall health, psychological well-being and self-fulfillment".[4] Toward this end, gender confirmation surgery provides the appropriate physical morphology and alleviates the extreme psychological discomfort of the patient. Furthermore, as discussed by Meyer *et al.* in 2001 and Cohen-Kettenis in 1984, adjusting the mind to the body is not an effective treatment, while adjusting the body to the mind is the best way to assist severely gender dysphoric persons.

Congruent genitalia allows an individual to experience harmony between one's body and self-identity, appear nude in social situations without violating taboos (i.e., health clubs, physician offices, etc.), and have legal identification concordant with one's physical appearance.

Surgical goals

A successful surgical result involves:

Transwomen

The creation of a natural-appearing vagina and mons pubis that is both sensate and functional. This includes a feminine-appearing labia majora and minora, removal of the stigmatizing scrotum, a sensate neoclitoris, and adequate vaginal depth

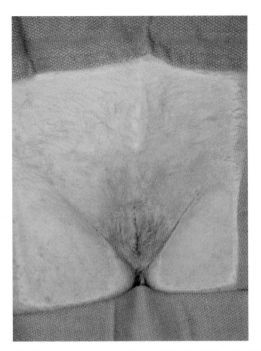

Fig. 15.1 Postoperative appearance following single-stage vaginoplasty.

and introital width for intercourse. Additional desirable qualities include a moist appearance to the labia minora, clitoral hooding, and lubrication for intercourse (Figs. 15.1 & 15.2).

Aside from genital reconstruction, breast augmentation, thyroid chondrolaryngoplasty ("tracheal shave"), and facial feminization offer additional procedures designed to feminize one's appearance.

Transmen

While phalloplasty represents the most complete genito-perineal transformation, the need for complex, staged procedures, the use of tissue from remote sites resulting in scarring

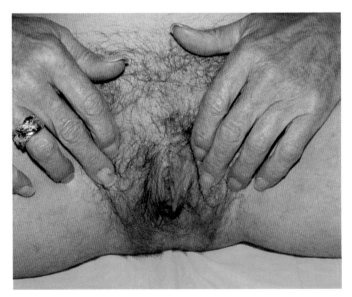

Fig. 15.2 Postoperative appearance following second-stage labiaplasty. Note the neoclitoris and prepuce formed by the glans penis and urethra. Additionally, a moist appearance of the labia minora is provided by the use of a urethral flap.

at the donor site, and potential complications associated with urethral reconstruction and implantable prostheses has led some individuals to forego this procedure. The alternative, a metoidioplasty, entails lengthening of the virilized clitoris and may be performed with, or without, urethral lengthening.

Chest surgery, involving bilateral subcutaneous mastectomies and contouring of the chest, is commonly performed prior to genital surgery. Chest surgery also includes repositioning and re-sizing of the nipple–areola complex when necessary. Several different techniques are employed, and the choice of technique depends upon the volume of breast parenchyma, degree of breast ptosis and position of the nipple–areola complex, and degree of skin elasticity.

Definitions

Pyschosexual development and differentiation entails three major components:

i. **gender identity**, referring to one's sense of belonging to the male or female sex category, both or neither
ii. **gender role,** sexually dimorphic behaviors and psychological characteristics within the population, such as toy preferences and mannerisms
iii. **sexual orientation,** one's pattern of erotic responsiveness.

As noted by the Institute of Medicine's 2011 report, *The Health of Lesbian, Gay, Bisexual, and Transgender People*, "transgender people are defined according to their gender identity and presentation. This group encompasses individuals whose gender identity differs from the sex originally assigned to them at birth or whose gender expression varies significantly from what is traditionally associated with or typical for that sex (i.e., people identified as male at birth who subsequently identify as female, and people identified as female at birth who later identify as male), as well as other individuals who vary from or reject traditional cultural conceptualizations of gender in terms of the male–female dichotomy. The transgender population is diverse in gender identity, expression, and sexual orientation. Some transgender individuals have undergone medical interventions to alter their sexual anatomy and physiology, others wish to have such procedures in the future, and still others do not. Transgender people can be heterosexual, homosexual, or bisexual in their sexual orientation. Some lesbians, gay men, and bisexuals are transgender; most are not. Male-to-female transgender people are known as MtF, transgender females, or transwomen, while female-to-male transgender people are known as FtM, transgender males, or transmen. Some transgender people do not fit into either of these binary categories".[5]

While **gender nonconformity** describes a difference between an individual's gender identity, role, or expression and that of cultural norms, **gender dysphoria** describes the discomfort or distress experienced by an individual due to a discrepancy between one's gender identity and the sex assigned at birth.[4]

Some gender-nonconforming individuals experience gender dysphoria, and treatment is available to assist these people. As noted in the *Standards of Care*, "transsexual, transgender, and gender-nonconforming individuals are not inherently disordered…the distress of gender dysphoria…is the concern that might be diagnosable and for which various treatment options are available".[4]

Epidemiology

Gender dysphoria

While early estimates on the prevalence of gender identity disorders were focused on identification of individuals for gender confirmation surgery, it was later realized that some individuals neither desired, nor were candidates, for reassignment surgery.[6] Early estimates of the prevalence of transsexualism were 1 in 37 000 biologic males and 1 in 107 000 biologic females.[6] Interestingly, approximately three times as many biologic males as compared to biologic females seek genital surgery. This discrepancy may exist for multiple reasons, including accessibility, cost, and surgical options available for biologic females. However, with the increase in third party coverage of gender confirmation surgery, there has been a corresponding increase in the number of biologic males seeking genital surgery.

Disorders of sex development

Distinct from gender identity disorders are disorders of sex development (DSD). DSDs represent congenital conditions in which development of chromosomal, gonadal, or anatomic sex is atypical.[7] This terminology replaces terms such as "intersex", "pseudohermaphroditism", "hermaphroditism", and "sex reversal". DSDs include a group of conditions interfering with normal sex determination and differentiation in the embryo and fetus. Although data on the prevalence and incidence of DSDs is limited, it is estimated that the incidence is 1 in 550.[8] Congenital adrenal hyperplasia is the most common cause of ambiguous genitalia, followed in frequency by mixed gonadal dysgenesis. Gender dissatisfaction occurs more often in individuals with DSDs as compared with the general population, but it is difficult to predict, based upon karyotype, prenatal androgen exposure, degree of genital virilization, or assigned gender. A summary of DSDs is included in Table 15.1.[8]

The birth of a child with ambiguous genitalia is distressing to families, and management of children with DSDs benefits from a multidisciplinary approach. Clinical management includes (1) avoidance of gender assignment prior to expert evaluation; (2) evaluation and management by a multidisciplinary team; (3) receipt of a gender assignment in all individuals; (4) communication with patients and families, as well as their participation and inclusion in decision-making; and (5) respect for patient and family concerns with strict adherence to patient confidentiality.[7] In discussions involving the

Table 15.1 Summary of the various types of disorders of sex development	
Revised nomenclature	**Types**
Sex chromosome, DSD	45,X Turner syndrome (mosaic, isodicentric Xq, ring chromosome, etc.)
46,XY DSD	Defects in testicular development 　　Complete gonadal dysgenesis (Swyer syndrome) 　　Partial gonadal dysgenesis (WT1, SOX9, SF-1 mutations) 　　Gonadal regression 　　Ovotesticular DSD Disorders in androgen synthesis or action 　　Androgen biosynthesis defects (e.g., 17-HSD, 5α-RD, StAR, POR, 3β-HSD, 17,20 lyase, Leydig cell hypoplasia or aplasia) 　　Defects in androgen action (CAIS, PAIS) Others 　　Hypospadias, micropenis, cloacal exstrophy, congenital anomaly syndromes 　　Persistent Müllerian duct syndrome
46,XX DSD	Defects in ovarian development 　　Ovotesticular DSD 　　Gonadal transformation (e.g., SRY translocation) 　　Gonadal dysgenesis Disorders of androgen excess 　　Fetal: CAH (11 hydroxylase deficiency, 21 hydroxylase deficiency, 3β-HSD, POR) 　　Fetoplacental: aromatase deficiency, POR 　　Maternal: luteoma of pregnancy, exogenous androgen Others 　　Congenital anomaly syndromes, vaginal atresia, cloacal exstrophy, MURCS
Ovotesticular DSD	46,XX/ 46,XY (chimeric) 45,X/46,XY (mixed gonadal dysgenesis)
46,XX Testicular DSD	XX sex reversal (SRY translocation)
46,XY Complete gonadal dysgenesis	XY sex reversal (SF1, WT1, SOX9) Swyer syndrome

CAIS, Complete androgen insensitivity; DSD, disorder of sex development; 17-HSD, 17-hydroxysteroid dehydrogenase; 3β-HSD, 3β-hydroxysteroid dehydrogenase; MURCS, Müllerian, renal, cervicothoracic somite abnormalities; PAIS, partial androgen insensitivity; POR, P450 oxidoreductase; 5α-RD, 5α-reductase deficiency; SF1, splicing factor 1; SOX9, sex determining region box 9; StAR, steroidogenic acute regulatory protein; WT1, Wilms tumor gene.
(From Nabhan ZM, Lee PA. Disorders of sex development. *Curr Opin Obstet Gynecol.* 2007;19:440-445.)

parents of newborns with DSDs, the description of the child's genitalia should include both the bipotential of the initial genital organs in addition to a discussion that the usual genetic and hormonal controls many not be fully functional. Children with DSDs may have conditions that result in excessive stimulation of female genitalia, leading to masculinization, or inadequate androgen stimulation of male genitalia resulting in incomplete formation or underdevelopment. Following appropriate testing and assessment of completeness of development of female and male structures, information should be provided to the parents so as to assist the family and physicians with the most appropriate sex assignment. Subsequent clinical discussions with the family include the need for, and benefits of, surgery, predicting future hormone production, and the projection of potential fertility.[8]

The surgical management of the genitalia of children with DSDs is made by the parents and, when appropriate, the patient. The goal of surgery is to achieve genitalia compatible with sex; prevent urinary obstruction, urinary incontinence, and infection; and provide good adult sexual and reproductive function.[9] Although controversy exists on the timing of genital surgery in girls with congenital adrenal hyperplasia (CAH), surgery is typically considered in cases of severe virilization and, when necessary, in association with repair of a common urogenital sinus. Surgery should be anatomically based so as to preserve erectile function and innervation of the clitoris. While the American Academy of Pediatric guidelines recommend genitoplasty between 2 and 6 months of age,[10] it is recognized that revision vaginoplasty will be performed at the time of puberty. For male newborns with hypospadias, standard techniques for chordee repair and urethral reconstruction apply. In patients requiring phalloplasty, the magnitude and complexity of the procedure must be discussed, especially if sex assignment depends upon it.[7] In individuals with 46, XY gonadal dysgenesis raised as females, testes or fragments of Y-chromosome material should be removed to prevent testicular malignancy. Gonadectomy is generally advised soon after diagnosis so as to initiate estrogen replacement when desired. In individuals with gonadal dysgenesis and scrotal testes, the current recommendation is to perform testicular biopsy at puberty to assess for malignancy. In females with ovotesticular DSD and functional ovarian tissue, early separation and removal of the testicular component is advised in an attempt to preserve fertility.[8] DSDs can be managed such that children can mature into well-adjusted individuals with a potential for sexual expression and, in select cases, reproductive potential.[8]

Etiology

The etiology of transsexualism remains unknown[21] and has included genetic links, the hormonal milieu, family dynamics, and psychoanalytic observations.[1] Early theories were based largely in psychoanalytic contexts, followed by attempts to define transsexualism in a biologic context. There are essentially three theories relating to the etiology of transsexualism: a psychological or sociological etiology, a biologic etiology, or some combination thereof.

Psychoanalytic explanations have ranged from an inability to separate on the part of the mother and child, psychotic disorders, and an unconscious motivation to discard bad and aggressive features.[21] As such, psychoanalysts viewed sex reassignment surgery as "psychosurgery" and argued that treatment of transsexualism could only be achieved through psychoanalysis.[21]

Proponents of a biologic explanation have examined a variety of theories including anatomic differences in the brains of transsexuals as well as hormonal influences on brain development at critical gestational stages. Paralleling advances in radiographic brain imaging, early biologic theories, referred to as gender transposition, examined hormone-induced cephalic differentiation.[21] This concept relied on the "default theory": in the absence of androgens, an embryo will feminize, and in the presence of androgens, testicles develop. However, many of these theories rested upon extrapolation from animal studies. Subsequent research later demonstrated important differences between hormone secretions in humans and animals.

Some of the most recent theories have focused attention on an attempt to identify a genetic link explaining transsexualism. However, at this time, no genetic markers have been identified that explain transsexualism. Therefore studies have used differences in physical characteristics between transsexuals and nontranssexuals as indirect evidence of a genetic etiology. These studies include such factors as the observation of a high prevalence of left-handedness in transsexuals, height differences between male-to-female transsexuals and nontransgendered males, the presence of an anomalous inframammary ligament in female-to-male transsexuals, a higher rate of polycystic ovaries in female-to-male transsexuals, and differences in bone proportion and fat distribution.[21] Still other theories have examined differences in autopsied brains of male-to-female transsexuals. These differences were noted in the region of the hypothalamus, an area of the brain involved in sexual behavior. The study noted that genetic females and male-to-female transsexuals had similar and smaller volumes of the central sulci of the stria terminalis compared to both homosexual and heterosexual males.[21]

However, in spite of continued research in this area, it must also be recognized that a spectrum of gender variance exists. Additionally, both cultural and social constructs play a significant factor in gender role. For example, while most of the studies compare transsexuals to nontranssexuals, these studies do not account for biologic explanations as to crossdressing heterosexual males or children with a history of gender identity disorder who become gender typical as adults. As Dr. Randi Ettner concludes, "…the etiology of transgenderism remains unknown. The goal of treatment, however, is known and is indisputable: to assist gender-variant patients who request medical interventions by providing state-of-the-art treatment".[21]

Diagnosis

Transgender is not a formal diagnosis.[4] When individuals possess concerns, uncertainties, and questions about gender identity, which persist during their development, become the most important aspect of their life, or prevent the establishment of an unconflicted gender identity, they have passed a clinical threshold. When such an individual meets the specified criteria in one of the two official nomenclatures, the *International Classification of Diseases – 10th edition* (ICD-10) or the *Diagnostic Statistical Manual of Mental Disorders – 5th edition* (DSM-5), they are diagnosed as having a Gender Identity Disorder (GID) or Gender Dysphoria.

The ICD-10[22] provides five diagnoses for gender identity disorders (F64):

- Transsexualism (F64.0), which has three criteria:
    i. The desire to live and be accepted as a member of the opposite sex, usually accompanied by the wish to make his or her body as congruent as possible with the preferred sex through surgery and hormone treatment.
    ii. The transsexual identity has been present persistently for at least 2 years.
    iii. The disorder is not a symptom of another mental disorder or a chromosomal abnormality
- Dual-role transvestism (F64.1)
- Gender identity disorder of childhood (F64.2)
- Other gender identity disorders (F64.8)
- Gender identity disorder, unspecified (F64.9)

In 1994, the DSM-IV committee replaced the diagnosis of "transsexualism" with "gender identity disorder". Incorporate to DSM-IV, individuals must demonstrate a strong and persistent cross-gender identification and a persistent discomfort with their sex or a sense of inappropriateness in the gender role of that sex. It is important to realize that the DSM-IV and ICD-10 are designed to guide research and treatment. The designation of gender identity disorders as mental disorders is not a license for stigmatization, or for the deprivation of gender patients' civil rights.[4] In DSM-V, published in 2013, the term "gender identity disorder was replaced with the term "gender dysphoria".

After the diagnosis of gender dysphoria is made, the therapeutic approach commonly included three phases (triadic therapy): a real-life experience in the desired role, hormones of the desired gender, and surgery to change the genitalia and other sex characteristics.

Multidisciplinary treatment

While the goals of surgery include a successful cosmetic and functional result with minimal complications, surgery is only one determinant in the overall therapeutic process.[23] As such, the surgeon performing gender confirmation procedures must assume an active and integral role in the overall care of the patient. It is the responsibility of the operating surgeon to understand the diagnosis that has led to the recommendation for genital surgery, medical comorbidities that may impact the surgical outcome, the effects of hormonal therapy on the patient's health, and the patient's ultimate satisfaction with the surgical result.[24] Furthermore, the surgeon should assist with the coordination of the patient's postoperative care in order to assure appropriate continuity.

Recognizing that, in appropriately selected individuals, gender reassignment surgery is the best way to normalize the lives of transgender individuals,[2] the question of how best to integrate the surgeon in the multidisciplinary team continues to undergo investigation. Although typically introduced to the patient only after diagnosis and hormonal therapy, the surgeon must actively participate in understanding the patient's diagnosis and hormonal and medical therapies. In order to do

so, a collaborative effort between the surgeon, mental health professional, and medical physician responsible for hormonal therapy is recommended. Understanding the limitations in access to formal multidisciplinary gender teams, the WPATH *Standards of Care* provides recommendations designed to standardize the process of surgical evaluation, treatment, and postoperative care of transgender individuals.[4] This standardized process of surgical management will, hopefully, lead to uniform and consistent surgical results worldwide.

Embryology

Genetic sex is determined at fertilization, either XX or XY. For the first six weeks of development, gender is not distinguishable, and this is known as the indifferent period. Characteristic external genitalia begin to form beginning about the ninth week of gestation.

Sexual differentiation of the internal and external female genitalia requires no active intervention. However, for development of the male external genitalia, androgen production by the Leydig cells and Müllerian inhibiting hormone (MIH) production by the Sertoli cells is required. Ovarian activity is not required for development of female internal genitalia.

The internal genitalia can only develop into one gender and are therefore termed unipotent. In the male, the Wolffian duct develops from the mesonephric duct, and in the female, the Müllerian ducts develop from the paramesonephric duct. In the male, MIH and androgens prevent development of female internal genitalia. Additionally, androgens actively maintain the Wolffian ducts, while MIH induces the regression of the Müllerian ducts. In the female, Wolffian ducts regress in the absence of androgens, while the Müllerian ducts persist.

External genitalia have the potential to be either male or female and are therefore termed bipotential. In order to develop male external genitalia, testosterone is required. In about the fourth week of development in both sexes, the genital tubercle develops and elongates to form the phallus. In a developing male, androgens induce the urethral folds to fuse to form the urethra. Additionally, the genital tubercle enlarges to form the glans penis. Midline fusion of the genital swellings results in formation of the scrotum. Alternatively, female development occurs in the absence of testosterone, independent of ovarian activity. The urethral folds and genital swellings remain separate to form the labia minora and majora, while the genital tubercle forms the clitoris.

In constructing the appropriate physical morphology, the relevant homologous structures are used to create "like-with-like".

Preoperative evaluation

Prior to performing gender confirmation surgery, the surgeon must be satisfied that the diagnosis of gender dysphoria has been established. Although the diagnosis is typically made by the behavioral scientist, the surgeon must be convinced that the diagnosis is accurate. As noted by Dr. J.J. Hage, "the surgeon remains responsible for any diagnosis on the basis of which he performs surgical interventions".[24] Direct communication between the surgeon and mental health professional(s) is both encouraged and recommended. This serves to educate the surgeon and to aid with his or her understanding of each patient's unique needs. It also helps to prevent possible falsification of letters of recommendation. The surgeon must be willing to personally communicate with other healthcare providers when questions or concerns regarding a patient's appropriateness for surgery exist. However, this communication should not be limited to the evaluation phase. It is the responsibility of the surgeon to communicate pertinent operative findings as well as postoperative instructions with the relevant members of the healthcare team.[25]

Although multiple studies conducted at a variety of international centers confirm the efficacy of surgery and low complication rates,[2,26-31] the surgeon must be familiar with preoperative psychosocial risk factors that may increase the risk of postoperative complications. It is incumbent upon the surgeon to actively investigate these potential risk factors prior to proceeding with surgery. In a study investigating the standards and policies of 19 gender clinics in Europe and North America, a high degree of consistency regarding policies and criteria for approval of reassignment surgery was identified.[32] Based upon questionnaire data, conditions that could result in delay or denial of surgery included psychosocial instability, married status, substance abuse, chronic or psychotic illness, and antisocial behavior. In addition, in a retrospective review of 136 patients who underwent sex reassignment in Sweden, several preoperative factors were identified and reported to be associated with higher rates of unsatisfactory surgical outcomes. These included personal and social instability, unsuitable body build, and age over 30 at operation. Additionally, in this study, adequate family and social support were noted to be important for adequate postoperative functioning.[23]

Though understanding potential preoperative risk factors is important, their presence is not necessarily a contraindication to surgery. In a retrospective review of 232 male-to-female transsexuals, Lawrence[28] noted that no participants regretted sexual reassignment surgery outright and only 6% were occasionally regretful. In this study, dissatisfaction was associated with unsatisfactory surgical results, not other indicators of transsexual typology, such as age at surgery, previous marriage or parenthood, or sexual orientation. This serves to reinforce the concept that the *Standards of Care* are intended to provide flexible direction for the treatment of transgender individuals. It is generally recognized that individual centers may vary with regard to specific hormonal regimens and time requirements for the real life test. It must be emphasized that the *Standards of Care* are not intended as barriers to surgery, but rather as a means of identifying patients who would benefit from surgical reassignment.

Hormone regimen

Upon completion of the first or diagnostic phase, the patient is referred to a medical physician for hormonal therapy. Though specific hormonal regimens may vary between centers, the surgeon should be familiar with the possible side effects of hormonal therapy and how they relate to the surgical care of the transgender patient. These include issues related to liver function, risk of venous thromboembolism, electrolyte imbalance, drug–drug interactions, and possible malignancy (i.e., breast cancer). It is helpful if the medical physician is a member of the multidisciplinary team. If not, the medical physician should have substantial experience in the field of transgender medicine.[24] Medical comorbidities should be investigated and, if possible, treated prior to

surgery. In patients with chronic medical conditions, the surgeon should work closely with medical colleagues to optimize and manage these conditions prior to surgery.

The goal of endocrine therapy is to change secondary sex characteristics in order to reduce gender dysphoria and/or facilitate a physical presentation consistent with the individual's sense of self.[33] Hormonal therapy is typically individualized to the needs and desires of the patient based upon their goals, associated medical conditions, and consideration of social and economic issues. The *Standards of Care* indicate the physician prescribing the hormones should:

1. Perform an initial evaluation that includes health history, physical examination, and relevant laboratory tests
2. Explain what feminizing/masculinizing medications do and the possible side effects/health risks
3. Confirm that the patient has the capacity to understand the risks and benefits of treatment and to make an informed decision about medical care
4. Inform the patient of the *Standards of Care* and eligibility/readiness requirements
5. Provide ongoing medical monitoring, including regular physical and laboratory examination to monitor hormone effects and side effects.

Feminization through hormonal therapy is achieved by two mechanisms: suppression of androgen effects and induction of female physical characteristics. Androgen suppression is achieved by using medications that either suppress gonadotropin releasing hormone (GnRH) or are GnRH antagonists (progestational agents), suppress the production of luteinizing hormone (progestational agents, cyproterone acetate), interfere with testosterone production or metabolism of testosterone to dihydrotestosterone (spironolactone, finasteride, cyproterone acetate), or interfere with the binding of androgen to its receptors in target tissues (spironolactone, cyproterone acetate, flutamide). Additionally, estrogen is used to induce female secondary sex characteristics, and its mechanism of action is through direct stimulation of receptors in target tissues (Table 15.2).[33]

Within the first 6 months of therapy, there is a redistribution of body fat, decreased muscle mass, softening of skin, and decreased libido. Breast growth may be expected after 3–6 months of therapy and continue for ≥2 years. Over a period of several years, body fat and facial hair become finer, although they are not completely eliminated by hormonal therapy alone. Progression of male pattern baldness may slow; however, hair does not typically regrow in bald areas. Many of the changes, perhaps with the exception of breast growth, are reversible with cessation of therapy.[33]

Masculinization through hormonal therapy for transmen follows general principles of hormone replacement for treatment of male hypogonadism. Both parenteral and transdermal testosterone preparations are available and may be used to achieve testosterone values in the normal male range.[34] Testosterone therapy results in increased muscle mass and decreased fat mass, increased facial hair and acne, male pattern baldness, and increased libido. In reference to male-to-female individuals, testosterone results in clitoromegaly, temporary or permanent decreased fertility, deepened voice, vaginal atrophy, and cessation of menses. If uterine bleeding continues, a progestational agent may be added. GnRH

Table 15.2 Hormone regimen

Agent	Estrogen			Androgen antagonist		
	17β-estradiol			Spironolactone		Finasteride
	Transdermal[a]	*or*	Oral	Oral	*and/or*	Oral
Pre-orchiectomy	Start at 0.1 mg/24 h applied twice a week; gradually increase up to maximum of 0.2 mg/24 h applied twice per week		Start with 1–2 mg daily; gradually increase up to maximum 4 mg daily	Start with 50–100 mg daily; increase by 50–100 mg each month up to average 200–300 mg daily (maximum 500 mg daily). Modify if there are risks of adverse effects[b]		Use 2.5–5.0 mg daily for systemic anti-androgen effect; use 2.5 mg every other day if solely for alopecia androgenetica
Post-orchiectomy	0.375–0.1 mg/24 h applied twice per week		1–2 mg daily	25–50 mg daily		2.5 mg daily

[a]Use transdermal estradiol if the patient is >40 years of age or is at risk for DVT. Oral estradiol is an option if the patient is <40 years of age and is low risk for DVT.
[b]If taking ACE-inhibitors or other potassium-sparing medication, spironolactone should not go above 25 mg daily and serum potassium should be closely monitored. If the patient has low blood pressure or renal insufficiency start at 50 mg and increase by up to 50 mg per week to a maximum of 300 mg daily, with a renal function test 1–2 weeks after each increase.
(From Dahl M, Feldman JL, Goldberg JM, Jaberi A. Physical aspects of transgender endocrine therapy. *Int J Transgenderism*. 2006;9:111–134.)

analogs or depot medroxyprogesterone may be used to stop menses and to reduce estrogen levels to those found in biologic males.[34] Individuals should be routinely monitored so as to maintain testosterone levels in the physiologic normal male range and avoid adverse events such as erythrocytosis, liver dysfunction, hypertension, excessive weight gain, salt retention, lipid changes, cystic acne, and adverse psychological changes.[34]

Adolescent therapy

Over the past decade, an emerging area of clinical interest involves the treatment of transgender adolescents. Adolescents with gender dysphoria may consider the physical changes of puberty unbearable. In an effort to prevent psychological harm, some centers have initiated treatment of adolescents with puberty-suppressing medications, such as a GnRH analog, before development of irreversible secondary sex characteristics. Potential benefits of this approach to pubertal suppression may include a relief of gender dysphoria and better psychological and physical outcome.[34]

The physical changes of puberty result from maturation of the hypothalamo-pituitary-gonadal axis and development of secondary sex characteristics. In girls, the first physical sign of puberty is breast budding, while in boys, an increase in testicular volume heralds the onset of puberty. Pubertal suppression may aid with management of gender dysphoria, and the hormonal changes are fully reversible.[34] Hormone-treated adolescents may be referred for surgery when the real-life experience has resulted in a satisfactory social role change, the individual is satisfied about the hormonal effects, and the individual desires definitive surgical changes.[34] Surgery is typically considered at 18 years of age, although individual exceptions may be appropriate.

Feminizing surgical therapy

Once the surgeon is satisfied that the diagnosis has been established, a hormonal regimen has been instituted and followed, and the patient has successfully completed the second stage or real-life test, surgical therapy is considered. A preoperative surgical consultation is obtained. During this consultation, the procedure and postoperative course are described, the potential risks and benefits of surgery are reviewed, and the patient's questions are answered. Equally important is a discussion of the patient's expectations as well as an understanding of the limitations of surgery. In a follow study of 55 transsexual patients treated in Belgium, De Cuypere *et al.*[27] noted that the transsexual person's expectations were met at an emotional and social level, but less so at the physical and sexual level. This occurred despite an indicated improvement in sex life and sexual excitement after reassignment surgery.[27] Based upon these findings, it was recommended that discussion regarding sexual expectations be entertained prior to surgery. After deciding to proceed with surgery, written documentation of informed consent should be included in the patient's chart.

Surgical conversion of the genitalia in transwomen has evolved since the use of skin grafts for creation of a neovagina in cases of vaginal agenesis.[35] The use of pedicled penile and scrotal flaps was described over 40 years ago, and despite technical refinements, remains the mainstay for neovaginal construction.[36–38] The vascular basis of these flaps is derived from one of two sources: 1) the femoral artery (deep and superficial external pudendal arteries) and 2) the internal pudendal artery (perineal branches).

A successful surgical result involves the creation of a natural-appearing vagina and mons pubis. This includes a feminine-appearing labia majora and minora with removal of the stigmatizing scrotum, a sensate neoclitoris, and adequate vaginal depth and introital width for intercourse (Figs. 15.3–15.5). Although a functional vaginoplasty is performed in a single stage, further feminization of the mons pubis can be performed at a second surgical stage. The labiaplasty, which can be performed under local anesthesia as an outpatient procedure three months after vaginoplasty, creates a convergent anterior commissure and provides additional clitoral hooding. However, with recent trends towards hair removal

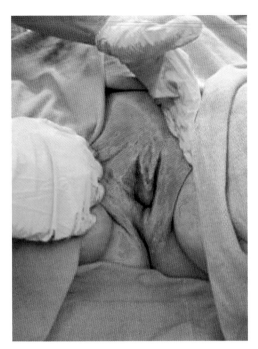

Fig. 15.3 Postoperative appearance following single-stage vaginoplasty, prior to labiaplasty. Note the width of the introitus provided by the perineal–scrotal flap and resection of the superficial muscles. Adequate introital width is essential for vaginal intercourse.

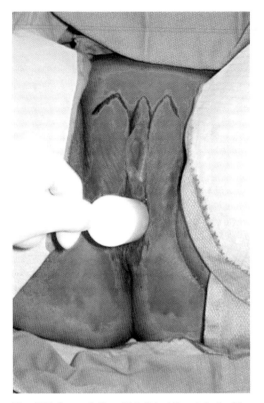

Fig. 15.5 Demonstration of introital width and depth of the neovaginal cavity. Markings on the mons pubis delineate the local tissue rearrangement for the labiaplasty. The labiaplasty will provide convergence to the labia majora as well as additional definition of the prepuce of the neoclitoris.

of the mons, fewer individuals opt to proceed with the vaginoplasty.

The surgical options for feminizing genital surgery consist of one of three options: penile inversion vaginoplasty, intestinal transplantation, or nongenital flaps. Most centers perform primary vaginoplasty with the penile inversion vaginoplasty using an anteriorly pedicled penile skin flap combined with a posteriorly based scrotal–perineal flap and/or skin graft. However, intestinal transposition, typically reserved for revision cases, is a first-line surgical therapy at some centers. The advantage of intestinal transposition is the creation of a vascularized 12–15 cm vagina with a moist lining. This may lessen the requirements for postoperative vaginal dilation as well as the need for lubrication during intercourse. However,

the drawbacks of intestinal transposition include the need for an intra-abdominal operation with a bowel anastomosis and the potential for excess neovaginal secretions with a malodorous discharge. Nongenital flaps are typically considered for reconstruction following oncologic resections, traumatic repair, or reconstruction following infection. Regardless of which technique is utilized, a preoperative bowel preparation is administered. Additionally, hair removal, whether by electrolysis or laser, is completed as thoroughly as possible from the penile shaft and central perineum and scrotum (Fig. 15.6) prior to surgery. Preoperative depilation helps to prevent

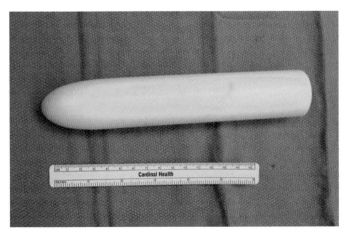

Fig. 15.4 Rigid dilator used for intraoperative blunt dissection of the neovaginal cavity.

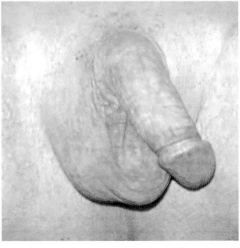

Fig. 15.6 Preoperative depilation of the penile shaft and scrotum.

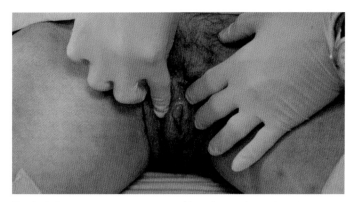

Fig. 15.7 Postoperative appearance: the labia majora are formed from the scrotum, the neoclitoris is formed from the dorsal glans penis, the labia minora are formed with a urethral flap, and the native penile urethra is shortened and spatulated to form the neo-urethra.

intravaginal hair growth. Finally, hormones are discontinued approximately two weeks prior to surgery to reduce the risk of venous thromboembolism.

Penile inversion

Primary vaginoplasty surgery most commonly involves penile disassembly and inversion with an anteriorly based pedicled penile flap. Although a variety of technical modifications are described in the literature, the penile disassembly and inversion technique utilizes the penile skin and a second, posteriorly based, scrotal–perineal flap to construct the vaginal cavity.[39] The author's preferred technique is described herein: the labia majora are formed from the lateral aspects of the scrotum, the neoclitoris is formed from the dorsal glans penis, and the labia minora are formed with the creation of a urethral flap. The penile urethra is shortened, spatulated, and everted to create the neo-urethral meatus (Fig. 15.7). Depending upon the length of the penis and previous surgical history (i.e., circumcision), skin grafts may be required

for additional vaginal depth. Full-thickness skin grafts may be harvested from discarded portions of the scrotum. If this is insufficient, additional full-thickness skin grafts may be harvested with a Pfannenstiel incision.[40] Alternatively, split-thickness skin grafts may also be harvested from the lower abdomen or mons region. However, the donor site of the split-thickness skin grafts may be left with areas of hypopigmentation depending upon depth of harvest and patient's skin tone.

Prior to surgery, sequential compression devices are placed and intravenous antibiotics are administered. Following induction of general anesthesia, chemoprophylaxis for VTE is administered subcutaneously (either fractionated or unfractionated heparin depending upon institutional policies), the patient is positioned in lithotomy, and an indwelling urinary catheter is placed under sterile conditions after the patient is prepped and draped.

The procedure is begun with the creation of a posteriorly based scrotal–perineal flap. This flap, which measures approximately 15 cm in length and 8 cm in transverse dimension, requires sufficient width so as not to limit the vaginal introitus. Additionally, the lateral aspect of the flap is designed in a "V"-shaped fashion so as not to create a circular introitus, thereby minimizing the chance of introital contracture (Fig. 15.8A). The flap is centered cephalad to the anus and dissected to the level of the anal sphincter, with care taken not to injure the external anal sphincter (Fig. 15.8B).

An incision is made on the ventral penis along the midline raphe (Fig. 15.8C). This allows access to the testicles for the performance of bilateral orchiectomies. The orchiectomy, including resection of the spermatic cords, is performed at the level of the inguinal ring. This allows the spermatic cord to retract within the inguinal canal and prevents a palpable bulge in the groin area. The skin of the penile shaft is then circumferentially incised at the junction of the glans and penile shaft. This facilitates separation of the penile skin from the underlying corpora cavernosa and corpora spongiosum, as well as the overlying muscles, the ischiocavernosus, and bulbospongiosus muscles, respectively (Fig. 15.8D).

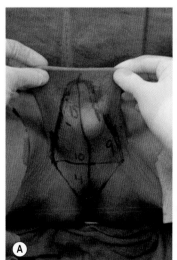
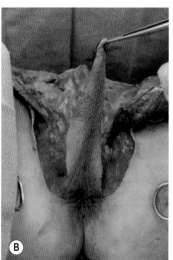
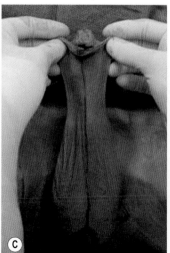
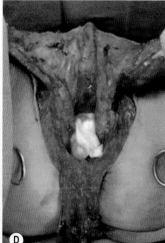

Fig. 15.8 (A) Design of the perineal–scrotal flap. Note the "V"-shape of the lateral aspect of this flap. This design assists with widening of the introitus and lessening the risks of introital scar contracture. **(B)** Elevation of the posteriorly based perineal–scrotal flap. **(C)** Incision of the ventral penile skin along the midline raphe. **(D)** Exposure of the corpora spongiosum and ischiocavernosus muscles with underlying corpora cavernosa. A sponge is placed in the neovaginal cavity.

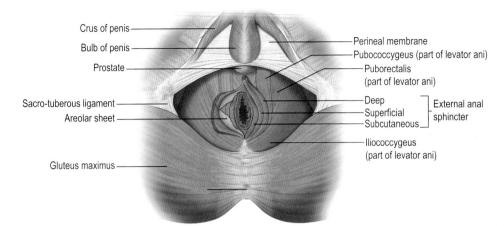

Crus of penis

Bulb of penis

Prostate

Sacro-tuberous ligament

Areolar sheet

Gluteus maximus

Perineal membrane

Pubococcygeus (part of levator ani)

Puborectalis (part of levator ani)

Deep
Superficial
Subcutaneous

External anal sphincter

Iliococcygeus (part of levator ani)

Fig. 15.9 The release of levator ani to aid with maintenance of neovaginal cavity.

At this point, the vaginal cavity is developed by dissection between the prostate and rectum. Care must be taken to avoid inadvertent entry into the rectum. Dissection follows Denonvilliers' fascia until the peritoneal reflection is reached. Most of the dissection is performed bluntly; however, release of the attachments between the prostate and rectum may require sharp division. The levator ani are then scored with electrocautery to further expand the neovaginal cavity (Fig. 15.9). Adequate dissection of the neovaginal space is essential in creating and maintaining adequate vaginal depth. Once the vaginal cavity is created, the superficial perineal muscles are resected. Resection of the ischiocavernosus muscles aids with creation of the introitus and exposure of the corpora cavernosa. At this point, the corpora spongiosum is separated from the corpora cavernosa. The corpora spongiosum is resected from the bulb of the penis in order to further open the vaginal cavity. If excess erectile tissue is not removed, this tissue may become engorged during sexual arousal and restrict entry to the vaginal cavity.[41]

The neoclitoris is then fashioned from the dorsal glans penis and dissected on the dorsal neurovascular bundle (Figs. 15.10 & 15.11A). The dissection of the dorsal vein and paired dorsal arteries and nerves is performed deep to Buck's fascia along the corpora cavernosa.[42] Dissection of the neurovascular pedicle is performed to the pubic symphysis, exposing the divergence of the underlying corpora cavernosa. The corpora cavernosa are resected at the pubis, leaving a short remnant of corpora on either sided. The retained corpora will be sutured together to form a base, upon which the neoclitoris will be attached (S. Monstrey, pers. comm).

In order to aid with the advancement of the penile flap, the skin of the mons and lower abdomen may be elevated to the umbilicus (Fig. 15.11B). In some individuals, this facilitates intravaginal positioning of the penile flap.[43] Depending upon the length of the penile flap, skin grafts may be required to increase vaginal depth. These may be harvested as full-thickness grafts from the non-used scrotum, groin crease, or lower abdomen. Additionally, split-thickness grafts may be

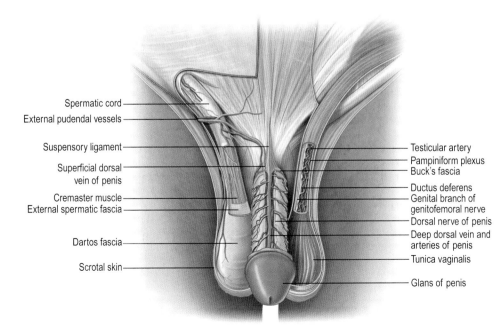

Spermatic cord

External pudendal vessels

Suspensory ligament

Superficial dorsal vein of penis

Cremaster muscle

External spermatic fascia

Dartos fascia

Scrotal skin

Testicular artery

Pampiniform plexus

Buck's fascia

Ductus deferens

Genital branch of genitofemoral nerve

Dorsal nerve of penis

Deep dorsal vein and arteries of penis

Tunica vaginalis

Glans of penis

Fig. 15.10 Dissection of dorsal glans penis on dorsal neurovascular bundle.

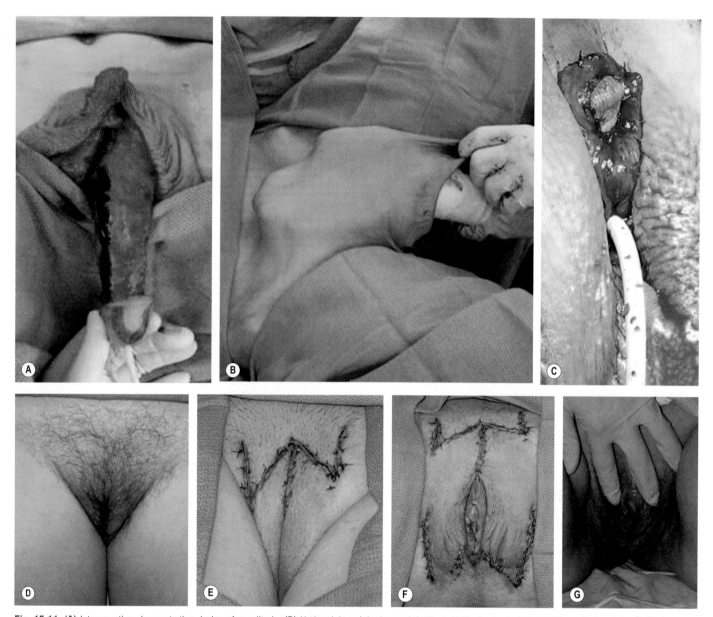

Fig. 15.11 **(A)** Intraoperative: demonstrating design of neoclitoris. **(B)** Undermining of the lower abdominal skin to the level of the umbilicus. Undermining facilitates advancement of the penile flap into the intravaginal position. **(C)** Design of the urethral flap to form the labia minora and prepuce of the neoclitoris. **(D)** Postoperative: after single-stage vaginoplasty. **(E)** Postoperative: following second-stage labiaplasty. Note the convergence of the labia majora in the mons pubis. **(F)** Postoperative: following second-stage labiaplasty. Note the prepuce of the neoclitoris. **(G)** Postoperative: demonstrating moist appearance of labia minora and neoclitoris with associated prepuce.

harvested from the mons or lower abdominal region.[44] The scrotal–perineal flap is sutured to the penile flap over a silastic stent and advanced into the intravaginal position. A "Y"-shaped incision is made in the penile flap in order to create the urethral meatus. The penile urethra is shortened and incised ventrally. This creates a urethral flap through which the glans penis will be placed, thereby creating the labia minora and providing a prepuce to the neoclitoris (Fig. 15.11C). The scrotal skin is then tailored to form the labia majora, and the incisions are closed in a layered fashion with absorbable sutures. Drains are placed on either side of the vaginal cavity (Fig. 15.11D).

Although most surgeons perform a single-stage vaginoplasty, an optional second stage, referred to as a labiaplasty, may be performed for further feminization of the mons pubis. This procedure is performed approximately 3 months after the vaginoplasty. The labiaplasty involves a local tissue rearrangement, frequently in the form of multiple "Z"-plasties, so as to create convergence of the labia majora and provide for additional clitoral hooding (Fig. 15.11E–G).

Technical variations include the use of a urethral flap inset within the penile skin designed to either lengthen or provide lubrication to the vaginal cavity.[45] Additionally, intravaginal placement of the glans penis to act as a neocervix has been described.[46]

The postoperative care consists of a variable period of bedrest, typically 4–5 days, during which a silastic stent is used to maintain the vaginal cavity. Additionally, a urinary catheter remains in place until the vaginal packing is removed and ambulation is initiated, typically 5–6 days after surgery. Once the vaginal stent is removed, a regimen of vaginal dilation with a rigid prosthesis is begun. Initially, dilation of the neovaginal cavity is performed 3–4 times daily for 6 weeks. The frequency of dilation is reduced over a period of 2–3 months, ultimately requiring dilation two to three times per week. This schedule may be varied depending upon the frequency of vaginal intercourse.

Additionally, intermittent vaginal douching with a dilute povidone-iodine solution is performed to remove intravaginal debris. This is initially performed two to three times per week beginning three to four weeks after surgery. Vaginal intercourse may begin 6–8 weeks after surgery. An annual speculum and prostate exam are also recommended.

Intestinal vaginoplasty

In the event that vaginal depth is inadequate, revision vaginoplasty typically requires either skin grafting, local and regional nongenital flaps, or intestinal transposition. While a skin graft may alleviate the need for an intra-abdominal procedure, the dissection of the previously operated upon vaginal cavity may be difficult. Visualization and protection of the urethra and bladder anteriorly and rectum posteriorly may be limited. Additionally, donor sites for full-thickness skin grafts may be limited, and hypopigmentation from split-thickness skin graft donor sites may be undesirable. Furthermore, skin grafts require regular postoperative dilation so as to prevent contraction of the neovagina. Local and regional nongenital flaps include the use of various thigh or perineal-based flaps. The advantages of these nongenital flaps include less risk of postoperative contraction. However, many of these flaps are bulky, limit the size of the neovagina, and provide no intrinsic lubrication. The advantage of intestinal transposition, especially in revision cases, is the provision of a reliable length of vascularized tissue with mucus secretion providing lubrication for vaginal intercourse. Intestinal transposition may utilize either the small or large intestine; however, the sigmoid colon is the most commonly used. The advantage of the sigmoid colon is the larger luminal diameter and less copious secretions as compared to that of jejunum or ileum.

Prior to performing the sigmoid vaginoplasty, a preoperative colonoscopy is performed so as to evaluate for colorectal malignancies. As with a primary procedure, a bowel preparation is prescribed preoperatively. The sigmoid vaginoplasty is also performed in the lithotomy position in conjunction with general surgery. A combined abdominal and perineal approach is utilized and allows visualization and protection of the bladder and urethra anteriorly and the rectum posteriorly. The sigmoid colon is harvested by the general surgery team, and the perineal dissection is performed concurrently by the plastic surgery team. A 12–15 cm segment of sigmoid colon is transferred in an isoperistaltic fashion (Figs. 15.12–15.14). The defunctionalized sigmoid colon is sutured to the introitus of the neovagina with a single layer of absorbable sutures. In order to prevent contraction of the introitus, several Z-plasties are used when insetting the distal bowel segment with the perineal skin (Fig. 15.15 ◉). Additionally, the mesentery of the defunctionalized sigmoid colon is gently sewn to the pelvis to prevent torsion of the vascular pedicle. An end-to-end colonic anastomosis is performed to restore intestinal continuity, and the distal stump of the neovagina is separated from the colorectal anastomosis so as to reduce the risk of fistulization. Intravenous antibiotics are maintained for 24 hours postoperatively.

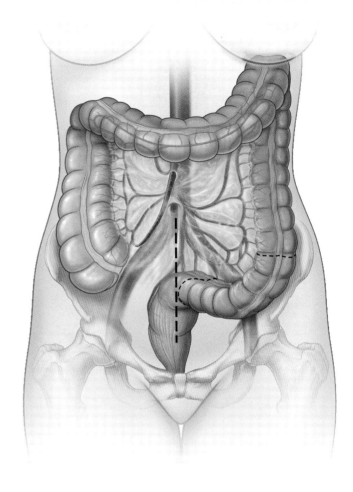

Fig. 15.12 Incision along mesentery of colon and development of the vascular pedicle.

Fig. 15.15B appears online only.

The neovagina is packed for 3–4 days with a soft stent, and the patient remains on bedrest with a urinary catheter. Upon return of bowel function and oral intake, the patient is discharged from the hospital.

The potential drawbacks of intestinal-based flaps include copious secretions, most notably with the small intestine, and possible malodorous discharge with the large intestine. Additional concerns include the possibility of diversion colitis in the defunctionalized sigmoid colon, as well as the risk of GI malignancies. Finally, the colonic mucosa may be somewhat friable, and small amounts of postcoital bleeding may occur.

Complications

Early postoperative complications include bleeding, infection, and delayed wound healing. Additional early or late complications include rectovaginal fistula, urinary stream abnormalities, inadequate vaginal depth or constricted introitus, partial flap loss, loss of neoclitoral sensation, and unsatisfactory cosmetic appearance.

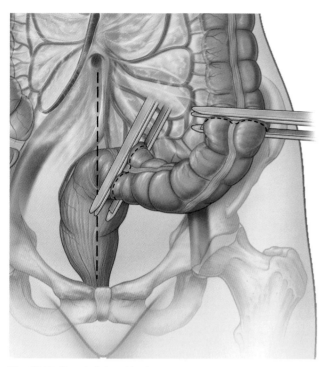

Fig. 15.13 Harvest of sigmoid colon.

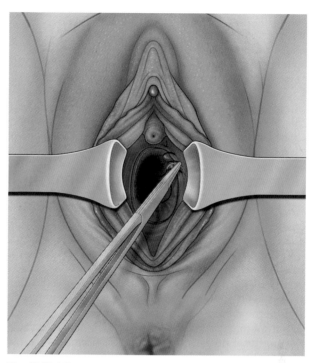

Fig. 15.15 (A) This figure demonstrates insetting of sigmoid colon. The use of laparoscopic instruments facilitates insetting several centimeters cephalad to the introitus.

In the event that a rectovaginal fistula is recognized intraoperatively, the rectum is closed in a layered fashion and may be left to heal. Because the patient has undergone a preoperative bowel preparation, the rectum may heal without further intervention. However, there is the potential need for diversion with a colostomy, as well as the risk of neovaginal stenosis. Although minor urinary stream abnormalities are not uncommon, the risk of stenosis of the neo-urethral meatus may be reduced by spatulation and eversion of the urethra. It is also

imperative that the individual continue routine dilation so as to prevent the risk of vaginal stenosis. Although the frequency of dilation may be reduced with sexual intercourse, pedicled penile flaps and skin grafts still require compliance with vaginal dilation.

Routine medical care of the transgender individual is recommended and includes clinical and laboratory monitoring. This allows assessment of the beneficial, as well as possible adverse, effects associated with cross-sex hormonal therapy. Monitoring of weight and blood pressure, directed physical examinations, complete blood counts, renal and liver function tests, and lipid and glucose metabolism should be considered.

Additional monitoring considerations for transwomen on estrogen therapy include measurement of prolactin levels, evaluation for cardiac risk factors, screening guidelines for prostate disease as recommended for biologic males, and screening guidelines for breast cancer as recommended for biologic females.[34] For transmen, additional monitoring considerations include evaluation of bone mineral density if risk factors for osteoporotic fracture are present, and, if mastectomy/hysterectomy/oophorectomy are not performed, mammograms and annual Pap smear, as recommended by the American Cancer Society and American College of Obstetricians and Gynecologists, respectively.[47]

Additional feminizing procedures

Additional procedures include both facial feminization as well as breast augmentation. The goal of these procedures is to remove the secondary sexual characteristics and stigmata associated with the male appearance. The timing of these surgeries in relation to genital surgery may vary between centers as well as within individual centers. It is not

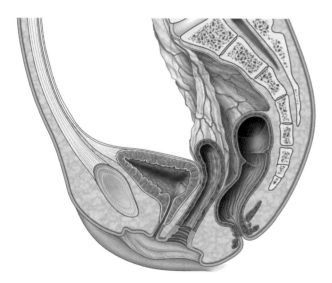

Fig. 15.14 This figure demonstrates placement of defunctionalized sigmoid colon to position of neovagina. The colorectal anastomosis is isolated from the sutured stump of the defunctionalized sigmoid colon.

uncommon for these procedures to be performed prior to genital surgery so as to improve the individual's sense of well-being and facilitate the real life test.[2]

Following hormonal therapy, there is frequently some breast growth in the transwomen. However, the degree of breast growth is oftentimes inadequate, and individuals continue to wear external prostheses or padded bras. As such, augmentation mammaplasty is a frequently requested procedure. Anatomic differences between the male and female chest are relevant as to implant selection, incision choice, and pocket location.[48]

The male chest is not only wider than the female chest, but the pectoral muscle is usually more developed. Furthermore, the male areola is smaller than the female areola, the distance between the nipple and inframammary crease is less, and there is less ptosis in the natal male breast, even after hormonal therapy.[49] Based upon these characteristics, a larger implant is commonly chosen. In addition, silicone implants are usually requested. Pocket location and incision choice depend upon the individual and the degree of breast growth in response to hormonal therapy. Either a subglandular, subfascial, or subpectoral pocket may be used. The potential issues associated with a subpectoral pocket are implant displacement due to the activity of the overlying pectoralis muscle. However, potential concerns with the subglandular pocket include capsular contracture and palpability of the implant due to less soft-tissue coverage. In terms of incisions, transaxillary, peri-areolar, or inframammary crease approaches may be used and are tailored to the requests and anatomy of the individual (Fig. 15.16).

Facial features may also be typically male or female. As such, surgery to "feminize" the face of transwomen is frequently requested. A variety of characteristics have been identified as male and are often associated with the forehead, nose, malar region, mandible, and thyroid cartilage. These differences include more pronounced supraorbital bossing in the male and a more continuous forehead curvature in the female.[50] The malar region is also more prominent in the female, and the female nose tends to be smaller, with a less acute glabellar angle than the male.[50,51] In addition, qualitative and quantitative differences in the skin, subcutaneous tissue, and hair also exist.[52]

Because the female eyebrow is located above the supraorbital rim and has a more arched appearance than the male, typical procedures for facial feminization include a brow lift with advancement of the frontal hairline and frontal bone reduction. Although the brow lift may be performed with an

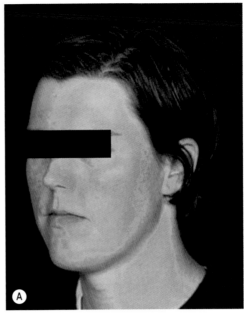
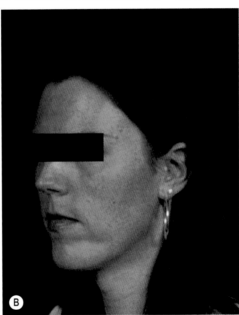

Fig. 15.17 (A) Preoperative: prior to brow lift and frontal bone reduction. **(B)** Postoperative: following brow lift and frontal bone reduction performed through an open, anterior hairline approach.

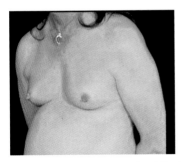
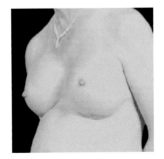

Fig. 15.16 Pre- and postoperative: following subpectoral silicone gel augmentation mammaplasty performed through an inframammary crease incision.

endoscope, reduction of the frontal bone and lateral brow is facilitated with the open approach. In addition, the open approach, performed through an anterior hairline incision, allows advancement of the frontal hairline, if desired (Fig. 15.17). Prior to proceeding with reduction of the frontal bone, lateral skull films are obtained in order to assess the thickness of the anterior table of the frontal sinus. Depending upon the thickness of the anterior table in relation to the degree of frontal bossing, craniofacial techniques may be employed for the desired correction.

A feminizing rhinoplasty typically involves dorsal hump reduction, cephalic trim, elevation of the nasal tip, and osteotomies to narrow the nasal pyramid. The chin and mandible represent additional anatomic sites that may require treatment. Based upon the individual's anatomy, either chin implants or osteoplastic genioplasty may be required. In addition, reduction of the masseter muscle or contouring of the mandibular angle may be performed through intraoral incisions. Other procedures, such as upper lip shortening, facelift (Fig. 15.18), blepharoplasty, malar implants, hair transplantation, injectable fillers, and skin resurfacing may also be requested.

Reduction thyroid chondroplasty is frequently requested to reduce the appearance of the "Adam's apple" or prominent thyroid cartilage (pomus Adamus). The procedure is typically performed as an outpatient under general or local anesthesia

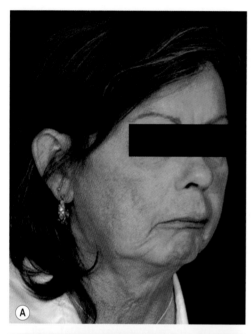

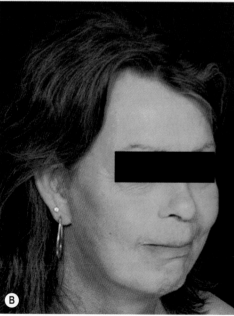

Fig. 15.18 **(A)** Preoperative: prior to facelift, upper eyelid blepharoplasty, and TCA chemical peel. **(B)** Postoperative: following facelift, upper eyelid blepharoplasty, and TCA chemical peel.

with sedation. The procedure is performed through a transverse incision in a naturally occurring skin crease. Following vertical division of the middle cervical fascia, the sternothyroid and thyrohyoid muscles are retracted laterally. The perichondrium is incised and a subperichondrial dissection is performed with care so as to enter the thyrohyoid membrane. On the posterior surface of the cartilage, subperichondrial dissection is performed inferiorly to the thyroepiglottic ligament. Dissection stops at this point so as not to injure the insertion of the vocal cords or destabilize the epiglottis. Identification of the insertion of the vocal cords may be facilitated with fiberoptic laryngoscopy by the anesthesiologist. Resection of the thyroid cartilage is performed between the superior thyroid notch in the midline and the superior thyroid tubercle superolaterally. The perichondrium is reapproximated, and the incision is closed in a layered fashion.[53]

Voice surgery, designed to raise vocal pitch, may be requested by individuals following voice therapy. Hormonal intervention does not commonly affect vocal pitch, and this may represent a residual stigma of masculinity. As such, various techniques to shorten the vocal cords, increase vocal cord tension, or reduce vibrating vocal cord mass may be performed.[21]

Masculinizing surgical therapy

Chest surgery

Chest-wall contouring is an important early surgical step in the process of gender confirmation for transmen. The goals of chest surgery include the aesthetic contouring of the chest by removal of breast tissue and skin excess, reduction and repositioning of the nipple–areola complex, release of the inframammary crease, and minimization of chest scars.[54]

Chest surgery in transmen presents an aesthetic challenge due to breast volume, breast ptosis, nipple–areola size and position, degree of skin excess, and potential loss of skin elasticity. Breast binding, commonly performed by female-to-male transsexuals, may lead to loss of skin elasticity, thereby necessitating additional skin removal. Both skin quality and elasticity are important determinants in the choice of surgical technique.[54] Technical considerations related to the subcutaneous mastectomy include preservation of subcutaneous fat on the skin flaps, preservation of the pectoralis fascia, and release of the inframammary crease and sternal attachments.

Choice of incision is largely determined by degree of breast ptosis and skin quality/elasticity as well as position of the nipple–areola complex. Incisions may range from a periareolar incision in small breasts with a small areola and good skin elasticity, to circumareolar incisions, to transverse inframammary crease incisions with free nipple grafts. Liposuction may be used as an adjunct to excisional techniques. The decision as to maintenance of the nipple–areola complex on a dermoglandular pedicle versus a free nipple–areola graft must also be considered. In positioning the nipple–areolar complex, the patient is sat upright and clinical judgment is used. In general, the nipple–areola is positioned just medial to the lateral border of the pectoralis major muscle, approximately 2–3 cm above the inferior insertion of the pectoralis major muscle (Fig. 15.19 ●). Postoperative management includes

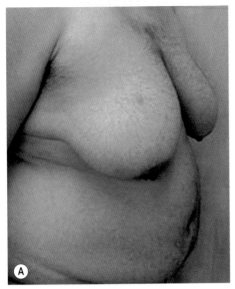
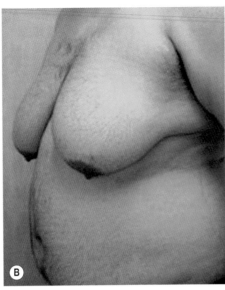
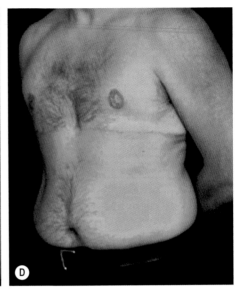

Fig. 15.19 **(A)** Preoperative: prior to chest surgery (right side). **(B)** Preoperative: prior to chest surgery (left side). **(D)** Postoperative: subcutaneous mastectomy with free nipple graft.

drains and elastic compression. Secondary revisions related to the scar and/or nipple–areolar complex are not uncommon.

Fig. 15.19C & E appear online only.

Genital surgery

The goal of genital surgery in transmen may range from clitoral release with or without urethral lengthening and capable of allowing voiding while standing, to a complete penis, capable of sexual penetration.[55]

Metoidioplasty

Metoidioplasty, described in 1196 by Hage, has been offered as an alternative to microsurgical or pedicled flap phalloplasty in transmen. The term, coined by Laub, is based upon the Greek prefix *meta-*, relating to change, and *aidoio*, relating to the genitals.[56] The procedure entails lengthening the hormonally hypertrophied clitoris by release of the suspensory ligament and resection of the ventral chordee and lengthening of the female urethra with the aid of labia minora and/or vaginal musculomucosal flaps.[57] Additionally, buccal mucosa grafts have been utilized to aid with urethral extension. Urethral reconstruction is the major challenge associated with metoidioplasty, and most complications involve either urethral fistulae and/or strictures.

The operative technique may involve concomitant removal of the female genitalia (vaginectomy) in addition to metoidioplasty.[58] Most often, a hysterectomy and oophorectomy are performed prior to the metoidioplasty. A caudally based anterior vaginal wall flap incorporating the muscularis of the ventral vaginal wall may be used. This flap can be used to reconstruct the fixed portion of the neo-urethra.[56] If a vaginectomy is not performed, the vaginal donor site is closed, thereby narrowing the retained vagina. The clitoral shaft is degloved and released by detaching the suspensory ligament from the pubic bone. On the ventral aspect of the clitoris, the urethral plate is dissected from the clitoral bodies. The urethral plate is divided so as to release the ventral clitoral curvature allowing straightening and lengthening of the

clitoris.[58] Additional lengthening of the urethra is performed with flaps developed from the labia minora. The vaginal mucosa and labial flaps are sutured to each other in a beveled fashion over a urinary catheter (Fig. 15.20).

Fig. 15.20 appears online only.

Scrotoplasty, constructed with bilateral labia majora flaps, may be performed at the time of metoidioplasty. Testicular implants are placed at a secondary surgical procedure so as to reduce the risk of infection and urethral complications (see Fig. 15.20C).

Conclusion

A letter addressed to the relevant governmental agencies petitioning for a change of legal "sex" status may be requested by the individual following surgery. This letter may be important for the individual's legal documents (i.e., driver's license, passport, social security, etc.) and should include the nature of the treatment rendered. Individual state laws may vary in regard to the requirements for change of legal documents.

Continued collaboration between the surgeon, mental health professional, and medical physician is important in providing comprehensive care to the transgender individual. In addition, continued research focused on objective parameters and reporting of outcomes data will foster innovation and continued improvements in surgical techniques.

🌐 **Bonus images for this chapter can be found online at**
http://www.expertconsult.com

Fig. 15.15 (B) Postoperative: intestinal vaginoplasty
Fig. 15.19 (C) Preoperative: limited incision chest surgery. **(E)** Postoperative: limited incision chest surgery.
Fig. 15.20 Metoidioplasty preoperative and postoperative photos.
(A) Preoperative: metoidioplasty. **(B)** Intraoperative: metoidioplasty.
(C) Postoperative: metoidioplasty.

Access the complete reference list online at **http://www.expertconsult.com**

2. Monstrey S, Hoebeke P, Dhont M, et al. Surgical therapy in transsexual patients: a multi-disciplinary approach. *Acta Chir Belg.* 2001;101:200–209. *Excellent review article on the care of transgender individuals.*

7. Lee PA, Houk CP, Ahmed SF, et al. in collaboration with the participants in the International Consensus Conference on Intersex. Consensus statement on management of intersex disorders. *Pediatrics.* 2006;118:e488–e500. *Review article on disorders of sexual development.*

21. Ettner R. The etiology of transsexualism. In: Ettner R, Monstrey S, Eyler E, eds. *Principles of Transgender Medicine and Surgery.* New York: Haworth Press; 2007:1–14.

25. Schechter L. The surgeon's relationship with the physician prescribing hormones and the mental health professional: review for version 7 of the World Professional Association for Transgender Health's Standards of care. *Int J Transgend.* 2009;11:222–225.

26. Bowman C, Goldberg J. Care of the patient undergoing sex reassignment surgery. *Int J Transgend.* 2006;9:135–165.

33. Dahl M, Feldman JL, Goldberg JM, et al. Physical aspects of transgender endocrine therapy. *Int J Transgend.* 2006;9:111–134. *Guidelines for endocrine therapy for transgender individuals.*

34. Hembree WC, Cohen-Kettenis P, Delemarre-van de Waal HA, et al. Endocrine treatment of transsexual persons: an endocrine society clinical practice guideline. *J Clin Endocrinol Metab.* 2009;94:3132–3153.

37. Edgerton MT, Bull J. Surgical construction of the vagina and labia in male transsexuals. *Plast Reconstr Surg.* 1970;46:529–539.

41. Karim RB, Hage JJ, Bouman FG, et al. The importance of near total resection of the corpora cavernosa in the surgery of male to female transsexuals. *Ann Plast Surg.* 1991;26:554–557.

45. Perovic SV, Stanojevic DS, Djordjevic MI. Vaginoplasty in male transsexuals using penile skin and a urethral flap. *BJU Int.* 2000;86:843–850.

51. Hage JJ, Vossen M, Becking AG. Rhinoplasty as part of gender-confirming surgery in male transsexuals: basic considerations and clinical experience. *Ann Plast Surg.* 1997;39:266–271.

52. Hage JJ, Becking AG, de Graf FH, et al. Gender-confirming facial surgery: consideration on the masculinity and femininity of faces. *Plast Reconstr Surg.* 1997;97:1799–1807.

16

Pressure sores

Robert Kwon, Juan L. Rendon, and Jeffrey E. Janis

 Access video lecture content for this chapter online at expertconsult.com

SYNOPSIS

- Pressure sores are a common problem associated with great morbidity and cost.
- They have been recognized since antiquity, though effective surgical treatment did not evolve until the 19th century.
- Originally thought to result from direct pressure to soft tissue exceeding the pressure found in the blood vessels supplying the affected area, pressure sores are now considered multifactorial entities involving friction, shear, moisture, nutrition, and infection.
- Successful treatment of pressure sores requires a multidisciplinary evaluation in order to accurately stage wounds, identify/eradicate wound/bone infection, minimize risk factors for recurrence, and optimize wound healing potential.
- Prevention and treatment of pressure sores should focus on correcting these risk factors, reserving operative intervention until the patient is optimized.
- As with any wound, pressure sores involving infected soft tissue and/or bone must be thoroughly debrided prior to definitive closure.
- Locoregional fasciocutaneous and musculocutaneous flaps remain workhorse flaps as they can provide enough viable tissue for large defects and allow for revision in the event of recurrence.
- Prevention remains the most effective treatment of pressure sores. More recently, the Hospital Acquired Conditions Initiative has led to the implementation of programs aiming to prevent complications, such as pressure sores, through promotion of thorough risk assessment and early identification.

 Access the Historical Perspective section online at
http://www.expertconsult.com

Introduction

Terminology

Though technically and semantically inaccurate, the terms "decubitus ulcer", "bedsore", and "pressure sore" are often used interchangeably. Decubitus ulcers – derived from the Latin *decumbere*, to lie down – occur over areas that have underlying bony prominences when the subject is recumbent, e.g., the sacrum, trochanter, heel, and occiput. Technically, sores resulting from pressure breakdown in areas that bear seated weight, such as the ischial tuberosities of spinal injury patients, and ulcers due to devices, such as splints, ear probes, or rectal tubes, are not decubitus ulcers. Nonetheless, "pressure sores" is likely the best term to use when describing these lesions, which all involve pressure as a key etiologic factor. Pressure sores are now recognized as multifactorial conditions, with pressure being only one of the many factors that contribute to their development.

Epidemiology

Over 500 English-language articles analyzing the incidence and prevalence of pressure sores have been published in the last 5 years. These studies not only examine the prevalence and incidence of pressure sores across multiple healthcare settings – general acute care, long-term care, and home care – but also among specific patient populations – including infants and children, the elderly, patients with hip fractures, and terminally ill patients. Given these disparate populations and the substantial variation across individual institutions, precise determinations of incidence and prevalence are challenging.

In 1999 Amlung *et al.*[1] performed a one-day pressure ulcer prevalence survey of 356 acute care facilities and 42 817 patients. The overall pressure ulcer prevalence rate was 14.8%; facility-acquired ulcers accounted for 7.1%. Ten years later, VanGilder *et al.*[2] reviewed the results of the International Pressure Ulcer Prevalence Survey (IPUPS) and found overall prevalence and facility-acquired ulcer rates of 12.3% and 5%, respectively. Overall prevalence rates were highest in long-term acute care facilities (22%), while facility-acquired rates were highest in adult intensive care units (ICUs), ranging from 8.8% in general cardiac care units to 12.1% in medical ICUs. A total of 3.3% of ICU patients developed severe ulcers, while 10% were device-related. A broader inquiry,[3] reviewing over

400 000 records from the survey between 1989 and 2005, found overall and nosocomial pressure ulcer prevalence rates of 9.2% in 1989 and 15.5% in 2004. Rates were higher in long-term acute care facilities, at 27.3%. Overall, pressure ulcer prevalence appears relatively stable despite significant advances in treatment and prevention.

The prevalence of pressure ulcers in the nursing home population has been reported to be anywhere from 2% to 28%.[4,5] Data from the 2004 National Nursing Home Survey revealed an overall 11% prevalence rate, with elderly residents, residents with recent weight loss, and short-term residents being at even higher risk.[6] The reported prevalence of pressure ulcers in long-term acute care facilities is likewise variable, ranging from 5% to 27%,[7,8] while the IPUPS reported an overall 22% rate in this setting.

Particular populations have been identified at particularly high risk. There is a strong association between hip fractures and pressure sores, though incidences have been reported from 8.8% to 55%. A large European study[9] revealed an overall prevalence of 10% on arrival and 22% at discharge in this population, with dehydration, advanced age, moist skin, higher Braden scores, diabetes, and pulmonary disease all associated with higher rates of ulceration. The majority were stage I, and none was stage IV. Baumgarten et al.[10] reported an 8.8% incidence of hospital-acquired pressure sores in a study involving multiple centers in the US. Another study by the same group,[11] with rigorous surveillance for ulcers in a slightly older population, revealed an incidence of 36.1%. Incidence was highest in the acute care setting and associated with longer wait before surgery, ICU stay, longer surgery, and general anesthetic.

Spinal cord injury (SCI) patients are at particular risk for pressure sores due to the combination of immobility and insensitivity. Rates have been reported to be 33–60%,[12–14] and it is the second leading cause of rehospitalization after SCI. Gelis et al.[15] reviewed pressure ulceration in the SCI population and noted a 21–37% prevalence in the acute stage, a 2% rate leaving a rehabilitation center, and a 15–30% rate in the chronic stage. Identified risk factors included race, history of previous ulceration, and tobacco use.

Anatomic distribution

In 1964, Dansereau and Conway[16] published the results of their evaluation of 649 patients from the Bronx Veterans Administration Hospital with 1604 pressure sores among them. The authors noted that the vast majority of pressure sores developed in the lower part of the body, the ischial tuberosity being the most common site, accounting for 28% of all ulcers. In Meehan's 1994[17] review of 3487 patients with 6047 pressure sores, the most common site of occurrence was the sacrum (36%), followed by the heel (30%). More recently VanGilder et al.[2] reported that the sacrum (28.3%) and the heel (23.6%) were the most common sites for pressure ulceration, followed by the buttocks (17.2%).

Classically, in the early acute phase after SCI, the sacral area tends to be the most common site of pressure sores as patients are stabilized and treated for concomitant injuries in the supine position. In the subacute and chronic phases after SCI, the ischial area becomes the predominant site of pressure sores as the patient begins to sit up in a wheelchair during rehabilitation. However, as will be discussed later in this chapter, this division is not absolute.

Costs

Calculating the costs associated with pressure sores is complex. Monetary figures are subject to inflation and variation over time. While patients admitted with a primary diagnosis of pressure sore are simple to analyze, patients are often admitted with pressure ulcer-related problems, such as septicemia, and carry pressure sore as a secondary diagnosis. However, despite the uncertainty, it is clear pressure sores are a costly problem for the healthcare system.

The National Pressure Ulcer Advisory Panel (NPUAP) has estimated the cost to treat and heal hospital-acquired pressure sores to be up to $100 000 per patient.[18] If the additional costs, both surgical and nonsurgical, of managing pressure sores at nursing homes and home care facilities are considered, the financial burden is estimated by the Agency for Healthcare Research and Quality at approximately 11 billion dollars in 2006.[19]

A review from 2006 of the Healthcare Cost and Utilization Project[19] revealed 503 300 hospital stays during which pressure sores were noted. Patients with pressure sores were inpatients nearly three times longer than patients without such a diagnosis (14.1 days versus 5.0 days). Patients with pressure sore as a primary diagnosis cost an average of $1200 a day, while patients with pressure sore as a secondary diagnosis cost an average of $1600 a day, compared with an average of $2000 a day for all other conditions. Mean cost per hospitalization was $16 800 and $20 400 for stays with a principal and secondary diagnosis of pressure sore, versus only $9900 for all other conditions. Aggregate costs were calculated to be $752 million and $10.2 billion for stays with primary and secondary diagnosis of pressure sore, respectively.

In response to a growing body of literature demonstrating the economic consequences of pressure sores and other hospital-acquired conditions, the Center for Medicare & Medicaid Services (CMS) identified eight hospital-acquired complications as never events. In 2008, CMS implemented the Hospital-Acquired Conditions (HACs) initiative, a policy that denies reimbursement for several preventable conditions, including pressure sores.[20] Since then, Waters et al. utilized the National Database of Nursing Quality Indicators (NDNQI) to perform a quasi-experimental study of adult nursing units (ICU and non-ICU) from 1381 US hospitals between July 2006 and December 2010 to determine the rate of stage III/IV pressure sores before and after the implementation of the HACs initiative.[21] Unfortunately, nonpayment did not affect the rate of pressure sores noted between 2006 and 2010.[21] While it is unclear whether this is due a concomitant increase in early diagnosis, pressure sores remain prevalent and continue to be a large economic burden.

Basic science

Multiple studies describe risks associated with the development of pressure sores.[32–34] Fisher et al. utilized a logistic regression analysis to identify risks for pressure sores and found that increased age, male sex, friction, shear, moisture, malnutrition, immobility, and altered sensorium all independently place patients at risk of developing pressure sores.[33] More recently, these observations were re-demonstrated in a prospective cohort study of 3233 patients admitted to a single hospital where 201 were diagnosed with a hospital-acquired pressure sore. In their analysis, Baumgarten *et al.* also found that increased age, male sex, moisture caused by incontinence, poor nutrition, and immobility limiting turning in bed all correlated with the diagnosis of pressure sores.[34] Recognition of these factors has led to the understanding of pressure sores as multifactorial entities and provide the basis for basic science research to further our understanding of these processes.

Pressure

As mentioned previously, Paget described the connection between pressure and decubitus ulcers as early as the 19th century. Though many other factors may contribute to their formation, pressure sores are thought to result from pressure applied to soft tissue at a level higher than that found in the blood vessels supplying that area for an extended time period. In 1930 Landis performed a classic series of experiments and found that the average capillary closing pressure is approximately 32 mmHg.[35] Fronek and Zweifach reported similar findings in their study, noting perfusion pressures between 20 and 30 mmHg (Fig. 16.1).[36]

Lindan *et al.*[37] documented the human distribution of pressure points by means of a "bed of springs and nails". With the subject supine, the points of highest pressure were the sacrum, buttocks, heel, and occiput, all of which were subject to pressures of roughly 50–60 mmHg. When sitting, pressures up to 100 mmHg were recorded over the ischial tuberosities. Subjects in Lindan's study were tested on surfaces that were significantly softer than comparable wheelchair seats of beds, but even on padded surfaces with wide load distributions, all major weight-bearing areas sustained pressures in excess of end-capillary pressures (Fig. 16.2).

However, simply applying pressure in excess of these levels does not necessarily result in tissue ischemia. Much of the pressure applied to tissues is carried by the connective tissues surrounding the blood vessels. Furthermore, autoregulation of local blood flow will tend to increase blood pressure in response to applied pressure within a certain range.[35,38]

Efforts have been made to quantify the degree of pressure necessary to cause tissue damage. Dinsdale[39] found that pressure roughly double capillary closing pressure, applied for 2 hours, resulted in irreversible ischemic damage to tissue.

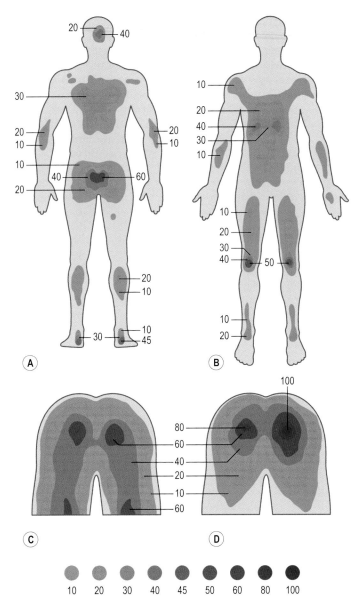

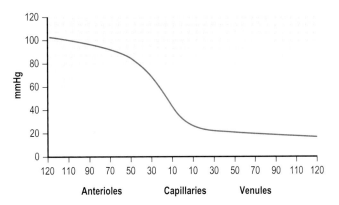

Fig. 16.1 Pressure in various components of the tissue microcirculation (diameter in μm). *(Data from Fronek K, Zweifach BW. Microvascular pressure distribution in skeletal muscle and the effects of vasodilation. Am J Physiol. 1975;228:791; reprinted with permission from Woolsey RM, McGarry JD. The cause, prevention, and treatment of pressure sores. Neurol Clin. 1991;9:797.)*

Fig. 16.2 Distribution of pressure in a healthy adult male while **(A)** supine, **(B)** prone, **(C)** sitting with feet hanging freely, and **(D)** sitting with feet supported. Values expressed in mmHg. *(Adapted with permission from Lindan O, Greenway RM, Piazza JM. Pressure distribution on the surface of the human body I. Evaluation in lying and sitting positions using a "bed of springs and nails". Arch Phys Med Rehabil. 1965;46:378.)*

Pressures below this threshold were unlikely to cause tissue necrosis, while increased pressures were correlated with increased likelihood of ulceration. Kosiak *et al.*[40] noted similar findings in dog tissues, but noted that if the pressure was released every 5 minutes, few changes occurred. Groth[41] published a detailed study on the relationship between applied pressure and the onset of tissue damage in a rabbit model, noting an inverse relationship wherein higher pressures caused damage in less time. Husain[42] had similar results in a rat model, also noting that pressure applied over a large area was less injurious than when applied over a smaller one.

Furthermore, various tissues have different susceptibility to pressure. Nola and Vistnes[43] noted that pressure on skin over a bone is more injurious than pressure on skin over muscle. On the other hand, Daniel *et al.*[44] noted that muscle was more susceptible to injury than skin, requiring less pressure for a shorter duration likely due to its increased metabolic activity.

Friction

Friction is the force resisting relative motion between two surfaces and is the precursor to shear. It develops between the patient's skin and any number of contact surfaces, including the patient's bedding, transfer devices such as sheets, rollers, or slide boards, various appliances and orthotics, and mobility devices such as wheelchair cushions. Excess friction may result in superficial skin injury such as abrasions, blisters, and even skin tears in patients with fragile skin.[45,46] While relatively minor in isolation, such injuries may potentiate further damage. As the integrity of the skin is compromised, transepidermal water loss increases and allows moisture to accumulate. Moisture in turn increases the coefficient of friction and promotes adherence to sheets and other contact surfaces.[47]

Shear (Fig. 16.3)

Reichel[48] was one of the first authors to describe shear as a risk factor for developing decubitus ulcers, noting that patients developed more sacral pressure sores when the head of their bed was elevated. Shear develops when friction adheres skin and superficial tissues to sheets or bedding, which are then stretched tightly over deeper structures. The underlying blood vessels are then stretched, angulated, and may be injured by this stress. Subcutaneous tissue in particular lacks tensile strength and is particularly susceptible to shear stress.[49]

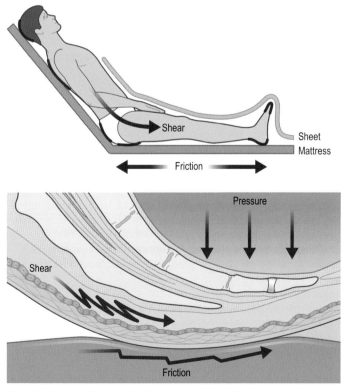

Fig. 16.3 Pressure, shear, and friction are related but distinct forces which contribute to pressure sore development.

Dinsdale[39] noted that addition of shear forces greatly decreased the amount of pressure needed to cause ulceration in a pig model, concluding that "a shear force is more disastrous than a vertical force". Goossens *et al.*[50] noted similar results in human subjects, finding that the addition of a small shear component drastically reduces the level of pressure needed to cause critical ischemia over the sacrum.

Patient transfers, sliding or dragging the patient in bed, "boosting" patients up in bed, or allowing patients to elevate themselves in bed by pushing with elbows and heels all cause significant shear.[46] Certain positions also cause elevated levels of shear: patients in the semi-Fowler's position or sliding down in a wheelchair both experience significant shear over the lower back and buttocks.[51] This can explain why wheelchair-bound patients may still develop a sacral pressure sore if they are not sitting upright in their chair, despite the fact that theoretically the ischial tuberosities should be bearing the majority of their weight.

Moisture

Excessive moisture is not only a risk factor for pressure sores but may also result in a separate pathology inclusive of incontinence dermatitis, perineal dermatitis, and moisture lesions.[52] Whether a separate entity resulting in skin breakdown due primarily to moisture and irritation as opposed to pressure is a legitimate or useful distinction is a matter of some debate.[53,54] However, it is clear that moisture is an important factor to consider when evaluating pressure sores, and pressure relief should not be neglected even if lesions are thought to be primarily due to moisture. Moist skin has a higher coefficient of friction and is prone to maceration and excoriation.[49]

Though excess moisture can have many causes, urinary and fecal incontinence is of particular concern in the etiology of pressure sores. Incontinence is common in the elderly, and rates are even high in the institutionalized population, with rates from 20% to 77% for urinary incontinence[55,56] and from 17% to 50% for fecal incontinence.[57] In addition to causing excess moisture, urine also negates the acidic pH of skin through the introduction of nitrogen derivatives. Fecal contamination introduces a large bacterial load. Lowthian[53] noted a fivefold increase in pressure sores in patients who were incontinent, though he did not distinguish between urinary and fecal incontinence. While some studies have found a relationship between urinary incontinence and pressure sores,[58] others have failed to find a correlation while noting a significant correlation with fecal incontinence.[59–61]

While excess moisture is clearly deleterious, the opposite is also true. Excessively dry skin is prone to cracking, has decreased tensile strength and lipid content, and impaired barrier function, and appears to be an independent risk factor for pressure ulceration.[62,63]

Malnutrition

Patients who are chronically ill and debilitated frequently have accompanying nutritional deficiencies that manifest as low serum albumin, prealbumin, or transferrin levels. Prevalence rates range from 1% to 4% in elderly patients living at home, versus 20% in hospitalized patients and 37% in institutionalized patients.[64] The deleterious effects of poor nutrition include weight loss, negative nitrogen balance, poor wound healing, and immunosuppression.[65] Several studies have documented a clear association between protein malnutrition and wound healing,[66–68] and patients who are severely malnourished are at increased risk of sepsis, infection, in-hospital mortality, and longer hospital stays.[69,70] However, the relationship between malnutrition and pressure sore prevention, as opposed to treatment, is not entirely clear. There is certainly a strong correlation between malnutrition and pressure sores,[71–73] but a clear causal link remains elusive.

Neurological injury

Despite extensive recommendations aimed at addressing the issue, pressure sores remain the most common complication[74,75] and the second most common cause of hospital admission[76] in the SCI population. Immobility, either in bed or in a wheelchair, leads to increased pressure, friction, and shear that is a causative factor in all pressure sores. However, SCI eliminates the protective sensation that would normally stimulate them to alter their position in response to prolonged pressure, particularly during sleep. Pressure that would be innocuous with intermittent relief leads to pressure sore development.[51]

In addition to the obvious problems of immobility and decreased sensation, incontinence, spasticity, and psychosocial issues are common problems in this population. Spasticity, a common but not inevitable sequela of SCI, is a problem unique to the SCI population, affecting 65–78% of patients one year postinjury.[77] Spasticity is characterized by hyperreflexia, clonus, and increased muscle tone. While it is not included in most pressure sore risk scales, it has effects due to direct increase in mechanical stress and altered weight distribution, as well as complicating patient positioning, skin inspection, and hygiene.[78]

Inflammatory milieu

The role of the local inflammatory milieu within the wound bed has gained significant attention but remains to be elucidated.[32] In 1994 Cooper et al. measured levels of multiple cytokines in pressure sore wound beds from 20 patients with stage III/IV wounds and found decreased levels of platelet-derived growth factor (PDGF), basic fibroblast growth factor (bFGF), epidermal growth factor (EGF), and transforming growth factor-Beta (TGF-B).[79] These cytokines play major roles in the progression of wound healing; thus a more comprehensive understanding of the normal temporal characterization of these molecules may facilitate novel therapeutic agents. Matrix metalloproteinases (MMPs) seem to play a role in healing of chronic pressure sores. MMPs are zinc-dependent proteases, which are capable of degrading various extracellular matrix proteins, and more recently been shown to play a role in cell proliferation, differentiation, apoptosis, angiogenesis and host immunity.[80] Under homeostatic conditions, a balance must be maintained between MMPs and their counterparts, namely tissue inhibitors of metalloproteinases (TIMPs) in order to maintain orderly formation/degradation of extracellular matrices. In chronic wounds from 56 patients with Stage III/IV pressure sores, Ladwig et al. found that as chronic wounds heal, the ratio of MMP-9:TIMP-1 decreases, thus suggesting that higher levels of MMP-9 and TIMP-1 are

necessary for appropriate healing of chronic wounds and may service as markers of healing/non-healing.[81] While MMP-9 and several other proteinases and their inhibitors have been studied in various kinds of wounds, human studies within the arena of pressure sores remain limited.

Diagnosis
Classification

Multiple classification systems exist to describe pressure sores. The most commonly used system is the NPUAP staging system,[82] a modification of Shea's original classification,[82,83] most recently revised in 2007 (Fig. 16.4). Though used in basic form for many years, two additional classifications, suspected deep-tissue injury and unstageable, have been added relatively recently to the NPUAP system.

"Stage" is somewhat of a misnomer, as it implies a progression that does not reflect reality. Stage IV ulcers do not necessarily start as stage I ulcers, a fact emphasized by the addition of the suspected deep-tissue injury classification. Likewise, healing pressure sores do not progress in reverse order but instead granulate and close by secondary intention in the absence of surgical treatment. Though panel members were aware of these issues, the term "stage" was retained due to its historical use and widespread adoption.

Patient evaluation

When evaluating a new patient with a pressure sore, a wide variety of factors must be considered. Both the wound and the patient should be meticulously examined. A wound history, noting the onset, duration, prior treatments and procedures, and wound care regimen, should be documented. Wounds should be measured in three dimensions, with notes made regarding any tunneling or undermining. The tissue at the margins of the wound should be examined for any signs of occult deep-tissue injury, infection, and scarring. The base of the wound should be characterized, noting the presence of eschar, slough, or other necrotic tissue. If necrotic material obscures the base of the wound, it should be debrided until a full assessment can be performed. Granulation should be noted in terms of both character and percentage of the wound bed covered. Exposed tissues, such as bone, tendon, or joint, should be noted. If easily accessible the bone can be characterized as hard, soft, or obviously necrotic. The amount and character of the wound exudate should be documented as well. A measuring tape and camera can improve documentation and make tracking progression easier.[84]

In addition to a thorough general history and physical, some attention should be paid to the risk factors specific to pressure sores. An attempt should be made to identify the etiology of the patient's pressure sore, though it is often multifactorial. Sources of friction, shear, and pressure should be evaluated and recommendations for proper pressure relief surfaces and skin care regimens made as appropriate. If incontinence is present an effort should be made to control this, possibly involving the assistance of other specialties if needed. Likewise, spasticity should be evaluated and if needed controlled medically or surgically. Nutrition should be evaluated with serum albumin and prealbumin. If needed, nutrition should be supplemented and progress of therapy monitored with weekly serum studies. Any underlying medical problems, such as hypertension, diabetes, or history of cardiac disease, should be investigated and optimized.

A reasonable initial set of studies would include a complete blood count, basic metabolic panel, creatinine, and blood urea nitrogen. Albumin and prealbumin should be obtained at the initial consult and regularly thereafter to evaluate for malnutrition and follow the progression of therapy. C-reactive protein and erythrocyte sedimentation rate (ESR) can be obtained to evaluate for osteomyelitis, though they will almost certainly be positive in deeper ulcers. The evaluation of the pressure sore patient for osteomyelitis is discussed in the next

section. Wound cultures of the open pressure sore are of little value and should not be used to direct antibiotic therapy,[85] as opposed to needle or surgical bone biopsy.

Osteomyelitis

In 1970 Waldvogel *et al.*[86] recognized that osteomyelitis is responsible for wound infection and breakdown after reconstruction of stage III and IV pressure sores (Fig. 16.5). Patients with pressure sores complicated by osteomyelitis have significantly longer hospitalizations than those who do not.[87] Establishing the diagnosis of osteomyelitis is essential before embarking on definitive surgical treatment of pressure sores.

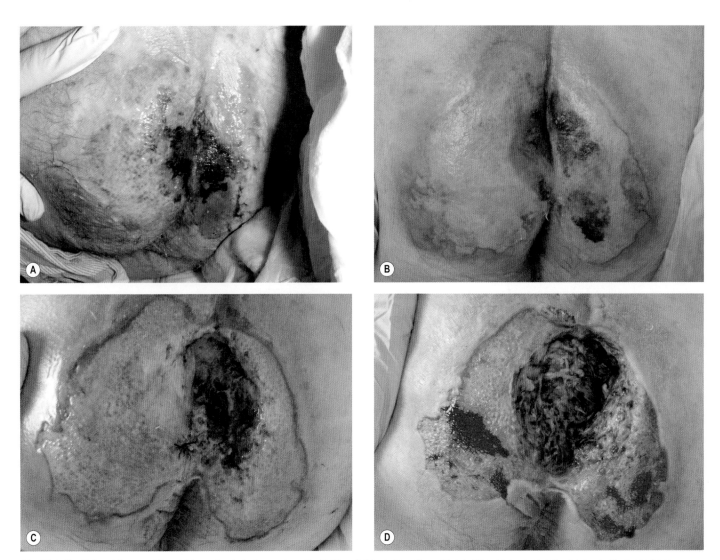

Fig. 16.4 The National Pressure Ulcer Advisory Panel staging system. **(A, E)** Stage I: Intact skin with nonblanchable redness of a localized area usually over a bony prominence. Darkly pigmented skin may not have visible blanching; its color may differ from the surrounding area. **(B, F)** Stage II: Partial-thickness loss of dermis presenting as a shallow open ulcer with a red pink wound bed, without slough. May also present as an intact or open/ruptured serum-filled blister. This should not be used to describe skin tears, tape burns, perineal dermatitis, maceration, or excoriation. **(C, G)** Stage III: Full-thickness tissue loss. Subcutaneous fat may be visible, but bone, tendon, or muscle is not exposed. Slough may be present but does not obscure the depth of tissue loss. May include undermining and tunneling. **(D, H)** Stage IV: Full-thickness tissue loss with exposed bone, tendon, or muscle. Exposed bone is sufficient but not necessary to define a stage IV pressure sore. Slough or eschar may be present on some parts of the wound bed. Often includes undermining or tunneling. May extend into muscle and/or supporting structures (e.g., fascia, tendon, or joint capsule), making osteomyelitis possible. Bone/tendon is visible or directly palpable. **(I)** Suspected deep-tissue injury: Purple or maroon localized area of discolored intact skin or blood-filled blister due to damage of underlying soft tissue from pressure and/or shear. The area may be preceded by tissue that is painful, firm, mushy, boggy, warmer, or cooler as compared to adjacent tissue. The wound may evolve and become covered by thin eschar. Evolution may be rapid, exposing additional layers of tissue even with optimal treatment. **(J)** Unstageable: Full-thickness tissue loss in which the base of the ulcer is covered by slough (yellow, tan, gray, green, or brown) and/or eschar (tan, brown, or black) in the wound bed. Until the base of the wound is exposed, the true depth, and therefore stage, cannot be determined.

Continued

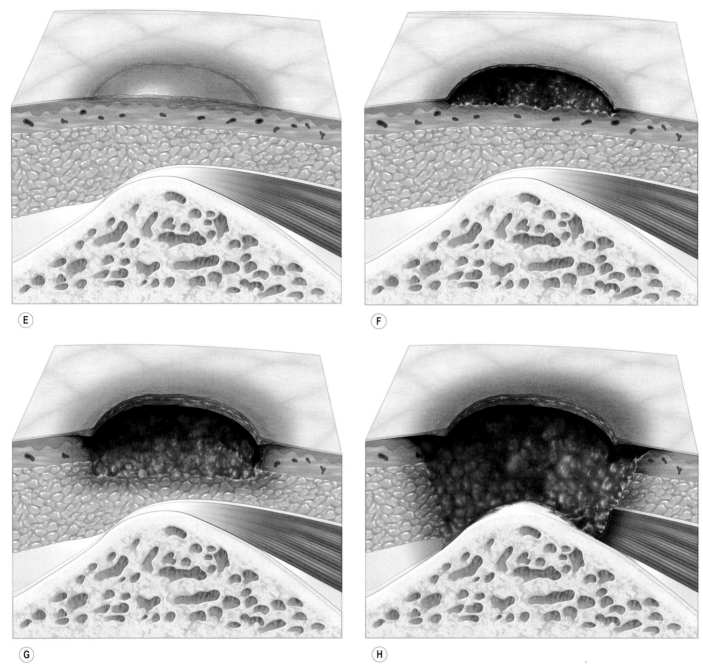

Ⓔ   Ⓕ

Ⓖ   Ⓗ

Fig. 16.4, cont'd

Unrecognized osteomyelitis is a major source of morbidity and increased costs.[87]

In 1988 Lewis *et al.*[88] tried to assess the value of some common tests in diagnosing osteomyelitis by following 61 patients with pressure sores, 52 of whom eventually had confirmed histopathologic diagnosis of osteomyelitis from surgical specimens. This prospective trial examined white blood cell count, ESR, plain X-ray, technetium-99m bone scans, computed tomography (CT) scan, and Jamshidi-needle bone biopsy. The authors felt that the most practical, revealing, and least invasive preoperative workup involved a combination of white blood cell count, ESR, and two-view X-ray. Only one positive test was needed to make the diagnosis. Sensitivity was 89% and specificity 88% using this protocol.

Bone scans and CT scans were expensive and not very sensitive. Needle bone biopsy had a sensitivity of 73% and a specificity of 96%. Of note, magnetic resonance imaging (MRI) was not included in this analysis.

MRI has taken on a larger role in the diagnosis of osteomyelitis. Huang and colleagues[89] analyzed 59 consecutive MRIs in 44 paralyzed patients and found an overall accuracy of 97%, sensitivity of 98%, and specificity of 89%. The authors concluded that not only was MRI accurate, it helped define the extent of infection, which may help limit the surgical resection. Ruan *et al.*[90] independently confirmed these findings and feel that MRI is superior to CT for the evaluation of osteomyelitis.

Han *et al.*[87] reviewed their series of press ulcers and noted that their high osteomyelitis-related complication rate – largely

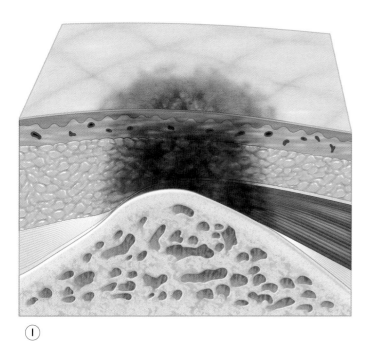

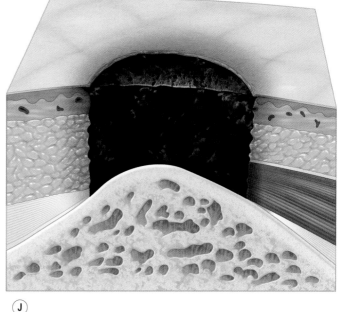

Fig. 16.4, cont'd

consisting of deep abscess and sinus tracts – was a result of their inability to diagnose osteomyelitis accurately preoperatively. Their group moved to a two-stage procedure, performing wound debridement and Jamshidi core needle bone biopsy at the first operation (Fig. 16.6). If the biopsy results were positive, closure was delayed for 6 weeks while the osteomyelitis was treated with antibiotics; otherwise the wound was closed with a musculocutaneous flap. The authors also noted that bone cultures alone were not as useful as bone cultures and histopathology of the bone biopsy together, and found that the biopsy had a positive and negative predictive value of 93% and 100%, respectively.

These results are in keeping with several other studies that support the utility of bone biopsy in the diagnosis of osteomyelitis.[91–94] Marriott and Rubayi[95] have used the results of bone biopsy to determine the duration of antibiotic therapy, in some cases truncating treatment if pathology reveals only chronic osteomyelitis.

Ultimately, MRI appears to be accurate and noninvasive, while providing detailed anatomic information. Bone biopsy likewise has admirable accuracy and, perhaps most importantly, is the only method that can be used to direct antibiotic therapy. Though local factors such as the availability of equipment and economic factors should be considered, used in conjunction MRI and bone biopsy allow for comprehensive evaluation of osteomyelitis in the pressure sore patient.

Psychological evaluation

Psychological problems are common in the pressure sore population. Langer[96] finds 22% of patients with SCI had diagnosable depression, considerably higher than found in the general population. Frank et al.[97] report 37.5% of patients with SCI had a diagnosis of major depression. Akbas et al.[98] report 47.4% of patients with pressure sores fulfilled the diagnostic criteria for major depression. In their prospective study, they found the depression rates to be higher in women,

younger patients, and those who had undergone multiple operations for their pressure sores. The authors recommend "intensive psychological counseling" in the treatment of the pressure sore patient. Foster et al.[99] suggest that psychological factors play a significant role in predicting pressure sore recurrences.

Patient selection

All patients with pressure sores should be optimized with regard to the risk factors already enumerated. It is worth remembering that pressure sores are rarely life-threatening, and there is no need to rush to treatment or surgery if the patient has not been optimized. Many more superficial wounds will heal with conservative therapies if correctable risk factors are identified and addressed. On the other hand, a patient who is malnourished, bedbound on an inappropriate mattress, with undiagnosed osteomyelitis, is doomed to failure regardless of the surgical technique used.

A judgment must be made regarding whether a wound is likely to heal successfully by secondary intention or whether a flap is required to resurface the wound and/or fill dead space left after debridement. In general, stage I and II pressure sores can be treated nonoperatively, while stage III and IV ulcers require flaps. Patients with suspected deep-tissue injury and unstageable ulcers should be debrided until they can be clearly staged. While surgical debridement is the gold standard, other methods can be used as appropriate.

While operative treatment is often delayed while the patient is optimized and risk factors corrected, it is a rare patient who does not qualify for any attempt at reconstruction. Obviously critically ill patients who cannot tolerate surgery should be stabilized before any sort of reconstruction is entertained. More uncommon is the patient with multiple severe comorbidities whose risk factors cannot be easily corrected, due to either medical or social factors. In such cases,

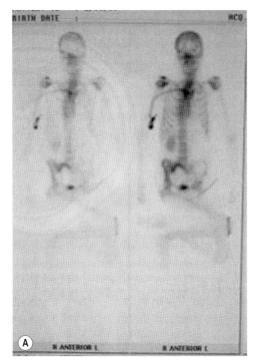

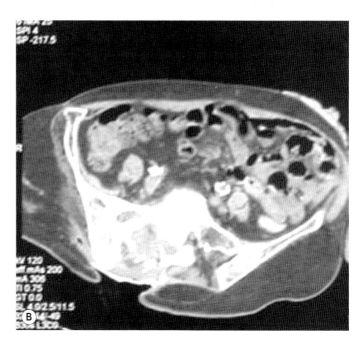

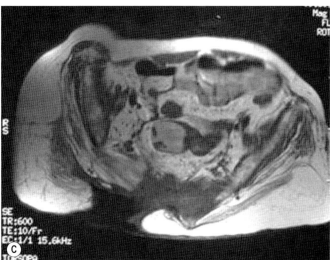

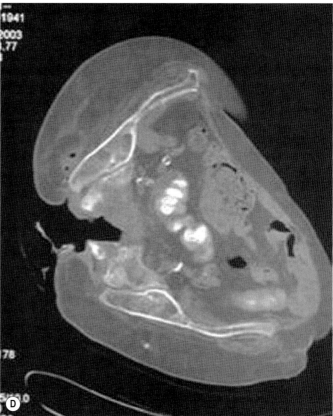

Fig. 16.5 (A–D) Bone scan, computed tomography, and magnetic resonance imaging of severe sacral osteomyelitis.

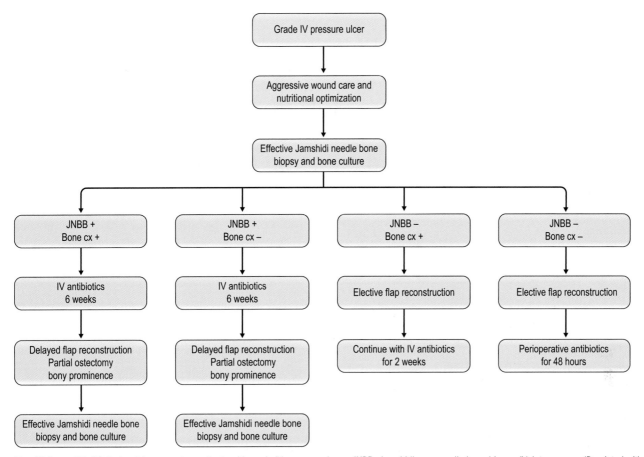

Fig. 16.5, cont'd (E) Protocol for managing patients with grade IV pressure ulcers. JNBB, Jamshidi core needle bone biopsy; IV, intravenous. *(Reprinted with permission from Han H, Lewis VL, Weidrich VA, et al. The value of Jamshidi core needle bone biopsy in predicting postoperative osteomyelitis in grade IV pressure ulcer.* Plast Reconstr Surg*. 2002;111:118.)*

chronic wound care may be preferable to attempted reconstruction that is doomed to failure and recurrence.

Treatment

Prevention

Obviously, prevention of pressure sores is preferable to treatment. As healthcare moves towards nonpayment for nosocomial pressure sores, there is an ever-greater incentive to avoid these lesions. However, despite extensive study and recommendations, overall pressure sores rates have changed little in recent years.[3,100,101]

Some pressure sores may not be preventable,[102–104] and using pressure sores as an indicator of quality is a contentious issue, particularly in light of possible negligence litigation.[105] However, though no strategy has been found that reduces pressure sore rates to zero, there are several measures, many of which now constitute standard care, that may contribute to pressure sore prevention.[63]

For the surgeon who is often consulted only after a pressure sore has developed, knowledge of prevention strategies is still critical not only to advise the consultation but also to optimize the patient before surgery, prevent additional pressure sores from developing, and, perhaps most critically, to prevent postoperative recurrence.

Risk assessment

The first step in pressure sore prevention is risk assessment. Multiple assessment scales have been devised, including those by Braden, Gosnell, Knoll, Norton, Waterlow, and Douglas.[106] Several are designed for specific subpopulations, and each has its merits. All suffer from potential inaccuracies as their use is dependent on the competence of its assessor and the setting in which it is used.

Norton[107] developed an assessment scale for use in geriatric patients. The scale incorporates general physical condition, mental status, activity, mobility, and incontinence and ranges from 5 to 20, with lower scores associated with greater risk. Patients with a score of 11 or less had a 48% incidence of pressure sores, while those with a score of 18 or greater had a 5% incidence. Gosnell[108] added nutritional status as a variable to his method, which is often referred to as the "modified Norton scale".

The most widely used pressure sore assessment tool is the Braden scale[109] (Table 16.1). The Braden scale incorporates six subscales that assess sensory perception, skin moisture, activity, mobility, friction and shear, and nutrition. Scores range from 6 to 23, with higher scores associated with an increased

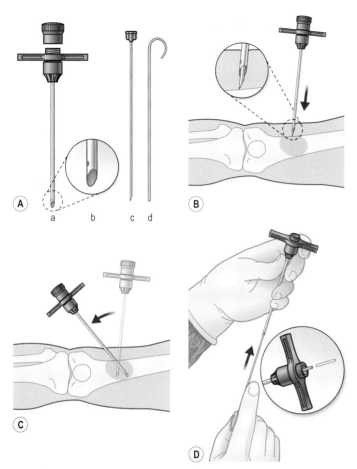

Fig. 16.6 (A) The Jamshidi bone biopsy needle, cannula, and screw-on cap (a), tapered point (b), pointed stylet to advance cannula through soft tissues (c), and probe to expel specimen from cannula (d). **(B)** With the stylet locked in place, the cannula is advanced through the soft tissue until bone is reached. The *inset* is a close-up view showing stylet against bone cortex. **(C)** The stylet is removed, and the bone cortex is penetrated with the cannula. The cannula is withdrawn, and the procedure repeated with redirection of the instrument to obtain multiple core samples. **(D)** The probe is then inserted retrograde into the tip of the cannula to expel the specimen through the base (inset). *(Reprinted with permission Powers BE, LaRue SM, Withrow SJ, et al. Jamshidi needle biopsy for diagnosis of bone lesions in small animals. J Am Vet Med Assoc. 1988;193:206–207.)*

risk of developing pressure sores. The original study noted a score of 16 to be the threshold for pressure sore development,[109] though a different cutoff score may be more appropriate in different settings.[110,111]

Multiple studies have examined the validity, sensitivity, specificity, and predictive value of the various scales. Generally, assessment scales are superior to nurses' clinical judgment when predicting future pressure ulceration.[106] However, there is no evidence that use of risk assessment decreases pressure sore incidence.[112–114] Whether this is because interventions are not instituted or are ineffective is unclear.[113] Given the recent efforts to improve healthcare quality, Bergman *et al.* analyzed one institution's National Surgical Quality Improvement Program (NSQIP) database to determine adherence to multiple process-based quality indictors, including pressure ulcer risk assessment. While this study only looked at 143 consecutive elective abdominal surgery admissions, authors note an adherence rate of only 35% in the risk assessment for pressure ulcers, supporting the notion

that interventions designed to stratify risk remain poorly utilized.[115]

Skin care (Box 16.1)

Ideal skin care encompasses cleaning, hydrating, protecting, and replenishing the skin as needed. Proper skin care can be time- and labor-intensive and is at times neglected by physicians and nurses alike.[116]

Common recommendations for skin cleansing involve the use of warm soap and water followed by drying by rubbing or patting.[117] Washing involves the use of soap and surfactants, which, while effective at removing debris, have the potential to be irritants.[118] The alkaline nature of soap also negates the protective natural acidity of the skin, which in turn alters the balance of resident flora on the skin.[119] Drying the skin by patting may cause less trauma,[120,121] though if it leaves excess moisture on the skin, this can lead to maceration and increased vulnerability to friction injuries.[122] Many alternative cleansers have been marketed that address the shortcomings of soap and water, but little data exist to recommend any particular product at this time.[123]

Maintaining proper skin hydration is most often achieved through the use of emollients, which occlude the skin surface with a hydrophobic layer, and humectants, which attract and absorb water from their surroundings. Numerous formulations exist, many with additional surfactants and emulsifying agents, which vary somewhat in their effectiveness, greasiness, and potential for skin irritation. While the theoretic advantages of treating dry skin are well established,[60,62,124] as with cleansers, few data exist to recommend any one hydrating product over another.[125,126]

Barrier products protect the skin, particularly in the setting of incontinence or in the presence of stomas, fistulas, or wounds. Many preparations consist of a lipid/water emulsion that forms a protective film over the skin. Newer barrier products incorporate a polymer that forms a thin semipermeable membrane over the skin.[127] Many incorporate an antiseptic agent such as cetrimide or benzalkonium as well. Again, despite their widespread use and the proliferation of products, data on their effectiveness are scant.[128]

While data on individual agents are not very robust, there is evidence that a clear skin care protocol can benefit patients. Multiple authors have found instituting such protocols results in reduction in pressure sore incidence rates.[129] Cole and Nesbitt[130] found a reduction from 17.8% to 2% over a 3-year period, whereas Lyder *et al.*[131] noted an 87% reduction in a nursing home setting. Based on the available data, the

---

BOX 16.1 General skin care principles

Assess the patient's skin daily

Cleanse skin when indicated using a pH-balanced cleanser

Avoid soap and hot water

Avoid friction and scrubbing

Minimize exposure to moisture (e.g., incontinence, wound leakage)

Use skin barrier product to protect vulnerable skin

Use emollients to maintain skin hydration

Table 16.1 The Braden scale for predicting pressure sore risk				
Sensory perception Ability to respond meaningfully to pressure-related discomfort	1. Completely limited Unresponsive (does not moan, flinch, or grasp) to painful stimuli, due to diminished level of consciousness or sedation or Limited ability to feel pain over most of body	2. Very limited Responds only to painful stimuli. Cannot communicate discomfort except by moaning or restlessness or Has a sensory impairment which limits the ability to feel pain or discomfort over half of body	3. Slightly limited Responds to verbal commands, but cannot always communicate discomfort or the need to be turned or Has some sensory impairment which limits ability to feel pain or discomfort in one or two extremities	4. No impairment Responds to verbal commands. Has no sensory deficit which would limit ability to feel or voice discomfort
Moisture Degree to which skin is exposed to moisture	1. Constantly moist Skin is kept moist almost constantly by perspiration and urine. Dampness is detected every time patient is moved or turned	2. Very moist Skin is often, but not always, moist. Linen must be changed at least once a shift	3. Occasionally moist Skin is occasionally moist, requiring an extra linen change approximately once a day	4. Rarely moist Skin is usually dry; linen only requires changing at routine intervals
Activity Degree of physical activity	1. Bedfast Confined to bed	2. Chairfast Ability to walk severely limited or nonexistent. Cannot bear own weight and/or must be assisted into chair or wheelchair	3. Walks occasionally Walks occasionally during day, but for very short distances with or without assistance. Spends majority of shift in bed or chair	4. Walks frequently Walks outside room at least twice a day and inside room at least once every 2 hours during waking hours
Mobility Ability to change and control body position	1. Completely immobile Does not make even slight changes in body or extremity position without assistance	2. Very limited Makes occasional slight changes in body or extremity position but unable to make frequent or significant changes independently	3. Slightly limited Makes frequent though slight changes in body or extremity position independently	4. No limitation Makes major and frequent changes in position without assistance
Nutrition Usual food intake pattern	1. Very poor Never eats a complete meal. Rarely eats more than half of any food offered. Eats two servings or less of protein (meat or dairy products) per day. Takes fluids poorly. Does not take liquid dietary supplement or Is NOP and/or maintained on clear liquids or IVs for more than 5 days	2. Probably inadequate Rarely eats a complete meal and generally eats only about half of any food offered. Protein intake includes only three servings of meat or dairy products per day. Occasionally will take a dietary supplement or Receives less than optimum amount of liquid diet or tube feeding	3. Adequate Eats over half of most meals. Eats a total of four servings of protein (meat, dairy products) per day. Occasionally will refuse a meal, but will usually take a supplement when offered or Is on a tube-feeding or TPN regimen which probably meets most of nutritional needs	4. Excellent Eats most of every meal. Never refuses a meal. Usually eats a total of four or more servings of meat and dairy products. Occasionally eats between meals. Does not require supplementation
Friction and shear	1. Problem Requires moderate to maximum assistance in moving. Complete lifting without sliding against sheets is impossible. Frequently slides down in bed or chair, requiring frequent repositioning with maximum assistance. Spasticity, contractures, or agitation leads to almost constant friction	2. Potential problem Moves feebly or requires minimum assistance. During a move skin probably slides to some extent against sheets, chair, restraints, or other devices. Maintains relatively good position in chair or bed most of the time but occasionally slides down	3. No apparent problem Moves in bed or chair independently and has sufficient muscle strength to lift up completely during move. Maintains good position in bed or chair	
				Total score

NPO, nil per os; IV, intravenous; TPN, total parenteral nutrtion.
(Reproduced from www.bradenscale.com.)

American Wound Ostomy and Continence Nurses Society has recently updated their guidelines for skin care.[132]

Incontinence

As noted previously, the relationship between urinary incontinence and pressure sore incidence is not clear, with limited evidence to suggest a causal relationship. Currently, the use of diapers or sanitary pads in conjunction with meticulous skin care is a reasonable option when compared to the risks associated with extended use of a urinary catheter.[133]

Fecal incontinence, on the other hand, has been shown to be a risk factor for pressure sores. At times fecal incontinence is due to factors that are not easily correctable: cognitive impairment, history of colorectal surgery, radiation proctopathy, inflammatory bowel disease, and various neurological or myogenic disorders of sphincter function are not easily correctable. The bladder and bowel dysfunction of SCI patients requires specific regimens and is generally managed by a specialist.[134]

However, many measures can be instituted to decrease the impact of fecal incontinence. Possibly the most common predisposing condition to fecal incontinence is fecal impaction, which is common in older adults and may lead to overflow incontinence.[135] Conservative measures include diet modification and a wide variety of antimotility agents, including clonidine, cholestyramine, loperamide, codeine, diphenoxylate, and atropine.[136,137] Diarrhea may be due to infection, which should be ruled out and treated prior to using antidiarrheal agents. If medical management is unsuccessful, surgery may be considered, ranging from attempts at sphincterplasty to elective colostomy when other options fail.[138] Though patients and families are often reluctant to proceed with colostomy, there is evidence overall quality of life is improved in patients with severe fecal incontinence.[139]

Spasticity

Control of spasticity may not only reduce the risk of pressure sores, but may also improve patient reports of pain and ability to perform activities of daily living (ADL).[140] However, it is worth noting that in some cases spasticity may increase stability in positioning, facilitate some transfers and ADLs, and prevent osteopenia.[141,142] Taken as a whole, the impact of spasticity on quality of life is not straightforward and should be considered before instituting treatment.

Physical therapy is the first step in treating spasticity and an important component of care in SCI patients in general.[143] Pharmacologic treatment is the next step. Diazepam, baclofen, clonidine, tizanidine, gabapentin, and dantrolene are commonly used agents.[144–147] Each has the potential for side effects, including sedation, nausea, diarrhea, muscle weakness, and cognitive effects, and treatment must be tailored to the individual patient.[147,148]

Patients who cannot tolerate or do not respond to oral therapy may benefit from intrathecal administration of baclofen.[146,149] As the drug directly accesses the central nervous system, systemic side effects are minimized at the cost of the risks of surgery and possible mechanical complications with the pump. Injection with chemodenervation agents, including phenol, ethanol, and botulinum, can be effective.[150,151] Reported complications include systemic side effects, vascular complications, skin irritation, and tissue necrosis. Though the effects

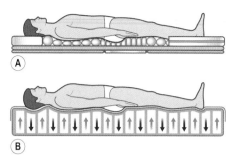

Fig. 16.7 (A) Constant low-pressure surfaces seek to distribute pressure statically, while **(B)** alternating-pressure surfaces vary applied pressure over time.

are temporary, long-term use of chemodenervation agents will result in denervation atrophy.

Surgical management of spasticity is an option when medical therapy is insufficient. Baclofen pump implantation is the most common surgical procedure for spasticity in individuals with SCI and has a history of success.[147,152] In select, refractory cases, orthopedic and neurosurgical techniques may be of benefit, though such procedures are unlikely to have pressure sore prevention as their primary indication. Local tenotomy or tendon transfer has had mixed results in the treatment of spasticity.[153] Rhizotomy has been complicated by both inadequate treatment of spasticity[154] and severe atrophy,[155] depending on the technique employed. Myelotomy and T-myelotomy involving direct sectioning of the spinal cord have been reported to be effective in several case series[156,157] in patients who did not have hope of regaining motor function, though the benefits did decrease over time.[158]

Pressure relief

As befits its primary role in pressure sore pathogenesis, extensive efforts have been made in modulating the pressure through the use of various surfaces and products as well as protocols mandating patient repositioning. Though numerous support surfaces exist, most can be divided into two general categories. Constant low-pressure (CLP) devices distribute pressure over a large area and include devices such as static air, water, gel, bead, silicone, foam, and sheepskin supports (Fig. 16.7). Alternating-pressure (AP) devices vary the pressure under the patient, avoiding prolonged pressure over a single anatomic point[159] (see Fig. 16.7).

Two particular types of CLP device deserve special mention, as they are commonly used in the prevention and treatment of pressures sores. Low air loss (LAL) beds float the patient on air-filled cells through which warm air circulates (Fig. 16.8). The circulating air both equalizes pressure exerted on

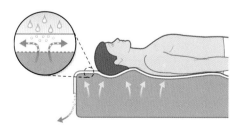

Fig. 16.8 Low air loss mattress concept.

the patient and keeps the skin dry. Properly utilized, LAL surfaces exert less than 25 mmHg on any part of the body.[160,161] Air-fluidized (AF) beds circulate warm air through fine ceramic beads, creating a unique support surface, while having a drying effect similar to LAL beds (Fig. 16.9). With proper use these beds exert less than 20 mmHg on the patient, but are expensive, heavy, and cumbersome.[162]

Within these classifications are a multitude of beds, mattresses, overlays, pads, and cushions, each with slightly different designs by different manufacturers. There is a daunting body of literature comparing various specific products to one another and with standard hospital beds. Evaluating this literature is challenging given the often small sample sizes, poor experimental design, and lack of generalizability common in these studies. Moreover, as new products are developed and old ones are phased out, many studies refer to products no longer in production or use. Despite these limitations, some general conclusions can be drawn from the literature.[163]

Considerable evidence exists that the use of a pressure-relieving overlay is superior to a standard bed in preventing pressure sores. Multiple studies have found decreased incidence and severity of pressure sores in high-risk patients with the use of constant low-pressure devices such as overlays[164–166] or sheepskin[167–169] when compared to a standard hospital foam mattress. Pooled analysis reveals a relative risk of 0.32.[163] Data also support the use of AP devices when compared to standard mattresses. Both Andersen et al.[166] and Sanada[170] noted a significant reduction in pressure sore incidence with the use of active devices, with a pooled relative risk of 0.31.[163] Though several studies have compared CLP and AP devices,[166,171–173] no clear advantage has been identified, despite attempts at pooled analysis.[163]

LAL, like other CLP surfaces, has been shown to be effective at preventing pressure sores,[174,175] with a relative risk estimated at 0.08.[163] Comparisons with other CLP devices in regard to prevention are limited, and no clear advantage for either has been demonstrated.[176,177] Likewise, though AF beds are perhaps the most effective pressure-relieving devices in widespread use, virtually no data on its role in prevention are available, perhaps because these expensive devices are reserved for treatment. Regardless of the type of mattress used, they lose their ability to disperse interface pressure as the head is elevated to 45° or higher.[178] As such, patients should avoid prolonged periods of sitting while on these mattresses.

Given the wide array, yet variable, data on the use of protective surfaces in high-risk patients, the American College of Physicians has formalized recommendations.[101] These clinical practice guidelines were developed after critical evaluation of the quality of evidence and strength of recommendations of the available literature. While there is moderate-level evidence demonstrating improved outcomes with the use of static mattresses or overlays (CLPs not including LAL beds), there is

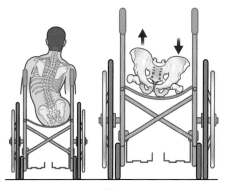

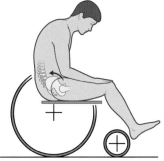

Fig. 16.10 Hammocking effect of wheelchair sling seat producing pelvic obliquity. Paraplegics lack innervation of the lower trunk muscles and sit on their coccyx, with exaggerated posterior pelvic tilt. *(Reprinted with permission from Letts RM. Principles of Seating the Disabled. Boca Raton, FL: CRC Press; 1991.)*

only low-level evidence supporting the use of LAL mattress or AP devices.[172,175,179–182] Moreover, in addition to the increased costs associated with the use of LAL and AP devices, the literature on LAL and AP devices demonstrate no difference or mixed results when compared to static mattresses/overlays. Therefore the American College of Physicians now recommends that all patients identified as being at increased risk for developing a pressure sore be placed on an advanced static mattress, but recommends against the routine use of AP devices in these patients.[101]

In addition to support surfaces, patient repositioning is often used in an attempt to prevent pressure sores, though the data are limited. Defloor et al.[183] found a significant reduction in pressure sore incidence when turning every 4 hours combined with a specialized foam mattress was compared to every 2 hours on a regular mattress. Given the study design it is difficult to determine the relative contributions of the pressure relief surface and the turning regimen. The ideal interval and posture for repositioning are not clear given the current data.[63,184] It bears mention that repositioning is not without its costs, both in terms of nursing time and effort, patient discomfort, and possible dislodgement of catheters and lines, and there is no evidence that more frequent repositioning reduces rates of pressure sores.

Cushions for wheelchairs filled with gel, foam, air, or water are available to relieve pressure. A typical wheelchair sling seat exerts a "hammocking" effect that can produce abnormal scoliotic posture and pelvic obliquity (Fig. 16.10). This in turn causes asymmetric pressure on both trochanter and ischium that requires specialized cushions for prevention.[185] Hip adduction and internal rotation of thighs, with consequent reduction in stability, are also seen in most paraplegics, who lack trunk or pelvic muscle innervation and tend to sit on their

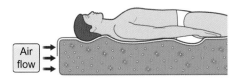

Fig. 16.9 Fluidized bed.

coccyx. Rigid-base cushions provide lumbar support and decrease ischial pressure by allowing wider weight distribution on the posterior thighs.[185] A direct correlation between buttock–cushion interface has been noted[186] (Fig. 16.11).

Houle[187] and Souther et al.[188] studied the effects of various wheelchair seats and found decreased pressures over the ischium, although none was below the capillary pressure benchmark. The authors recommend additional measures for pressure relief to prevent ulceration. Ragan et al.[189] studied seat interface pressures on wheelchair cushions of various thicknesses. They found the highest subcutaneous stress concentrated within 2 cm of the ischial tuberosity. The subcutaneous pressures decreased with thicker cushions, with the maximum effectiveness obtained with an 8-cm cushion. Increasing the thickness beyond 8 cm did not give further benefit in reducing subcutaneous stress. As with pressure relief mattresses, no data exist to recommend a particular type of cushion over another at this time.[163,171,190,191]

The development of pressure consciousness by the patient is an essential part of pressure sore prevention.[192] Pressure release maneuvers are reinforced to patients and should be performed at least every 15 minutes while the patient is seated.[193]

Nutrition

Multiple studies have examined the effect of nutritional supplementation on pressure sore prevention. Despite improvement in secondary measures such as caloric intake, body weight, and serum nutritional markers, most studies have failed to find reduction in pressure sore rates.[194–196] Bourdel-Marchasson and Rondeau[197] found a modest reduction in pressure sore rates when patients were given oral dietary supplementation. A more recent meta-analysis by Stratton et al.[198] found a modest reduction in pressure sore rates in patients treated with enteral tube feeds, estimating that 19.25 patients would need to be given enteral nutritional support to prevent one pressure sore. Overall, the evidence that pressure sores can be prevented by nutritional supplementation, much less specific formulations or micronutrient additives, is limited.[199]

Nonsurgical management

Limited wounds may heal spontaneously without surgical intervention so long as the wound is cleansed meticulously, pressure is avoided, and risk factors are corrected. The

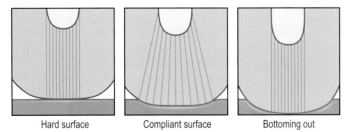

Hard surface   Compliant surface   Bottoming out

Fig. 16.11 Compressive force exerted on tissue by bone in an individual lying or sitting on (left) a hard surface; (center) an effective pressure-reducing device; and (right) an ineffective pressure-reducing device that "bottoms out". *(Reprinted with permission from Woolsey RM, McGarry JD. The cause, prevention, and treatment of pressure sores. Neurol Clin. 1991;9:797.)*

measures implemented in pressure sore prevention become doubly important once the transition is made to treating an established ulcer.

Pressure relief

Pressure relief continues to be critical in the treatment of pressure sores. While more advanced LAL and AF surfaces would in theory be preferred in the treatment of established pressure sores, the literature is mixed on this point. Ferrell et al.[200] found similar results when comparing LAL beds to foam mattresses. Ochs et al.[201] in turn found AF beds to be superior to both standard overlays and LAL beds. On the other hand Branom and Rappl[176] found LAL mattresses inferior to an advanced foam surface, while Economides et al.[202] failed to find any superiority of an AF bed over a foam overlay. Nonetheless, as mentioned previously current recommendations support the use of low cost static mattresses overlays over high cost LAL and AP devices.[101,163,203]

Spasticity

Spasticity should be addressed not only to improve patient positioning, weight distribution, and hygiene but also to prevent tension on the healing wound, particularly if surgical intervention is planned.[204,205] Spasticity treatment may be complicated by a reluctance to perform surgery or implant devices in a patient with an open wound, though this has been reported with favorable results.[205] If pump implantation is not an option, then temporary chemodenervation should be considered, with delayed pump placement once the wound is healed.[78]

Malnutrition

While the role of nutritional status on the risk of developing pressure sores remains unclear, its role in treatment of pressure sores is better described. In 2010, Keys et al. found that albumin levels below 3.5 g/dL were associated with ulcer recurrence within 1 year;[206] thus malnutrition should be corrected and nutritional markers, including albumin and prealbumin, followed and trended. While many small studies have been published examining the effect on nutritional supplementation of the healing of pressure sores, many suffer from design flaws that limit their application, prohibiting the development of specific guidelines. In 2003, Langer et al.[199] felt the quality of the existing literature was inadequate to perform a meta-analysis and that no firm conclusions could be drawn. More recently, both Heyman et al.[207] and Frias Soriano et al.[208] found improved wound healing with oral supplementation, but did not include controls in their studies. Van Anholt et al.[209] and Lee et al.[210] both found accelerated healing with the use of oral nutritional supplement in randomized control trials. Taken together, the American College of Physicians now recommends protein or amino acid supplementation in patients with pressure sores.[211] From a surgeon standpoint, optimizing nutritional status to an albumin of at least 3.5 g/dL will minimize chances of flap failure and recurrence.

In regards to micronutrient supplementation, there is still little evidence to support routine supplementation of micronutrients such as vitamin C or zinc in the absence of a specific deficiency state.[199,211,212] Though small, a randomized control trial of 88 patients failed to demonstrate an increase in rate of healing of pressure sores.[213] Similarly, a double blind study of 14 patients treated with oral zinc failed to demonstrate any clinical benefit in the treatment of pressure sores.[214] Until larger studies are conducted to elucidate the role of micronutrient supplementation in the treatment of pressure sores, routine supplementation is not necessary.

Infection

Osteomyelitis is a common complication of deep pressure sores and, as previously mentioned, often mandates operative therapy. Many authors rightly emphasize the importance of adequate debridement in the treatment of osteomyelitis.[215] However, biopsy-directed antibiotic therapy is still an important adjunct to surgery.[87] While traditional therapy calls for 6 weeks of intravenous antibiotic therapy, there is some evidence that shorter courses many be effective.[95]

Wound care

Debridement, regardless of the method used, should be the first step in the care of pressure sores. Only once the wound is thoroughly debrided can the full extent of the wound be examined and staged. Necrotic material impedes wound healing and acts as a nidus for infection. Traditional wet to dry dressing may debride effectively but may remove healthy tissue and granulation in addition to necrotic tissue.[216] They may also aerosolize bacteria from the wound.[217] Allowing the wound to desiccate despite evidence that wound healing proceeds best in a moist environment is also counterproductive.[218] Enzymatic debridement can be effective, though papain preparations are no longer available in the US. Biologic debridement is enjoying something of a resurgence, using maggots that consume necrotic material while sparing living tissue. Currently no evidence suggests superiority of one agent over another.[219] Ultimately, though many complementary methods of debridement are available, they are no substitute for proper sharp debridement.[84]

Selection among the many available dressings must be guided by the characteristics of the wound. Lionelli and Lawrence[219] review the multitude of dressings available. In the context of pressure sores, occlusive films and hydrocolloids are frequently used on more shallow ulcerations while alginates find use in deeper, heavily exudating wounds (Fig. 16.12). It is worth noting that, even within a classification, individual products may differ widely in their capacity for absorption, occlusion, permeability, and cohesion.[219] There exists little evidence to recommend a particular dressing in this context. When Bradley et al.[220] performed a meta-analysis of the various dressings and topical agents used for pressure sore treatment, no significant differences were found.

As with dressings, numerous topical agents are used in the hopes of improving wound healing. Antiseptic solutions are commonly used in hopes of reducing the bacterial burden of a wound. However, while mafenide,[221] acetic acid,[222,223] Dakin's solution,[224] and iodine preparations[225] have broad-spectrum antibacterial activity, they have all been shown to kill fibroblasts and impede wound healing.[226] If they are used at all, they should be reserved for instances of active infection. Silver sulfadiazine and other silver agents may be less toxic to fibroblasts.[227,228] A review by Reddy et al.[203] failed to find any convincing data to support a particular dressing or topical agent, which correlates with the results of multiple Cochrane

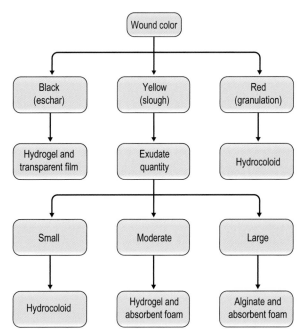

Fig. 16.12 Suggested guidelines for the use of wound products in the full-thickness, noninfected, chronic wound. *(Reprinted with permission from Ladin DA. Understanding dressings.* Clin Plast Surg. *1998;25:433.)*

reviews that also failed to identify a superior dressing for arterial ulcers,[229] venous stasis ulcers,[230] or surgical wounds.[231] Ultimately the dressing selection should be guided by the characteristics of the wound and should balance moisture, bacterial control, and debridement.

Negative-pressure wound therapy

Negative-pressure wound therapy (NPWT) entails applying topical negative pressure to a wound. The most common commercially available system, the vacuum-assisted closure (VAC) system, consists of an open-cell polyurethane or polyvinyl alcohol foam sponge with a pore size ranging from 400 to 600 μm in diameter. This sponge is cut to the appropriate dimensions to fill the entire wound. Suction is then applied to the sponge after it is covered with an adhesive drape to create an airtight seal. This suction can be adjusted in intensity and frequency. The most common settings are 125 mmHg negative pressure and either continuous or intermittent frequency.

The NPWT dressing has been applied to a multitude of clinical problems,[232] and its mechanism of action[233] has been extensively studied. Given its success in multiple arenas, pressure sores seem a task to which it is well suited. Evidence for its use is somewhat limited, however. Deva et al.[234] noted positive results in treated grade III ulcers but did not utilize any controls. Ford et al.[235] reported improved healing with VAC dressings when compared to standard wound care, but results did not reach significance. Joseph[236] noted a greater decrease in wound depth with NPWT dressing when compared to saline dressings, but had limited follow-up and endpoints did not include wound closure. On the other hand, Wanner et al.[237] failed to find any advantage to NPWT therapy in treating pressure sores, a finding echoed in a larger review by Reddy et al.[203] It is perhaps surprising that more evidence does not support the use of NPWT in this clinical scenario, but is unclear whether this is due to inadequate data or a reflection of the altered physiology associated with pressure sores, which at times may render them resilient to closure by secondary intention.

Manipulating the local wound milieu

Several studies propose the use of biologic and recombinant agents as possible modalities for the nonsurgical treatment of pressure sores. Robson *et al.* performed a double blind randomized control trial in which 50 patients with stage III/IV pressure sores were treated with recombinant bFGF; notably, samples from patients treated with recombinant bFGF demonstrated significantly increased fibroblast and capillary formation than other groups.[238] Similarly, Rees *et al.* found that application of recombinant human platelet-derived growth factor-BB to pressure sore wounds resulted in increased healing as compared to placebo. Despite the high cost of recombinant proteins, Robson *et al.* suggest that treatment with recombinant cytokines may actually result in a cost reduction as compared to surgical treatment.[239] While it remains unlikely that this will become a mainstay therapy, recombinant agents may become an option of patients unable to undergo surgery or as a temporizing treatment until medically optimized for surgical treatment.

Surgical treatment

Surgical guidelines

The basic tenets of surgical treatment of pressure sores remain essentially unchanged since they were enumerated in Conway and Griffith's report[240] over half a century ago:

- Excision of the ulcer, surrounding scar, underlying bursa, and soft-tissue calcifications, if any
- Radical removal of underlying bone and any heterotopic ossification
- Padding of bone stumps and filling dead space
- Resurfacing with large regional pedicled flaps
- Grafting the donor site of the flap, if necessary.

The authors also stressed two points of flap design that are still applicable today. First, the flap should be designed as large as possible, placing the suture line away from the area of direct pressure. Second, the flap design should not violate adjacent flap territories so as to preserve all options for coverage in the event that breakdown or recurrence dictates further reconstruction.

Debridement

Complete debridement is the crucial first step in the operative treatment of these lesions. Chronic pressure sores will generally have a relatively well-defined bursa in continuity with the base of the ulcer. Application of methylene blue can make dissecting around the margins of the bursa easier. The bursa and any surrounding scarred tissue, calcifications, or heterotopic ossification should be excised completely, leaving only healthy, pliable tissues (Fig. 16.13). The bursa commonly extends much farther than the surface wound would indicate. Taking a small skin margin around the wound and following the contours of the bursa as it undermines adjacent tissues ensures it is entirely excised. After the initial excision the

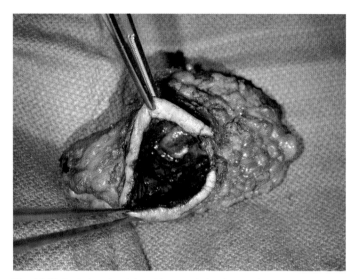

Fig. 16.13 Depiction of excision of bursa and chronic scar tissue.

wound base should be palpated to identify any residual areas of woody, scarred tissues, which require excision.

Once the soft tissue has been debrided, the underlying bone must be evaluated and, if necessary, debrided. There should be a very low threshold to debride back to healthy, hard, bleeding bone using an osteotome or rongeurs. A bone biopsy can also be taken at this time if desired.

Debridement should never be compromised to facilitate wound closure, as incomplete debridement is a common cause of flap failure. The affected tissue must be debrided radically and flap coverage designed as appropriate to fill the resulting defect, even if this may require larger, or even multiple, flaps for complete obliteration of dead space and wound closure.

Procedure selection

Once the wound has been adequately debrided, a reconstruction method must be selected. Options for surgical coverage of pressure sores include random skin flap, myoplasty plus skin graft, pedicled muscle, myocutaneous, fascial, or fasciocutaneous flap, free flaps, and tissue expansion. The choice of flap depends on many factors, including location of the ulcer, the patient's level of spinal injury, history of prior ulceration and surgery, ambulatory status and potential, daily habits, educational status, motivational level, and associated medical problems.

Muscle flaps

The indications for using muscle in pressure sore surgery remain poorly defined. As previously noted, muscle is more susceptible to ischemic necrosis than either skin or subcutaneous tissue,[40] at times resulting in necrotic muscle under intact overlying skin.[241] On the other hand, interposing muscle between skin and bone resulted in a decreased rate of skin ulceration in a rat model,[43] presumably because the increased mass of muscle can help diffuse the effects of pressure on the skin.

Compared with skin grafts and flaps, muscle flaps have the advantages of greater bulk for filling the wound cavity and obliterating dead space,[240] the ability to cover larger wounds, and a better local vascular supply.[242,243] Despite their theoretic advantages, whether the improved vascularity of muscle flaps results in clinically significant effects on infection and wound healing when compared to other options has not been determined.[244]

Anthony and associates[245] reviewed their experience with pressure sore therapy in 60 consecutive patients treated between 1979 and 1990, during which time their practice transitioned toward an increased use of muscle and musculocutaneous flaps. During this interval the number of operations per ulcer declined from 1.9 to 1.1 and the time to complete healing dropped from 12.8 to 4.8 weeks. Though they recognize that advances in supportive care certainly have played a role, the authors conclude that widespread use of muscle flaps, which allow debridement and wound closure at a single operation, is the single most important factor contributing to the improved outcome.

Musculocutaneous flaps

Bruck et al.[246] raised random skin flaps and latissimus dorsi musculocutaneous flaps in pigs, which were then transferred for coverage of iatrogenically created pelvic pressure sores. The wounds were subsequently inoculated with *Staphylococcus aureus* and *Escherichia coli*, and the flaps evaluated for their resistance to infection-induced necrosis. Only the skin flaps showed necrosis, leading the authors to conclude that the muscle acts as a barrier for vertical spread of infection and strongly recommend their use in patients with a history of osteomyelitis.

Perforator flaps

In a break from previous literature to that point, Kroll and Rosenfield[247] challenged the assumption that muscle is necessary when reconstructing pressure sores. In 1988 they reported favorable results using fasciocutaneous flaps based on parasacral perforators to cover midline and sacral wounds. Koshima et al.[248] developed the superior gluteal artery perforator flap, which they used to cover trochanteric and ischial pressure sores with good results.

Advocates of perforator flap techniques argue that such flaps not only preserve muscle but also conserve future reconstructive options and adhere to the basic tenet of placing suture lines away from areas of direct pressure. Higgins et al.[249] state that, until further studies are performed, "muscle sparing should always be a goal in the ambulatory and sensate patient, as it may prevent some functional loss and potentially reduce postoperative pain".

Free flaps

Though not a common option, several authors have described free tissue transfer in the reconstruction of pressure sores, with and without preservation of sensation. Nahai et al.[250,251] and Hill et al.,[252,253] among others, have described transferring the tensor fasciae latae muscle–skin unit as a free flap for lower trunk reconstruction. Sensation is maintained by including the lateral femoral cutaneous nerve in the neurovascular pedicle.

Chen et al.[254] reported coverage of multiple extensive pressure sores with a single filleted lower leg musculocutaneous free flap, with satisfactory results. Yamamoto et al.[255] report successful coverage of a sacral pressure sore with a free lateral thigh fasciocutaneous flap based on the first and third direct cutaneous branches of the deep femoral vessels. A second successful reconstruction involved an ischial pressure sore covered with a free medial plantar fasciocutaneous flap based on the posterior tibial vessels.

Sekiguchi et al.[256] confirm the value of free sensory plantar flaps in the treatment of paraplegic patients who have ischial ulcers. They reason that "while the ischial region is being subject to enormous pressure, the plantar region with its more resilient skin pad is no longer functioning as a weight-bearing area. Thus [transferring] a plantar flap on to the ischial region [...] offers a long-term solution to the problem of chronic pressure sores".

Tissue expansion

Expanders are tolerated very well in SCI patients. According to Esposito et al.[257] the main advantage of tissue expansion is the advancement of sensitive skin that can be used for pressure awareness and future ulcer prevention. Tissue expansion is also useful in the event of an unstable wound secondary to previous skin graft or secondary healing. Multiple reports by Braddom and Leadbetter,[258] Yuan,[259] Esposito et al.,[257] Neves et al.,[260] and Kostakoglu et al.[261] attest to the success of tissue expansion in the treatment of recalcitrant ulcers in paraplegics.

Kostakoglu et al.[261] also described pre-expansion of tensor fasciae latae and lumbosacral fasciocutaneous flaps in 6 patients. The authors felt expansion allowed the closure of large wounds while still allowing for primary closure of the donor site, while speculating that "additional benefits may include a reduction in the mechanical shear potential for these flaps and an improvement in their vascularity".

Critics question the wisdom of placing a foreign body (the expander) into a contaminated wound (all pressure sores). At this time, the primary indication for skin expansion is to cover shallow ulcers with no dead space to fill, particularly if sensate skin can be used to resurface a previously insensate area.

Single- versus multiple-stage reconstruction

Several reports in the literature describe single-stage surgical management of pressure sores.[262,263] Most of these reports involved few patients, however, until a retrospective analysis of 120 patients operated on during a 10-year period was published in 1999.[264] Although there was a large discrepancy between the number of patients treated in a single stage versus the number treated in multiple stages (120 versus 10), the hospital stay was decreased by an average of 10 weeks in the single-stage group – 9.5 weeks versus 19 weeks. This led to a considerable cost savings per admission. The authors list the disadvantages of single-stage surgical management as longer operative time and higher intraoperative blood loss. The advantages of single-stage pressure sore management include fewer anesthetic episodes, shorter hospital stays, earlier rehabilitation, and lower costs. The authors reserve multistage procedures for patients who have concurrent pressure sores on the anterior and posterior trunk that are difficult to address simultaneously.

Reconstruction by anatomic site

Many of the published descriptions of musculocutaneous flaps offer considerable flexibility in flap design to allow subsequent re-rotation of the cutaneous component. In most cases this involves expanding and reshaping the skin margins towards a more rotational flap design and away from the limitations imposed by transposition and island flaps.

A number of techniques are available for closure of sacral pressure sores, including wide undermining and primary closure, random skin flaps, gluteus myoplasty, advancement flaps, pedicle island flaps, fasciocutaneous flaps, musculocutaneous flaps, and free flaps[240,247,248,265–288] (Table 16.2). Though dozens of variations have been described, musculocutaneous rotation and advancement flaps based on the gluteus maximus remain a proven option in this area.

Parry and Mathes[280] reported favorable results after sacral coverage of pressure sores with bilateral gluteus maximus musculocutaneous advancement flaps in ambulatory patients. Foster et al.[289] had high success rates with V–Y gluteus maximus flaps (36/37 or 97%) as well as with gluteal island flaps (20/22 or 91%). When the patient is ambulatory, the authors recommend closure by means of bilateral V–Y gluteus maximus advancement flaps based on the superior half of the gluteus muscle to preserve muscular function.

Borman and Maral[265] describe a modification of the gluteal rotation flap, incorporating a V–Y closure, allowing closure of defects up to 12 cm with a unilateral flap. The suggested advantages include a smaller incision compared to a class V–Y advancement and the ability to convert to a musculocutaneous V–Y advancement if necessary. Though quite hardy in thinner patients, it can be unreliable in obese patients with abundant presacral subcutaneous tissue. Additional modifications include the expansive gluteus maximus flap described by Ramirez and colleagues,[281] which is advanced in a V–Y fashion either unilaterally or bilaterally to cover sacral ulcers.

Multiple authors have reported their success with gluteal artery perforator flaps, and variations abound.[290–292] Wong et al.[293] modified the classic gluteal rotation flap to spare the perforators down to the level of the piriformis. Xu et al.[294] designed a multi-island perforator propeller flap for use in large sacral defects. Cheong et al.[295] described an innervated variant of the superior gluteal artery perforator flap for sacral coverage.

Moving superiorly, both Hill et al.[273] and Vyas et al.[284] described random flaps from the thoracolumbar area to close sacral wounds. Hill et al.[273] described the transverse lumbosacral back flap, which is based on the contralateral lumbar perforators. The donor site is most commonly skin grafted. Vyas et al.[284] described the thoracolumbar sacral flap, which is a very large rotational flap based on thoracolumbar perforators, which may or may not require back grafting.

Kroll and Rosenfield[247] and Koshima et al.[248] described perforator-based flaps from the parasacral area for coverage of low posterior midline defects. Kato et al.[277] took this concept a step further in their anatomic study on the lumbar artery perforator-based island flap, identifying the second lumbar

Table 16.2 Reconstructive options in sacral pressure sores

Primary closure White and Hamm, *Ann Surg 124: 1136, 1946*	Gluteal fasciocutaneous rotation-advancement flap with V-Y closure Borman and Maral, *Plast Reconstr Surg 109: 23, 2002*
Reverse dermal graft Wesser and Kahn, *Plast Reconstr Surg 40: 252, 1967*	Bilateral gluteus advancement flap Parry and Mathes, *Ann Plast Surg 8: 443, 1982*
Interiorly based random skin flap Conway and Griffith, *Am J Surg 91: 946, 1956*	Gluteus plication closure Buchanan and Agris, *Plast Reconstr Surg 72: 49, 1983*
Tranverse lumbosacral arterial and random flap Hill, Brown, and Jurkiewicz, *Plast Reconstr Surg 62: 177, 1978*	Sensory island flaps Snyder and Edgerton, *Plast Reconstr Surg 36: 518, 1965* Dibbell, *Plast Reconstr Surg 54: 220, 1974* Daniel, Terzis, and Cunningham, *Plast Reconstr Surg 58: 317, 1976* Little, Fontana, and McColluch, *Plast Reconstr Surg 68: 175, 1981*
Thoracocolumbar-sacral arterial/random flap Vyas, Binns, and Wilson, *Plast Reconstr Surg 65:159, 1980*	Gluteal thigh arterialized flap Hurwitz, Swartz, and Mathes, *Plast Reconstr Surg 68: 521, 1981*
Superior gluteus myoplasty Ger, *Surgery 69:106, 1971* Ger and Levine, *Plast Reconstr Surg 58: 419, 1976*	Expansive gluteus maximus flap Ramirez, Hurwitz, and Futrell, *Plast Reconstr Surg 74: 757, 1984*
Turnover gluteus myopathy Stallings, Delgado, and Converse, *Plast Reconstr Surg 54: 52, 1974*	Parasacral perforator-based musculocutaneous flap Kroll and Rosenfield, *Plast Reconstr Surg 81: 561, 1988* Koshima et al., *Plast Reconstr Surg 91: 678, 1993*
Gluteus maximus musculocutaneous flap Minami, Mills, and Pardoe, *Plast Reconstr Surg 60: 242, 1977*	Parasacral peforator-based fasciocutaneous flap Kato et al., *Br J Plast Surg 52: 541, 1999*
Gluteus maximus musculocutaneous island flap Maruyama et al., *Br J Plast Surg 33: 150, 1980* Stevenson et al., *Plast Reconstr Surg 79: 761, 1987* Dimberger, *Plast Reconstr Surg 81: 567, 1988*	Parasacral peforator-based fasciocutaneous flap Kato et al., *Br J Plast Surg 52: 541, 1999*
Gluteus maximus fasciocutaneous flap Yamamoto et al., *Ann Plast Surg 30: 116, 1993*	

perforator as the preferred vessel. Advantages of this flap include sparing of the muscle, a large arc of rotation, and a donor site that can be closed primarily.

Unless the skin flaps have been reinnervated at a preliminary operation or are harvested from a site that has intact sensation,[296] the reconstructed sites will not be sensible. The advantage of using sensory flaps for pressure sore coverage in patients with distal SCI is the hope that sensation will prompt behavior modifications by the patient to avoid pressure on ulcer-prone areas and prevent recurrent ulceration. Dibbell[269] and Daniel et al.[267] describe intercostal island flaps to bring sensation to the sacral area. Other reports by Coleman and Jurkiewicz[297] and Mackinnon et al.[298] discuss various techniques for reinnervation of the intercostal flap and the tensor fasciae latae flap, including nerve grafts to the intercostal muscles and to the territory of the lateral femoral cutaneous nerve.

Prado et al.[299] also described innervation-sparing bilateral perforator fasciocutaneous and myocutaneous V–Y flaps for the closure of large sacral wounds. Though they demonstrated no recurrence at 1.5 years and sensation was preserved with this technique, it has the drawbacks of placing scars over the ischium as well as preventing further readvancement of the gluteal muscles.

DeWeerd and Weum[268] modified Kato's lumbar perforator island flap design to include two lumbar artery perforators as well as the intermediate nerve to preserve protective sensation. The flap is drawn as a butterfly design. At 8 weeks postoperatively, good protective sensation was documented over most of the flap by Semmes–Weinstein monofilament testing.

Selected technique: myocutaneous gluteal rotation flap (Fig. 16.14 and Box 16.2)

One of many options based on the gluteus maximus muscle, the myocutaneous gluteal rotation flap is technically straightforward, keeps scars off pressure-bearing surfaces, and is easily revised or re-rotated. The muscle is useful for obliterating the dead space, which is often significant after the preparatory bursectomy and ostectomy.

The vascular supply is based on the superior gluteal artery perforator. This vessel can easily be identified in the plane beneath the gluteus maximus immediately superior to the piriformis muscle.

Skin incision is marked to follow the contour of the iliac crest and descends inferiorly, staying posterior to the greater trochanter and the footprint of the tensor fasciae latae flaps. Dissection is carried down through the thick subcutaneous tissues of the hip to the level of the muscle fascia.

The fascia and muscle are then divided. It can be helpful to bevel the incision so the muscle and fascia are divided more

---

BOX 16.2 Myocutaneous gluteal rotation flap

As always, complete debridement is the key to any flap surgery.

This flap can survive entirely on its major vascular pedicle. The muscle can be disinserted and the skin and fascia divided circumferentially without compromising the vascularity of the flap. Creating an island design without tension is preferable to leaving a skin bridge, which results in tension.

---

peripherally than the skin. This both accounts for some degree of muscle retraction and provides extra soft tissue to obliterate dead space and additional fascia for added security and ease of wound closure. The flap should then be undermined in the plane beneath the gluteus maximus. The pedicle can usually be identified at this time with relative ease as it passes superior to the piriformis. It may be easier to proceed from lateral to medial, as scarring and inflammation near the ulcer can impede dissection, and the separation between the hip muscles becomes more distinct as they approach their insertion on the trochanter.

If additional length is needed or tension is excessive, the flap can be partially delaminated at either the fascial or subcutaneous level, so long as the major perforators are identified and protected. The flap is then closed in multiple layers over drains using long-lasting absorbable sutures in the muscle and superficial fascial system and either staples or nonabsorbable sutures in the skin.

Drains remain in place until output is less than 20–30 cc/day, though some may opt to use drains for an extended period.

Ischial ulcers

Multiple techniques have been described to cover these defects, including inferior gluteal rotation flaps, island flaps, posterior V–Y advancement flaps, gluteal thigh flaps, perforator flaps, and free flaps[274,281,289,300–311] (Table 16.3).

One of the most common options in ischial pressure sore coverage is the posterior V–Y advancement flap. This flap can be based on the biceps femoris muscle in ambulatory patients or on the hamstring muscle in SCI patients. This flap is able to fill the dead space with viable muscle and can be readvanced quite easily in the case of recurrence.

Some authors, however, prefer fasciocutaneous flaps over musculocutaneous flaps in this region.[312–314] Homma et al.[312] reported using a posteromedial thigh fasciocutaneous flap based on the perforators from either the gracilis or the adductor magnus muscles in the treatment of ischial pressure sores. In 11 patients with variable follow-up, they noted two flaps with distal necrosis.

The posterior thigh skin can be transferred based on perforating vessels from a cutaneous branch of the inferior gluteal artery that accompanies the posterior femoral cutaneous nerve between the semitendinosus and biceps femoris muscles.[247,302,309] The flap can be used repeatedly in the event of recurrences. When the descending branch of the inferior gluteal artery is absent – a common vascular anomaly in this region[274] – the flap can be elevated as a superiorly based random fasciocutaneous unit supplied by multiple perforators from the cruciate anastomosis of the fascial plexus.[315]

In addition to the gluteal rotation flap, the superior and inferior gluteal arteries provide multiple options for reconstruction for ischial ulcers. The pedicle of the superior gluteal artery perforator flap is suboptimal for reaching the ischial region and is more useful in the coverage of sacral and trochanteric ulcers. The inferior gluteal artery perforator flap, on the other hand, is well suited to ischial reconstruction, with multiple authors reporting results comparable to existing methods.[249,316,317] It has the advantage of sparing muscle for future use, is associated with minimal morbidity, and has a donor site that can often be closed directly.[311]

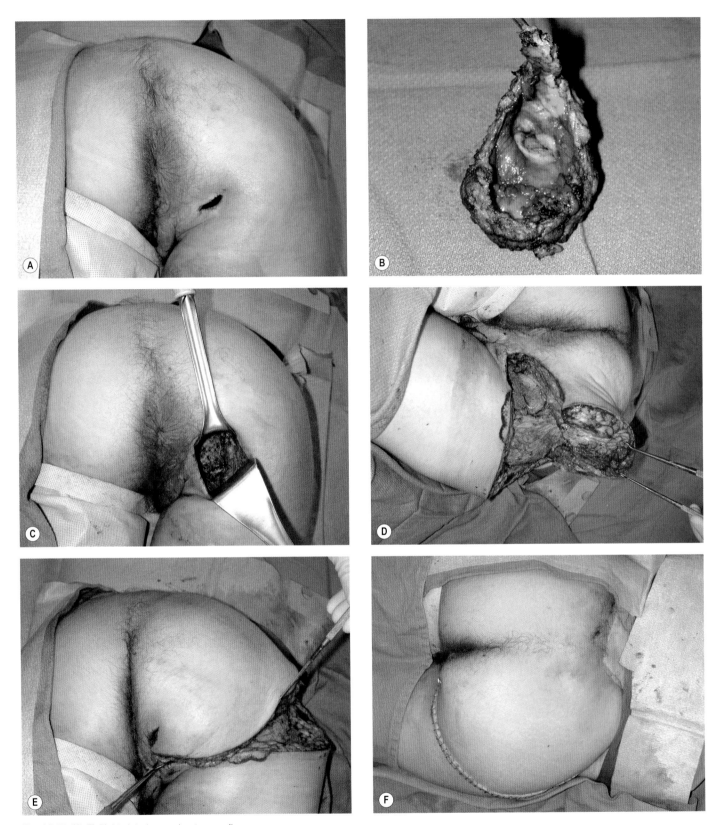

Fig. 16.14 (A–F) Right gluteal musculocutaneous flap.

Table 16.3 Reconstructive options in ischial pressure sores

Primary closure Arregui et al., *Plast Reconstr Surg 36: 583, 1965*	Biceps femoris musculocutaneous flap Tobias et al., *Ann Plast Surg 6: 396, 1981* Kauer and Sonsino, *Scand J Plast Reconstr Surg 20: 129, 1986*
Random posterior thigh flap ± biceps femoris myoplasty Campbell and Converse, *Plast Reconstr Surg, 14: 442, 1954* Conway and Griffith, *Am J Surg 91: 946, 1956* Baker, Barton, and Converse, *Br J Plast Surg 31: 26, 1978*	Gluteal thigh flap Hurwitz, Swartz, and Mathes, *Plast Reconstr Surg 20: 129, 1986*
Inferior gluteus maximus musculoplasty Ger and Levine, *Plast Reconstr Surg 58:419, 1976*	Sliding gluteus maximus flap Ramirez, Hurwitz, and Futrell, *Plast Reconstr Surg 74: 757, 1984*
Inferior gluteus musculocutaneous flap Minami, Mills, and Pardoe, *Plast Reconstr Surg 60: 242, 1977*	Tensor fasciae latae + vastus lateralis Krupp, Kuhn, and Zaech, *Paraplegia 21: 119, 1983*
Interior gluteus musculocutaneous island flap Rajacic et al., *Br J Plast Surg 47:431, 1994*	Lateral thigh fasciocutaneous flap Maruyama, Ohnishi, and Takeudhi, *Br J Plast Surg 37: 103, 1984* Hallock, *Ann Plast Surg 32: 367, 1994*
Gracilis musculocutaneous flap Wingate and Friedland, *Plast Reconstr Surg 62:245, 1978* Lesavoy et al., *Plast Reconstr Surg, 85: 390, 1990*	Anterolateral thigh fasciocutaneous island flap Yu et al., *Plast Reconstr Surg 109: 610, 2002*
Gracilis musculocutaneous flap (with sartorius as a double muscle unit) Apfelberg and Finseth, *Br J Plast Surg 34:41, 1981*	Rectus abdominis musculocutaneous flap Bunkis and Fudem, *Ann Plast Surg 23: 447, 1989* Mixter, Wood, and Dibbell, *Plast Reconstr Surg 85: 437, 1990*
Hamstring musculocutaneous flap Hurteau et al., *Plast Reconstr Surg 68: 539, 1981*	Inferior gluteal artery perforator flap Higgins et al., *Br J Plast Surg 55:83, 2002*

(Reproduced from Janis JE, Kenkel JM. Pressure sores. In: Barton FE Jr., ed. *Selected Readings in Plastic Surgery*, vol. 9, no. 39. Dallas, TX: Selected Readings in Plastic Surgery; 2003:27.)

Alternatives for coverage of ischial pressure sores include gracilis musculocutaneous flaps,[318–321] lateral thigh fasciocutaneous flaps,[315,322] anterolateral thigh fasciocutaneous island flaps,[319,323,324] and rectus abdominis musculocutaneous flaps transferred through the space of Retzius to the perineum.[325–327] However, because the rectus initiates vertebral flexion and aids in respiration, urination, defecation, and vomiting, Bunkis and Fudem[325] speculate the muscle is more important, and thus less expendable, in paraplegics than in neuromuscularly intact patients.

Nahai et al.[250,253,328] introduced the sensate tensor fasciae latae flap for coverage of ischial and trochanteric pressure sores. The flap provides protective sensation in paraplegic patients to help avert recurrence of pressure sores, sharpens sensation of rectal filling, and enhances sitting control in a wheelchair. Dibbell et al.[329] as well as Luscher et al.[330] report successful experiences with the extended sensory tensor fasciae latae flap, which is innervated by the lateral femoral cutaneous nerve, for pressure sores in patients with meningomyelocele and paraplegia, respectively. At follow-up of 1–10 years no new or recurrent sores were noted in Luscher's series.

Foster et al.[289] reviewed their experience with ischial pressure sore coverage from 1979 to 1995. During this time, 114 consecutive patients with 139 ischial pressures sores were treated. Analysis of these cases showed significant differences in healing rates and complications according to the flaps used. The inferior gluteus maximus island flap and the inferior gluteal thigh flap had the highest success rate, 94% (32/34) and 93% (25/27), respectively, while the V–Y hamstring flap and tensor fasciae latae flap had the poorest healing rates, 58% (7/12) and 50% (6/12), respectively. When Ahluwalia et al.[331] reviewed their series of 72 ischial wounds, the authors found an overall complication rate of 16% and a recurrence rate of 7%. After reviewing their results the authors felt their best results were obtained with medial thigh and biceps femoris flaps.

Selected flap: V–Y hamstring advancement (Fig. 16.15)

Flaps from the posterior thigh are common options for ischial reconstruction. They have the advantage of leaving the lateral hip and buttock for use in trochanteric and sacral reconstruction. The V–Y hamstring advancement is a robust flap that is relatively easy to raise and can be readvanced if necessary.

The vascular supply to the hamstring flap is based on perforators of the profunda femoris, with minor contributions from the inferior gluteal, medial circumflex, and superior geniculate arteries. These vessels are generally not specifically identified when elevating the flap, as they are well protected on the deep surface of the muscle.

Superiorly the flap is bounded by the gluteal crease or the inferior border of the ulcer. Laterally the flap extends to the posterior border of the tensor fasciae latae, while medially the dissection extends to the adductor magnus. Inferiorly the flap can be extended to the popliteal fossa, though a lesser flap can be designed as needed.

The flap is incised and dissection carried down the level of the fascia. The muscles are divided distally at the musculotendinous junction and proximally by elevating the muscles from the ischium, though this step is often partially

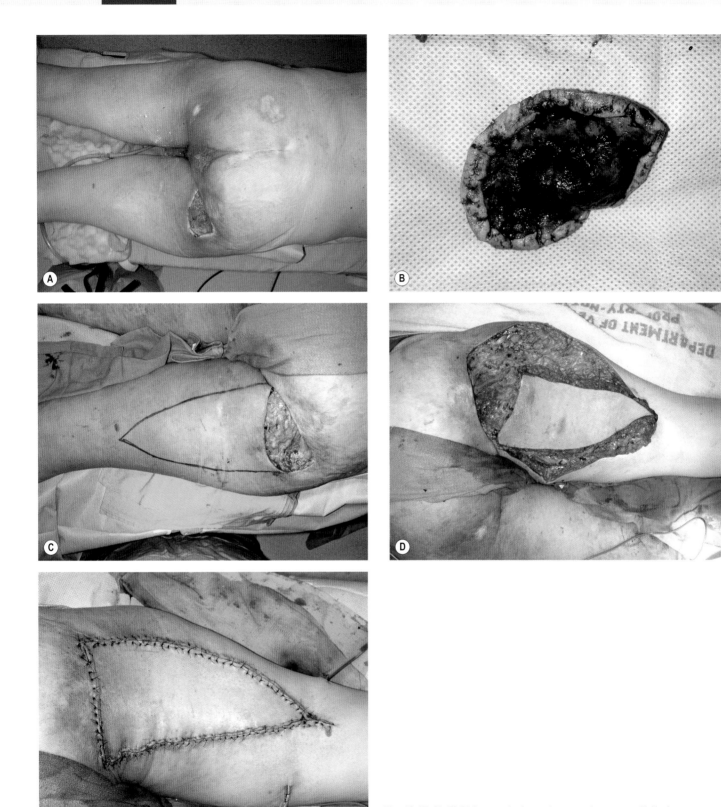

Fig. 16.15 (A–E) Right posterior hamstring musculocutaneous V–Y advancement flap.

accomplished during bony debridement of the ischium. Minimal blunt dissection may be performed at the lateral and medial margins to mobilize the flap, but it is generally not necessary to perform a complete dissection on the undersurface of the muscle or to identify the major pedicle of the flap.

As with the gluteal rotation flap, it is inset in layers over drains and the donor site is closed in linear fashion.

Trochanteric ulcers

Trochanteric ulcers are generally closed with tensor fasciae latae[250,253,328–330,332–335] or vastus lateralis flaps[336–339] (Table 16.4). The tensor fasciae latae can be transferred as muscle only, as skin and muscle, with the skin of the anterolateral mid and lower thigh, as an island flap, or as a free flap. For details regarding this flap's anatomy, vascularity, design, and elevation, the reader is referred to Nahai's publications on the subject.[250,253,329] Lewis et al.[333,340] described a modification of the standard tensor fasciae latae musculocutaneous flap, the tensor fasciae latae V–Y retroposition; this appears to be as durable and versatile as its predecessor.

While the tensor fasciae latae is a workhorse option in this region, multiple alternative and secondary options exist. Flaps based on the gluteus maximus[341–343] or medius[344] can be used to reconstruct this region. Ramirez[341] recounts his experience with 20 distal gluteus maximus posterior thigh flaps.

A profusion of perforator flaps have found use in trochanteric reconstruction as well. The anterolateral thigh flap provides an option with considerable flexibility, allowing the option of taking chimeric flaps if necessary.[345,346] Flaps based on the gluteal,[347] ascending circumflex,[348] or adductor[349] perforators all share the advantages of minimal donor morbidity and sparing of muscle for further reconstruction. The

adductor perforator flap also has the advantage of being medially based and often outside the field of previous operations.

Foster et al.[289] noted a success rate of 93% (68/73) when covering trochanteric ulcers. Their most frequently used flap was the tensor fasciae latae flap, particularly in the V–Y design. Complications occurred in 15%, the most common being wound dehiscence.

If more radical treatment of the trochanter is required, e.g., a Girdlestone procedure, then the vastus lateralis becomes the flap of choice, either as a muscle or musculocutaneous flap[350–352] (Fig. 16.16).

Selected procedure: V–Y tensor fasciae latae flap (Fig. 16.17); tensor fasciae latae rotation flap

The many variations on the tensor fasciae latae flap are common options for dealing with trochanteric ulcers. A fasciocutaneous or musculocutaneous rotation flap is technically straightforward, can reach a variety of defects, and may be readvanced if necessary.

The blood supply to the tensor fasciae latae is from branches of the lateral circumflex femoral artery, which enter the deep surface of the muscle anteriorly. The proximal, muscular portion of the tensor fasciae latae is relatively small. The distal portion of the muscle consists almost entirely of fascia but still provides perforators to the overlying skin. If necessary, the flap can be extended just proximal to the knee and rotated to cover ischial or even sacral defects, though such extended flaps are not entirely reliable unless delayed. A much more limited dissection is possible when addressing trochanteric ulcers.

Though the blood supply to this flap is robust and relatively reliable, minor variations are common. If necessary, the flap

Table 16.4 Reconstructive options in trochanteric pressure ulcers

Anteriorly based random thigh flap Vasconez, Schneider, and Jurkewicz, *Curr Probl Surg 14: 1, 1977*	Tensor fasciae latae musculocutaneous flap, island Kauer and Sonsino, *Scand J Plast Reconstr Surg 20: 129, 1986*
Random bipedicle flap Conway and Griffith, *Am J Surg 91: 946, 1956*	Vastus lateralis myoplasty Minami, Hentz, and Vistnes, *Plast Reconstr Surg 60: 364, 1977* Dowden and McCraw, *Ann Plast Surg 4: 396, 1980*
Tensor fasciae latae musculocutaneous flap Nahai et al., *Ann Plast Surg 1: 372, 1978* Hill, Nahai, and Vasconez, *Plast Reconstr Surg 61: 517, 1978* Withers et al., *Ann Plast Surg 4: 31, 1980*	Vastus lateralis musculocutaneous flap Bovet et al., *Plast Reconstr Surg 69: 830, 1982* Hauben et al., *Ann Plast Surg 10: 359, 1983* Drimmer and Krasna, *Plast Reconstr Surg 79:560, 1987*
Tensor fasciae latae musculocutaneous flap, bipedicle Schulman, *Plast Reconstr Surg 66: 740, 1980*	Gluteus medius tensor fasciae latae musculocutaneous flap Little and Lyons, *Plast Reconstr Surg 71: 366, 1983*
Tensor fasciae latae musculocutaneous flap, V–Y advancement Lewis, Cunningham, and Hugo, *Ann Plast Surg 6: 34, 1981* Siddiqui, Wiedrich, and Lewis, *Ann Plast Surg, 31: 313, 1993*	Distally based gluteus maximus flap Becker, *Plast Reconstr Surg 63: 653, 1979*
Tensor fasciae latae musculocutaneous flap, innervated Dibbell, McCraw, and Edstrom, *Plast Reconstr Surg, 64: 796, 1979* Nahai, Hill, and Hester, *Plast Reconstr Surg 7: 286, 1981* Nahai, *Clin Plast Surg 7: 51, 1980* Cochran, Edstrom, and Dibbell, *Ann Plast Surg 7: 286, 1981*	Gluteal thigh flap Hurwitz, Swartz, and Mathes, *Plast Reconstr Surg 68:521, 1981*
	Expansive gluteus maximus flap Ramirez, Hurwitz, and Futrell, *Plast Reconstr Surg 74: 757, 1984* Ramirez, *Ann Plast Surg 18:295, 1987*

(Reproduced from Janis JE, Kenkel JM. Pressure sores. In: Barton FE Jr., ed. *Selected Readings in Plastic Surgery*, vol. 9, no. 39. Dallas, TX: Selected Readings in Plastic Surgery; 2003:29.)

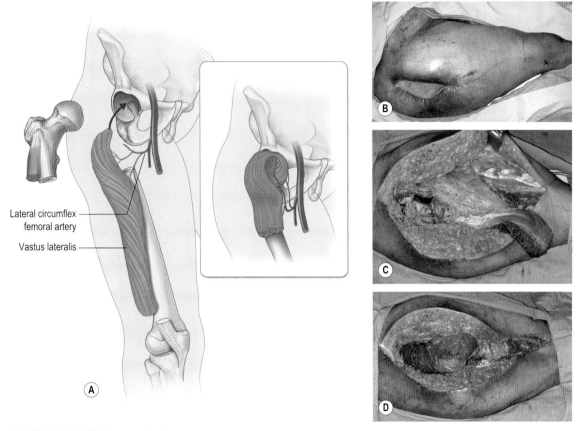

Lateral circumflex
femoral artery

Vastus lateralis

Fig. 16.16 (A–D) Girdlestone arthroplasty.

may be based on alternate branches of the circumflex vessels. If the perforators to the muscle are not usable, dissection of the descending branch of the lateral circumflex allows relatively simple conversion to a pedicled anterolateral thigh flap.

The ulcer will generally define the posterior margin of the flap. A line from the anterior superior iliac spine to the knee marks the anterior border of the flap. Flaps up to 15–20 cm proximal to the femoral condyle are very reliable without delay. The inferior point of the flap can be taken just short of the condyle if preferred. Though it may be excessive for single-stage ulcer coverage, a lengthier flap is easier to readvance if necessary. The pedicle is generally roughly 10 cm inferior to the anterior superior iliac spine and 10–15 cm lateral to the pubic tubercle.

After incising the skin down to fascia, dissection is easiest distally, where the tensor fasciae latae is essentially entirely fascia. Dissecting under the fascia, it is generally easy to identify the pedicle as the tensor fasciae latae transitions to muscle proximally. The fascia and muscle can then be completely divided and the flap rotated to fill the defect. As with the other flaps discussed in this section, the flap is then inset in layers over drains and the donor site closed in linear fashion.

Bone resection

Kostrubala and Greeley[28] first suggested removing the underlying bony prominences as an adjunct to the treatment of patients with pressure sores. The authors initially recommended excision of the posterior sacral promontories and

greater trochanters when these areas were exposed, and subsequently expanded the resection to encompass the entire ischium. Conway and Griffith[240] noted a decrease in recurrence from 38% after partial ischiectomy to 3% after total ischiectomy.

Although total ischiectomy minimizes ipsilateral recurrence, secondary problems are frequent. Arregui et al.[353] evaluated 94 patients with pressure sores treated by total ischiectomy over a 10-year period. Despite "good" results in 81%, there was a 16% complication rate and a 28% occurrence of contralateral ischial ulcer. The authors subsequently recommended contralateral ischial resection on a prophylactic basis.

After total bilateral ischiectomy, however, weight is transferred to the pubic rami and perineum as well as the proximal femur. When sitting, pressure is borne directly by the membranous and proximal bulbous urethra.[354] Perineal ulcers, urethrocutaneous fistulas,[355] and perineourethral diverticula[30] have been reported in up to 58% of patients after complete bilateral ischiectomy. Given the high incidence of serious complications, total ischiectomy should be reserved for deep, extensive, recurrent ischial pressure sores.

Proximal femoral resection with muscle flap coverage may be indicated in instances of large and/or recalcitrant trochanteric ulcers complicated by osteomyelitis and ulcers involving the hip joint.[351] Patients who undergo proximal femoral resection may experience a piston effect that prevents the obliteration of dead space. Klein et al.[352] addressed the issue through the use of an external fixator for 2–3 weeks, and reported all 10 of their patients' wounds healed, despite a 50% incidence

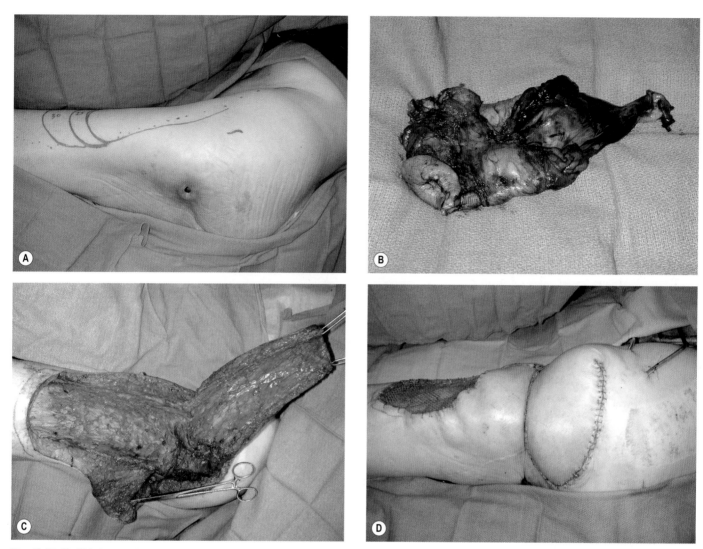

Fig. 16.17 (A–D) Left tensor fasciae latae flap with backgrafting.

of pin loosening. Rubayi et al.[356] prefer to use an abduction pillow and antispasmodic drugs to control femoral motion. A total of 24 of 26 wounds healed in the hospital, and all wounds healed eventually.

Patients with proven osteomyelitis in the bone underlying their pressure sore should be treated with at least partial ostectomy. Although in principle osteomyelitis should be treated by radical excision,[215,357] the endpoint of all bony debridement should be healthy bleeding bone,[84] and osteopenia in paraplegics may cloud this goal. In these cases, preoperative imaging may be helpful in determining the extent of bony involvement. The identified areas can then be resected down to bleeding, healthy-appearing bone and cultures taken from the depths of the wound. Postoperative antibiotic therapy should be guided by the results of deep bone cultures and biopsies.[358]

Postoperative care

The care of patients after pressure sore surgery has been reviewed by multiple authors, including Vasconez et al.,[359] Conway and Griffith,[240] Stal et al.,[360] Hentz,[361] Constantian,[362] and Disa et al.[363] The measures used to address pressure relief, shear, friction, moisture, skin care, incontinence, spasticity, and nutrition should be continued aggressively through the postoperative period, in addition to standard postoperative care. Two additional issues that need to be addressed prior to discharge are length of immobilization and when to restart sitting protocols and therapy.

Traditionally pressure sore patients were kept in bed for 6–8 weeks based on experimental data indicating that wounds reached maximum tensile strength after this period.[364] More recent studies have advocated a more rapid progression to sitting. In a prospective, randomized trial Isik et al.[365] found equivalent complication rates when comparing 2 and 3 weeks of immobilization, though overall length of stay was similar and long-term follow-up was deemed inadequate to draw any firm conclusions. Likewise, Foster et al.[289] began a sitting regimen at 10–14 days and had postoperative hospital stays averaging 20 days, with short-term success rates of 89%.

Regardless of how long patients are kept in bed, they should begin active and passive range-of-motion exercises of the uninvolved extremity early in the postoperative course,[193] while the affected extremity can be ranged just prior to initiation of a sitting protocol. A typical regimen involves having

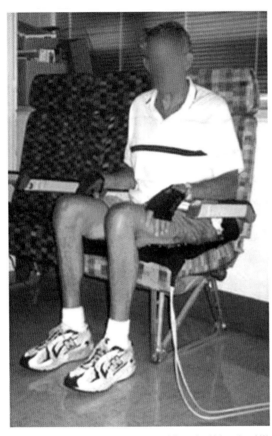
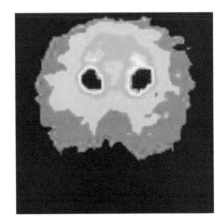
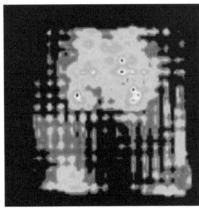

Fig. 16.18 Seat mapping. *(Reproduced from the University of Washington PM&R website: http://sci.washington.edu/info/forums/reports/pressure_map.asp.)*

the patient sit for 15-minute intervals once or twice a day, then gradually increasing the length and frequency of sitting periods until discharge.[365] Pressure release maneuvers are performed at least every 15 minutes while the patient is seated, and the surgical site is carefully monitored for signs of recurrence.[193]

Prior to discharge, patients should have their support surfaces re-evaluated (Fig. 16.18). This assessment is particularly important in patients who have had bony resections or multiple procedures that may result in altered weight-bearing or pelvic and truncal instability.[366] An appropriate seat cushion should be selected, ideally with the assistance of seat mapping. Maximum recommended pressures are 35 mmHg for patients unable to relieve pressure themselves by lifting or leaning and 60 mmHg for those who can.[367]

Patient education should also be emphasized postoperatively. Though studies have demonstrated a positive effect of education on patient knowledge,[368,369] research relating education to recurrence rates is lacking at this time. However, given the evidence that recurrence rates are associated with poor patient compliance, social factors, and communication barriers,[193,370] attempts at addressing these issues through education seem reasonable.

Outcomes, prognosis, and complications

Long-term outcome studies of patients with pressure sores are difficult to conduct, and the existing literature reports a wide

variation in recurrence rates, ranging from as low as 3–6%[300,361,371] to as high as 33–100%.[301,313,363,372]

The most extensive published experiences with pressure sore treatment are those of Conway and Griffith[240] (1000 cases) and Dansereau and Conway's[16] update of the Bronx Veterans Administration Hospital data (2000 cases). In their follow-up article from 1961, Griffith and Schultz[373] categorized the therapeutic history of the earlier series as follows:

- Sacral ulcers: Nonsurgical treatment succeeded in 29%, split-skin grafts in 30%. Excision of bone with the ulcer and closure by large rotation flap achieved healing in 84%.

- Trochanteric ulcers: 41% of patients were adequately treated without surgery; 33% needed split-thickness skin grafts. When ulcer, bursa, and trochanter were excised and the wound simply sutured, 83% healed but 20% recurred. When the trochanter was more thoroughly removed and the site reconstructed with a rotation flap, 92% healed and only 6% recurred.

- Ischial ulcers: Conservative therapy was successful in 18% of cases, skin graft in 17%, and partial ischiectomy with primary suture in 46% (but with 54% recurrence). Total ischiectomy lessened the number of recurrences to 22%, and when combined with muscle flap and regional rotation flap, it further decreased the recurrence rate to 3%.

In 1994 Evans *et al.*[374] reviewed their experience with the surgical treatment of pressure sores in both paraplegic and nonparaplegic patients. Among paraplegics the recurrence rate was 82% with an average time to recurrence of 18.2

months. In contrast, the nonparaplegic group had no recurrence of ulceration.

Relander and Palmer[372] reviewed their experience with 66 flaps for primary coverage of pressure sores and noted a 43% recurrence rate with cutaneous flaps and a 33% recurrence rate with musculocutaneous flaps at 2–12-year follow-up, a nonsignificant difference.

Disa et al.[363] evaluated 40 consecutive patients with 66 pressure sores and, despite a cure rate of 80%, noted a 69% recurrent rate within 1 year. Two subgroups with higher recurrence rates were identified. The young, post-traumatic paraplegic subgroup demonstrated a recurrence rate of 79% at a mean of 10.9 months. The cerebrally compromised elderly subgroup had a 69% recurrence rate at a mean of 7.7 months. The authors conclude that surgical treatment of pressure sores among patients in these subgroups may not be warranted given the high recurrence rates, which they felt resulted from poor patient compliance. The ultimate causes of noncompliance were individual personalities, an unsteady social situation, and inadequate family network.

Tavakoli et al.[370] studied 27 patients with 37 ulcers who underwent musculocutaneous flap coverage of their ischial pressure sores with a mean follow-up of 62 months. Overall ulcer recurrence was 41.4% and overall patient recurrence rate was 47.8%. The recurrences were attributed by the authors to psychological and behavioral factors, such as lifestyle activities that led to neglect of skin care, drug and alcohol abuse, cultural barriers, and neglect of appropriate seating practices.

Kierney et al.[193] reported a lower recurrence rate in 268 pressure sores treated over a 12-year period. Mean postoperative follow-up was 3.7 years, and overall recurrence rate was 19%. Unlike Evans et al.,[374] Kierney et al. did not find an association between pre-existing pressure sore risk factors and recurrence. Instead, the authors emphasize the importance of collaboration between plastic surgeons and physical medicine rehabilitation physicians as a major determinant of outcome.

In 2002 Singh et al.[375] published one of the few studies examining the outcome of surgical reconstruction of pressure sores in children. The records of 19 patients in 25 pressure sores with an average follow-up of 5.3 years were reviewed. Site-specific and patient recurrence were 5% and 20%, respectively, considerably lower than generally reported in adults with similar follow-up.

Clearly, variable patient populations, risk factors, and follow-up periods make comparisons difficult. With such a wide range of outcomes, assigning a single value for recurrence is virtually impossible. Some question the wisdom of surgical intervention if the higher range of recurrence rates is legitimate.[374] It may be that select subpopulations are not good surgical candidates given their poor prognosis. However, a thorough evaluation of a patient's risk factors and a multidisciplinary approach to treatment should be routine even for patients who initially seem like poor candidates.[193]

Complications

Common postoperative complications of pressure sore surgery include hematoma, seroma, infection, and wound dehiscence. A breakdown in the suture line should heal with local wound care within a week. If slough persists, then the wound debridement, particularly of bone, was likely inadequate.[95] The patient should be re-evaluated for risk factors and optimized, prior to return to the operating room for complete debridement, followed by flap advancement or alternative flap for coverage.[99,289]

Every chronic wound exposed to continuous trauma carries the risk of malignant degeneration.[376] Benign-appearing ulcerations are a frequent problem in our population and are usually treated conservatively, yet the suspicion of malignancy in these lesions must always be entertained, especially if the margins of the ulcer are verrucous. The term "Marjolin's ulcer" is used to describe malignant degeneration in burn scars, chronic venous ulcers, pressure sores, and sinuses from osteomyelitis. Malignant transformation is heralded by increased pain or discharge, foul odor, and bleeding. The latency period of carcinomas arising from pressure sores is approximately 20 years, compared with 30 years or more for carcinomas arising from burn scars and stasis ulcers.[377] Biopsy is indicated in all chronically draining ulcers and tracts, especially those with recent change in appearance or drainage, and should include the central area of the ulcer as well as the margins. Early recognition and proper staging offer the best chance for cure.[378]

Secondary procedures

It is critical that, before embarking on revision or repeat flap surgery, the patient be fully re-evaluated. Assuming proper surgical technique, the same risk factors that led to the patient's original ulcer are likely to be at least partially responsible for recurrence, and neglecting them will reliably result in poor outcomes.

Every pressure sore surgery should allow for the possibility of future secondary procedures. Despite favorable initial healing rates, long-term recurrence is common, even in the most favorable series. Assuming basic principles have been adhered to, multiple options should still exist, even in cases of multiple recurrences.

The simplest option may involve readvancing a previously performed flap (Fig. 16.19). Flaps can often be readvanced multiple times, but, as always, excessive tension must be avoided. If tension is an issue, a change of plane, such as advancing a fasciocutaneous flap over a previous musculocutaneous flap, can provide additional length without violating another anatomic region or flap design. If a particular flap has already been readvanced or the tissue is of poor quality due to recurrent ulceration or scarring, a new, preferably virgin, anatomic area should be used to address the wound. For example, while flaps from the thigh area are commonly used to address ischial ulcers, a superiorly based gluteal flap can afford coverage if the posterior thigh is no longer a viable option.

Amputation or salvage flaps should be reserved for recalcitrant pressure sores where the ulcer is extensive to the point of precluding closure with standard flaps, or for patients who are severely ill because of uncontrollable infection, as these flaps are associated with high morbidity.[379–381] Likewise, hemicorporectomy is a highly morbid[382] last-resort measure reserved for potentially life-threatening and incurable conditions, as in patients with multiple, large, confluent ulcers in the setting of malignancy or extensive pelvic osteomyelitis[383,384] (Fig. 16.20).

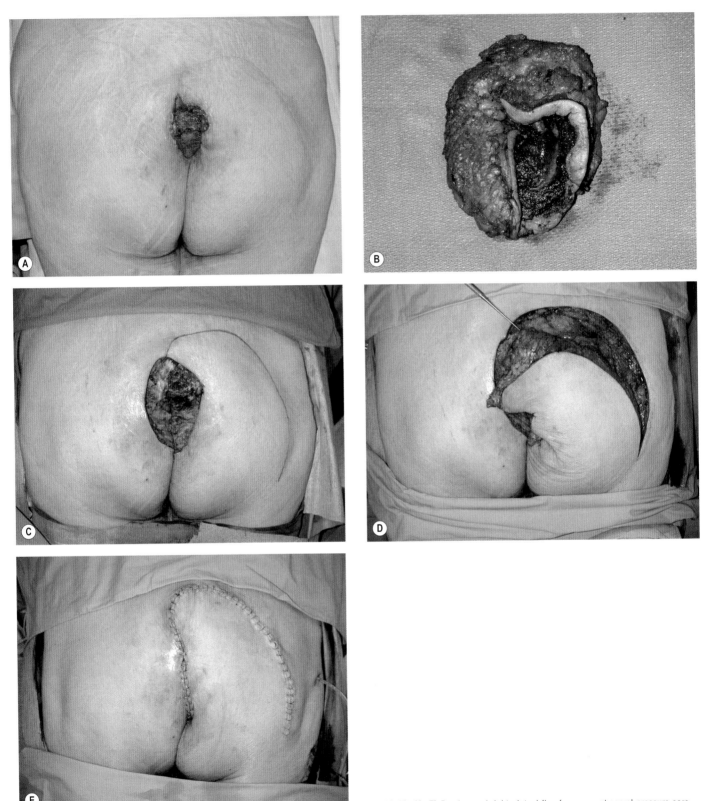

Fig. 16.19 (A–E) Readvanced right gluteal flap for recurrent sacral pressure sore.

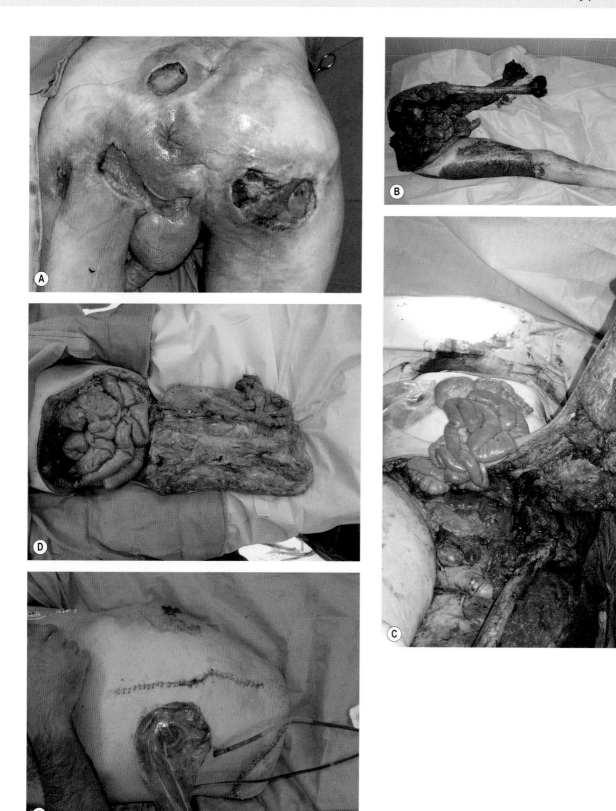

Fig. 16.20 (A–E) Hemicorporectomy with right subtotal thigh flap.

4. Cuddigan J, Frantz RA. Pressure ulcer research: pressure ulcer treatment. A monograph from the National Pressure Ulcer Advisory Panel. *Adv Wound Care (New Rochelle)*. 1998;11:294–300, quiz 302.

21. Waters TM, Daniels MJ, Bazzoli GJ, et al. Effect of Medicare's nonpayment for hospital-acquired conditions: lessons for future policy. *JAMA Intern Med*. 2015;175:347–354.*This article examines the effect of Medicare's non-payment policy for Hospital-Acquired Conditions on the rate of never events, including hospital acquired pressure sores. Overall, since implementation of this policy in 2008, there has been no improvement in the rate of hospital acquired pressure sores, highlighting the continued challenge pressure sores place on our healthcare system and the need for further advancement in the prevention and treatment of pressure sores.*

32. Cushing CA, Phillips LG. Evidence-based medicine: pressure sores. *Plast Reconstr Surg*. 2013;132:1720–1732. *This article provides an evidence-based update regarding the pathophysiology, risk factors, as well as non-surgical and surgical treatments for all types of pressure sores.*

36. Fronek K, Zweifach BW. Microvascular pressure distribution in skeletal muscle and the effect of vasodilation. *Am J Physiol*. 1975;228:791–796.

39. Dinsdale SM. Decubitus ulcers: role of pressure and friction in causation. *Arch Phys Med Rehabil*. 1974;55:147–152. *This classic article establishes a role for pressure and friction in the development of pressure sores.*

63. Reddy M, Gill SS, Rochon PA. Preventing pressure ulcers: a systematic review. *JAMA*. 2006;296:974–984. *This article provides a comprehensive review of randomized controlled trials examining interventions to prevent pressure sores. Notably, this review highlights evidence for the use of support surfaces, repositioning, nutritional optimization, and moisturizing sacral surfaces.*

87. Han H, Lewis VL Jr, Wiedrich TA, Patel PK. The value of Jamshidi core needle bone biopsy in predicting postoperative osteomyelitis in grade IV pressure ulcer patients. *Plast Reconstr Surg*. 2002;110:118–122.

132. Wound, Ostomy and Continence Nurses Society. *WOCN Policy and Procedure Manual*. Mount Laurel, NJ: WOCN Society; 2015. *The WOCN policy and procedure manual remains the authority in accurate diagnosis and standard of care treatment for pressure sores.*

211. Qaseem A, Humphrey LL, Forciea MA, et al. Clinical Guidelines Committee of the American College of Physicians. Treatment of pressure ulcers: a clinical practice guideline from the American College of Physicians. *Ann Intern Med*. 2015;162:370–379. *The American College of Physicians examined a multitude of pressure sore treatment strategies to evaluate comparative effectiveness for improved clinical outcomes and potential harms in order to provide treatment guidelines based on evidence.*

240. Conway H, Griffith BH. Plastic surgery for closure of decubitus ulcers in patients with paraplegia; based on experience with 1,000 cases. *Am J Surg*. 1956;91:946–975.

245. Anthony JP, Huntsman WT, Mathes SJ. Changing trends in the management of pelvic pressure ulcers: a 12-year review. *Decubitus*. 1992;5:44–47, 50–51.

247. Kroll SS, Rosenfield L. Perforator-based flaps for low posterior midline defects. *Plast Reconstr Surg*. 1988;81:561–566.

17

Perineal reconstruction

Hakim K. Said and Otway Louie

Access video lecture content for this chapter online at expertconsult.com

SYNOPSIS

- The surgical site is typically hostile after resection and/or radiation for an underlying condition.
- Healthy tissue transfer is usually necessary to mitigate wound-healing challenges.
- A proactive surgical approach can help lessen impact of complications.

Introduction

Perineal reconstruction poses the challenge of healing a problem area despite a number of site-specific obstacles. Although a number of benign conditions exist that can require resurfacing perineal skin, more frequently reconstruction is needed after treatment of underlying cancer. Modern treatment of malignancies in this region has evolved to consistently use neoadjuvant radiation therapy, which can yield a high rate of complications at the time of surgical intervention. Local effects of radiation therapy and close proximity (combined in many cases with ostomies) to bowels, reproductive organs, and bladder can all complicate reconstructive flap inset, contaminate the surgical site, and threaten surgical outcomes. Successful reconstruction takes into account these impediments and minimizes the consequences of complications in this hazardous region.

 Access the Historical Perspective section online at
http://www.expertconsult.com

Basic science/disease process

The processes requiring reconstruction of the perineum can broadly be broken into superficial and deep processes (Table 17.1). Benign conditions primarily include hidradenitis suppurativa, infectious destructive processes such as fasciitis or Fournier's gangrene, and trauma, but can range to other rarer dermatologic conditions such as pyoderma gangrenosum and vasculitic ulcers. Malignant superficial lesions usually include vulvar cancers and cutaneous lesions in the area. These entities have in common the depth of involvement, which typically leaves only an external cutaneous deficit on the perineum (see Figs. 9.13 & 9.18). Also, radiation treatment is unusual, so the surrounding skin is typically healthy. Once the primary process is addressed and resolving, the defect can begin secondary healing. Negative pressure therapy and skin grafts can often play a useful role in shortening the time to healing. Some authors advocate locoregional flaps to hasten treatment for superficial defects, although this has yet to gain universal use.[17] Challenges to healing in this area include a high bacterial bioburden in many of the causative etiologies, an inherently moist surgical site, and pressure, tension, and shearing forces, which threaten to disrupt the site as the patient begins to mobilize. Outcomes are more favorable in this group.

Deep defects are primarily the result of malignancy, including colorectal cancer, urologic, and gynecologic cancers, most of which originate from and involve pelvic structures (see Figs. 9.11 & 9.12). Abdominoperineal resection or exenteration has been demonstrated to provide the best cure in these cases. Typically, this extensive resection is accompanied by perioperative radiation therapy. Treatment of these more complex defects must be individualized for the missing and exposed structures. The bony pelvis effectively splints open the pelvic outlet, so contraction cannot occur, and seromas are common. Further impediments to healing such as fistulas and radiation changes in the area generally mean these defects are frequently contaminated, prone to infection, and will not heal without the addition of a non-radiated tissue transfer. After extensive resection, large areas of dead space and loss of support allow the abdominal viscera to fall into the irradiated pelvic basin. This can lead to pelvic hernias, adhesions, obstruction, and fistulas, all of which can be disastrous to treat secondarily.

Table 17.1 Processes requiring reconstruction of the perineum

Process	Etiology	Complicating factors	Reconstructive options
Superficial (simple, mostly benign)	Hidradenitis suppurativa Necrotizing fasciitis Fournier's gangrene Trauma Autoimmune ulcers Vulvar cancer	Bacterial bioburden Moisture Mobility	Secondary healing Negative pressure therapy Skin graft Fasciocutaneous perforator flaps
Deep (complex, malignant)	Colorectal cancer Vulvar cancer Vaginal cancer Uterine cancer Bladder cancer	Radiation Ostomies Contamination Dead space Pelvic hernia Moisture Mobility	Rectus abdominis flap Gracilis flap Anterolateral thigh flap Singapore flap Fasciocutaneous perforator flaps Free flap

Nearby organs such as the bladder or vagina may also be resected in part or whole as part of the treatment course. Finally, the surgical incision is inherently moist, and mobilizing the patient can cause pressure or shearing stresses, further compounding the difficulty of healing a radiated closure at that location. Surgical outcomes reflect the many challenges posed in this group.

Diagnosis/patient presentation

Patients with superficial disease may present at various stages in their treatment. As a rule, reconstruction should not be initiated until the primary process is identified and resolved with repeated surgical debridements or excisions; underlying medical conditions or autoimmune disorders should be treated. Typically, areas of external pudendal skin are involved and will require resurfacing in some fashion (Fig. 17.1).

Patients with deep disease are typically treated in conjunction with a multidisciplinary oncologic team for an underlying malignancy. Often the extent of the defect is not obvious until after the surgical resection is performed, and must be anticipated in advance. Preoperative consultation is important to manage patient expectations, outline the possible extent of surgery, and prepare for postoperative adversity. Such cases may involve more extensive external pudendal defects (Figs. 17.2 & 17.3) or deeper structures (Fig. 17.4). In the event that vaginal resection is necessary, preferences regarding vaginal versus simple perineal reconstruction should be discussed, along with a thorough dialogue about sexual function. Further details and management of vaginal reconstruction are discussed in depth in Chapter 14.

Patient selection

Patients with superficial defects are more straightforward in management; as their underlying process resolves, the defect begins to heal secondarily, even in response to a conventional wet to moist dressing regimen. Typically a modest, shallow

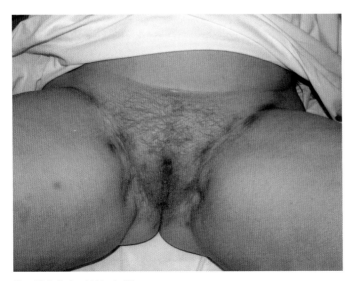

Fig. 17.1 Perineal hidradenitis.

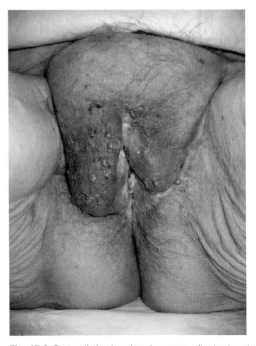

Fig. 17.2 Post-radiation lymphangiosarcoma after treatment of vulvar cancer.

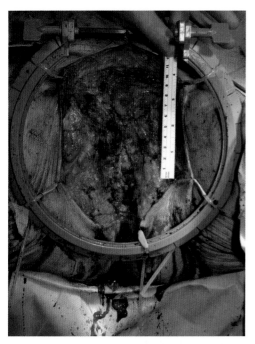

Fig. 17.3 External perineal skin and soft-tissue loss.

perineal defect is left. A number of publications support the use of a negative pressure therapy plan to accelerate the healing process. Within a matter of weeks, a healthy wound bed can be established, confirming the suitability of these patients for skin grafting. If the wound fails to begin the healing process despite wound healing optimization, a more complex approach and tissue transfer might be warranted. Especially for superficial malignancies such as vulvar cancer, reconstruction at the time of resection is feasible, and standard in many centers. Application of microsurgical principles for perforator flap dissection has been proposed in that setting.

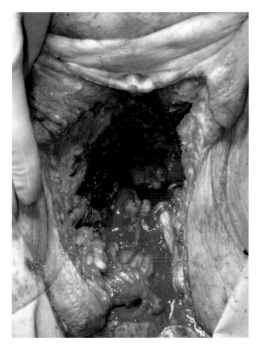

Fig. 17.4 Complex perineal defect involving external skin, soft tissues, vagina, and pelvic floor.

In the case of deeper malignancies, such as colorectal, gynecologic, or urologic cancer, radiation therapy is part of the preoperative routine in most centers. This factor alone is the most significant indication for flap reconstruction at the time of resection. Large prospective series suggest that abdominal based flaps demonstrate the most favorable outcomes and mildest complication profile in this setting, even compared to thigh flap reconstruction.[18] This must be balanced with the abdominal morbidity of the harvest. Some surgeons prefer to avoid using abdominal flaps if ostomies are necessary on both sides, although these can be inset through the external oblique musculature with no additional morbidity. A vertical skin pedicle provides the most discreet scar, but an oblique paddle can provide more tissue by extending off the muscle, effectively also extending its reach. Pre-existing abdominal wall defects might direct some surgeons to alternative flap options. Nevertheless, Butler has shown no increased incidence of abdominal wall problems after abdominal flap harvest.[18,19] Rarely, perineal resection can be performed without laparotomy, and this might predispose toward use of a non-abdominal flap option.

The complication profile of the gracilis flap is also reasonable and represents a dramatic improvement over primary closure under these circumstances. Early studies comparing gracilis reconstruction to primary closure demonstrate a dramatic reduction in infectious complications from 46% to 12% with flap reconstruction.[20]

The anterolateral thigh flap represents an alternative option with documented excellent reliability for many applications, but with less support for its use in this setting at this point. One recent study suggests it has reliability comparable to abdominal flaps, and other studies may corroborate this in time.

Some surgeons favor a posterior thigh flap, harvested in similar fashion to the anterolateral thigh flap, but the axial nature of the perfusion off the inferior gluteal artery has been called into question. Recent series document a wound healing complication rate of over 50% using this method,[21] which does not compare favorably to abdominal flaps.

For defects with less dead space or requiring less bulk, skin flap reconstruction (e.g., Singapore or perforator flaps) can be used, although outcome data are more mixed and overall less favorable compared to abdominal flaps. Complications are reported to range from 7% to 62%.[22-24] Recent outcome studies are not available directly comparing this method to other options in a head-to-head fashion.

Massive defects in pelvic support may in fact require multiple flaps. Occasionally, pelvic floor support is needed in the form of mesh reinforcement. In a hostile, radiated, often contaminated surgical site, prosthetic mesh is contraindicated. Newer bioprosthetic options provide a reinforcement alternative that is more robust in the face of complications.[25]

Finally, if the two abdominal flaps and eight thigh-based flaps are unavailable or insufficient for the defect, there are several reports of distant flaps used in conjunction with microsurgical transfer. Composite thigh tissues can be transferred *en bloc*, and large surface area flaps such as the latissimus dorsi have been reported in extreme cases.

Laparoscopic or robotic techniques represent a new frontier in both extirpative and reconstructive surgeries. Performing the entirety of an abdominoperineal resection is now possible through incisions that total 2 cm in length. As techniques are developed for resection without an open laparotomy, the necessity for harvesting non-radiated tissue to fill the radiated pelvic basin remains. Typically this entails harvest of the rectus muscle through the posterior sheath using either a laparoscopic or robotic approach. Laparoscopic tools are widely available, but the robotic equipment is less widely available, and surgeons trained in using that for reconstruction are rarer still. This will undoubtedly change as the growing field of minimally invasive reconstruction matures.

Treatment/surgical technique

Skin graft reconstruction

Benign, uncomplicated wounds of the perineum that granulate in response to dressing changes or negative pressure therapy can usually be treated in a staged fashion with split-thickness skin grafts.

Regional skin flaps

Processes such as Fournier's gangrene may leave more extensive but still subcutaneous defects that can be reconstructed with local flaps. Exposed subcutaneous structures such as testes can be buried under nearby intact skin if available. These adjacent areas of intact skin on the thighs or perineum can also be advanced using a V–Y pattern, rotational or keystone design to provide resurfacing (Figs. 17.5, 17.6). Some authors have described tissue expansion in conjunction with regional flaps to augment the amount of subcutaneous coverage available, for example in the case of missing scrotal coverage.[26] Perforator-based flaps have been described for superficial defects using medial circumflex femoral vessels,[17,27] profunda femoris perforating branches,[28] and almost any vascular axis in the region.[15]

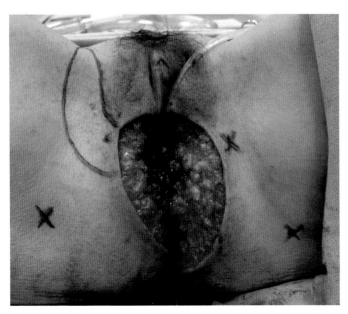

Fig. 17.5 Extensive but subcutaneous defect of the external perineal skin.

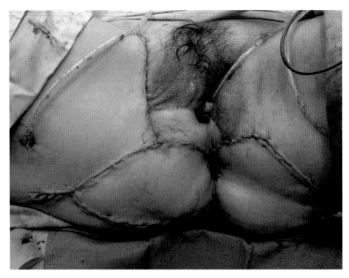

Fig. 17.6 Multiple regional flaps for reconstruction. Right Singapore flap used in conjunction with bilateral V–Y advancement flaps. *(Courtesy of Peter C. Neligan, MD).*

Rectus-based reconstruction

Rectus-based flaps have emerged as workhorses for more complex perineal reconstruction. These flaps provide well-vascularized tissue with adequate bulk to fill dead space. In addition, lining for external or vaginal wall coverage can be obtained if harvested as a musculocutaneous flap. They are known for having a wide arc of rotation with a reliable pedicle. They have been shown to decrease the risk of perineal complications in irradiated APR defects.[29] When compared to thigh-based flaps, rectus-based flaps had lower major complications without increased abdominal morbidity.[18]

The rectus flap can be muscular or myocutaneous, depending on whether external skin or vaginal lining is needed for reconstruction. The right rectus is typically used, saving the left rectus for a colostomy if needed. After the resection is complete, the deep inferior epigastric vessels are examined to confirm they are patent, undamaged by the resection, and preferably pulsatile before proceeding with flap design. The skin paddle is based on the periumbilical perforators of the deep inferior epigastric vessels,[51] and can be oriented in vertical, transverse, or oblique directions (Figs. 17.7 & 17.8; see Figs. 14.6 & 14.7). The vertical design theoretically includes more perforators as the skin paddle overlies the length of the rectus; however, its arc of rotation is limited by the muscle itself, and the bulk of the muscle itself can make insetting difficult, particularly in a narrow male pelvis. The transverse paddle has been well described for perineal reconstruction as well, and provides excellent cosmesis for the donor site.[30] Dumanian and others have had success with an oblique design for the rectus flap, noting the long, excellent arc of rotation and thin, reliable skin paddle obtained.[31,32,53] In addition, cadaver injection studies have shown flow in a lateral and superior oblique direction from the periumbilical perforators. After marking the periumbilical perforators with a Doppler, a skin paddle is designed with an axis towards the ipsilateral tip of the scapula, ending at the anterior axillary line. Flaps up to 12×30 cm can be obtained with this design.

Once the skin paddle has been marked in one of these orientations, the skin incisions are made and dissection carried

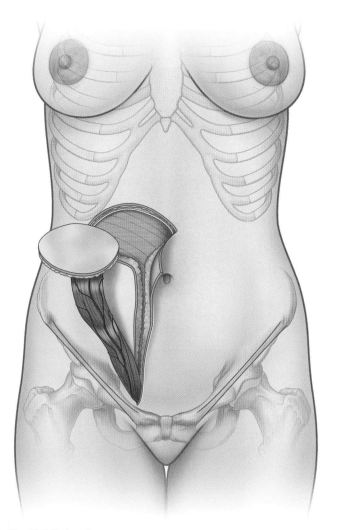

Fig. 17.7 Design of transverse rectus abdominis myocutaneous (TRAM) flap for perineal and pelvic reconstruction.

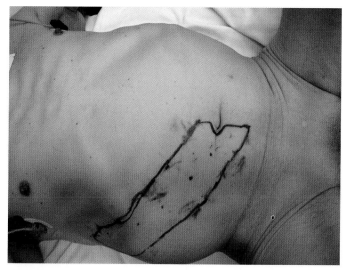

Fig. 17.8 Design of oblique rectus abdominis myocutaneous (ORAM) flap for perineal and pelvic reconstruction. Note skin paddle designed around periumbilical perforators, extending toward ipsilateral scapular tip.

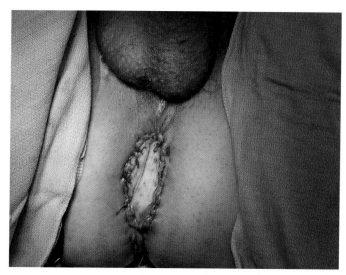

Fig. 17.9 Cutaneous paddle inset for external perineal skin reconstruction.

down to the external oblique and rectus fascia. The skin paddle is dissected circumferentially, approaching the deep inferior epigastric perforators coming through the rectus muscle. The fascia immediately adjacent to these perforators is opened, and the anterior sheath elevated off the rectus muscle. The muscle is then dissected free of the rectus sheath, working down toward the deep inferior epigastric vessels. These are identified lateral to the rectus beneath the arcuate line. The superior rectus is divided, and the muscle transposed out of the rectus sheath. The vascular pedicle can be mobilized but does not need to be skeletonized. The insertion of the rectus on the pubis typically does not need to be divided completely and is left intact at least in part to help prevent traction injury to the pedicle.

The flap is then delivered down through the pelvis and out to the perineum (see Fig. 14.7). The requisite skin for external lining or vaginal reconstruction is marked, and the remainder of the skin paddle de-epithelialized and inset under the radiated skin edges (Fig. 17.9). The skin paddle may be tubed if needed for total vaginal reconstruction (Fig. 17.10). The flap

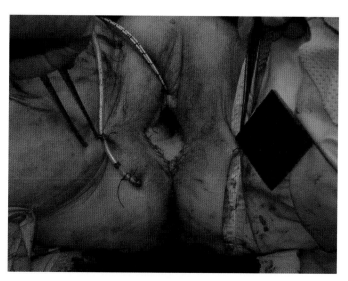

Fig. 17.10 Cutaneous paddle inset for vaginal and perineal reconstruction.

is then inset with a layered closure. The fascial donor site is closed primarily if possible, or the remaining anterior and posterior sheaths are sewn together and used to span the fascial defect. Bioprosthetic mesh may be used to repair extensive anterior sheath defects. The abdominal skin is closed primarily over closed suction drainage.

Gracilis flap

The gracilis flap was first introduced in its myocutaneous form by McCraw and used as a healthy tissue to augment genital reconstruction.[33] As described, it was based on the medial circumflex femoral vessels to the gracilis muscle, and to the overlying skin. Subsequent studies have shown that the perforators originating from the deep femoral system only pass reliably through the gracilis muscle proximally. To consistently capture the perfusion to distal portions of a longitudinal skin paddle, the fasciocutaneous vascular network around the gracilis muscle must be widely harvested intact from proximal to distal as described by Whetzel.[34]

A line is drawn from the adductor insertion on the pubis to the semitendinosus muscle at the medial condyle of the knee. Centered on this axis at the anterior edge of the gracilis muscle, the skin flap is designed as a 6–10 cm wide ellipse that can reach up to 30 cm in length (see Fig. 14.9A). This position is slightly more anterior than the traditional design, which failed to harvest peri-gracilis fascia and was associated with a less reliable skin paddle. The skin pattern is incised distally to identify the thin, round gracilis muscle near the knee, and a bowstring technique is used to confirm its course. If necessary, the skin design is adjusted to overlie the anterior edge of the muscle. The paddle is then incised anteriorly, and beveling dissection outward ensures that the gracilis is harvested encased within its surrounding fat, vessels, and fascia, essentially denuding the sartorius and adductor musculature (Fig. 17.11; see Fig. 14.9B). The perforating branches off the superficial femoral vessels are divided very close to their take-off, preserving the longitudinal arcade of fasciocutaneous vessels in communication with the primary pedicle off the deep femoral system proximally. The greater saphenous vein is divided proximally and distally and preserved within the substance of the flap as an additional venous conduit. The flap is isolated back to its pedicle off the medial circumflex femoral vessels, usually at 7–10 cm distal from the pubis (see Fig. 14.9F). Upgoing adductor branches are divided to yield extra length. The muscular origin is exposed and divided off the pubis to allow rotation of the flap 180 degrees into the perineum. To reduce the chance of flap ptosis, the flap is suspended from high within the perineal defect, or into the pelvis if possible. Layered closure over drains completes the inset (Figs. 17.12 & 17.13).

Anterolateral thigh flap

The anterolateral thigh flap was first described by Song in 1984.[35] Since that time it has become a valuable tool in the armamentarium of the reconstructive surgeon, with extensive uses in head and neck, trunk, and lower extremity reconstruction.[36] Luo first described its use in perineal reconstruction after failed gracilis flaps in 2000.[37] Increasing experience with it in perineal reconstruction has confirmed its utility in complex pelvic defects.[12,13] It provides a regional flap that can

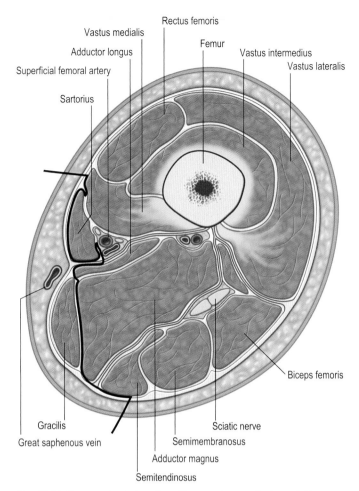

Fig. 17.11 Cross-sectional view of gracilis myocutaneous flap harvest. The fasciocutaneous vascular network around the gracilis muscle must be widely harvested to preserve perfusion to the distal tip of the skin. Adductor magnus, vastus medialis, sartorius, and semitendinosus muscles are denuded by the harvest, as described by Whetzel.[34] *(Adapted from Whetzel TP, Lechtman AN. The gracilis myofasciocutaneous flap: vascular anatomy and clinical application. Plast Reconstr Surg. 1997;99:1642–1652; discussion 1653–1655.)*

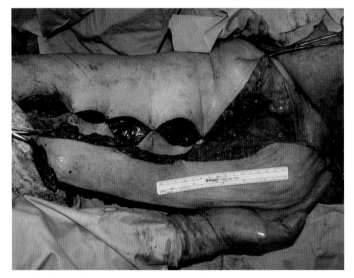

Fig. 17.12 Gracilis myocutaneous flap elevated before inset. Pedicle is visible 7–10 cm from pubis.

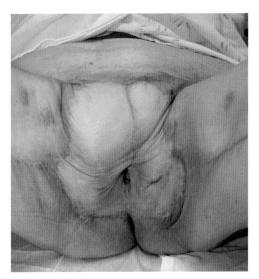

Fig. 17.13 Bilateral gracilis myocutaneous flaps for large area external perineal defect.

provide large, reliable skin paddles and muscle in the form of the vastus lateralis as well.

With the patient in a supine position, a line connecting the anterior superior iliac spine with the superolateral patella is marked (Fig. 17.14). A circle with a 3 cm radius is marked at the center of this longitudinal axis, delineating the most

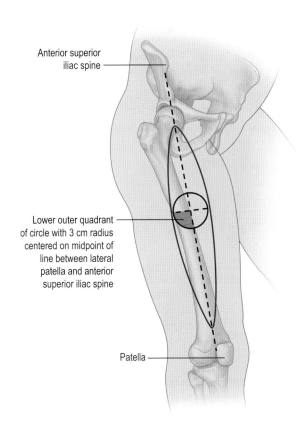

Fig. 17.14 Design of anterolateral thigh flap, centered midway along an axis between the anterior superior iliac spine (ASIS) and the superolateral corner of the patella.

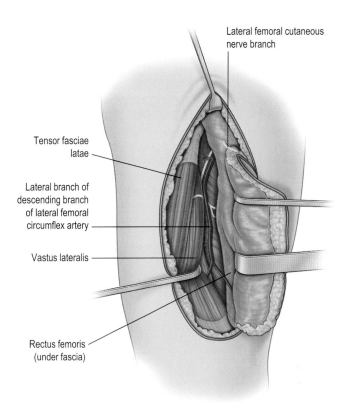

Fig. 17.15 Elevation of anterolateral thigh flap, including skin, soft tissue, fascia, and occasionally a small cuff of muscle. Perforators are pursued toward the septum between the vastus lateralis and rectus femoris, and then followed superomedially up to the descending branch of the lateral circumflex femoral vessels.

common location of perforators of the descending branch of the lateral femoral circumflex vessels. Locations of perforators are confirmed by Doppler, and the skin paddle is designed as an ellipse centered on these perforators.

The anterior incision is made first, dissecting down to the fascia overlying the rectus femoris muscle (Fig. 17.15). Dissection proceeds laterally, either in a subfascial or suprafascial plane, looking for septocutaneous perforators, which are then followed superomedially back to the descending branch of the lateral femoral circumflex vessels. Intramuscular perforators can be harvested with a small cuff of vastus lateralis muscle to minimize risk of injury to the perforators. The posterolateral incision is subsequently made and the harvest completed.

The flap can be delivered through either a perineal or inguinal route, as elegantly described by Yu.[38] If a perineal skin defect exists, the flap is delivered under the rectus femoris and through a subcutaneous tunnel in the medial thigh to reach the perineum (see Fig. 17.9). If the perineal defect can be closed primarily, the inguinal ligament can be divided and the vastus lateralis muscle delivered intraperitoneally through the abdominal wall to fill any dead space in the pelvis (Fig. 17.16). The flaps are then inset with layered closure and ample drainage.

Singapore flap

First reported by Wee, Singapore flaps are fasciocutaneous flaps harvested from the groin ideally using non-hair-bearing skin just lateral to the labia majora.[11] These flaps are based on

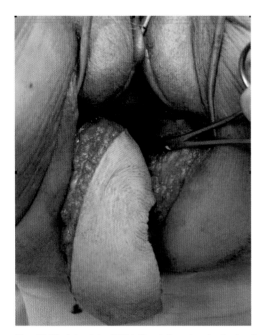

Fig. 17.16 Anterolateral thigh flap delivered under the inguinal ligament into the pelvis, then out through the pelvic defect to fill the pelvic dead space and reconstruct the perineal skin defect. The flap can be tunneled subcutaneously across the thigh if no pelvic defect is present.

the posterior labial arteries, tracing back from the perineal arteries, which in turn originate from the internal pudendal vessels. A horn-shaped flap up to 15×6 cm is designed lateral to the labia majora and harvested to include deep fascia and adductor epimysium to preserve dermal blood supply. The original description divided the dermis at the base of the design and tunneled the flap into the defect. In order to maximize perfusion under the most adverse circumstances, Woods subsequently described a modification to avoid dividing the skin at the base of the flap.[39] This design added an incision made at the posterior base of the labia majora in order to avoid dividing the dermal circulation to the flap entirely. The released labia are allowed to shift anteriorly, and the flaps are transposed 70 degrees through the release incision into the defect (Fig. 17.17; see Fig. 14.4). Although this method is well established, in some patients it may transpose hair-bearing skin, which can be a liability, especially in vagino-perineal reconstruction. Some populations are less hirsute, and this issue is less important. For use in European populations, however, some groups advocate depilatory treatments prior to this surgery. Newer methods using fasciocutaneous flaps based on other perforators (see perforator flaps below) eliminate this issue and are becoming a preferred solution.

Posterior thigh flap

Although this flap has been described based on axial flow from the inferior gluteal artery,[52] this pattern of perfusion has been called into question. A significant number of flaps in this distribution are actually based on perforators from the profunda femoris vessels,[28] which are frequently divided using the flap design as traditionally described.[40,41] This may relate to the high wound healing complication rate (53%) recently reported in a series of these flaps.[21] There are settings where this flap can be useful, especially when an abdominal approach

is contraindicated and the previous flaps are not available. In such cases, using a profunda femoris perforator flap design is recommended (see perforator flaps, below). Not all surgeons are comfortable with this style of dissection, and the literature shows far fewer reports of its use in this manner. These various issues prevent it from being a first-line choice in comparison with the better-established and supported flaps above.

Perforator flaps

As the use of perforator-based techniques becomes more widespread, a number of fasciocutaneous perforator or free-style flaps have been described with good success in perineal reconstruction. Originally described for vulvar cancer, which results in external cutaneous defects without radiation treatment, a number of authors have reported their usefulness even in settings of deeper resection and radiated tissues. Mostly based on perforators from the internal pudendal artery, these include the Singapore flap, pudendal thigh flap, lotus leaf flap, and gluteal fold flap.[15,16,42,43] The latter of these are more recent designs, which are less prone to hair-bearing, thus eliminating the most significant liability of the Singapore flap. Also described are local perforators from the thigh vessels, either the profunda femoris or medial circumflex femoral arteries (Fig. 17.18). Many of these flaps can be designed remotely enough to yield non-radiated tissue for transposition into the defect. For both deep and superficial resection defects, bilateral flaps can be employed to provide tissue with minimal morbidity. As surgeons become more comfortable with perforator flaps, the prevailing algorithms for perineal reconstruction may evolve, although the strong, reliable record of the muscle flaps still leaves them as the first line option in most cases.

Free flap

Given the number of reliable local flap options, microsurgical tissue transfer is rarely indicated. In extenuating circumstances, however, large composite flaps of skin and muscle from the thigh can be elevated and re-anastomosed using gluteal recipient vessels.[14] Alternatively, the latissimus dorsi muscle can be harvested on the thoracodorsal vascular system and anastomosed to the gluteal vessels.

Minimally invasive flap harvest

The rectus flap has emerged to be a workhorse in perineal reconstruction in these settings, as it brings in well-vascularized tissue to an often-irradiated bed with a large amount of dead space. However, the traditional rectus flap harvest involves a midline laparotomy. Minimally invasive abdominoperineal resections and pelvic exenterations are increasingly being used to limit morbidity. In these settings, some groups have explored the possibility of harvesting the rectus flap in a similarly minimally invasive manner. Early experiences focused on endoscopic-assisted harvests. In 1996, Bass described using a balloon dissector to create a plane between the posterior sheath and rectus muscle, followed by CO_2 insufflation and rectus harvest.[44] Subsequently, Friedlander *et al.* utilized a tripod device to improve visualization during minimally invasive rectus harvest in cadavers.[45] Both of these techniques utilized incisions through the anterior sheath. The first clinical case of laparoscopic harvest was performed by Greensmith in

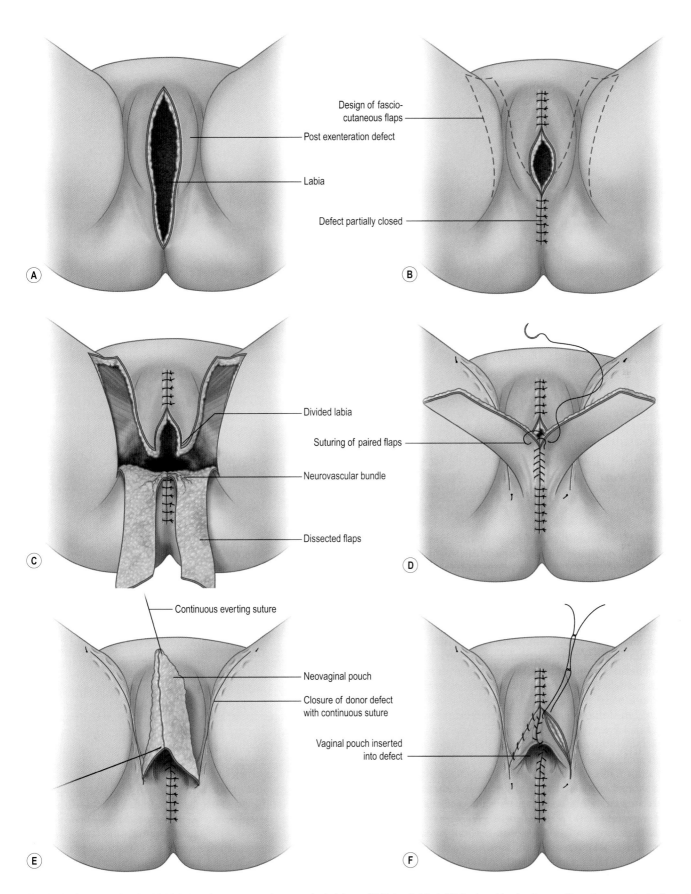

Fig. 17.17 Elevation of pudendal thigh flaps for more extensive, or vaginal, defects. **(A)** Perineal defect. **(B)** Design of fasciocutaneous flaps along vascular territory of perineal arteries. **(C)** Primary closure of donor sites and suturing of flaps together. **(D)** Inset of flaps into pelvic and perineal defect.

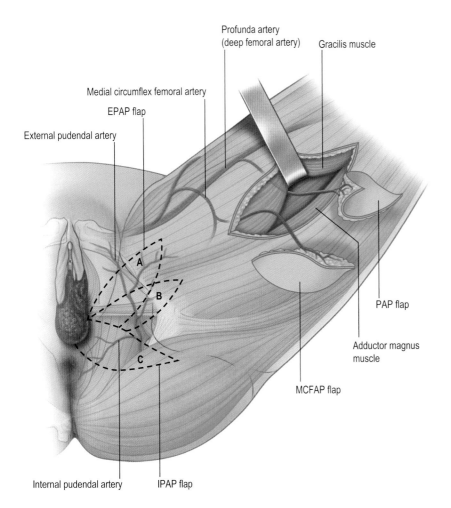

Profunda artery
(deep femoral artery)   Gracilis muscle

Medial circumflex femoral artery

EPAP flap

External pudendal artery

A

B

C

PAP flap

Adductor magnus
muscle

MCFAP flap

Internal pudendal artery   IPAP flap

Fig. 17.18 Perforating vessels in the vicinity of the perineum. Several flaps shown based on internal or external pudendal vessels, and the profunda femoris and medial circumflex femoral vessels. EPAP, external pudendal artery perforator; IPAP, internal pudendal artery perforator; MCFAP, medial circumflex femoral artery perforator; PAP, profunda artery perforator.

2000.[46] In their transperitoneal approach, the rectus is harvested by taking down the posterior sheath. Therefore no incisions were made in the anterior sheath, decreasing the risk of hernia formation. More recently, Winters *et al.* reported on the results of robotic total pelvic exenteration in conjunction with a laparoscopic harvested rectus flap.[47] Yet another advancement is the use of the robot in rectus flap harvest. Selber reported their experience with the Intuitive Surgical robot, with harvest times of 45 minutes and incisions limited to 3 ports, totaling 2 inches in length.[54] As experience builds in other disciplines with minimally invasive techniques, it is likely that flap harvests will continue to be refined in plastic surgery as well.

Special considerations – sphincter reconstruction

For treatment of rectal cancers in patients seeking to avoid colostomy, some centers have advocated resection with sphincter reconstruction as a strategy. In such cases, functional transfer using one or two gracilis muscles wrapped around a perineal colostomy has been described with some success, although the morbidity of this approach is high.[55] Early authors in the 1950s encountered issues generating resting sphincter tone when using a voluntary muscle to perform an autonomic smooth muscle function. This was addressed using an implantable electrical stimulator (electrically stimulated dynamic graciloplasty), but a high

complication rate ultimately led the manufacturer to withdraw the device from the US market in 1999.[48] Evolution of this approach has continued in Europe where the device is still available, but one meta-analysis has shown more favorable results using an artificial bowel sphincter (Acticon Neosphincter™, American Medical Systems, Minnetonka, MN).[49] All methods of sphincter preservation or reconstruction carry a significant (30–100%) risk of complications, and a consensus is still not available on the best of these alternatives. Despite these newer options, in a recent review the traditional abdominal colostomy has been advocated as still having the lowest complication rate for this group of patients.

Postoperative care

The management of these patients follows the basic tenets of surgical postoperative care. A key principle is to avoid excessive pressure on the flap, as this can lead to venous congestion and flap loss. The authors have the patients on bed-rest for several days, followed by progressive ambulation. However, the patients are instructed not to sit upright for several weeks. Drains are typically placed in both the donor site and the perineum. Deep venous thromboprophylaxis in the form of sequential compression devices and subcutaneous heparin is used. Nutrition must be optimized. The patient is seen regularly by all involved teams postoperatively.

Outcomes, prognosis, complications

It is important to emphasize that reconstruction of the perineum cannot eliminate complications. In fact, multiple series highlight complications even in the best of circumstances; what has improved with advances in the state of surgical treatment has been the complication profile. In earliest descriptions, extensive abdominoperineal resections and exenterations were accompanied by significant mortality, small bowel obstruction, small bowel fistulae, pelvic abscesses, perineal hernias, and profound interstitial fluid losses through what frequently became a chronic draining perineal wound.

In contrast, when flaps are used, the small bowels are separated from the radiated pelvic basin, which dramatically reduces or eliminates all these major sequelae in every major series.[18,19,29,50] Complications remain at a significant incidence of 5–33% overall, but these manifest a shift toward minor complications. Still present are delayed wound healing at the inset incisions, seromas, or superficial dehiscence or infection, but none of these normally requires re-operation. Understanding the vulnerabilities of the surgical site and the clinical outcome data makes it possible to employ a reconstructive plan that can limit complications and make perineal reconstruction a relatively safe, reliable process.

Access the complete reference list online at **http://www.expertconsult.com**

11. Wee JT, Joseph VT. A new technique of vaginal reconstruction using neurovascular pudendal-thigh flaps: a preliminary report. *Plast Reconstr Surg.* 1989;83:701–709.

18. Nelson RA, Butler CE. Surgical outcomes of VRAM versus thigh flaps for immediate reconstruction of pelvic and perineal cancer resection defects. *Plast Reconstr Surg.* 2009;123:175–183. *The largest series of prospectively collected cases comparing abdominal vs thigh flap reconstruction in perineal reconstruction, demonstrating most favorable complication profile after abdominal flap use (M.D. Anderson Cancer Center).*

19. Butler CE, Gündeslioglu AO, Rodriguez-Bigas MA. Outcomes of immediate vertical rectus abdominis myocutaneous flap reconstruction for irradiated abdominoperineal resection defects. *J Am Coll Surg.* 2008;206:694–703. *Documented improvement in outcomes using flaps in radiated perineal reconstruction.*

20. Shibata D, Hyland W, Busse P, et al. Immediate reconstruction of the perineal wound with gracilis muscle flaps following abdominoperineal resection and intraoperative radiation therapy for recurrent carcinoma of the rectum. *Ann Surg Oncol.* 1999;6:33–37. *Early evidence that flaps can reduce complication rate from 46% to 12% in radiated perineal reconstruction.*

29. Chessin DB, Hartley J, Cohen AM, et al. Rectus flap reconstruction decreases perineal wound complications after pelvic chemoradiation and surgery: a cohort study. *Ann Surg Oncol.* 2005;12:104–110. *Documented improvement in outcomes using abdominal flaps in radiated perineal reconstruction (Memorial Sloan-Kettering Cancer Center).*

31. Lee MJ, Dumanian GA. The oblique rectus abdominis musculocutaneous flap: revisited clinical applications. *Plast Reconstr Surg.* 2004;114:367–373. *Variation in skin paddle design, expanding the size and the reach of the rectus abdominis myocutaneous flap.*

34. Whetzel TP, Lechtman AN. The gracilis myofasciocutaneous flap: vascular anatomy and clinical application. *Plast Reconstr Surg.* 1997;99:1642–1652, discussion 1653–1655.

38. Wong S, Garvey P, Skibber J, Yu P. Reconstruction of pelvic exenteration defects with anterolateral thigh-vastus lateralis muscle flaps. *Plast Reconstr Surg.* 2009;124:1177–1185.

51. Lefevre JH, Parc Y, Kernéis S, et al. Abdomino-perineal resection for anal cancer impact of a vertical rectus abdominis myocutaneus flap on survival, recurrence, morbidity, and wound healing. *Ann Surg.* 2009;250:707–711.

18

Acute management of burn and electrical trauma

Raphael C. Lee and Chad M. Teven

SYNOPSIS

- Review of the pathogenesis of various burn-related injuries
- Review of the classification and diagnosis and of cutaneous burn injuries
- Review of the first aid management of burn patients
- Develop insight between extent of burn injury and physiologic stress response
- Review acute management of burn patients, including fluid, nutritional, and wound care
- Review state of the art wound management of burn patients
- Learn indications for wound debridement, wound dressing and splinting, and skin grafting

 Access the Historical Perspective section online at
http://www.expertconsult.com

Aims of burn care

Rescue: Stop the burn injury process and provide life support.

Resuscitate: Immediate support must be provided for any failing organ system.

Refer: After initial evacuation to emergency department, some patients with burns may need transfer to a burn center for multidisciplinary intensive care.

Resurface: Close open wounds as soon as possible.

Reconstruct: Replace damaged anatomic structure needed for normal function.

Rehabilitate: Recover, as far as is possible, physical, emotional, and psychological well-being.

Epidemiology

Burn trauma incidence has a cyclical pattern with the peak incidence during holidays and vacations. According to the most recent statistics compiled by the World Health Organization and the World Fire Statistics Center (WFSC), fire cause roughly 6.6 million major burn injuries and 400 000 deaths every year.[1] In economically developed nations, 1–2% of the population receives a burn injury annually and 10% of those require professional medical attention. Roughly 10% of those requiring medical attention have major burns that require burn center management. Major burn trauma is a disease of the poor and disabled, as the majority of cases occur in poor neighborhoods and in low-income countries where prevention programs are almost nonexistent. A practical indication of fire mortality risk is the international median death rate which is 0.9–1.2 per 100 000 inhabitants by country. In addition, the cost to society in terms of lost wages, acute medical care, and rehabilitation is enormous. In 2009, the WFSC noted that the cost of direct fire losses ranged from 0.06–0.26% of countries' gross domestic product (GDP) and the cost of indirect fire losses ranged from 0.002–0.95% of countries' GDP.

Risk factors

In addition to poverty, major burns are more common in populations that have some predisposing factor such as mental illness and substance abuse. For adults, predisposing factors to burns include alcoholism, senility, psychiatric disorders, and neurological disease such as epilepsy.[2] Children under 5 years old are also particularly vulnerable to burns. Among all children, scald burns account for about two-thirds of burn injuries. For children less than 5 years of age, they account for 75% of all pediatric burns.

Definition of burn injuries

Stedman's medical dictionary list more than 22 types of burn injury including thermal, chemical, electrical, friction, cement, and other "burns".[3] The pathogenesis of these burn injuries is quite different which causes some confusion. What they have in common is that the injury process begins with damaging molecular structure of tissue. Although the treatment of these different injuries would have aspects in common, there are differences that address the specific pathogenesis.

Thermal burns occur when the tissue temperature exceeds the chemical bond energy thresholds stabilizing molecular structure. This happens when tissue comes in contact with a thermal energy source that results in heat transfer by conduction, convection, and/or radiation. When tissues are heated to supraphysiologic temperatures for long enough, molecular alterations result that do not spontaneously reverse. The extent of tissue damage resulting from heat exposure depends on the tissue type and recent history of heat exposure. Cells have some capability to repair such molecular damage. The amount of molecular damage tolerated by cells is dependent on the history of trauma exposure. Cells adapt to repetitive trauma by upregulating stress proteins that repair or remove damaged molecules. In effect, tissue exposure to sub-lethal injury increases cellular injury repair rates, thus allowing tissues to subsequently survive greater thermal burn injury. This is called thermal preconditioning. When the extent of damage exceeds cellular repair capabilities, then loss of cell and subsequent tissue viability results, which manifests as a "burn".[4]

The extent of thermal burn injury scales with both the tissue temperature and duration of exposure (Fig. 18.1). Characteristic molecular alterations include disruption of cell membranes, aggregation of unfolded proteins, curling of collagen and other structural macromolecules, activation of degradative proteases, and dehydration. A basic comparison across modes of cell injury due to burns can be appreciated in Fig. 18.2. Cell membrane disruption is common to all forms of trauma because membranes are the most vulnerable vital cellular structure.[5]

Contact with electrical power sources may cause injury by both thermal and non-thermal processes. The injury mode(s) depend on the voltage, current capacity, and frequency of the

power source. In addition, other parameters such as the duration of electrical contact and the anatomic path of the current through the body are deterministic. For example, although static electrical shocks involve more than 1000 volts, they do not injure tissue because the current is small and it only passes on the outer surface of the body.

Frequency is a measure of how often the current changes direction. The abbreviation "DC" (i.e., direct current) indicates the current frequency to be zero (i.e., constant voltage), and "AC" (i.e., alternating current) indicates that the current is changing direction of flow (i.e., alternating polarity) with time. Tissue damage can result from electrical energy at any frequency in the electromagnetic spectrum (Table 18.1). But the exact molecular details of the injury is quite frequency dependent. The frequency of the change is measured in cycles per second and is called Hertz (Hz). Commercial electrical power usually operates in the 50–60 Hz range meaning it changes direction every 8.4 milliseconds.

Radiation injury can result from either ionizing or non-ionizing electromagnetic waves. Ionizing is higher energy and shorter wavelength radiation. Ionizing radiation is absorbed at the atomic level to disrupt the electron structure around

Table 18.1 Electrical shock by frequency

Frequency range	General applications	Tissue injury pathway
"Low" (DC – 10 kilohertz)	Commercial electric power; batteries.	Joule heating; cell membrane electroporation
"Radiofrequency" (10 kilohertz to 10 megahertz)	Radio-communication; diathermy; electrocautery	Joule heating; dielectric heating of proteins
"Microwave" (10 megahertz to 10 gigahertz)	Microwave heating	Dielectric heating of water
"Light and ionizing" (10^{15} hertz and higher)	Photo-optical and ionizing irradiation (ultraviolet, X-ray, gamma, etc.)	Heating and direct protein damage; oxidative damage

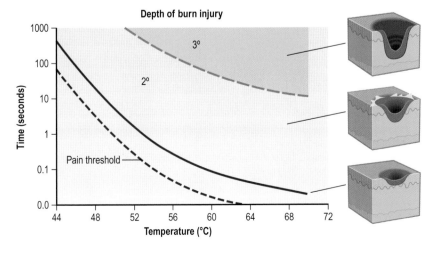

Fig. 18.1 The importance of both temperature and time in determining the depth and extent of injury is illustrated by this curve. The threshold for feeling pain precedes injury and sensation is lost once all cutaneous pain receptors are burned. The data is adapted from various models.

Before injury

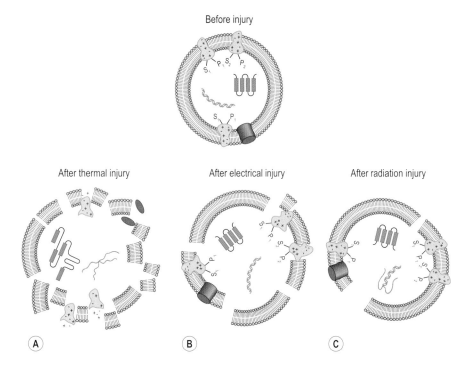

After thermal injury   After electrical injury   After radiation injury

(A)   (B)   (C)

Fig. 18.2 Schematic illustration of the different molecular manifestations of thermal, electrical, and radiation burn trauma.

molecules or atoms. This leads to chemical reactions that damage. In tissue, water is the primary absorber. Ionizing irradiation causes water and molecular oxygen to bind and produce hydroxyl radicals with an unpaired electron in the valence shell. Unpaired electrons on the outer shell are very reactive with other biomolecules causing damage to DNA, proteins, lipids, etc.

Burn trauma classification

Clinically, thermal burns are classified according to depth of penetration from the epithelial surface into the tissue. This stratification was historically labeled "degree of burn wound", but more recently by fractional thickness of injury (Table 18.2).

Flash and flame burns

Although the mechanisms of "flash" and "flame" burns are similar, there are some differences. Both flame and flash phenomena pertain to hot, electricity-conducting gases emanating from a fire that emit light and radiation. Typically, a flame burn implies that an individual was exposed to flames in an ongoing fire, whereas a flash burn implies that the individual was exposed to an explosion (e.g., gasoline) or an electrical arc (Fig. 18.3). Flash and flame burn injuries are very common cause of adult burn admissions. Ambient air temperatures associated with flash exposures are typically 10-fold higher than flame exposures and have a significant radiation heat energy component. Fortunately, flames and flashes are composed of gases with very low heat capacity. Flash burns usually result in less deep burns than flame burns because flash heating is usually quite brief. In general, flash burn depth relates the amount and type of fuel that explodes. Unlike flash injuries, flame burns are often associated with inhalational injury and other concomitant trauma.

Scald burns

Scald burns result from skin contact with hot liquid or steam. Scald burn depth is often more difficult to clinically judge than flame burn depth because it is a low temperature burn (Fig. 18.4). Tissue structural changes are less noticeable compared to flame burns. The depth of scald injuries are often not apparent for 48–72 hours. The skin temperature changes in scald burns depend on geographic location, being less severe in high mountainous regions than at sea level. Unless superheated at high pressures, the maximum skin temperature reached in scalding water can be 100°C. Because water has a very high heat capacity and also cools by evaporation, the duration of tissue contact with damaging temperatures

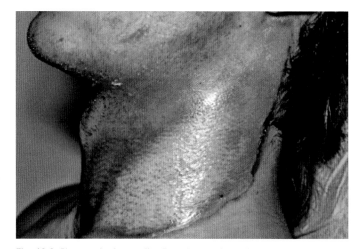

Fig. 18.3 Photograph of a gasoline flame burn to the neck and face illustrating the non-uniform heat exposure corresponding to depth of injury from deep partial to epidermal.

Table 18.2 Clinical presentation of thermal burn wounds

Depth of burn	Skin involvement	Examples	Signs	Sensation	Self-healing capacity	Skin healing time	Visible scarring
Epidermal burn	Epidermis	Brief flame or flash; Sunburn	Dry and red, blanches with pressure, no blisters	Tender and painful when exposed to air.	Excellent with use of occlusive dressing	Within 7 days	Unusual
Superficial partial-thickness burn	Epidermis and part of the papillary dermis	Scald (spill or splash), short flash	Pale pink with fine blistering, blanches with pressure	Very painful	Excellent with proper management.	Within 14 days	Can have color match defect. Low to moderate risk of hypertrophic scarring
Deep partial-thickness burn	Epidermis, the entire papillary dermis down to reticular dermis	Scald (spill), flame, oil or grease	Dark pink to blotchy red, capillary refill sluggish to none. In child, may be dark lobster red with mottling	May be painful or reduced/absent sensation	Should not be left to heal by itself, but instead should probably be submitted to surgery	14 to over 21 days	Moderate to high risk of hypertrophic scarring
Full-thickness burn	Entire thickness of the skin and possibly deeper	Scald (immersion), flame, steam, oil, grease, chemical, high-voltage electricity	White, waxy or charred, no blisters, no capillary refill. May be dark lobster red with mottling in child	Insensate	No healing capacity and as such should always be submitted to surgery	Never. Replaced by scar and contracture	Yes.

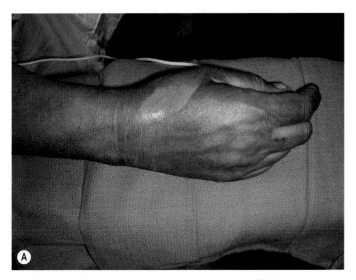

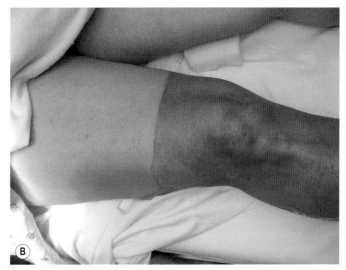

Fig. 18.4 Typical appearance of superficial skin burns from **(A)** low energy electical arc flash and **(B)** sunburn.

depends on factors like clothing or other vapor barriers. The water temperature is also important. Skin surface contact with 60°C water creates a deep dermal burn in 3 seconds but will cause the same injury in 1 second at 69°C. If the water contains oils or lipids, as in soups, evaporation is slowed, resulting in longer burn duration and a deeper skin injury.

Hot object "contact burns"

Contact burns occur when tissue is exposed to a hot, thermally-conducting object (e.g., cooking pan or radiator). Burn depth depends on the thermal energy storage capacity and thermal conductivity of the object. Thus a hot metal rod would produce a deeper burn than a hot plastic rod. Contact burn injuries are often associated with workplace-related hand burns, patients prone to seizures, and intoxicated individuals. They are also seen in elderly people after a loss of consciousness; such a presentation requires a workup of the cause of syncope. Contact burns commonly result from mechanical contact with hot metals, thermoplastic composites, glass, or coals in an industrial setting. Because the heat energy transfer is large, contact burns often involve full-thickness skin and subcutaneous tissue.

Tar and asphalt burns

Tar and asphalt burns occur in workers engaged in surfacing pavement and roads, roofing, and other industrial applications. Tar is a wax and oil composite that is difficult to remove from skin without causing injury. When hot tar makes contact with skin, it solidifies and sticks. The tar usually retains sufficient heat to produce prolonged heat transfer to the skin resulting in deep skin burns. Once cooled, tar strongly adheres to the tissues and is chemically damaging. In order to expedite the cooling and solidification process one should apply cold water. Often, the tar is cool by the time the patient arrives at the medical facility. Injuries typically occur on the exposed skin of the face and extremities, and the burn is of variable depth ranging from deep partial to full thickness.

Electrical injury/"electrical burns"[6,7]

Extent of injury depends on the amount of current and the anatomic path of the current. Contact with an electrical power source results from both direct electrical force injury and heat generation. Commercial electrical power operates in the narrow frequency range of DC to 150 Hz. Electrical shocks in this frequency range are clinically most common is the second most common cause of workplace injury. Because of the electrolytes content in tissue fluids, the body is a good conductor of electricity. With wet skin, the DC resistance of a current path from one hand to the other is about 1000 ohms and from hand to both feet is about 750 ohms. At frequencies greater than 100,000 Hz electrical power can radiate across air gaps from the power source into the body. Microwave (10^9 Hz) and infrared heating (10^{19} Hz) used for cooking is a common example (see Table 18.1).

Sometimes electrical shock injuries are categorized as low or high voltage depending on whether the voltage is below or above 1000 volts, respectively. Practically when the contact voltage is less than 1000 volts, direct mechanical contact is usually required to initiate current flow. Once mechanical contact with the power source occurs, it is can be impossible

Table 18.3 Thresholds for electrical current effects	
Threshold effect of 60 Hz current (Path: hands to feet)	Threshold current (milliamps)
Tingling sensation/perception	1–4
"No let go" (i.e., skeletal muscle tetany)	16–20
Respiratory muscle paralysis	20–50
Ventricular fibrillation	50–120

to voluntarily release the contact. Thus shock times are typically longer in low-voltage shocks with higher risk of cardiopulmonary arrest (i.e., electrocution). For high voltages (>1000 volts), electrical arcing initiates the electrical current flow before mechanical contact. High-voltage electrical shocks are associated with more severe extremity damage, but lower rates of electrocution. Also, high-voltage contact arcs can reach very high temperatures leading to corneal burns and clothing ignition.

As the current passes through the body, injury may result from either heat generation in the tissue or from strong electric forces that rupture cell membranes. Electrical shock by commercial electrical power can produce a range of neuromuscular effects (Table 18.3). Of course, the most life threatening is the immediate risk for cardiopulmonary arrest when the current passes through the heart, especially during the myocardial repolarization phase.

Factors that determine the relative contribution of heat versus direct electrical damage include the amount of current, anatomic location, and the contact duration. The type of clothing, use of protective gear, and the power capability of the electrical source also make a difference. So knowing just the voltage of contact is not enough to estimate the injury.

Because the epidermal layer of the skin is very resistive, it is instantly destroyed in contact with electrical power sources greater than 100 volts. Contact with commercial AC electrical power does not cause "entrance" and "exit" wounds because the current goes in and out of every contact point (Fig. 18.5). If the skin is wet, extensive subcutaneous tissue damage can occur without skin burns. For electrical shock injury, the skin surface area damage is not reflective of the injury extent. The damage is more volumetric and scattered along the current path, often requiring CT or MR imaging to quantify (Fig. 18.6).

Peripheral nerve and skeletal muscle tissues are most vulnerable to non-thermal damage during electrical shock. Just 14–16 milliamperes of current passing through the forearm induces tetanic contractions of muscles controlling handgrip, which may prevent a person from voluntarily releasing the electrical conductor (see Table 18.3). Joint dislocations and fractures may result from the muscle spasm as well. A current of 50 milliamperes or more passed through the chest can result in cardiopulmonary arrest. Non-thermal electric injury to nerves and muscles can occur in milliseconds while taking seconds for burns to occur. Thus brief shocks commonly result in neuromuscular function disturbances in the absence of thermal burns.

Disruption of skeletal muscle membranes leads to release of myoglobin and hemoglobin that enter the circulation and muscle edema. Skeletal muscle damage and edema lead to secondary compartment syndromes, leading to further

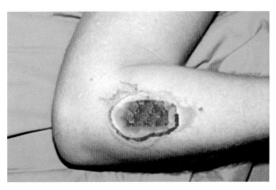
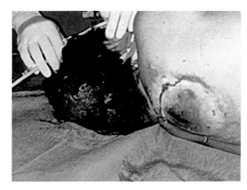

Fig. 18.5 Appearance of a full-thickness electrical contact burns resulting from contact with AC electrical power. All contacts are entrance points and all are exit points because the current is alternating direction of flow during the shock.

ischemic injury. Release of myoglobin from muscle into the circulation and then into the urine is a characteristic feature of severe electrical shock injury. Renal failure can result from intrarenal aggregation of myoglobin. Direct electrical shocks to the head may cause increased intracranial pressure as well.

Lightning is another common form of electrical shock. Most of the lightning current passes around the body via the lightning arc to ground. There are often superficial epidermal burn marks that do not penetrate into the dermis. Cardiac and central neurological arrest often occurs due to the magnetically induced electrical currents. Because signs of brain damage are unreliable, they cannot be used to guide CPR efforts. In both high-voltage electrical contacts and lightning strikes, ignition of the electrical arc can produce a strong thermo-acoustic blast wave resulting in barotrauma. The flash generated radiant heat injury associated with arc-mediated electrical current can lead to eye injury. Table 18.1 presents a classification of electrical injury according to frequency regime.

Frostbite

Frostbite results from tissue exposure to lethally cold or freezing temperatures. Loss of circulation, and the reperfusion consequences on rewarming, are major pathogenic features of clinical frostbite injury. Demographically, distal extremities, ears, and other ambient air exposed areas of the face are involved.[8] Tissue tolerance to cold (above freezing) temperatures is also very tissue type specific. Brain and cardiac function does not tolerate temperatures less than 21°C for more than 20–30 minutes. Skin tolerates it better but not for more than 19–24 hours. Freezing with ice formation in any tissue creates a severe injury. Ice formation in tissues concentrates electrolytes around proteins that leads to unfolding and aggregation. Tissue freezing also dehydrates cells in addition to promoting ice crystal propagation through cell membranes. The thaw cycle also causes injury by osmotic rupture of tissue cells. The majority of frostbite cases arise from homeless or disabled populations in climates with cold winters. Ethanol consumption predisposes to cold injury by vasodilatation and rapid heat loss.[8]

Radiation burns

The most common cause of radiation burn is heavy sun exposure. Sunlight produces a wide spectrum of radiating energy from infrared to cosmic energies. In typical sunburn, it is the heavy dose of the infrared heating and ionizing ultraviolet (UV) that does the most damage. UV radiation produces oxidative free radicals in the epidermis and dermis.

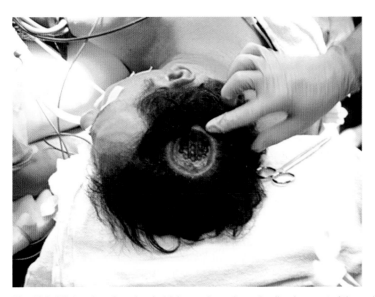
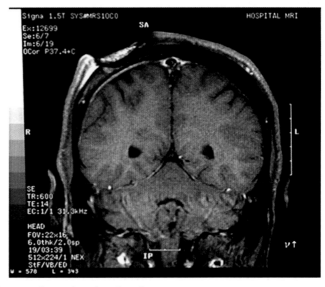

Fig. 18.6 MR imaging of an electrical injury to the scalp to visualize the extent of tissue damage and secondary edema formation.

When free radical scavenging mechanisms are exceeded, damage occurs. It is rare that the burn depth is greater than epidermal or superficial dermal. Clinical manifestations are painful partial-thickness burns and blistering. Sunscreen lotions absorb the UV and increase the amount of sun exposure required to cause a burn. However, until recently they did not totally shield the entire UV range. There is some evidence that use of narrow-band (i.e., UVB) sunblock is associated with other long-term consequences related to prolonged exposure to DNA reactive irradiation outside of the blocked UVB band.

Radiation injuries also occur from therapeutic, accidental, space travel, or military use of ionizing irradiation. The molecular target of the radiation depends on the type of radiation.[9] Most commonly, the damage is caused by generation of hydroxyl (OH*) free radicals in oxygenated water. The higher the water and oxygen in the tissue, the greater the radiation injury to cells. Under conditions of tissue water and oxygen content, doses of radiation less than 5 Gray (Joules/kilogram) create protein and DNA cross-links that destroy the body's most rapidly dividing cell lines. Severe immune compromise due to neutropenia and bleeding secondary to thrombocytopenia are seen over a period of 3–5 weeks. At higher levels of exposure (30–100 Gy), the membranes of cells, even non-proliferating nerves and muscle, are damaged leading to tissue death within 6–24 hours. Non-ionizing radiation such as that from a hot fire or an electrical arc can cause transfer of thermal energy to the body by non-ionizing irradiation. This is similar to infrared heating.

Deliberate burn injury

Up to 10% of pediatric burns are due to non-accidental injury. Detecting these injuries is important, as many children who are repeatedly abused eventually suffer a fatal injury. Usually children less than 3 years old are affected. As with other non-accidental injuries, the history and the pattern of injury may arouse suspicion (Fig. 18.7). A social history is extremely important. Abuse is more common in poor households with single or young parents. Such abuse is not limited to children: elderly and other dependent adults are also at risk, and a similar assessment can be made in these scenarios.

Chemical injuries and burns

See Chapter 22 for details of chemical burns.

Clinical features of thermal burn injury

The skin is the largest organ of the body and serves multiple functions essential to our survival including (1) transport barrier against evaporative fluid and heat losses; (2) thermal regulation; (3) immune barrier against microbes and foreign chemicals; and (4) sensory receptors that provide information about environment. Burn injuries often disrupt the skin barrier functions, and the secondary effects of large burn injury result in systemic stress responses.

Burn survival associated with burn injuries is strongly dependent on the age of the patient, the percentage of the body surface burned, and the presence or absence of smoke-inhalation injury. Without the support of modern medical facilities, individuals who suffer a major burn injury are

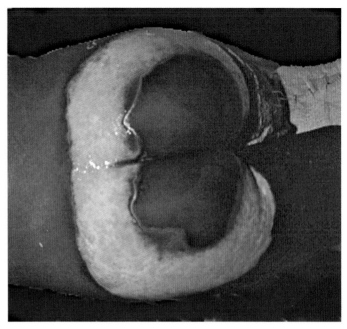

Fig. 18.7 The anatomic pattern of injury often provides clues to the cause of injury. The burn tideline associated with sitting in a bath of hot water. The non-burned in the center of the ring results from contact with the ceramic in the tub that is a poor conductor of heat.

unlikely to survive more than a few days. In the United States, only 25% of burn-related deaths occur after the patient arrives in the burn center. In remote locations without access to an acute care medical center, death results from acute dehydration and hypothermia. In such locations, initial burn management must control this dehydration and hypothermia until the patient arrives at a hospital.

Zones of burn tissue injury

Skin burns resulting from contact with a heat source usually result in a non-uniform injury depth (Fig. 18.8). The pattern of thermal burns has been traditionally divided into three zones: (1) coagulation, (2) stasis, and (3) hyperemia. The three zones of a burn were initially described by Jackson, Topley, and Cason in 1947.[10]

The zone of coagulation represents the most severely burned tissue with extensive aggregation of intracellular and extracellular matrix proteins, dehydration due to protein coagulation, and loss of vascular perfusion. Historically, the damage is thought to be irreversible and requires surgical or enzymatic removal.

Moving away from the heat source contact area, the next zone of injury is the zone of stasis, which is characterized by cellular swelling, partial extracellular matrix denaturation, and decreased vascular perfusion. Initial resuscitation timing and strategy can influence the survival of tissue in the zone of stasis. Additional insults, such as ischemia infection, or edema, can push tissue in this zone toward necrosis. With proper resuscitation and wound care, however, cell recovery can occur and matrix molecular changes may be reversed.

The next adjacent zone is the zone of hyperemia. In this outermost zone, vascular perfusion is increased in response to inflammatory cytokines released from the zone of stasis.

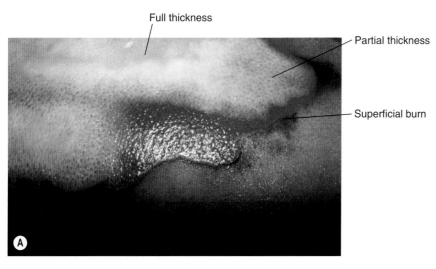

Full thickness

Partial thickness

Superficial burn

(A)

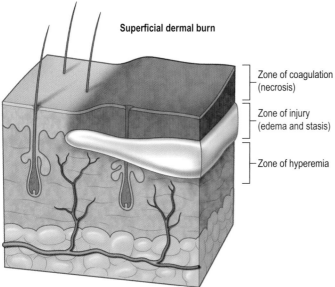

Superficial dermal burn

Zone of coagulation
(necrosis)

Zone of injury
(edema and stasis)

Zone of hyperemia

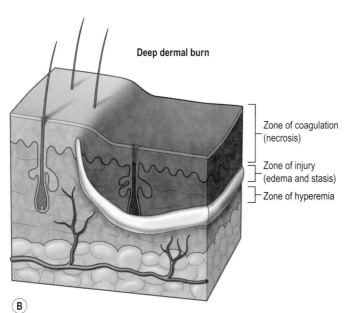

Deep dermal burn

Zone of coagulation
(necrosis)

Zone of injury
(edema and stasis)

Zone of hyperemia

(B)

Fig. 18.8 (A) Flame burn on abdomen showing zones of injury. Dry full-thickness thermal burn coagulation is in the upper aspect of the wound. Away from the coagulation zone, the injury severity becomes progressively less. **(B)** Schematic showing zones of injury in deep and superficial dermal burns.

Histopathology in this zone reveals swollen cells and capillaries, suggestive of cell membrane disruption. The tissue here will invariably recover unless the burn victim suffers prolonged hypotension and/or sepsis.

Estimating the depth of a skin burn on the basis of clinical exam is difficult. The depth of a skin burn is not always obvious initially, and experienced experts often disagree. This is particularly true for scald or other low temperature burns in patients with dark skin. Many methods have been proposed to predict the depth of the injury immediately or soon after injury (ultrasound examination, intravenous fluorescent probes), but none has been as reliable as serial examination of the wound. The final depth of the injury typically becomes obvious 48–72 h after injury. Rarely, the thermal injury penetrates into the subcutaneous or deep tissue.

Local injury progression

Burn tissue damage activates inflammatory mediators, especially in the perfused subsurface, which degrade and extend the volume of injury. Release of mitochondria, xanthine oxidase, and other intracellular substances into the circulation generates destructive reactive oxygen species in the tissue as well as the local circulation. This causes thrombosis that potentiates ischemic tissue necrosis. Both complement activation and intravascular stimulation of neutrophils add to small vessel injury. Increased histamine activity, enhanced by the catalytic properties of xanthine oxidase, further increases in vascular permeability. As a general rule, the volume of tissue necrosis after an uncomplicated burn injury progresses over 48 hours.

One important goal of resuscitation is to minimize the injury extension. Edema formation often follows a biphasic pattern. An immediate and rapid increase in the water content of burn tissue is seen in the first hour after injury. A second and more gradual increase in fluid flux of both the burned skin and non-burned soft tissue occurs during the first 12–24 h following burn trauma. The rate of progression of tissue edema is dependent upon the adequacy of resuscitation that is determined by both rate and composition of the fluid administered.

Systemic injury progression

Thermal burn trauma produces an inflammatory cytokine storm of local and system mediators that are released into the circulation. These inflammatory cytokines mediate generalized stress responses including altered capillary permeability and total body interstitial edema. This is mediated by numerous vasoactive inflammatory mediators, including serotonin, bradykinin, prostaglandins, and leukotrienes produced by calcium influx into thermally disrupted cells. Inflammatory cytokines also trigger generalized proteolysis, lipolysis, gluconeogenesis, and an increased metabolic rate. Severe burn injury also depresses the function of the heart, large vessels, and lungs.

Cardiovascular responses to the burn often result in hypotensive shock once the burn reaches 20–30% of the total body surface area (TBSA). Shock is a pathophysiologic condition characterized by high sympathetic neurovascular responses such that brain and cardiovascular perfusion is prioritized over other tissues. Splanchnic vasoconstriction

and gut ischemia are features. Adding to this can be a delay or inadequate fluid resuscitation resulting in increased hematocrit values that increase the blood viscosity and hamper perfusion.

As in the treatment of hypovolemic shock, the primary initial therapeutic goal is to quickly restore vascular volume and to preserve tissue perfusion to minimize tissue ischemia. Burn shock is not easily or fully repaired by isotonic electrolyte fluid resuscitation. Large volumes of resuscitation solutions maybe required to maintain vascular volume during the first several hours after an extensive burn. Burn shock evolves through a dynamic pathophysiologic process even if hypovolemia is corrected. Increases in pulmonary and systemic vascular resistance (SVR) occur despite adequate preload and volume support. Such cardiovascular dysfunctions can further exacerbate tissue ischemia resulting in a vicious cycle of accelerating organ dysfunction. The critical concept in burn shock is that massive fluid shifts can occur even though total body water remains unchanged.

Hints and tips

- Thermal burn results in three distinct zones: coagulation, stasis, and hyperemia.
- One goal of burn resuscitation is to maintain perfusion of the zone of stasis.
- Major burns (>15–20% TBSA) require burn center admission (see Box 18.1).
- Different burn mechanisms lead to different anatomic injury patterns.

BOX 18.1 Burn injuries that should be referred to a burn unit

- Partial-thickness burns >10% TBSA and patients requiring burn shock resuscitation
- Burns that involve the face, hands, feet, genitalia, perineum, or major joints
- Deep partial-thickness burns and full-thickness burns in any age group
- Circumferential burns in any age group
- Electrical burns, including lightning injury
- Chemical burns
- Burns with a suspicion of inhalation injury
- Burns of any size with concomitant trauma or diseases that might complicate treatment, prolong recovery, or affect mortality
- Diseases associated with burns such as toxic epidermal necrolysis, necrotizing fasciitis, staphylococcal scalded child syndrome, etc., if the involved skin area is 10% for children and elderly and 15% for adults or any doubt of treatment
- Burned children in hospitals without qualified personnel or equipment for the care of children

(Modified from: American Burn Association.)

Acute burn trauma management

Initial evaluation and treatment in the field

Treatment of a burned patient starts with the removal of the patient to a safe environment where first aid can be rendered. In all cases (especially chemical or electrical injuries), care must be taken to avoid personal injury by ensuring that the area is safe and that appropriate protective clothing is worn. Basic trauma victim life support protocols should be used to assess and stabilize the patient. Top priority should be given to assessing the airway, breathing, and circulation, and presence of any coexisting injuries that may require more urgent treatment than the burn. Clothing should be removed. If the burn occurred in a closed space, inhalation injury should be ruled out by inspecting the oropharyngeal airway for soot and carbon particulate. Supplemental oxygen is given if signs of hypoxia exist.

Substantial evidence demonstrates the beneficial effects of cooling on reducing tissue damage and wound healing time.[11] Although immediate burn wound cooling is preferable, application of cooling after a delay of more than half an hour is still beneficial to the burn wound.[11] While transporting the patient to a medical center, cooling the burn wound by wrapping in a hydrogel blanket or room temperature water-soaked gauze is useful. Cooling for 20 minutes should achieve near maximum benefit. However, systemic hypothermia and hypotension must be avoided. The patient should be triaged to a level 1 trauma center, stabilized, and then transported to the nearest burn unit for definitive management (Box 18.2).

Initial hospital burn management

Once the patient arrives at the emergency room, the primary survey should focus on the ABCs of trauma management (i.e., *Airway*, *Breathing*, and *Circulation*). It is also important to exclude associated trauma and inhalation injury (see below). Once the life-threatening problems are stabilized, a secondary survey should be done including relevant history (i.e., time, location, and circumstances of the injury), where the patient was found, and their condition. Past medical and social history, current medication usage, drug allergies, and tetanus status should be determined. It is also important to consider the possibility of non-accidental burns or scalding.

A thorough assessment of a person with a burn should then take into account:

- The type of burn (e.g., flame, scald, electrical, radiation, or chemical)

- The depth and TBSA of the burn, and therefore the severity
- Signs of inhalation injury (singed nasal hair, black carbon in the sputum, or carbon in the oropharynx)
- Any coexisting medical conditions (e.g., cardiac, respiratory, or hepatic disease; diabetes; pregnancy; or immunocompromised state)
- Any predisposing factors that may require further investigation or treatment (e.g., a burn resulting from a fit or faint)
- The possibility of non-accidental injury
- The person's social circumstances (e.g., ability to self-care or need for admission).

The airway should be secured because upper airway obstruction can develop quickly. Smoke inhalation causes more than 50% of fire-related deaths. Patients sustaining an inhalation injury may require aggressive airway intervention. Most injuries result from the inhalation of toxic smoke; however, super-heated air may rarely cause direct thermal injury to the upper respiratory tract (see complications, below). Patients who are breathing spontaneously and at risk for inhalation injury should be placed on high-flow humidified oxygen. Patients trapped in buildings or those caught in an explosion are at higher risk for inhalation injury. These patients may have facial burns, singeing of the eyebrows and nasal hair, pharyngeal burns, carbonaceous sputum, or impaired mentation. A progressive change in voice quality or hoarseness, stridorous respirations, or wheezing may be noted. The upper airway may be visualized by laryngoscopy, and the tracheobronchial tree should be evaluated by flexible bronchoscopy. Patients who have suffered an inhalation injury are also at risk for carbon monoxide poisoning.

Chest radiography is not sensitive for detecting inhalation injury. The pulse oximeter is not accurate in patients with carbon monoxide poisoning because only oxyhemoglobin and deoxyhemoglobin are detected. CO-oximetry measurements are necessary to confirm the diagnosis of carbon monoxide poisoning. Other pulmonary assessments include arterial blood gas measurements and bronchoscopy. Patients exposed to carbon monoxide should receive 100% oxygen using a non-rebreather facemask.

The secondary survey must include assessment of the location, depth, and fractional TBSA burned. Tetanus prophylaxis should be administered as appropriate for immunization history. Tetanus immunization or vaccine prophylaxis must be administered according to standard practice guidelines, particularly in elderly patients (Box 18.3).

Initial wound management

In the hospital setting, initial wound management is focused on documenting the extent of injury, removing harmful wound contaminants, reducing the rate of bacterial colonization, and preventing evaporative water loss. Assessment of burn depth and size on admission is important in making decisions about fluid resuscitation requirements, type of topical antimicrobial agents to use, splints, dressings, and surgery (see Table 18.2).

Appropriate wound care reduces morbidity and mortality. It also shortens the time for healing and return to normal function and reduces the need for secondary reconstruction.

BOX 18.2 Field management of a major burn

Perform an ABCDE primary survey:

A – Airway with cervical spine control

B – Breathing

C – Circulation

D – Neurological status and pain control

E – Environment (heat loss) control

F – Initiate fluid resuscitation

- Stop the burning process
- Rough estimate of % body surface area burned
- Establish peripheral intravenous access and start lactated Ringer's; in children, the interosseous route can be used for fluid administration if intravenous access cannot be obtained
- Pain management as needed
- Catheterize patient or establish fluid balance monitoring
- Take baseline blood samples for investigation (full blood count; urea and electrolyte concentration; clotting screen; blood group; and save or cross-match serum)
- Electrical injuries:
  - 12-lead electrocardiography
  - cardiac enzymes
- Inhalational injuries:
  - chest X-ray
  - arterial blood gas analysis
- Clean and dress wounds
- After completion of the primary survey, a secondary survey should assess the depth and TBSA burned, reassess, and exclude or treat associated injuries
- Arrange safe transfer to specialist burns facility

Epidermal (superficial) burns

These burns involve only the epidermis. They do not present with blisters, but are hyperemic and tender. Sunburn is the most common example. Over 2–3 days, the erythema and the pain subside. Protective occlusive dressing changes is usually all that is required, with analgesia and intravenous fluids for extensive injuries. By about day 4, the injured epithelium peels away from the newly healed epidermis underneath, a process which is commonly seen after sunburn. By day 7, healing is complete by regeneration from viable keratinocytes within dermal glands and hair follicles. The patient should be advised of measures to provide symptomatic relief, e.g., cover with occlusive dressing like petrolatum gauze or hydrogels, non-steroidal analgesia (e.g., ibuprofen), and avoid direct sun exposure. First-degree burns are not considered in calculation of the TBSA burned.

Superficial partial-thickness burns

These involve the epidermis and superficial dermis. Blistering is a characteristic feature. The exposed superficial nerves make these injuries painful. They leave behind epithelial-lined dermal appendages including sweat glands, hair follicles, and sebaceous glands. When thermal damaged superficial dermal tissue is removed, epithelial cells migrate from the lining of dermal glands and hair follicles, forming a new, fragile epidermis on top of a thin residual dermal bed.

Most superficial facial burns close well with an initial washing, immobilization, and proper physiologic dressing for healing. Progression to a deeper burn is unlikely unless it is allowed to dry, becomes edematous, and/or infected. Also, systemic problems such as hypotension and sepsis from a remote site may cause a partial-thickness wound to convert. Treatment is aimed at preventing wound progression by the use of occlusive dressings, since epithelialization progresses faster in a moist environment. Appropriate management of blisters is a subject of debate. Topical antimicrobials are useful if the patient is likely to be immune-compromised by a large TBSA burn or other comorbid condition.

Optimal burn care requires early excision and grafting of all burned tissue that raises the infection risk or will result in problematic scars, so a good estimation of burn depth in the first few days is crucial. The appearance of the wound – and the apparent burn depth – changes dramatically within the first 7–10 days. A burn appearing superficial on day 1 may appear considerably deeper by day 3. For superficial burns, wound closure with thin epithelium is expected within 14 days by regeneration of epidermis from keratinocytes within dermal glands and hair follicles.

Deep partial-thickness burns

Deep partial-thickness burns cause total or near total destruction of dermal glands and hair follicles. Closure by epithelialization takes much longer or does not occur. Distinguishing between deep partial-thickness burns that are best treated by early excision and grafting and superficial partial-thickness burns that heal spontaneously is never simple by physical examination. Many burn wounds have a mixture of superficial and deep partial-thickness burns, making precise classification of the entire wound difficult. They may initially seem superficial, with blanching on pressure or sweating on bright light exposure, but later progress to manifest fixed capillary staining on re-examination after 48 h.

Some deep partial-thickness injuries will heal if the wound environment is optimized to encourage endogenous healing. This includes keeping it warm, moist, and at reduced microbial colonization. Topical antimicrobials are important to use because immune function in the damaged dermis is compromised. Deep partial-thickness burns that require longer than 3 weeks to heal likely result in hypertrophic scars and scar contractures. This often results in functional impairment. Therefore large area deep partial-thickness burns, or those in highly mobile or cosmetically sensitive areas, should be excised as soon as possible to a viable depth and then skin grafted.

Full-thickness injuries

Full-thickness burns involve all layers of the dermis and often injure underlying subcutaneous adipose tissue as well. These burns are usually insensate because of destruction of nerve endings, but the surrounding areas are extremely painful. All regenerative elements are non-viable, and the dehydrated extracellular matrix will not support healing. Over days and weeks if left *in situ*, eschar separates from the underlying viable tissue, leaving an open, unhealed bed of granulation tissue. Without surgical intervention, wound healing occurs by eschar separation, granulation from the base, and wound contraction, leaving severe contracture deformities. Unless the burn wound is very small, optimum treatment of full-thickness burns involves early excision and grafting.

Extremities should be examined for existence of circumferential burns with distal vascular compromise. This problem is not to be confused with skeletal muscle compartment syndromes. In pure muscle compartment syndromes, the peripheral pulses are not reflective of severity of muscle perfusion compromise. With subtotal or total circumferential burned skin contraction, the perfusion to all tissues in the extremity at and distal to the site of compression are at risk for ischemic necrosis. In most cases it is best to prophylactically incise or "release" the deep burn tissue at the time of burn center admission to allow expansion and restoration of distal perfusion. This mitigates the risk. In borderline cases where it is not clear that vascular compromise will occur after adequate resuscitation, monitoring of distal arterial pulses is essential for early detection of ischemia. Doppler monitoring of distal pulses is commonly used to monitor, but this measurement is very qualitative. Pulse oximetry of digits distal to the possible site of constriction is useful as well, but changes in fingertip oxygenation occur late. Subcutaneous or muscle compartment pressures should be measured if there is doubt. Escharotomy should be performed for pressures >30 mmHg.

Important special considerations

For patients with facial burns, fluorescent staining of the cornea and ophthalmologic consultation are necessary. For patients with genital burns a urethral catheter should be placed. For patients with perineal burns a rectal catheter should be placed. Specific burn circumstances such as chemical and electrical burn injuries may dictate further diagnostic studies and treatments (see later).

Quantifying the burn size[12,13]

For several reasons, it is important to accurately estimate the fractional body surface area involved in a burn injury. It is useful to guide the initial fluid resuscitation rate and determine whether the patient should be admitted to a burn center or intensive care facility. For adults, Wallace's "rule of nines" is a simple and moderately accurate method of calculating TBSA burned. However, the Lund and Browder chart is slightly more accurate and widely accepted because it accounts for the different body proportions in infants and children (Fig. 18.9). For all patients, burn diagrams and photographs of the wounds should be placed in the medical record and updated if the burn wound extends. More precise methods require computer estimation (Fig. 18.10). The improved accuracy is valuable for more precisely stratifying burn injuries when investigating quality control or research outcomes.

Inhalation injury[14–16]

Upper and lower airway injuries can result from inhalation of chemically reactive smoke and/or other products of combustion. People burned in house or building fires are at high risk for inhaling smoke or fumes. Thermal injury from the flame or hot gases can damage the upper airway (supraglottic). This results in burns of the lips and oropharynx, leading to edema and airway obstruction. Heat rarely causes subglottic injury unless the inhalant is hot steam. The products of combustion

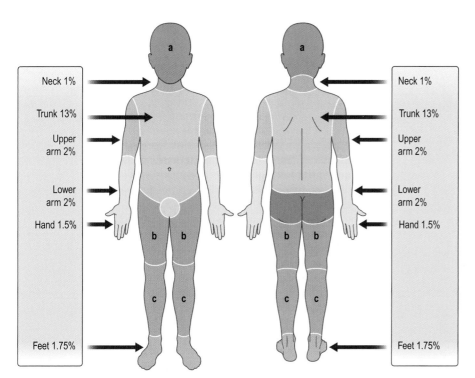

Body part	0 yr	1 yr	5 yr	10 yr	15 yr	Age
	relative % of body surface area					
a = 1/2 of head	9 1/2	8 1/2	6 1/2	5 1/2	4 1/2	
b = 1/2 of thigh	2 3/4	3 1/4	4	4 1/4	4 1/2	
c = 1/2 of lower leg	2 1/2	2 1/2	2 3/4	3	3 1/4	

Fig. 18.9 Estimation of burn size with the Lund and Browder method. Body surface area calculations in children must account for unique pediatric body proportions, here with the Lund and Browder method.

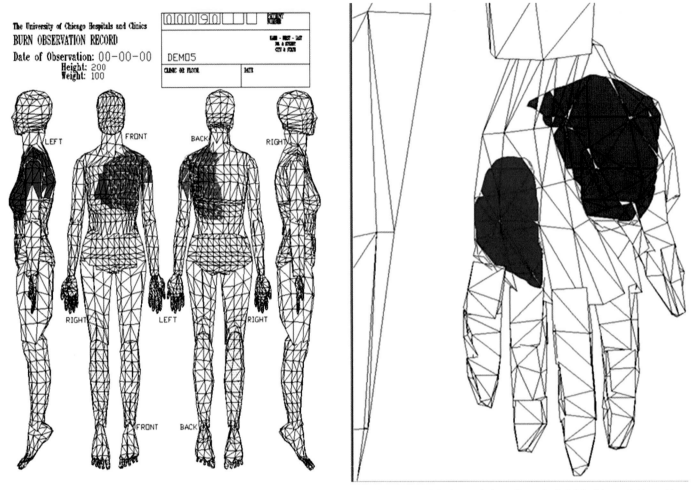

Fig. 18.10 Future burn charting will involve more precise digital technology and adjustable charts to match body morphology. *(From Orgill, DP. Excision and skin grafting of thermal burns. New Engl J Med. 2009;360:893–901.)*

are chemically reactive and are directly toxic to cells. The resulting chemical injury causes edema, bronchospasm, and bronchorrhea. The intrabronchial transudate is not cleared because of loss of mucosal ciliary action and atelectasis and potentially pneumonia follows. Bronchopulmonary inhalation injury releases inflammatory mediators that also depresses cardiac muscle function. Successful management involves delicate fluid resuscitation to avoid pulmonary edema and subsequent respiratory failure (Box 18.4).

Burn patients with inhalation injuries exhibit significantly higher mortality rates than comparable TBSA burn patients without inhalation injury. Consequences of smoke inhalation account for more than 50% of fire-related deaths. Most smoke inhalation victims are injured in closed space house fires. The

degree of respiratory injury depends on the type and properties of the toxic gases and chemicals emanating from burning carpets, furniture, and other domestic objects comprising the smoke to which the patient is exposed.

A high index of suspicion is needed to manage these patients. Inhalation victims may or may not have facial burns, erythema of mucous membranes, and soot in the airways. Examination of the pharynx for evidence of edema or particulate should be done as soon as possible after a patient is extracted from a closed space fire. Stridor, difficulty speaking, or history alone is enough to proceed with flexible bronchoscopy (gold standard for diagnosing inhalation injury).

Inhalation injury results in bronchial edema and sequestration of fluid in pulmonary alveolae. A strong indication that pulmonary edema is developing is when the resuscitation fluid requirement to maintain urine output far exceeds Parkland formula guidelines. The common clinical pattern of significant inhalation injury is large fluid requirements, high pulmonary artery pressures, and large ventilation–perfusion O_2 gradient. Early endotracheal intubation is important in patients with upper airway or inhalation injury to safeguard patency of the airway, to deliver mechanical ventilatory support, and to provide aggressive pulmonary toilet (Box 18.5).

BOX 18.4 Signs of inhalational injury

- History of flame burns or burns in an enclosed space
- Full-thickness or deep dermal burns to face, neck, or upper thorax
- Singed nasal hair
- Carbonaceous sputum or carbon particles in oropharynx

Carbon monoxide intoxication

Carbon monoxide (CO) is a combustion byproduct from the burning of biomaterials such as petroleum products, coal, and gas. CO binds to deoxyhemoglobin at 40 times greater affinity than molecular oxygen (O_2). It also binds to intracellular proteins, particularly those involved in handling oxygen for energy metabolism. These two effects lead to intracellular and extracellular hypoxia and a shift to inefficient anaerobic metabolism, resulting in metabolic acidosis. Closed space fires often have high CO levels. CO toxicity can occur with or without inhalation injury.

In the presence of carboxyhemoglobin, conventional electrode blood gas analyzers display erroneously high values for the calculated oxygen saturation and content. In these circumstances pulse oximetry is also inaccurate as it cannot differentiate between oxyhemoglobin and carboxyhemoglobin and may therefore give normal results.

A blood oximeter, however, accurately determines oxygen saturation and content and also rapidly measures carboxyhemoglobin concentrations. However, under conditions of CO intoxication, arterial blood gas analysis will reflect metabolic acidosis and raised carboxyhemoglobin levels but may not show hypoxia. Treatment is with 100% oxygen with a nonrebreather facemask, which displaces carbon monoxide from hemoglobin much faster than atmospheric oxygen.

The amount of carbon monoxide produced in a car engine can cause fatal carbon monoxide poisoning without producing enough particulate matter to cause inhalation pneumonitis. Also, some burning materials do not produce much CO. The half-life of carboxyhemoglobin is ≈1 hour at an FIO_2 near 100%.

Patients with carboxyhemoglobin levels greater than 25–30% have had clinically significant exposure to combustion products and should be ventilated (Table 18.4). When hyperbaric oxygen therapy is available, it can reduce the blood half-life of carbon monoxide to 23 minutes. Hyperbaric oxygen is recommended for patients with carboxyhemoglobin levels greater than 25%, myocardial ischemia, cardiac dysrhythmias, or central neurological abnormalities. Hyperbaric oxygen is also recommended for pregnant women and young children with carboxyhemoglobin levels of ≥15%.

Cyanide intoxication

Nitriles, which contain hydrogen cyanide (HCN), are commonly used in industrial solvents, polyurethanes, and vinyl plastic. They all release HCN during burning. HCN is rapidly absorbed in lungs or skin and contributes to the morbidity from smoke inhalation in industrial fires. Cyanide competitively inhibits oxygen binding to hemoglobin and inhibits the cytochromes of oxidative phosphorylation, resulting in cellular energy depletion. Dicobalt edetate is known treatment for massive cyanide poisoning in cases of ingestion or industrial explosion. In cases of inhaled cyanide products, the plasma concentrations of free cyanide is often low. Use of dicobalt edetate to treat low cyanide levels is risky because it is also toxic. A better approach is to use amyl nitrite inhalant or sodium nitrite intravenously. They convert hemoglobin to methemoglobin, which has a lower cyanide binding affinity.

Fluid resuscitation

Initiation of intravenous fluid administration should begin immediately in major burn resuscitation. Establishment of burn resuscitation IV fluid protocols should be reserved for burns involving greater than 20% TBSA (Table 18.5). In pediatric patients, fluid resuscitation should be initiated in all infants with burns ≥10% TBSA and in older children with burns ≥15% TBSA. Lactated Ringer's solution with or without colloid is the most commonly used fluid for burn resuscitation.

Patients undergoing post-burn fluid resuscitation should have a Foley catheter inserted in order to monitor urine output. Urine output should be used as a measure of renal perfusion and to assess fluid balance. In adults, a urine output of 0.5–1.0 mL/kg per hour should be maintained.

The color and consistency of the initial urine in patients with deep thermal burns or electrical injury should be monitored. The urine may be dark red, indicating hemoglobinuria or myoglobinuria. These heme-proteins can precipitate in the renal collecting ducts resulting in renal failure. If so, then osmotic or tubular diuretics should also be used to flush the renal collecting ducts to avoid renal failure.

In elderly patients, patients with cardiorespiratory disease, and patients who have delayed presentation, consider inserting a central venous pressure line. This can play an important part in the subsequent restoration of volume in a patient with a severe burn. The risks of infection related to a central line are small in the early stages. With current methods of line management these risks are outweighed by the importance of the line for monitoring and access.

Resuscitation fluid composition

Burn fluid resuscitation protocols vary considerably across different burn centers. The amount of replacement fluid is predicted from the extent of burn and size of the patient, and fluid replacement should proceed at the same rate as the loss. Fluid administered in excess of the capillary leak is excreted by the kidney or results in increased hydrostatic pressure and

Table 18.4 Clinical signs of carboxyhemoglobinemia	
Carboxyhemoglobin levels	**Symptoms**
0–10%	Minimal (normal level in heavy smokers)
10–20%	Nausea, headache
20–30%	Drowsiness, lethargy
30–40%	Confusion, agitation
40–50%	Coma, respiratory depression
>50%	Death

Table 18.5 Fluid resuscitation formulae

Formula	Electrolyte	Colloid	Glucose
Colloid formulae			
Brooke	Lactated Ringer's at 1.5 mL/kg/% TBSA burn	0.5 mL/kg/% TBSA burn	2 L 5% dextrose
Evans	0.9% NaCl at 1 mL/kg/% TBSA burn	1 mL/kg/% TBSA burn	2 L 5% dextrose
Slater	Lactated Ringer's 2 L/24 h	Fresh frozen plasma at 75 mL/kg/24 h	2 L 5% dextrose
Crystalloid formulae			
Modified Brooke's	Lactated Ringer's at 2 mL/kg/% TBSA burn		
Parkland	Lactated Ringer's at 4 mL/kg/% TBSA burn	20–60% estimated plasma volume	Titrated to urinary output of 30 mL/h
Hypertonic saline formulae			
Hypertonic saline solution (Monafo)	Maintain Urine output at 30 mL/h Fluid contains sodium 250 mmol/L		
Modified hypertonic (Warden)	Lactated Ringer's + 50 mmol/L NaHCO$_3$ for 8 h to maintain UO at 30–50 mL/h Lactated Ringer's to maintain UO at 30–50 mL/h beginning 8 h post-burn		
Dextran formula (Demling)	Dextran 40 in saline at 2 mL/kg/h for 8 h Lactated Ringer's titrated to maintain urine output at 30 mL/h	Fresh frozen plasma at 0.5 mL/kg/h for 18 h beginning 8 h post-burn	

extra interstitial edema. Lactated Ringer's solution most closely resembles the electrolyte content of normal body fluids.

Today, the Parkland formula (and its variations) is the most widely used burn resuscitation guideline. The Advanced Burn Life Support curriculum supports the use of this formula for initial resuscitation in burn injury. It is 4 mL/kg/% TBSA, describing the amount of lactated Ringer's solution required in the first 24 h after burn injury. Starting from the time of burn injury, half of the fluid is given in the first 8 h and the remaining half is given over the next 16 h. As an example, by the Parkland formula, a 70 kg patient with a 40% TBSA burn receives (70×40×4) = 11,200 mL of lactated Ringer's solution during the first 24 h after the burn (approx. 470 mL/h).

Crystalloids are the resuscitation fluids of choice given the lack of survival benefit and increased cost associated with albumin and a meta-analysis comparing albumin to crystalloid that showed a more than doubled mortality rate with albumin. Administration of albumin, and other colloids, are usually avoided in the first 24 h post-burn, but may have a role in severe burns (>50% TBSA) after the first 24 h.

Vital organ function monitoring

Heart rate and urine output are the primary modalities for monitoring fluid therapy in patients with large burns although there is a lack of evidence supporting them. Titrating intravenous fluid administration rate according to body weight is commonly practiced. A minimum of 0.5–1.0 mL/kg per hour urine output in adults and in children is recommended, but 1–2 mL/kg per hour urine output is preferred. Lesser hourly urinary outputs in the first 48 h post-burn almost always represent inadequate resuscitation. Hemodynamic monitoring and treatment of deviation from normovolemia are the

fundamental tasks in intensive care. A pulse rate ~110 beats/min or less for adults usually indicates adequate volume, with rates >120 beats/min usually indicative of hypovolemia. Narrowed pulse pressure provides an earlier indication of shock than systolic blood pressure alone.

Non-invasive blood pressure measurements by cuff are inaccurate due to the interference of tissue edema and read lower than the actual blood pressure. An arterial catheter placed in the radial artery is the first choice, followed by the femoral artery. The decision to perform invasive hemodynamic monitoring requires careful consideration. The lack of benefit associated with goal-directed supranormal therapy has resulted in waning enthusiasm for the use of pulmonary artery catheters.

Management of the burn wound

The priority in thermal burn wound management is to create a physiologic environment for healing and reduce evaporative losses. In a hospital setting, wounds should be washed and debrided of contaminants and loose non-viable tissue. For treatment of major burns or in cases of smaller deep burns, topical antibiotics are useful to control microbial invasion. This is followed by coverage with sterile dressings that serve as an evaporative barrier and as an immobilizer. Extremity splints also help immobilize and are helpful to reduce edema and pain. There is a wide range of wound products that subserve these purposes. Preferences vary from institution to institution.

Some practical first aid tips can make a significance difference to the burn outcome. Small superficial burns are reduced in severity by immediate rapid cooling with running cold water for 5 to 10 minutes. Subsequent careful cleaning, immobilization, and barrier protection are the next steps. Topical antibiotics are unnecessary unless there is contamination with foreign material or large surface area involvement.

In wilderness situations well away from medical facilities, the management priority for large surface area burn wound care is the control of evaporative and heat losses until evacuation. Cleaned and boiled leaves can block evaporative losses. The inner cambium layer of plants or trees can also be used to provide salicylates to control pain and reduce bacterial and fungal growth.

Topical antimicrobials

In the hospital setting, some formulation of topical silver is the most commonly used topical antibacterial. Historically, silver nitrate, as a 0.5% solution, was widely used to deliver silver ions. It is a liquid which can be poured into the gauze dressings on the patient to saturate them. It has excellent antibacterial properties but does not diffuse through eschar well. Therefore it was not too effective in reducing colonization beneath the eschar in deeper burns. Also, silver nitrate is not very popular with burn center staff because it discolors the bedding, floors, and uniforms. A more practical approach is to use nanocrystalline silver coated dressings like Acticoat (Fig. 18.11). When soaked in water, it releases mono- and di-atomic silver ions, which can penetrate burn tissue and provide broad-spectrum antibacterial coverage. This product does not discolor the skin as silver nitrate does. The Acticoat sheeting has enough silver to be effective for several days. It has to be moistened with pure water occasionally to release and transport the silver ions into the wound.

Silver, like many other transition metals, interferes with bacterial energy metabolism. Other antimicrobial transition metals clinically used are iodine, gold, titanium, platinum, and zinc, to name a few. Silver ions are particularly well tolerated by tissue and rapidly cleared in the urine. Another silver compound, silver sulfadiazine, is a very commonly used antimicrobial ointment because it combines the antimicrobial effects of silver and sulfur. It has intermediate eschar penetration and a large antibacterial spectrum. The antibacterial activity lasts 8–10 h, and the dressings are changed once or twice a day. Silver sulfadiazine causes an exudative reaction

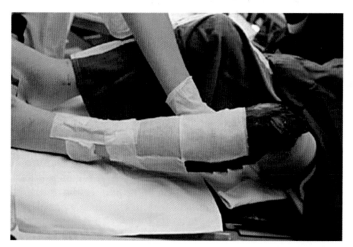

Fig. 18.11 Application of a topical antimicrobial silver dressing (Acticoat) is helpful to control bacterial proliferation in partial- to full-thickness burn injuries, large surface area burns, heavily contaminated or immunocompromised patients.

and discolors the wound, making it more difficult to evaluate burn depth. This exudative process is associated with a transient leucopenia in some patients when it is used on large open areas. A switch to a different topical agent for a few days allows the white blood cell count to recover. Restarting silver sulfadiazine rarely causes recurrent leucopenia. Silver sulfadiazine is best indicated for mid to deep partial-thickness burns that clearly require excision and grafting.

Mafenide acetate is also commonly used and looks similar. It has excellent eschar penetration and bacteriostatic action. Use of mafenide acetate on full-thickness burns prevents deeper infections. Often used on the ear, it helps against infection of the cartilage. Systemic absorption of mafenide acetate, when it is applied to large burns, produces a metabolic acidosis by inhibition of carbonic anhydrase. The effect is usually noted after 3–5 days. Use of the compound on open wounds also causes pain on initial application. The pain subsides after several minutes, but patients usually do not like it.

Another topical dressing uses Dakin's solution (0.25% sodium hypochlorite), which is an oxidizing solution that bleaches proteins and lipids. It is good for suppressing bacterial and fungal proliferation but is not effective against bacterial biofilms. Practically, it is useful as a three-times-per-day gauze dressing to reduce devitalized tissue. Dakin's solution-soaked gauze is often alternated with topical silver sulfadiazine to treat a wound heavily colonized with bacteria.

Agents such as povidone-iodine solution and nitrofurazone are still used but are becoming less popular. They are less expensive to use. However, efficacy and side effects limit acceptance. They are still widely used in many parts of the world where access to more expensive agents is limited.

Fortunately, wound infections have decreased dramatically during the last two decades largely due to a better understanding of their causes. Early tangential debridement and coverage of the wound with skin have markedly decreased the opportunity for burn wound infection. Despite meticulous wound care, and even under the most sterile conditions, the patient's own microbial flora quickly colonizes and then invades the non-perfused burned tissue. Only by removing the devitalized burn tissue and providing stable coverage is native immunity restored and risk of wound infection reduced.

Wound dressings[17]

Standard burn dressing consists of petrolatum or wax impregnated gauze, which effectively restores the transport barrier function of the epidermis and helps to prevent adherence to the wound. A topical antiseptic may be applied over this followed by cotton wool or gauze to absorb the exudate. Newer dressings have been introduced that are claimed to be less adherent and allow less water to be lost by evaporation from the wound while also protecting it from external pathogens. Some dressings are meant to provide temporary coverage while others are meant to be permanent. These may further be classified into two groups:

- *Biologic dressings*: These can be used either fresh or after storage following preparation by freezing in liquid nitrogen or rapid dehydration (lyophilization) and later reconstitution with saline.

- *Physiologic dressings*: These consist of synthetic materials such as polyethylene or silicone, which prevent adherence to the wound, and plastic films, which reduce evaporation and contamination.

Biologic wound dressings

Restoring immune defense boundaries to beyond the healing wound requires restoration of vascular perfusion superficial to the wound. This requires placement of a biologic dressing on the wound that is capable on inducing vascular ingrowth (Table 18.6). The most widely used biologic dressing remains fresh or frozen human cadaveric split-thickness skin. Properly handled, cadaveric skin remains viable and vascularizes ("takes") when it is placed on a healing wound bed. The allograft's dermal capillaries imbibe interstitial fluid, proliferate, and form channels with the wound bed 2–5 days after grafting. The process is called inosculation. Once taken, the wound beneath the allograft becomes sterile and less inflamed.

Of course, allografts contain foreign proteins that will trigger an immunologic rejection. The immunosuppression manifested in massively burned patients may delay the rejection process some, but eventually the grafts develop an abundant inflammatory cell infiltrate and the epidermis dies and sloughs from the patient. Loss of the epidermis requires replacement with another set of cadaveric grafts, or, it is hoped, the patient is ready for coverage with permanent autologous tissue. Disease transmission from the donor to the burn patient is possible but occurs rarely. After the epidermis is lost, much of the allograft dermis is remodeled by host cells and becomes permanent.

Porcine skin and freeze-dried human cadaveric skin were once routinely used to cover burn patients. But they do not take as well as properly preserved frozen cadaveric skin. Thus they tend to detach from the wound bed during dressing changes. However, they do help reduce evaporative fluid and heat loss while they are attached to the burn wounds.

Over the past 30 years, both cellular and acellular tissue-engineered biomaterials have served an increasing role in burn wound coverage (Table 18.7). Acellular matrices of collagen and proteoglycans were manufactured and marketed as the first "artificial skin" and is now sold under the name Integra. A thin porous polymer sheet, to serve as a barrier to the air, covers the surface. Engraftment of the material takes approximately 2 weeks, and any disturbance, such as excessive movement, fluid accumulation under the material, or infection, causes loss of the material. Once the matrix is incorporated, the polymer sheeting is replaced with a thin skin graft.

Replacement of lost dermis with Integra in deep partial- or full-thickness burns during the initial treatment of the wound may decrease the need for later reconstructive surgery by improving the elasticity of the grafted skin. Despite the technical problems with these materials, the advantage of reducing functional and cosmetic deformities from scar contractures makes their use worthwhile in many clinical situations.

AlloDerm is chemically treated human cadaver dermis produced from skin allograft in which most non-cross-linked proteins and lipids are removed. It is commercially available as dermal replacement. As with Integra, however, the engraftment process for the matrix is variable, and the matrix does not support the attachment of cultured epidermal autograft

(CEA) well. The rapidity of the engraftment process is likely to depend on growth factors in the matrix material as much as the wound bed on which it is placed.

Many burn centers do not routinely use dermal replacements for extensive coverage of acute burns because of the unpredictable engraftment rate. Large clinical trials have not demonstrated a survival advantage with use of any of these products or presented data to suggest that post-injury function is improved. Therefore most surgeons use dermal replacements for burn scar reconstruction when supplemental dermis improves functional and cosmetic outcomes of the grafting procedure and survival of the patient is not an issue.

The ability to grow and expand isogenic human keratinocytes in tissue culture has made survival possible for burn injuries above 90% TBSA that would not have survived previously. No longer was an adjacent skin source a major limitation for restoration of a keratinizing isogenic epithelial barrier. In a landmark case in 1984, twin children with burns over almost their entire bodies were treated at the Shriners Burns Institute in Boston with cultured keratinocytes taken from a small biopsy specimen of undamaged axillary skin. During the course of their treatment, the keratinocytes were successfully expanded in tissue culture and used to resurface some of their wounds. Survival of the patients was directly attributed to the use of the technique. Now several biotechnology companies offer the service for a fee. Skin biopsy specimens sent to the company are expanded in culture and returned to the patient, usually in 2–3 weeks. The sheets of CEA are placed directly onto a cleanly debrided wound bed. The grafts survive well, and wounds close much faster than without treatment.

Despite its theoretic advantages, CEA has not succeeded in solving wound coverage needs of massively burned patients. Covered by CEA, areas around joints and over muscles, such as the face, have little motion and poor function. CEA placed directly on muscle or subcutaneous tissue only gradually forms a basement membrane, in some cases during 6 months. Often a mechanically fragile and unstable epithelial barrier results, which requires replacement over time.

Physiologic wound dressings

Similar products like Biobrane are also available. These composite materials provide a matrix for vascular endothelial cell ingrowth and establishment of perfusion beyond the wound surface that effectively internalizes the wound surface. They can provide physiologic wound control in large percentage surface area burns while the process of autograft coverage takes place. Biobrane is also used to provide a physiologic environment for the healing of superficial burns and donor sites.

If applied correctly, Biobrane usually adheres to the wound bed. Left undisturbed, the dressing limits fluid loss and prevents stimulation of the wound. Epidermal regeneration is undisturbed beneath. The dressing falls off once the epithelial layer completely heals underneath; much like a scab falls off an open wound once it is healed. These materials work best on superficial partial-thickness burn wounds and skin graft donor sites that heal in 7–10 days. Placed on deeper wounds, the materials adhere poorly and as foreign material serve as a nidus for infection much like the burn eschar. These

Table 18.6 Temporary skin substitutes

Product	Source	Layers	Category	Uses	Advantages	Disadvantages
Human allograft	Human cadaver	Epidermis and dermis	Cryostored split-thickness skin	Temporary dressing of partial-thickness and excised burns before autografting or when there is a lack of autograft	A bilayer skin providing epidermal and dermal properties Revascularizes maintaining viability for weeks Dermis incorporates Antimicrobial activity	Epidermis will reject Risk of disease transfer Expensive Need to cryopreserve
Gammagraft	Human cadaver	Epidermis and dermis	Split-thickness skin	Temporary dressing of partial-thickness and excised burns before autografting or when there is a lack of autograft	A bilayer skin providing epidermal and dermal properties Revascularizes maintaining viability for weeks Dermis incorporates	Epidermis will reject Risk of disease transfer Expensive Store at room temperature
Human amnion	Placenta	Amniotic membrane	Epidermis Dermis	Temporary dressing of partial-thickness and excised burns before autografting or when there is a lack of autograft	Acts like biologic barrier of skin Decreases pain Easy to apply, remove Transparent	Difficult to obtain, prepare, and store Must change every 2 days Disintegrates easily Risk of disease transfer Expensive
Pig skin Xenograft	Pig dermis	Dermis	Dermis	Temporary dressing of partial-thickness and excised burns before autografting or when there is a lack of autograft	Good adherence Decreases pain More readily available compared to allograft Bioactive (collagen) inner surface with fresh product Less expensive than allograft	Does not revascularize and will slough Short-term use Need to keep the fresh product frozen
Oasis	Xenograft	Extracellular wound matrix from small intestine submucosa	Bioactive dermal-like matrix	Temporary coverage of superficial partial-thickness burns, although it has been used for coverage of autograft and for donor	Excellent adherence Decreased pain Provides bioactive dermal-like properties Long shelf-life, store at room temperature Relatively inexpensive	Mainly a dermal analogue Incorporates and may need to be reapplied
Transcyte	Allogenic dermis	Bilayer product Outer: silicone Inner: nylon seeded with neonatal fibroblasts	Bioactive dermal matrix components on synthetic dermis and epidermis	Temporary coverage of superficial partial-thickness burns, although it has been used for coverage of autograft and for donor	Bilayer analogue Excellent adherence to a superficial partial-thickness burn Decreases pain Provides bioactive dermal components Maintains flexibility Good outer barrier function	Need to store frozen until use Relatively expensive
Suprathel	Synthetic copolymer of polylactide, and ε-caprolactone	Monolayer	Synthetic epidermis and dermis	Temporary coverage of superficial partial-thickness burns, although it has been used for coverage of autograft and for donor	Long shelf-life, store at room temperature	Relatively expensive Not absorbent, requires fairly frequent replacement to obviate pooling of exudate and related problems

Table 18.7 Engineered skin substitutes or scaffolds

Product	Tissue of origin	Layers	Category	Uses	Advantages	Disadvantages
Apligraf	Allogenic composite	Collagen matrix seeded with human neonatal keratinocytes and fibroblasts	Composite: epidermis and dermis	Excised deep partial-thickness burn	Readily available	Expensive Vascularizes slowly No epithelial barrier No antimicrobial activity
Epicel	Autogenous keratinocytes	Cultured autologous keratinocytes	Epidermis only	Deep partial- and full-thickness burns >30% TBSA	Readily available Live cells	Expensive Vascularizes slowly No epithelial barrier No antimicrobial activity
Alloderm	Allogenic dermis	Acellular dermis (processed allograft)	Dermis only	Deep partial- and full-thickness burns	Readily available Live cells	Expensive Vascularizes slowly No epithelial barrier No antimicrobial activity
Integra	Synthetic	Silicone outer layer on bovine collagen GAG and shark chondroitin sulfate dermal matrix	Biosynthetic dermis	Full-thickness burns; definitive "closure" requires skin graft	Readily available Live cells	Expensive Vascularizes slowly No epithelial barrier No antimicrobial activity

materials have no antimicrobial activity and therefore should not be placed on a contaminated wound. Most of the newly developed synthetic biologic dressings are used mainly in developed countries because most of these products are extremely expensive.

Non-operative wound closure

For major burn patients, it is worthwhile to place these patients in protective isolation to limit contact with hospital-based pathogens, such as multidrug-resistant organisms. Despite these precautions, many have one or several bouts of infection through the course of their treatment. The skin and gut of the patient are common sources of microbial pathogens, and no known therapy can eliminate these sources of infection. Contamination and then overgrowth of burn wounds by pathogens causing a systemic picture of sepsis typically occur 2–3 weeks after injury. Early enteric feeding and early wound coverage with skin greatly reduce the incidence of burn wound infections.

Basically, most burn wounds eventually heal unless there is infection, lack of blood flow (tissue ischemia), or inadequate nutritional intake. Physiologic wound care helps minimize the chance of infection and maximize healing. The daily dressing changes in burn patients permit inspection of the wound to assess the need for further interventions but, more important, offer the chance to remove non-viable tissue. In burn centers, the providers dedicate a large part of the time to gently scraping off dead skin and proteinaceous debris that have gathered since the last dressing. This leaves a healthy bed for the migration of keratinocytes.

Conceptually, the approach to wound management is to create a healing environment that attempts to mimic the in

utero environment of a fetal wound. Typically, the wound is covered between dressings with a moist, antimicrobial covering to minimize microbial growth, fluid loss, and painful stimuli and to maximize skin regeneration. Superficial partial-thickness burns heal in a short time and with little pain or contracture with warm, moist and bacteria-free dressings.

For small deep partial- or full-thickness burns that could heal without causing functional limitations, the time for healing can be more than several weeks with high risk of infection. Fo r these wounds, it is far better to treat by surgical debridement and coverage with skin grafts or an engineered scaffold. For a deep burn over a small area or one with a patchy distribution, the time for healing by secondary intention may be no longer than the healing of a skin graft. For these wounds, surgical debridement and grafting may not be appropriate. After all, it takes a skin graft 7–10 days to stabilize on a wound and about the same amount of time for the donor site to heal.

Operative wound closure[18]

The main goals of surgical treatment of patients with burns are removal of damaged or devitalized tissue and replacement with viable tissue. It is well established that early removal of the necrotic tissue decreases wound infections and mortality. The tissue undergoing necrosis incites a local and systemic inflammatory response, serves as a growth medium for pathogens, and delays wound healing. Early closure reduces the time of inflammation. Open wounds lose heat and fluids, contributing to the patient's hyperdynamic and hypermetabolic state. To achieve early debridement and stable permanent coverage of the wound, the surgeon must overcome two main obstacles, the physical insult of the debridement process and, on occasion, the limited source of replacement skin for permanent coverage of large surface area burns.

Necrotic burn tissue is usually debrided in sequential layers until all tissue appears viable. In obvious full-thickness injuries, the burn can be excised to deep fascia in one stage to reduce blood loss. Optimal timing to accomplish debridement is within five days of injury to minimize blood loss. With major burns, treatment is directed towards preservation of life or limb, and large areas of deep burn must be excised before the burnt tissue triggers multiple organ failure or becomes infected. In such cases more superficial burns may be treated with dressings until healing occurs late or fresh skin donor sites become available.

The main limitation to removal of the burned tissue in large burns is the need to limit blood loss during the debridement. Blood platelet function often becomes less effective with repeated blood transfusions. Although some units practice large (>20% TBSA) debridement in one procedure, most burn units limit each operative session to debridement of 10–20% TBSA. This keeps blood replacement, fluid administration, and anesthetic requirements within the range of stress tolerance. Tangential debridement involves cutting the skin tissue at the depth of the dermal and subcutaneous capillary network (Fig. 18.12). Historically, before modern pharmacologic agents were available, tangential debridement of each square centimeter of burn would cause 1 mL of blood loss. Today, this amount of bleeding is uncommon due to use of pressure

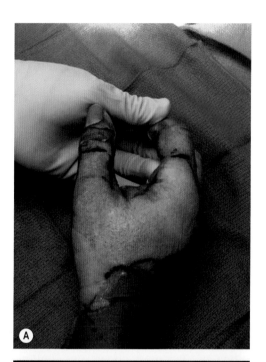

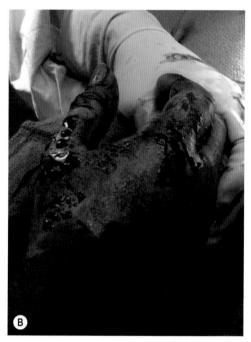

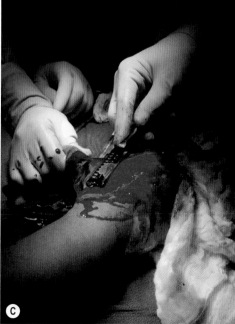

Fig. 18.12 (A) Burn wound is marked prior to debridement. **(B)** Hand scald burn post-debridement. **(C)** Using a Weck guarded knife for debridement of a hand scald burn.

dressings, hemostatic agents, electrocautery, avoidance of agents that interfere with the coagulation, and subcutaneous lactated Ringer's injection beneath the burned tissue all reduce blood loss. Although full-thickness excision to the level of muscle fascia with electrocautery minimizes blood loss, it requires skin grafts on fascia resulting in poor functional and cosmetic results.

Autologous split-thickness skin grafts from unburnt areas are the "gold standard" for definitive coverage of burn wounds if enough donor sites are available (Fig. 18.13). When available, the extremities, minus the hands and feet, are the best areas for harvesting of skin grafts (Fig. 18.14). The trunk is used next, but obtaining the grafts is technically more challenging because of contour irregularities. Tissue inflation with lactated Ringer's with 1 : 1 000 000 epinephrine allows harvesting of thinner grafts and minimizes blood loss. Hair-bearing scalp skin is a great but often underused donor site. The scalp skin is thick and re-epithelializes rapidly owing to the density of hair follicles. The scrotum can also be used. Regrowth of the hair is rarely a problem; thus, the donor site is well camouflaged after healing.

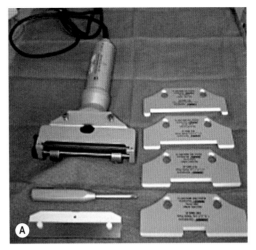

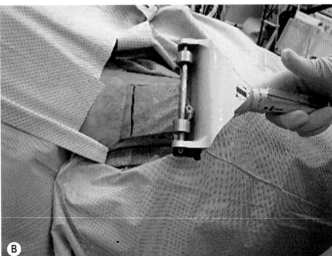

Fig. 18.14 (A) Commonly used powered dermatome used to harvest skin grafts. **(B)** Thin split-thickness autograft harvested.

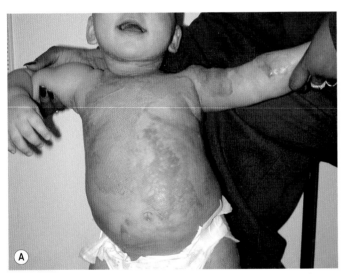

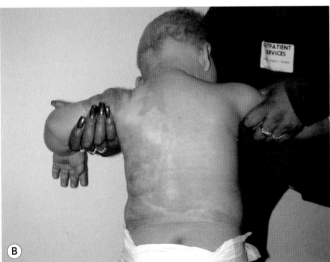

Fig. 18.13 (A) Healed split-thickness graft. **(B)** Donor site.

Repeated harvesting of skin graft donor sites multiple times is possible, but the donor site must allowed time to regenerate between harvest procedures. Donor sites should ideally be harvested from areas that optimize color match. Non-meshed ("sheet") grafts are preferred to improve the cosmetic and functional result. Meshing the skin grafts allows coverage of larger areas. Commercially available skin graft meshers allow expansion ratio of the skin graft either 1.5 : 1 or 3 : 1. Meshing improves graft "take" and faster burn coverage; the mesh pattern is permanent and unsightly. Sheet grafts are often used on hands and faces, and over any future site for intravenous central lines and tracheostomies to obtain rapid cover.

Allografts (Table 18.6) and skin equivalents (Table 18.7) have allowed rapid excisions of extremely large burns and still achieve physiologic closure, with potentially lower mortality in these injuries. Cultured epithelial autografts can also be used to provide temporary burn wound closure while the donor sites heal. The cultured cells can be applied as sheets (available after 3 weeks) or in suspension (available within 1 week). A few burns units use these cells for superficial skin loss or in combination with mesh graft to improve the cosmetic result.

Burn wounds are typically debrided and covered with skin grafts in one procedure. In large area burns, the patient may undergo skin grafting a few days after debridement. Between the time of excision and the skin grafting procedure, the wounds are covered with a biologic dressing (Integra or cadaver skin) (Fig. 18.15). Removing burned tissue reduces physiologic stress. This allows the wound bed and the patient to recover before harvesting the donor sites. Autograph skin coverage begins as soon as the debridement is complete. Although this is a more expensive approach to wound coverage, the improved functional outcome more than compensates for the investment. Donor sites harvested a second time can heal slowly, but the alternatives are limited in these patients with large burns. Unfortunately, this approach is not feasible in less developed countries.

A strategic plan directed toward achieving the best functional outcome should be used in planning skin graft coverage of large surface area burn patients. Most important is to cover joints and intravenous access sites, thereafter grafting large torso areas where skin grafts have a high probability for take to decrease the surface area of the injury and reduce physiologic stress. Burns to the hands, neck, and face warrant special consideration, however. To prevent excessive functional impairment to these areas after the burn wounds are healed, these areas should be grafted earlier rather than later. In full-thickness burns to the hands, neck, and face, delay in grafting will result in scar contractures and functional limitations that are difficult to overcome. Thus deep burns to these areas should be grafted early or closed with flaps so that range of motion and hypertrophic scar management can be started early (Box 18.6).

Management of tar burns[19–21]

Burns due to hot tar are difficult to manage because of the difficulty in removing the tar without inflicting further injury to the underlying burn. As it is difficult to remove the tar rapidly and there is no pressing medical need to do so, it is best to treat the injury as a deep burn with appropriate fluid resuscitation or preparation for skin grafting as needed. Removal of the tar is not essential, but it improves patient comfort and allows early assessment of the underlying tissue damage. This approach carries the risk of infection and the potential conversion of a partial-thickness injury to a full-thickness injury.

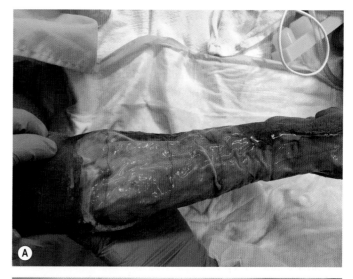

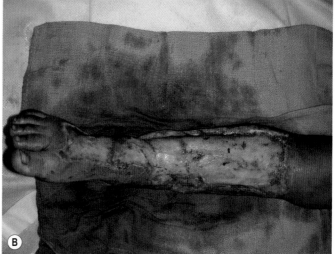

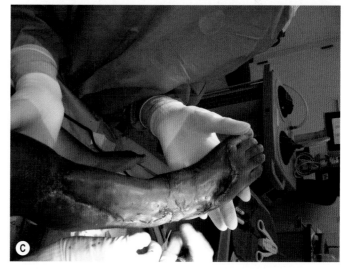

Fig. 18.15 (A) Integra acellular dermal matrix in place over a full-thickness wound. **(B)** Well-vascularized Integra graft. **(C)** Coverage of Integra.

BOX 18.6 Techniques for burn scar reconstruction

- Without deficiency of tissue
  - Excision and direct closure
  - Local tissue rearrangement
- With deficiency of tissue
  - Serial excision and direct closure
  - Split and full-thickness skin autografts
  - Local/regional flaps
  - Distant flaps
  - Tissue expansion
  - Free flaps

Numerous substances have been used in the past with variable results, and selection of the appropriate agent for the removal of adherent tar is still challenging. The detergent surfactant copolymers like polyoxyethylene–sorbitan or poloxamer 188, which are basically emulsifying agents commonly used as a wax base, when applied will separate the tar from the skin. Since they are water soluble, they easily wash off.

Alternatively silver sulfadiazine, neosporin (with polyoxyethylene sorbitan as a base), or polysorbate may be left under the bandage on the tar-contaminated burn. The tar comes away with the bandages when they are removed the next day. With some of these agents, it is recommended to leave it on for 12–48 h at a time until the tar has dissolved. Organic solvents, such as alcohol, acetone, aldehydes, ether, gasoline, and kerosene, are not recommended for removing tar from tissue. When these emulsifiers above are not available, common household agents, such as mayonnaise (15–30 min), butter (20–30 min), sunflower seed oil (20–30 min), and baby oil (1–1.5 h) placed on sterile gauze and onto the tar, should help to remove tar without further tissue damage, over the aforementioned time periods.

Mechanical debridement of tar burns is often painful, relatively ineffective, and results in the removal of underlying viable skin and hair follicles, thus extending the depth and area of the dermal injury. In addition, a degree of autodebridement will occur. If the skin has a light coat of tar and the patient does not complain about the underlying skin or surrounding tissue, leaving the asymptomatic tar in place may be acceptable.

Treatment of electrical injuries[22–24]

The majority of people that seek medical attention for electrical shock have experienced brief contacts with an electrically energized conductor. The presenting symptom is pain in the sensory distribution of the shock, a small contact burn, and perhaps soreness from falling. Very few have cardiac abnormalities. Electrical function of the heart should be assessed by an electrocardiogram. It is common practice to continuously monitor cardiac rhythm for the first 24 h after shock if the current passed through the chest or if the patient reports cardiac rhythm disturbance after the shock. This has proven to be unnecessary. If there are no cardiac abnormalities on admission, it is very unusual for it to develop. Fatal electrocutions occur at the time of shock. Because of significant risk of late onset neurological sequelae, these patients should follow-up with a trauma specialist or neurologist.

Patients presenting with cardiac arrhythmias or full cardiac arrest should undergo cardiac resuscitation procedures according to standard criteria and will likely need agents to reduce myocardial excitability in order to recover a functional rhythm. Once resuscitated, these patients should be admitted and evaluated for myocardial injury while being monitored in an inpatient monitored bed or ICU setting for several days.

Patients that have suffered major electrical injuries from high energy electrical power sources should be admitted to a specialty burn center to undergo appropriate care. Vital organ function should be stabilized as soon as possible. Thorough evaluation to determine the full extent of injury throughout the current path is the next priority while being constantly monitored and receiving fluid resuscitation. Diagnostic imaging is often essential to determine the extent and location of tissue damage. MRI without contrast is most accurate. However, in the setting of a severely injured patient, soft-tissue CT imaging is faster and more practical.

The surface area of burn usually does not factor into fluid resuscitation for electrical injury patients unless they have extensive skin burns as well. If the clinical exam indicates a significant injury, a Foley catheter should be placed. If the urine is clear, then fluid administration should be enough to maintain urine output at 0.5–1 mL times kg body weight/hour. After 3–4 hours, a judgement can be made about the severity of injury and whether the intravenous fluids can be reduced to maintain a baseline urine output of 20–30 mL/h. If on the contrary the urine is dark colored due to myoglobin, then intravenous fluid administered should be increased to keep the urine output at 2 mL per kg body weight. Sometimes an osmotic diuretic like mannitol is needed to increase urine output. Alkalinizing agents (e.g., bicarbonate) may prevent protein aggregation in the renal collecting ducts. Once the urine is clear, then the fluid administration can return to the level required to maintain a normal urine output.

Skin burns are managed the same as thermal injuries. Deep tissue injury, usually skeletal muscle, requires early diagnosis of deep muscle injury locations, compartment pressure monitoring, fasciotomies, and debridement of non-viable tissue. Manual testing of the compartment pressure is unreliable. Various ways can be used to measure the pressure. Elevated pressures over 30 mmHg requires fasciotomies of the fascia and epimysial layers in the muscle. Escharotomies and other releases needed to optimize perfusion should be done as soon as feasible. Most electrical shocks involve the hand. When hand edema is present, carpal tunnel Guyon's canal releases are needed. Doppler and pulse oximeter verification of perfusion in distal tissue is needed.

A second look operation at 48–72 hours is needed for a final muscle debridement. Deep wound cover with allograft or composite, with an aim to preserve vital structures, is indicated between debridements. Serial and multiple debridements of wounds, including superficial and deep muscles, must be performed, but nerves, tendons, joints and bones, even if partially damaged, can be preserved. Further assessment with time to guide reconstruction is appropriate.

Large blood vessels that are damaged should be bypassed by vascular grafting or removal. Injured nerves should be decompressed by tunnel releases and kept physiologically moist for later assessment. Allografts or biologic dressings can be used for interim coverage until the second look procedure and debridement are completed. If needed to fill dead space, vascularized coverage is beneficial but may be technically difficult to achieve in an unstable patient. The vascular damage and resulting thrombotic phenomenon abates during second week and tissues become less inflamed. This is the time when tissues around the wound withstand manipulation for a local, regional, axial, or free flap. The mortality rate of patients who suffer high-energy electrical burns is high with main cause of death being multi-organ failure.

Once wounds are closed, recovery of nerve and muscle function becomes the next challenge. Nerve releases, nerve grafts, and transfers are often necessary. Amputation and replacement with a prostheses is often the most cost-effective and rapid approach to regaining productivity. Months after wounds are closed, patients often develop neuromuscular coordination problems, pain syndromes, and neuropsychological disorders that require a team approach to manage.

Treatment of radiation injury[9,25]

Treatment of sunburn injury is to immobilize to speed edema resolution and apply a cool evaporative barrier. Dressings like Xeroform, AquacelAg, or hydrogel sheeting are excellent antimicrobial and evaporative barriers to maintain a physiologic environment for healing and substantially reduce pain. Non-steroidal anti-inflammatory medications reduce the inflammation and inflammation-driven pain.

Radiation-induced oxidative injury is the central mode of injury in ionizing radiation-induced injury. Therefore the administration of antioxidants, e.g., superoxide dismutase (Cu/Zn/Mn-containing SOD), nitroxides (tempol), and aminothiols (amifostine), represents a standard approach and a first-line treatment in clinical therapies for ROI-mediated injury. They scavenge free radicals, protecting cellular components against oxidative damage. N-acetylcysteine (NAC) is another thiol-containing antioxidant that replenishes cellular levels of reduced glutathione, an endogenous antioxidant, as well as scavenging aqueous phase free radicals. These mechanisms allow NAC to serve as a radioprotectant against the oxidative effects of gamma rays and other forms of ionizing radiation.

At high radiation doses, it is very difficult to completely block the effects of reactive oxygen intermediates (ROI) production throughout the intracellular water. Consequently, in parallel with the search for efficient antioxidants, sustained research efforts are currently focused on identifying critical targets of the ROIs at the cellular level and on developing effective treatments for restoring these damaged cellular components.

Effect of burn trauma on metabolism[26–28]

Extensive burns elicit a pronounced metabolic response to trauma causing physiologic derangements leading to the hypermetabolic state (Table 18.8). Over weeks post-burn, the hypermetabolic response involves severe catabolism, nitrogen depletion, and loss of lean body mass. This condition is associated with a progressive decline of host defenses that impairs the immunologic response and can lead to sepsis. The burn wound consumes large quantities of energy due the increased cost of thermal homeostasis, maintaining host defense barriers as well as protein biosynthesis.

Burn patients often increase the basal metabolic rate 50–100% of the normal resting rate. The main features include increased glucose production, insulin resistance, lipolysis, and muscle protein catabolism. Without adequate nutritional support, patients suffer delayed wound healing, decreased immune function, and generalized weight loss. Many formulas predict the nutritional needs of patients on the basis of lean body mass and percentage TBSA burned (Table 18.9). Increased intake of both nutritional calories and protein are needed to restore the deficit. Using the gut for providing nutrition has several benefits including reduction of translocation of gut microbes into the circulation.

Nutritional management[29–35]

Patients fed early have significantly enhanced wound healing and shorter hospital stays. Meeting the extensive calorie requirement by oral route alone is practically not possible in the major burn patients. Enteral nutrition through nasogastric or nasoduodenal transpyloric tubes are the preferred supplementary route of providing calorie deficit to the acutely injured burn patient. Patients with 20% TBSA burns will be unable to meet their nutritional needs with oral intake alone, and the transpyloric tube should be inserted at admission, as it is better tolerated than if inserted after the return of peristalsis. In the rare case that precludes use of the gastrointestinal tract, parenteral nutrition should be used only until the gastrointestinal tract is functioning.

Early enteral nutrition can relieve gastrointestinal damage and maintain the integrity of intestinal mucosa after severe burn. Gastrointestinal mucosal lesions take place during ischemia and reperfusion period after severe burns. Early enteral nutrition can relieve the ischemia and reperfusion injury by means of increasing the ability of eliminating oxygen free radical. The increase of intestinal permeability is one of the early features of intestinal mucosal barrier damage. Early enteral nutrition is an effective method to keep a normal intestinal permeability through the maintenance of blood circulation and the prevention of ischemia and reperfusion injury of intestine. Parenteral nutrition requires additional vascular access with its concomitant risks. It also lacks the beneficial effects of gut mucosal stimulation and protective effects against bacterial translocation and stress hemorrhage.

The rigorous schedule of dressing changes for burn wound care, operations, and rehabilitation sessions often interferes with meals. Diminished appetite from high-dose analgesics also contributes to poor feeding. Adequate nutritional support is so critical to recovery from burn injury that most clinicians will place feeding tubes in patients with inadequate oral calorie intake despite the risk of aspiration pneumonia.

Much like fluid resuscitation, the exact nutritional requirements are debatable. The clinical response of the patient remains the best indication of nutritional repletion during recovery from the injury. The rapidity of epidermal regeneration of superficial burns and donor sites and improving serum nutritional parameters are the best indicators of adequate nutrition. Measurement of the basal metabolic rate also guides nutritional replacement therapy. Measuring weight loss and gain during treatment is not useful because of the large fluid shifts. Even with adequate nutritional support, most patients lose muscle mass and weight. Optimizing nutrition to cover nutrient utilization is the fundamental goal. Over- or underfeeding increases the risks of complications.

Table 18.8 Percentage increase in metabolic rate versus burn size

% Burn (TBSA)	Metabolic rate (% increase)
20	30
30	50
40	75
50	100
60	100

Table 18.9 Formulae for estimating calorie and protein needs

Formula	Age (years)	% TBSA burn	Calories (kcal) per day	Protein
Adults				
Burke and Wolfe	>18	Any	2×BMR	Not calculated
Curreri	16–59	Any	(25 × body weight in kg) + (40 × % TBSA burn)	Not calculated
	>60	Any	(20 × body weight in kg) + (65 × % TBSA burn)	
Davies and Liljedahl	>18	Any	(20 kcal × body weight in kg) + (70 kcal × % TBSA burn) [>50% TBSA injuries are calculated as a 50% injury]	(1 g × body weight in kg) + (3 g × % burn)
Galveston I	>18	Any	(2100 kcal/m² × TBSA) + (1000 kcal/m² × % TBSA burn)	Not calculated
Ireton-Jones	>18	Any but must be ventilator-dependent	1784 − (11 × age in years) + (5 × weight in kg) + 244 (sex: male = 1; female = 0) + 239 (trauma: yes = 1; no = 0) + 804	Not calculated
Modified Harris-Benedict	>18	<40	Male = 1.5 × ([66 + (13.7 × weight in kg) + (5 × height in cm) − (6.8 × age)) Female = 1.5 × [655 + (9.6 × weight in kg) + (1.7 × height in cm) − (4.7 × age))	1.5 g×weight in kg
		≥40	Male = 2 × ([66 + (13.7 × weight in kg) + (5 × height in cm) − (6.8 × age)) Female = 2 × [655+(9.6 × weight in kg) + (1.7 × height in cm) − (4.7 × age)	2 g × weight in kg
Children				
Curreri Junior	0–1	Any	BMR + (15 kcal × % TBSA burn)	Not calculated
	1–3	Any	BMR + (25 kcal × % TBSA burn)	Not calculated
	4–15	Any	BMR + (40 kcal × % TBSA burn)	Not calculated
Davies Child	1–12	Any	(60 kcal × body weight in kg) + (35 kcal × % TBSA burn) [>50% surface injuries are calculated as a 50% injury]	(3 g × body weight in kg) + (1 g × % burn)
Galveston Infant	0–1	Any	(2100 kcal/m² × TBSA) + (1000 kcal/m² × % TBSA burn)	Not calculated
Galveston II	1–11	Any	(1800 kcal/m² × TBSA) + (1300 kcal/m² × % TBSA burn)	Not calculated
Galveston Adolescent	12–18	Any	(1500 kcal/m² × TBSA) + (1300 kcal/m² × % TBSA burn)	

1 g nitrogen = 6.25 g protein; BMR, basal metabolic rate.

Nutrition formulae

The main features include increased glucose production, insulin resistance, lipolysis, and muscle protein catabolism. Without adequate nutritional support, patients have delayed wound healing, decreased immune function, and generalized weight loss. Many formulas predict the nutritional needs of these patients on the basis of lean body mass and percentage TBSA burned. Increased intake of both total calories and protein (1.5–3 g of protein/kg/day) is needed to restore the deficit. Much like fluid resuscitation, the exact nutritional requirements are debatable. The clinical response of the patient remains the best indication of nutritional repletion during recovery from the injury.

Close glucose control of 80–110 mg/dL can be achieved using an intensive insulin therapy protocol, leading to decreased infectious complications and mortality rates. Burn centers continue to use a variety of formulae to estimate nutrient needs (see Table 18.9). The number of energy estimation formulas has increased in recent years

with many developed for specific patient populations. Burn-specific equations have been developed both for pediatric and adult populations. A study compared 46 published energy calculations with indirect calorimetry in burn patients and found none precisely estimated calorie needs and most demonstrated some inaccuracy for any given patient.

Several studies propose the use of anabolic steroids or growth hormone to reduce muscle catabolism and weight loss during the injury and to enhance weight gain during recovery. It appears that anti-catabolic and anabolic agents can markedly diminish the net catabolism of burn injury during the acute and recovery phases. These agents, in combination with optimum protein intake, appear to be of significant benefit in the metabolic management of the severe burn. Adequate nutritional support from the beginning of acute care is critical to burn patient survival.

Therapeutic strategies should aim to prevent body weight losses of more than 10% of the patient's baseline status because more profound weight loss is associated with significantly worse outcomes. Known consequences of catabolic disorders with loss of lean body mass above 10% include impaired immune function and delayed wound healing. Lean body mass reduction beyond 40% leads to imminent mortality. Therefore complications of ongoing catabolism remain a major cause of morbidity and mortality in severely burned patients.

Pain control

The adverse sequelae of inadequate pain in the burn population have been long recognized, yet control of pain remains inadequate globally. The dynamic evolution of the pain both centrally and peripherally, and the many factors that influence pain perception, illustrate the need for a therapeutic plan that is similarly dynamic and flexible enough to cope with the facets of background, breakthrough, procedural, and postoperative pain. Regular, ongoing, and documented pain assessment is key in directing this process.

Severe pain with burns is a major physiologic stress that can have a negative impact on the patient's recovery. Often, bedside procedures require high doses of anxiolytic and opiates. Particularly painful and anxiety-provoking is the first dressing change after skin grafting. In addition to significant pain, especially at the donor site, patients often experience great anxiety as they confront their new graft for the first time. Various approaches have been studied to provide sedation, comfort, and pain control. Conventional pharmacotherapy utilizes opioids for analgesia and benzodiazepines for sedation. The risk of apnea may cause the provider to err on the side of administering too little drug. To combat this, some centers offer patient-controlled analgesia (PCA) using propofol. PCS allows the patient to self-titrate to the comfort level desired, which may have the added benefit of allowing the patient to feel in control of the situation.

In general, it is helpful to have an anesthesiologist or pain specialist involved in the day-to-day management of burn patients. Providers caring for burn patients should keep in mind several key points in order to optimize pain control during dressing changes: optimize nutrition and hydration to stimulate the healing process; ensure the safety and comfort of sedated patients both during and post-procedure by frequently assessing pain level and vital signs; and control acute pain during the most painful stages of dressing changes (dressing removal and wound cleansing). Close monitoring of respiratory status is required when consciousness is diminished.

More emphasis on pain control not only helps the patient's psychological wellbeing but may significantly affect physical outcome as well. Painful stimuli influence the release of a number of circulatory factors that affect tissue perfusion, immune system function, and wound healing. Effect management of pain requires a working knowledge of pain neurophysiology and pharmacology. These skills are important for burn care providers.

Patients without a substance abuse problem before the injury typically do not develop opiate addiction even after receiving high doses for prolonged periods, but physical dependence often occurs after sustained treatment with opiates. Gradually reducing the doses of opiates as pain diminishes avoids opiate withdrawal.

Complications

Skin graft loss

Loss of skin graft is the most common operative complication and is caused by inadequate immobilization, inadequate wound debridement, or formation of blood clot beneath the graft. Infection is usually the direct consequence of failed graft take (Fig. 18.16). Thus careful placement of dressings to immobilize the graft relative to the wound bed is essential. Some burn surgeons spray freshly applied skin grafts with fibrin sealant to help immobilize the graft and accelerate vascular ingrowth. Unless carefully splinted, avoid circumferential compression dressings on a grafted extremity. Any movement in a grafted and circumferentially wrapped extremity will generate shear stress between underlying muscles and the overlying graft. Early graft inspection on day 2–3 after grafting should be encouraged with removal of any underlying hematoma. After day 3, capillary ingrowth has occurred and would be interrupted by graft movement. If examination shows that the skin grafts are grossly infected, then microbiologic cultures can be performed and appropriate antimicrobial therapy instituted.

Invasive wound infection

In burn patients, systemic antibiotic prophylaxis administered in the first 4–14 days significantly reduces all-cause mortality by nearly a half; limited perioperative prophylaxis reduces wound infections but not mortality. Topical antibiotic prophylaxis applied to burn wounds, commonly recommended, had no large beneficial effects. The methodologic quality of the evidence is weak, however, so a large, robust randomized controlled trial is now needed.

Wound infection should be suspected if the wound becomes increasingly uncomfortable, tachycardic, painful, or malodorous; if cellulitis is observed; or if the patient becomes febrile. Several biopsies from suspicious areas in the burn wound should be sent for microbiology. Since all wounds will be colonized after a few hours, it is best to measure the density of bacteria in the wound. This is called quantitative bacterial culture. Some experience, clean instruments, and training is

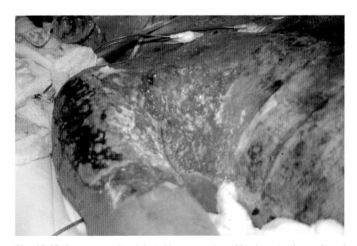

Fig. 18.16 Appearance of an infected burn wound resulting in systemic sepsis and loss of skin autografts and allografts.

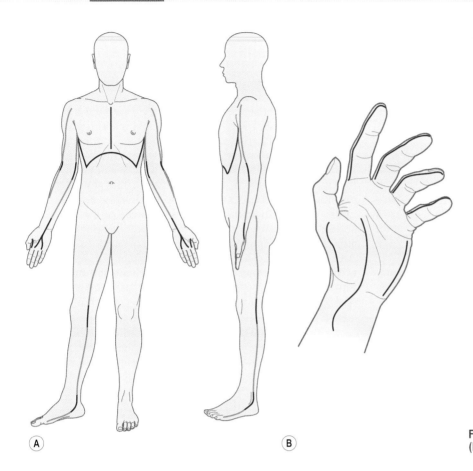

Fig. 18.17 (A) Escharotomy lines and relevant anatomy.
(B) Hand escharotomy incisions.

necessary to accurately perform the test. When the density of bacteria in the wound exceeds 100 000 colony-forming units per gram of tissue (equivalent to 10^5/gram), then host defense mechanisms are no longer effective. This condition permits invasive wound infection.

Treatment of invasive wound infections requires both antibiotics and excision of all infected tissue. Empiric broad-spectrum antibiotic treatment should be started after discussion with the microbiology team. The antibiotic treatment regime can be adjusted to be more specific according to the rapid-slide Gram stain results obtained in a few hours from the biopsy. In 24–48 hours, more specific identification of the bacteria and its antibiotic sensitivities can be used to decide on the antibiotic regime. The recommended choice of antibiotic is guided by the most likely cause of infection and local patterns of antibiotic resistance should also be considered.

Adrenal insufficiency

Some degree of adrenal insufficiency occurs in up to 36% of patients with major burns. Correcting for it is not as simple as administering corticotropin. Probably due to the variation in the stress responses across different patients, there is no statistically resolved association between response to corticotropin stimulation and survival. The clinical relevance of this finding has not been established.

Circumferential limb compression with vascular compromise

Patients may require escharotomies (Fig. 18.17), fasciotomies, or both (Fig. 18.18) for the release of extremity compartment

syndrome. Patients presenting with burns of neck, thorax, abdomen, extremities that are near circumferential, or greater full-thickness burns are likely to have obstructed blood flow to the extremity and require escharotomies. In extremities there is impaired capillary refill and paresthesia, and increased pain develops earlier than decreased pulses. Measurement of muscle or tissue pressures with a manometer and Doppler meter can be used to monitor tissue perfusion distal to the site. If tissue pressures are high, surgical release maybe indicated. If the pressures are moderately high, constant monitoring is indicated. The orbit is a compartment limited to expansion

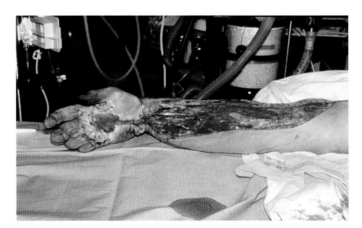

Fig. 18.18 Volar escharotomy and extensive fasciotomies of the volar forearm and hand with necrotic muscle debridement following electrical injury. The fasciotomy extended into normal skin above and below the skin contracture. The fasciotomies included the investing compartment fascia and epimysial layers.

and may require lateral canthotomy to successfully reduce intraocular pressure to normal.

Compartment syndromes

Compartment syndrome occurs when the tissue pressure within an enclosed space is elevated above venous pressure. If the pressure exceeds venous pressures, the result is decreased blood flow within the fascial compartment, decreased tissue oxygenation, and ischemia. Tissue hypoxia leads to intracellular edema and increase in compartment pressure. The final result without prompt treatment is tissue necrosis.

The occurrence of abdominal compartment syndrome has a similar pathophysiology. Because of the vital organs involved, it can become life-threatening. It often follows fluid extravasation/edema in a major burn patient with severe capillary leak. It is diagnosed by an intra-abdominal pressure >20 mmHg and at least one new organ dysfunction. It is associated with renal impairment, gut ischemia, and cardiac and pulmonary malperfusion. Clinical manifestations include tense abdomen, decreased pulmonary compliance, hypercapnia, and oliguria. Urine output monitoring is not sensitive or specific enough to diagnose abdominal compartment syndrome. Careful monitoring and aggressive treatment should be instituted to avoid this mortal complication. Appropriate intravascular volume, appropriate body positioning, pain management, sedation, nasogastric decompression if appropriate, chemical paralysis if required, and torso escharotomy are all interventions to increase abdominal wall compliance and decrease intra-abdominal pressures. Bladder pressure monitoring should be initiated as part of the burn fluid resuscitation protocol in every patient with 30% TBSA burn. Patients who receive >250 mL/kg of crystalloid in the first 24 h may require abdominal decompression. Percutaneous abdominal decompression is a minimally invasive procedure that should be performed before resorting to laparotomy. If less invasive maneuvers fail, decompressive laparotomy should be performed in patients with abdominal compartment syndrome that is refractory to other therapies.

Deep venous thrombosis

Deep venous thrombosis incidence ranges from 1% to 23% in burn patients and deep venous thrombosis chemoprophylaxis with heparin is recommended. Often coagulopathies develop after multiple transfusions. Alteration in clotting parameters can trigger intravascular thrombosis in low flow veins.

Systemic inflammatory response syndrome

There are standardized definitions for sepsis and infection-related diagnoses in burn patients. Patients with large burns have a baseline temperature reset to 38.5°C, and tachycardia and tachypnea may persist for months. Continuous exposure to inflammatory mediators leads to significant changes in the white blood cell count, making leukocytosis a poor indicator of sepsis. Use other clues as signs of infection or sepsis, such as increased fluid requirements, decreasing platelet counts >3 days after burn injury, altered mental status, worsening pulmonary status, and impaired renal function. The term "systemic inflammatory response syndrome" should not be applied to burn patients because patients with large burns are in a state of chronic systemic inflammatory stimulation.

Neutropenia

Transient leucopenia is common, primarily due to a decreased neutrophil count. Maximal white blood cell depression occurs several days after admission with rebound to normal a few days later. Use of silver sulfadiazine has been associated with this transient leucopenia; resolution is independent of continued silver sulfadiazine.

Sepsis[36–39]

Patients with large TBSA burns are immunosuppressed and at increased risk for infections, especially of the wounds, venous access sites, and lungs. Small injuries (<10% TBSA) heal rapidly, and infections are rare. Clinical surveillance for signs of infection is not simple because many burn patients have a fever and altered white blood cell counts without infections. Many burn patients exhibit a low-grade fever in the first week after injury due to chemical sepsis syndrome.

Common causes of infections in burn patient populations arise from translocation of gut flora in physiologically stressed patients and cross contamination. The first priority is to rule out central venous catheter sepsis and change the line if it is positive. Burn wounds become rapidly colonized with Gram-positive bacteria, mainly staphylococci from hair follicles and dermal glands. The moist burn eschar encourages microbial growth. Gram-negative bacterial infections result from translocation from the gut because of reduced mesenteric blood flow at the time of burn and subsequent insults. Finally, burn patients can incur hospital-acquired infections common to other patients in intensive care units, including intravascular catheter-related infections and ventilator-associated pneumonia, with an overall incidence of infection higher than that of other patients in intensive care units.

Current guidelines for management do not recommend continuous systemic antibiotic prophylaxis for burns patients, indicating lack of evidence for efficacy and induction of antibiotic resistance. A recent meta-analysis found that for burn patients systemic antibiotic prophylaxis administered over the first 4–14 days post-burn significantly reduced all-cause mortality by nearly a half and limited perioperative prophylaxis reduced wound infections but not mortality.[39] In addition, the study suggested that topical antibiotic prophylaxis applied to burn wounds, commonly recommended, had no beneficial effects. Because of the difficulty of multicenter clinical studies, methodologic quality of the data was weak, and they concluded that prophylaxis could not be recommended for patients with severe burns other than perioperatively and that there was a need for randomized controlled trials to assess its use. Prophylactic antibiotics are administered immediately prior to burn wound excision is commonly performed as a treatment to prevent burn wound infection. It is important to establish adequate blood levels at the time of the incision.

Patients with large surface area burn injuries that have failed coverage and remain open for long periods still develop wound infections and ultimately succumb to infection. Isolation of the patient in specialized unit beds along with infection precautions by the healthcare workers (handwashing, gloves, and gowns) reduces the transmission of pathogens from one patient to another. A high level of suspicion for wound infection must be kept when the patient's condition deteriorates rapidly. Wound cultures, particularly quantitative assessment, and biopsies for histologic examination help confirm the diagnosis and direct therapy. Prompt excision of necrotic or infected tissue, appropriate topical treatment, and systemic antimicrobial therapy are critical to survival of the patient.

The best clinical approach to prevent sepsis is to bolster the immune system with early nutritional support and re-establish the barrier function of the gut and skin. Treatment with an antibiotic usually controls the infections but alters the patient's microbial flora. Should the patient remain at risk for infections after the first infection is treated, a second, more drug-resistant infection often occurs. Should the burn be large enough that the patient remains at risk for a month or longer, systemic fungal infections become a major clinical problem. Treatment of fungal sepsis with less toxic fluconazole has greatly increased the therapeutic options.

Ventilator management

Inhalation injury and respiratory complications are still one of the major causes of mortality in severe burns. Ventilatory support and airway management in this situation are often challenging, and the need for prolonged endotracheal intubation is very common in patients affected by different degrees of respiratory distress syndrome. Despite the use of high-volume low-pressure cuffs, considerable controversy exists among burn surgeons as to whether to convert endotracheal tubes to tracheostomy in burns patients, particularly when ventilator support is prolonged beyond two weeks or when other airway complications occur, as many studies have recorded high mortality and high tracheostomy complications.

The pathogenesis of these entities is still unclear, but the combination of inhalation injury, infection, presence of an endotracheal tube, and individual factors play an important role in their development. Tracheostomies may provide a good portal of entry for microorganisms into the respiratory tract, with a high incidence of respiratory infection and sepsis. In addition, feeding aspirations, obstructive abnormalities, increased incidence of pneumonia and tracheo-innominate fistulas have been reported as high-morbidity complications of tracheostomies. Long-term sequelae are no less important. Stenosis of the airway, dysphagia, alterations of speech, tracheo-esophageal fistulas, and tracheomalacia can compromise the favorable outcome of this selected group of patients. Every effort should be made to maintain airway pressures at the lowest range, in order to prevent tracheomalacia. Advantages of tracheostomy include minimizing dead space, ease of suctioning, presence of a more secure airway, and ease of movement. Theoretically, it should prevent the appearance of subglottic stenosis.

The use of low-pressure balloons in modern endotracheal tubes has markedly decreased the incidence of tracheal erosion and life-threatening tracheo-innominate artery fistulas. Tracheostomies are still useful so patients can be gradually and safely weaned from prolonged dependence on mechanical ventilation and to decrease injury to vocal cords.

Thrombophlebitis

Venous thrombosis is a common problem in major burn patients, especially in the veins used for intravenous access. Heparin prophylaxis is routinely used in burn centers to reduce the incidence of this problem. Venous clots in large surface area burn patients serve as a rich culture media for bacteria. Many major burn patients who require many weeks of care require central venous lines at some point in their treatment because peripheral access sites are usually limited. Central line-related infections can cause major morbidity, and constant attention is given to changing catheters once a line infection is suspected. Septic thrombophlebitis is a common complication of venous thromboembolism in burn patients. It should be suspected and ruled out in burn patients with unexplained signs of sepsis. The evaluation begins by inspecting all sites of prior catheter access. Resection of the infected vein is often required for effective therapy.

Rehabilitation[40–44]

Major burn injuries create indescribable challenges for the patient to overcome. Alteration in body image, mechanical disabilities, increased risk of further injury, and pain are just a few of the problems. Burn trauma rehabilitation is the restoration of health and work capacity of a person incapacitated by burn injury. Achieving success in burns rehabilitation is often challenging.

Adaptation and regain of capability requires the investment of support groups, family, friends, and a multidisciplinary rehab team. Very few countries have the resources to support that level of investment. But effective rehabilitation can produce a gainfully employed and psychologically intact person. Burn patients have to recover mobility and balance to gain the confidence in their ability to work or engage in personal interactions.

Formulation of an optimal rehabilitation strategy begins in the first few days after hospital admission. Before the wounds are closed, therapy to prevent contractures by musculoskeletal dynamic therapy, traction, and splinting is of paramount importance especially for wounds surrounding joints. Splints are made preoperatively and placed in the operating room at the time of grafting. Some burn centers use hydrotherapy as a part of physical therapy to range extremities while the patient is in warm water. This reduces joint stiffness and pain.

Skilled physiotherapy is very important in the prevention of the burn contractures. Because the competing factors controlling scar and scar contracture as well as the incomplete information, debates over whether to rest or mobilize healing wounds continues. Recently, early motion has been strongly advocated to avoid joint contractures. Injured upper and lower extremities are elevated to allow adequate venous drainage and to reduce edema.

Experienced judgment is required to recognize the stages of wound healing and the relative importance of inflammation and mechanical tension in scar stimulation. A study has demonstrated that starting good burn physiotherapy on post-burn day 1 for non-grafted areas and post-burn day 3 for skin-grafted areas resulted in only 6% burn contracture. Early and proper splinting and stretching of flexion crease burns, such as the neck, axilla, and antecubital areas, reduce the extent of scar contractures and may prevent subsequent functional deformities and the need for reconstruction.

Plan for continuation of physiotherapy treatment after releasing the patient from hospital, for at least 18 months. In the acute and post-healing stages of recovery, the move out of the burn center is the first defining point in a patient's post-burn life. In addition to physical considerations, wound healing and recovery after burns is promoted by good nutrition, for initial wound healing and long-term scar reduction. Rehabilitation involves the whole burn team to collectively encouraging the patient to live as normal a life as possible between dressing changes and operations; the therapists take the lead in maintaining muscle strength, joint range, and activities of daily living.

In the chronic phase, the prevention and management of hypertrophic scarring and contractures are significant issues. Another important aspect of burn care is recognizing the psychosocial needs of burn patients. To facilitate this, many centers provide psychologists, social workers, and vocational counselors as part of the multidisciplinary team. The physiologic recovery of burn patients is divided into categories (critical stage, acute stage, long-term rehabilitation), each with unique psychosocial aspects to consider.

Psychological challenges in the critical stage are due to over- and understimulation, an uncertainty about and a struggle for survival, painful treatments, delirium and confusion, and impaired communication. At this stage, physical survival is the primary goal and psychological intervention may be of little value. During the acute or restorative phase of care, patients often display symptoms of depression and anxiety. Patients may also exhibit grief, impaired sleep, and acute stress disorder. Pharmacotherapy and counseling can help patients during this stage.

After discharge from the acute rehab program, long-term rehabilitation begins. There are several basic challenges to overcome. Anxiety and depression are common issues. Learning to cope with a potential decrease in physical function (i.e., due to deconditioning and scarring) is also important. Psychological factors such as sexuality and changed body image also require supportive management. Post-traumatic stress disorder is another common inexorable sequelae of burn trauma that requires early intervention to contain its consequences. Negative emotional interpersonal experiences only add to the severity. The direct involvement of psychiatric services is an invaluable aspect of burns rehabilitation.

Another post-healing concept is community outreach. It was introduced to try to overcome the gap recognized at this stage of recovery, to provide links with the community services and local hospitals. Rehabilitation centers start integration back into society in a protected environment with other people who had sustained physical trauma. They could receive the help in returning to work, to the home, hobbies, and to society, and if necessary return for "top up" help after reconstructive surgery.

For children, reintroduction to society that usually centers around school is more challenging especially during adolescence. Children's burn clubs go a long way in providing confidence-building support before and after hospital discharge. Issues related to a full return to the community, and their solutions such as partnership with teachers, behavior therapy, and adaptive equipment, may be outside the limits of this chapter. However, follow-up recommendations, including a more comprehensive checklist of potential areas of need, may be helpful.

Electrical injury patients have particularly difficult rehabilitation challenges.[41,42] Many of the widely reported neurological, neuromuscular, and neuropsychiatric complications manifest months after an electrical shock injury. These problems are common even in patients who have low-energy electrical shocks. In general, a multidisciplinary team of neurologists, neuropsychologists working in collaboration with the burn rehabilitation team is needed.[41,42] Intense and protracted physical and occupational therapy is required to regain normal balance and coordination.

Fortunately, severe radiation skin injury is not common. Wound closure with non-irradiated skin is required.[25] The non-irradiated cells in the autografted skin will gradually improve the quality and healing capacity of surrounding radiation-injured skin.[9] Adipose transfer into radiation-injured soft tissue has also been found to benefit radiated skin.[25]

Managing burn scar hypertrophy and contracture[45–50]

The ideal scar is strong enough to subserve the mechanical requirements and support epidermal functions. Ideally, just enough scar forms for this purpose. However, the wounds of burn patients often heal with excess (i.e., hypertrophic) scarring. There is no quantitative definition of hypertrophic scarring. Rather, the diagnosis is given to scars that are thicker than necessary. Hypertrophic scar formation after burn wound healing is a common obstacle to rehabilitation.

Several epigenetic causes of hypertrophic scarring are well known and important to consider. Basically, prolonged wound inflammation, dynamic tension (shoulders, chest, volar forearm, and dorsal legs) on the wound, endocrine or hormonal factors associated with rapid growth, pregnancy, and pigmented skin predispose to hypertrophic scar formation. Factors that increase inflammation include wound infection, prolonged healing by secondary intention, or immunologically foreign material present in the wound. It is postulated that hypertrophic scars begin as the result of an injury to the deep dermis. They are especially pronounced in wounds that have a prolongation of the inflammatory and proliferative phases of wound healing. The incidence of hypertrophic scars following burn wound healing is close to 90%.

Hypertrophic scarring also occurs as the result of dynamic mechanical skin tension acting on the healing wound. As a result of mechanical tension, scars located on certain areas of the body (e.g., sternum, deltoid, and upper back) are frequently hypertrophic, the typical appearance of which can be seen in Fig. 18.19. This anatomic dependency seems to correlate with patterns of skin tension. The natural history of hypertrophic scars is that they regress with time after injury, leaving behind, however, an unsightly wide gap of thinned dermis between wound edges.

A familial pattern in hypertrophic scarring is not described; however, populations with higher skin melanin content are known to have a higher incidence of hypertrophic scars. These populations include people of African, Asian, and Hispanic descent.

Hormonal influences are also known to be a factor, with hypertrophic scarring often initiated at the start of puberty or during pregnancy. Scar tissue cells are sensitive to the influences of the same growth factors that drive normal tissue growth and development. Schierle reported an increase in testosterone receptors in hypertrophic scars, which may

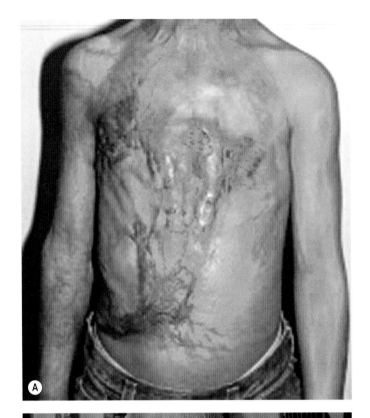

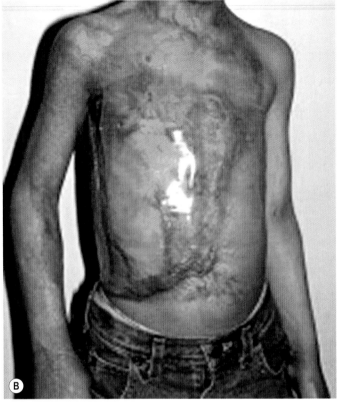

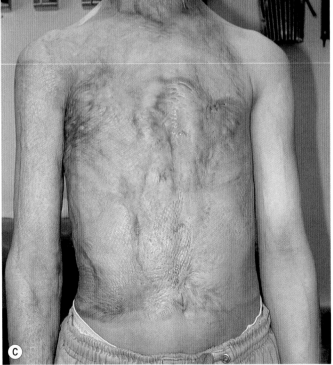

Fig. 18.19 **(A)** Hypertrophic burn scar 6 months after flame burn to chest and neck. **(B)** Application of hydrogel or polymer sheeting sheeting to scar to increase moisture content and comfort. **(C)** Scar appearance several months later.

contribute to the formation of these scars during adolescence. Hypertrophic scars occur in 60% of burned children aged under 5 years.

Hypertrophic scarring, unstable epithelium, and poor skin elasticity often occur when deep burns are allowed to heal without grafting. Initial therapy is focused on controlling scar pathogenesis. Effect treatments requires induction of scar remodeling and softening. Topical non-steroidal

anti-inflammatory agents, anti-histamines, and other immunomodulators are useful to downregulate scar inflammation, which often persists long after the wound is epithelialized. Ointments moisturize by blocking evaporation and reduce harmful scratching of healed skin grafts.

Typically, the rehabilitation team (occupational and physical) evaluates and formulates a treatment plan early to minimize scarring. Preventative therapy begins with pressure garments, moisturizers, anti-inflammatories, functional range of motion, splinting, edema control, and scar treatments while the scarring is in the immature phase, before it is hypertrophic or contracted. Hand scars are particularly important to address early. They often require splinting, message and range of motion exercises.

Management of mature scars that are hypertrophic on presentation is another level of challenge. For burns of the hand and extremities, physical and occupational therapists often use thermoplastic splints, serial casting, gel sheeting inserts, and pressure to decrease hypertrophic scars and joint contractures.

Major burn patients are known to be vitamin D deficient, in part, resulting from the skin damage. Vitamin D is an anti-inflammatory hormone that also regulates calcium metabolism. Normal Vitamin D levels are essential for normal healing.

⊕ Access the complete reference list online at **http://www.expertconsult.com**

2. Demling RH. Burns. *N Engl J Med.* 1985;313:1389–1398. *This article is an excellent early review of burns and burn management. It details acute resuscitation, burn-associated infection, metabolic aspects of burns, wound healing, and more.*

5. Despa F, Orgill DP, Neuwalder J, Lee RC. The relative thermal stability of tissue macromolecules and cellular structure in burn injury. *Burns.* 2005;31:568–577.

6. Lee RC, Parsons RW. Confusion in electrical trauma terminology. *Plast Reconstr Surg.* 1992;89:1020–1021. *This paper discusses the cellular structure of tissue macromolecules during burn injury. The authors suggest that strategies to minimize the damage in a burn injury should include the stabilization of the cellular membrane and membrane-bound ATPases.*

7. Cancio LC, Lundy JB, Sheridan RL. Evolving changes in the management of burns and environmental injuries. *Surg Clin N Am.* 2012;92:959–986. *This review of electrical shock trauma details the anatomic patterns of the resultant tissue injury from various modes of electromagnetic exposure. Also, the physics of tissue injury due to power lines, exposure to lightning and radio frequency, ionizing radiation, and microwave is discussed.*

10. Jackson D, Topley E, Cason JS, et al. Primary excision and grafting of large burns. *Ann Surg.* 1960;152:167–189.

11. Nguyen N, Gun R, Sparnon A, et al. The importance of immediate cooling – a case series of childhood burns in Vietnam. *Burns.* 2002;28:173–176.

12. Mankani MH, Kicska G, Lee RC. A three-dimensional computerized burn chart – stage II: assessment of accuracy. *J Burn Care Rehab.* 1994;15:191–193.

18. Orgill DP. Excision and skin grafting of thermal burns. *N Engl J Med.* 2009;360:893–901. *The clinical problem associated with thermal burns is reviewed. The author also discusses the benefits of skin grafting, clinical evidence associated with it, clinical use, and adverse events.*

23. Lee RC, Jang DJ, Hannig J. Biophysical injury mechanisms in electrical shock trauma. *Ann Rev Biomed Eng.* 2000;2:477–510.

31. Venter M, Rode H, Sive A, et al. Enteral resuscitation and early enteral feeding in children with major burns: effect on McFarlane response to stress. *Burns.* 2007;33:464–471. *This study discusses enteral resuscitation and early enteral feeding in children with major burns. The authors provide recommendations on the use of enteral resuscitation and early enteral feeding based on the clinical scenario.*

50. Edstrom LE, Robson MC, Macchiaverna JR, et al. Prospective randomized treatments for burned hands: nonoperative vs. operative. Preliminary report. *Scand J Plast Reconstr Surg.* 1979;13:131–135.

19

Extremity burn reconstruction

Lorenzo Borghese, Alessandro Masellis, and Michele Masellis

SYNOPSIS

- In electrical burn injuries, the patient's condition often seems less critical than it really is.
- Always consider burn-induced compartment syndrome (BICS) when limbs have extensive burns.
- When performing escharotomy on the limbs, pay attention to dangerous sites, such as the basilic or saphenous veins, and the radial or tibial nerves.
- The extremities are the most frequent areas affected by post-surgery scar contractures. Correct positioning of articulations, good management of scars, and postoperative care are mandatory.
- The Z-plasty technique (in all its variations) remains one of the most effective procedures for post-burn scar retractions.
- Reconstructive surgery of burn sequelae often needs "imagination". Due to the presence of scars, to the damaged tissues, and to the lack of good vessels, it is very hard to follow a single preoperative plan. You need many arrows in your quiver.

 Access the Historical Perspective section online at
http://www.expertconsult.com

Introduction

The upper and lower extremities are often involved in burn-related accidents. In particular, the arms, forearms, hands, and legs are the most exposed areas, as they constitute the first means of self-protection and are used to aid escape in accidents.

Most burn-related accidents involving the extremities occur at work, caused mainly by fire and electricity, and at home where the majority of victims are babies.[1,2] Extremity burns can be considered "difficult" burns, especially if they are extensive circumferential burns. Deep second- and third-degree burns, if not treated early and adequately in a well-equipped burn specialized facility, can result in severe *burn-induced compartment syndromes (BICS)*, which can cause death of viable tissues such as skin muscles and nerves and even the loss of the extremity involved.[3,4]

Knee and elbow joints are often prone to severe damage related to electrocution. In this type of accident, electricity often finds its entry or exit point in one of these joints, causing their explosion.

Extremities scarring often represents a challenge for the plastic surgeon. About 50% of Z-plasties, as well as other surgical techniques such as scar revision, involve the extremities. In developing countries, the percentage of scar retraction causing disabilities is significant. This results in a grotesque thoraco-brachial and brachio-antebrachial clinical picture, or severe leg adhesions and contractures.

While the patient is hospitalized, physical and occupational therapy is specifically aimed at maintaining mobility of the major joints. Even if they are only marginally involved in the accident, these parts are in fact often subject to arthritis, dysplasia, and joint calcification, which are not easy to treat.

Thus the reconstruction of the extremities, which are a person's main means of self-sufficiency, is not simply a matter of aesthetics but represents a real challenge for both the surgeon and the patient. For the sake of clarity, the following analysis will consider the upper and the lower extremities separately.

Basic science/disease process

Electrical burns

In cases of electrocution, the upper extremities are almost always involved, especially as entry or exit points of what is known as the *electric arc*.[15]

The electric arc mainly involves the wrist, elbow, and ankle joints with devastating effects on the joints themselves, the nervous structures, and the muscular masses. Often the most serious damage is to the wrist and ankle. Since the hands and feet are the most frequent entry and exit points, the wrist and ankle are the nearest points of electrical resistance. The patient's clinical condition on admission often looks less critical than it really is, since the cutaneous lesions may be misleading, with limited skin burn; in some other cases, ample charred areas can be witnessed. These are the electric current's entry and exit points. However, the underlying damage is always more extensive and may well involve the muscular fasciae. This is because nerves and vessels are very good conductors of electricity, and they may suffer damage a few days after the accident. Venous thrombosis or ischemia can be caused by internal destruction of the vessels catalyzed by the electric current. Peripheral neurological damage may occur with total *destruction of the nerve (neurotmesis)*, if close to the electricity entry and exit points, or with partial *axonal damage (axonotmesis)*, which often resolve in a few months.[16,17]

In cases of high-voltage electrical burns (over 1000 volts), muscles, bones, and nerve structures can be totally destroyed and complete destruction of the major joints is common.[18] In such cases, intervention should be performed within 3–5 days from the accident in order to save the affected joints and to remove destroyed muscular tissue. Myoglobinuria is closely linked to muscular damage, since the destruction of muscle cell causes the release of *myoglobin* and in turn catalyses myoglobinemia. This is a difficult condition to manage, and the first sign of this pathology is the dark pink color of the urine.[19,20] An accurate diagnosis of myoglobinuria can be provided only by serum differentiation between hemoglobin and myoglobin.

All patients with myoglobinuria should be treated with mannitol IV, bicarbonate IV, and Ringer's lactate therapy in order to obtain alkaline osmotic diuresis. This can minimize the precipitation of the pigment at the level of the renal tubules.

The damage caused by an electric current passing through the body, especially if of high voltage, depends not only on the characteristics of the electricity itself but also on the path it follows and on the characteristics of the tissues affected by the electricity. Even if adequate medical and surgical therapy is available, the risk of amputation of an extremity remains high, rated between 37% and 65%.[16,21]

From a surgical point of view, debridement of necrotic tissue plays a fundamental role in the very first phase after the electrical accident. As said, this can be very extensive compared to the skin lesion. Reconstruction in these cases is rarely limited only to skin graft coverage. It often also requires vascular reconstruction, nerve grafts, and the transposition of microvascular free flaps.

Vascular and neural reconstruction has to be carefully monitored, since late electricity-related damage affecting the neurovascular structures can occur even some days after the accident and the surgical procedures, due to irreversible endothelial damage, which affects small terminal vessels in particular. Hence, it is preferable in such cases to postpone the more complex reconstruction procedures.[22] During the acute phase, it is advisable to proceed by more limited simple debridement and temporary skin coverage with a free skin graft, isolating and preparing the vascular and nervous structures that will be treated in a secondary surgical stage.[23]

Diagnosis/patient presentation

Deep burns in the entire upper extremities are statistically infrequent. Areas most often affected by burns are the hands and the forearms. The involvement of any part of the upper arms may have negative consequences distally to the burn, even if the burn itself does not affect that area.

Patients affected by upper extremity burns often suffer other associated traumas because of work-related accidents, very frequent in this type of injury. An assessment of potential fractures, amputations, wounds, blast, and crush injuries is essential for planning subsequent reconstruction procedures. The function of the shoulder joints must be carefully examined, and the nervous function of the median, ulnar, and radial nerves should also be evaluated.[24]

After this first assessment, and after calculating the extent and depth of the burn surface area, it is of fundamental importance to assess whether an escharotomy is needed. This is an emergency procedure that should be executed as soon as possible with the objective to resolve/prevent the pathologic increased subcutaneous pressure that is the main pathophysiology of electrical current-induced compartment syndrome.

Fluid infusion and edema

Burn can be defined as a non-hemorrhagic hypovolemic shock with loss of water, sodium, and plasma proteins but not of corpuscular elements. In the first 24–48 h, fluid losses cannot be stopped but only replaced, though early colloid administration may attenuate it.

The objective of the treatment is to restore and preserve tissue perfusion and avoid ischemia. One of the biggest complications of burn shock is the increase of capillary permeability throughout the organism due to the effects of heat on the microcirculation. Edema reaches its maximum expression within 8–12 h of the accident in minor burns and within 12–24 h in major ones.

These phenomena, caused by endothelial damage and by hypoperfusion, lead to the liberation of vasoactive substances and cytotoxic free radicals, which in turn are responsible for cellular edema and the generalized inflammatory reaction.[17,19]

When burns exceed 20–30% of the total body surface area (TBSA), even unburned areas develop edema owing to the increase of vascular permeability secondary to hypoperfusion and because of the plasma protein deficit.

The first choice "emergency solution" is an IV administration within the first 8 h of crystalloids (Ringer's lactate). In patients with extensive burns in whom it is not possible to achieve adequate tissue perfusion, even by doubling the infusion volume normally prescribed, it is possible to use hypertonic solutions (Ringer's lactate + 50 mEq of $NaHCO_3$ + 40 mEq lactate). These solutions have to be used carefully, monitoring natremia (which must never exceed 160 mEq/dL) and plasma osmolarity. Note: hyperosmolar syndrome induces kidney failure.

The administration of colloids is not effective in the first 8 h post-burn; later on, it is possible to infuse solutions of albumin or fresh plasma. The quantity of colloids to infuse has to be defined: one can calculate 0.5–1 mL/kg/% TBSA in fresh plasma in the first 24 h, starting 8/10 h post-burn. Elderly patients and those with extensive burns (>50%) maintain better hemodynamic stability and develop less edema, thanks to the administration of colloids.

If no colloids have been used in the first hours after the trauma and oncotic pressure remains low because of the depletion of plasma proteins, it is necessary to return the losses: the 5% albumin. Albumin demand during the second 24 h is 0.3–0.5 mL/kg/% TBSA, attempting to keep its blood levels above 2 g/dL to reabsorb peripheral edema.

The volume of fluids indicated in the resuscitation of burn patients depends on the gravity of the burn, the age and general condition of the patient, and the presence of associated lesions. In patients with burns of more than 15% TBSA, the quantity of fluid to provide has to be calculated on the basis of the burned area and body dimensions (ABA Guidelines), being careful not to overload the patient, aggravating the swelling with secondary edema to systems such as the lungs, subcutaneous tissues and BICS, etc.[3]

Burn-induced compartment syndrome (BICS)[14]

Deep second-degree and third-degree circumferential burns can trigger a serious "burn-induced compartment syndrome" (BICS) (Figs. 19.1–19.6, Box 19.1), which if not adequately treated can easily result in the loss of the extremity involved.

Full circumferential burns, or burns involving at least three-quarters of the extremity's circumference, are liable to develop BICS. The clinical reaction that occurs when edema develops during the first hours post-burn triggers a pressure increase at the subcutaneous and at the muscular level of the extremities. The expansion of the subcutaneous tissues is blocked by the burned skin, which has no elasticity. After the initial restriction of venous outflow, if proper treatment is not given, there is the risk of a reduction in arterial flow, resulting in ischemic tissue distally to the burn. It is important to perform direct monitoring of compartment pressure or at least the subcutaneous tissue all providing the very first sign of the

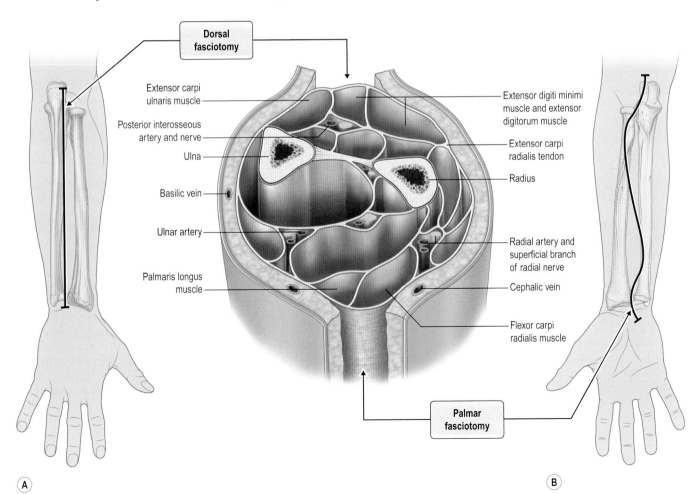

(A)   (B)

Fig. 19.1 Anatomy of forearm escharotomy incisions.

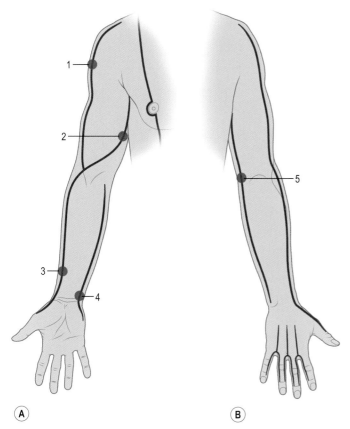

(A) (B)

Fig. 19.2 Recommended sites for upper extremity and chest escharotomies. Numbers 1 to 5 indicate dangerous incision sites.

This surgical procedure must involve all the burned tissues, skin, fat, and sometimes fasciae, until decompression of the compartment is observed. These escharotomies should follow the recommended procedures and be performed before the initial signs of either vascular (frozen hand) or neurological deficits occur. In cutaneous burns, the muscular and neural damages are secondary to the increased subcutaneous swelling; thus an early escharotomy of the skin may prevent or resolve BICS. In the later stages, when the muscles themselves are ischemic, they swell and a fasciotomy is needed. Escharotomies can be performed with an electrosurgical knife or a scalpel, ensuring complete release of the muscles (see Figs. 19.4B & 19.5).

When treating the upper extremity, particular attention should be paid to the blood flow through the cephalic and basilic veins and superficial branch of the radial nerve at the level of the wrist. In the most serious cases, it may be necessary to perform complete decompression of the carpal tunnel (see Figs. 19.1 & 19.2).

Escharotomy of the lower limb must be performed avoiding the tibial anterior nerve, the medial saphenous vein and nerve, the tibial posterior nerve, the fibular nerve, and the external saphenous nerve but not directly over the tibial plateau (see Figs. 19.3, 19.4, & 19.6).[28]

Recent reports indicate that an early on admission use of bromelain-based (NexoBrid) debriding enzyme can resolve or prevent BICS.[10–14]

Direct pressure measurement pre- and post-debridement/escharotomy should be performed after any procedure to ensure that the pressure did return to normal (Fig. 19.7).

Medication of the extremities should be carried out after careful cleaning and debridement of the affected surface.

developing danger. Main clinical signs of initial compartmental syndrome are the 5 Ps: diminished *Pulses* in distal arteries; *Pallor* and cold limb; initial intense *Pain* especially at passive flexion–extension, which then may decrease following muscular ischemia; under the subcutaneous *Pressure* the skin of the hand or the foot is very tight; *Paraesthesia*.[25] Screening with Doppler ultrasound could be useful during initial assessment, but this method cannot evaluate the exact compartment pressure. If laboratory values give high levels of creatinine phosphokinase (CPK), it may indicate severe muscle damage, or ischemia.

Direct measurement of compartment/subcutaneous pressure by hypodermic needle may provide the first measurable sign of imminent, developing BICS. One of the most common devices that allow a precise measurement of compartment pressure is the Stryker Set. This device includes a monitoring unit and a syringe with 3 mL of saline solution. The needle is introduced into the subcutaneous tissue or the muscular compartment that has to be monitored, and is flushed with 0.3 mL to re-equilibrate the pressure with interstitial fluids. After a few seconds the pressure level in mmHg appears on the monitoring unit. For measurements exceeding 35–40 mmHg (some claim even 30 mmHg), it is necessary to perform an emergency escharotomy and sometime fasciotomy or even canal release even in the very first hours in order to restore normal blood flow. In case of measures lower than 30 mmHg, it is possible to administer non-steroidal anti-inflammatory drugs combined with antioxidants to prevent progression.[26,27]

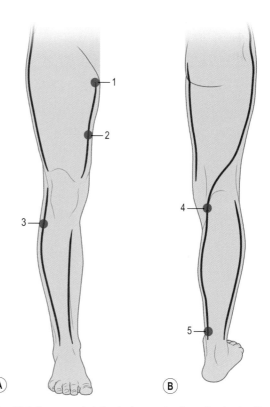

(A) (B)

Fig. 19.3 Recommended sites for lower extremity escharotomies. Numbers 1 to 5 indicate dangerous incision sites.

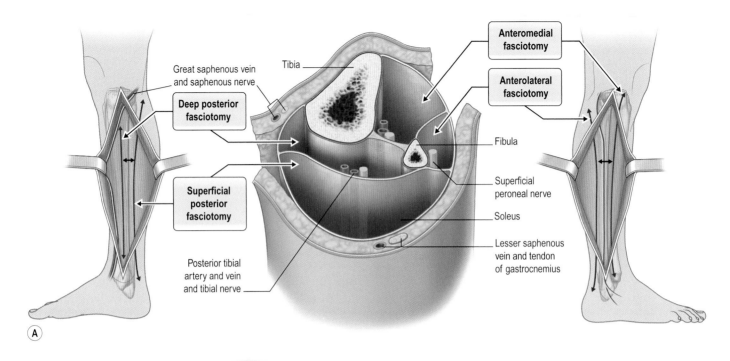

Great saphenous vein
and saphenous nerve

Tibia

**Deep posterior
fasciotomy**

**Superficial
posterior
fasciotomy**

Posterior tibial
artery and vein
and tibial nerve

**Anteromedial
fasciotomy**

**Anterolateral
fasciotomy**

Fibula

Superficial
peroneal nerve

Soleus

Lesser saphenous
vein and tendon
of gastrocnemius

(A)

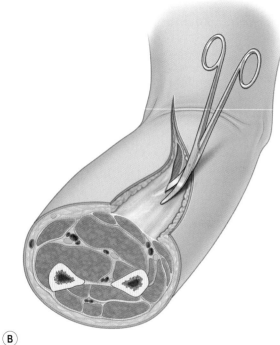

(B)

Fig. 19.4 (A) Anatomy of lower extremity escharotomy and fasciotomy incisions.
(B) Schematic of fascial release after escharotomy in the lower extremity.

Early mobilization of the joints is recommended unless otherwise specified. Nonadherent dressings such as Vaseline gauze are indicated for all burn-affected areas. For areas affected only superficially or at mid-dermal level, it is better to use primary biologic dressings/medications such as Biobrane, Mefix, or Aquacel-Ag to protect the exposed, raw wound bed ensuring good epithelialization. In areas that are deeply affected or clearly of third-degree, it is possible to proceed with protective biologic dressings until the time comes for surgical procedures. Early on admission enzymatic debridement can remove the eschar and serve as an escharotomy resolving/preventing BICS and preparing the patient for a scheduled surgical autografting operation or engraftment of skin substitute. During hospitalization it is fundamentally important to keep the upper and lower extremities of the patient in an elevated position in order to avoid the formation of new edema and reduce existing edema.

Surgery of the burn areas that will remove dead tissues (debridement) and cover the raw areas (engraftment) should be performed as early as possible in order to prevent the eschar-related inflammatory process. Inflammation that proceeds to granulation tissue formation leads to a greater incidence of hypertrophic scars, weaker scar tissues, and delays in prompt mobilization of the extremities.[29,30]

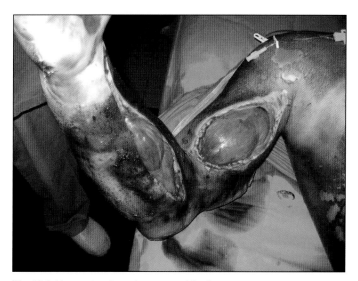

Fig. 19.5 Upper extremity escharotomy and fasciotomy.

Deep burned areas should be subjected to the earliest debridement (surgical or enzymatic) and cover treatment as soon as possible. Burns that do not heal within in 2 or 3 weeks should also be considered for surgical treatment. Depending on the burn area, regional or local anesthesia can be performed in the extremities, but preferably only in patients with relatively limited burn areas. The preferred treatment remains early debridement and autologous skin graft.

Related trauma

The local trauma most frequently associated with burns is bone fracture. In this case, close collaboration between the plastic and orthopedic surgeons is essential in order to choose the most appropriate surgical plan to follow. Stabilization of fractures contiguous to deeply burned areas should be performed early, preferably within the first 48 h after the accident, before bacterial colonization can hamper orthopedic

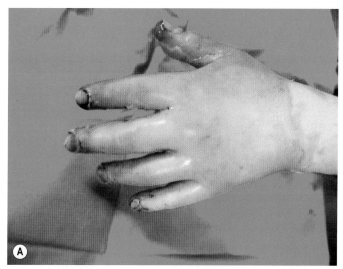

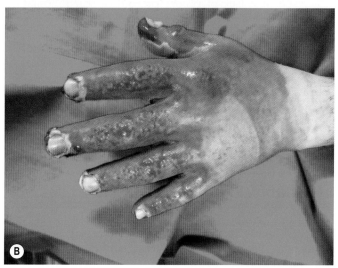

Fig. 19.7 (A) Admission, 4 hours post-injury, burns diagnosed as full-thickness, compartment interstitial pressure measured 80 mmHg. NexoBrid enzymatic dressing applied. **(B)** Immediately after removal of NexoBrid enzymatic dressing: pressure reduced to 20 mmHg, eschar wiped away revealing viable deep dermis. *(With the courtesy of Prof Lior Rosenberg.)*

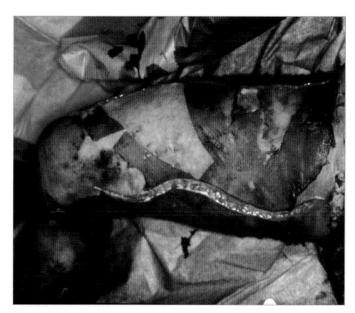

Fig. 19.6 Lower extremity escharotomy.

action. It has frequently been reported that the early stabilization of burn patients drastically decreases the onset of complications.

Various related trauma should be treated contextually or before their coverage with skin grafts, in order to avoid re-opening already treated burn areas.

In the deepest burn areas, especially if the result of electrocution or if accompanied by related trauma, the explosion of bones or tendons can occur, especially in major joints. This condition imposes an additional priority in the planning of the surgical procedures. The exposed tendons are liable to rapid dehydration and consequent necrosis, and prompt coverage is therefore essential. In the preparatory phase, cadaver skin or biologic medications can be useful, while in the surgical phase it is recommended to use dermal substitutes (such as Integra, Matriderm, etc.), which allow the formation of new tissue between the tendons and the grafted skin. Grafting directly on the exposed tendons is counter-indicated in terms of graft survival and functional results.

Also, exposed bone should be covered as early as possible, even though resistance to exposure is much higher and more easily resolved than in the case of tendons. Coverage can be performed at a second stage utilizing rotation or free flaps.[31]

Patient selection

Plastic/burn surgeons possess all the necessary tools and scientific know-how to treat burn patients. From intensive care to the surgical phase, they should be able to take the best decisions for the patient. He should decide the necessity, extent, and timing of surgery and, in some cases, also the choice to pursue a second intention healing process. The preoperative care plan for scars is also crucial and should be prepared by the same medical team that treated the patient during the previous acute phase. The extremities are the most frequent sufferers from post-surgery scar contractures, often as a result of a lack of proper preventive scar modulation measures (such as *massage therapy*, *elastic compression*, *kinesitherapy*, and *splinting*) aimed at preventing pathologic scarring. An assessment of the affected areas will suggest to the specialist whether to proceed with corrective measures or engage in additional surgical interventions.

Considering that importance of normal walking, physical autonomy, and self-dependence at home and work depend on the complete rehabilitation of the affected areas, the main objective of sequelae surgery is to re-establish the extremity's proper range of motion (ROM) and function.[32]

Treatment/surgical technique

Burn surgery can be subdivided into acute-phase surgery and sequelae surgery. Acute-phase extremity surgery is not fundamentally different from surgery in any other part of the body. Procedures such as fasciotomy, debridement, and coverage with autologous skin grafts, as previously described, follow the surgical guidelines of acute-phase general burns with special attention to prevention of BICS. Regarding sequelae surgery of the extremities, it must be noted that the majority of scar retractions here lead to disabilities, and localized burn-related joint contracture may occur.[17]

Acute-phase surgery

BICS and emergency procedures such as escharotomy and fasciotomy were largely dealt with in the foregoing section. Focusing only on the extremities, the commonest surgical procedures continue to be debridement and sheet or meshed free-skin graft of autologous skin. These procedures should preferably be performed as early as possible, i.e., before the 5th and 7th day post-injury. As previously said, some *ad hoc* surgical variations may be necessary, depending on the type of damage affecting the extremities and the kind of structures involved. In order to limit bleeding and thus operate in a condition of controlled hemostasis, tourniquet can be used. This procedure facilitates extremity surgery, reducing blood loss, but at the same time assessment of tissue viability and the limiting tourniquet-time are challenging. Debridement should be performed up to the viable tissues, after carefully removing necrotic eschar and paying special attention to the flexion–extension areas and the axillary hollow areas. In these

areas the necrotomy is more complex to perform. In deep or electrical burns, it is possible to avulse the entire skin and subcutaneous fat down to the muscular fascia in order to reduce blood loss and avoid the risk of incomplete eschar removal. Unlike the cutaneous dermis, the viable fat underneath is an unpredictable recipient bed for free skin grafts, often necessitating preparatory procedures such as temporary allo- or xenograft that, when removed a few days later, leaves an adequately perfused recipient bed.[33–36]

During debridement of more superficially burned areas that require surgical treatment, dermabrasion or hydrosurgery (with instruments like VersaJet) provide useful support as they minimize the waste of vital tissue and also permit careful debridement in non-flat surfaces, such as the extremities.[34]

Recently a new rapid and effective enzymatic debridement using bromelain-derived pharmaceutical gel-like agent (NexoBrid) allows the removal of the entire eschar early on admission day by a single, 4-hour, local application. This enzymatic debridement does not harm viable tissues, preserving the non-injured dermis, and has been found to act as an enzymatic escharotomy tool. Being eschar-specific it can be applied on all burns without committing to a specific diagnosis of the burn depth: the enzyme will dissolve only the dead eschar, leaving the viable tissue for healing by epithelialization or autografting. Being a topical agent, it can be easily applied by non-surgeons without initial burn depth diagnosis, independent of any surgical facilities even on difficult areas such as extremities and joints (including axillae). As in surgical debridement, the enzymatically debrided bed needs immediate cover to protect it from desiccation but, as much of the dermis is preserved, autografting is needed only for full-thickness areas and most of the burns (>70%) can heal spontaneously by epithelialization (see Fig. 19.7).[10–14]

Skin grafts

Skin grafts can be meshed with mesher 1:1 or 1.5:1, or even larger 2–5:1 if the patient does not have donor areas. Meshing the graft will facilitate adherence, drainage, and take besides increasing in size. The elbow joint and the axillary and popliteal cavities are preferably grafted with medium-thickness skin, which provides greater elasticity and resistance in areas subject to high mobility and trauma. All skin grafts should be positioned considering the least relaxed skin tension lines in order to obtain the aesthetically best results. In the specific case of the arms, it is recommended to position the skin grafts longitudinally for the best aesthetic outcome.

Skin grafts must be checked after 4–5 days and treated until full recovery is completed.

Skin substitutes

Over the last decade, the use of dermal substitutes in acute-phase burn surgery has become more frequent. In particular, this technique is now used in acute-phase burn surgery in cases of extensive deep burns with exposure of bones and tendons.

The characteristics of an ideal skin substitute were defined in 1978 by Tavis, but to date none of the available skin substitutes fulfil all those criteria.

The currently available products (Integra, Matriderm, allograft, Terudermis, etc.) have different characteristics, but they all aim for the same objective: re-establishment of a layer of dermis under a free skin graft. There is an ongoing debate as to whether these newly formed tissues can be considered dermis or not.

A fundamental prerequisite for valid results is that the application should be onto vital tissue that is free of any contamination or necrotic residue.

In acute burns of the extremities, the use of skin substitutes is extremely effective in the treatment of critical areas (axilla, elbow, popliteal cavity) and on exposed bones and tendons.

These products provide immediate coverage of the burned area, resulting in reduced risk of infection or tissue necrosis, and facilitate the regeneration of subcutaneous-like tissues between the deep structures and the skin graft.

Applying dermal substitutes is usually easy. However, when treating the extremities, some critical aspects should be considered, such as range of movement, the autonomy of the various segments, and perfect adherence between the product and the wound bed. In the post-surgical period it is recommended that the surgeon should be guided by the instructions of the manufacturer of the product together with personal experience.[35-37]

It is important to recall, however, that the commonest possible complication following their use in the acute phase is infection, which can lead to complete loss of the skin grafts applied in 30–40% of cases.

Negative pressure dressings (NPDs) (V.A.C., Renasys, etc.) are often used for a few days as primary dressing for skin grafts or skin substitute sheets. The use of negative pressure devices improve the graft take, perform its better adherence on the wound bed, prevent contamination, protect the graft from traumas, and finally create a good environment for skin graft taking or vascularization of skin substitute. It is possible to use these devices on meshed and unmeshed skin grafts, on single/double layer sheets with interposition of Vaseline gauze between the graft and the NPD gauze/sponge. Many authors suggest removing the dressing directly on the 6th/7th postoperative day, but it is possible to do so before. We found this kind of dressing very useful in critical areas such as hollows, axilla, popliteal region, and neck, giving much more stability and a perfect adhesion between the graft and the wound bed, but it is safer not to use it beyond the graft imbibition phase (3–5 days) as it may interfere with the graft's venous outflow and final vascularization. For the same reason, bulky gauzes, bolsters, and soft collars should not be used in these areas.

Flaps

There is a general hesitancy to perform early free tissue transfer in acute burns because of the concept of progressive tissue necrosis following electrical and thermal burns. Occasionally local flaps and free flaps may be utilized in primary reconstruction after electrical injuries in forearm and legs. Debridement in these areas often produces large tissue defects or large bone exposition. Fascial flaps may provide good coverage for the axilla and forearm. Recent studies have looked at the use of free flaps in primary reconstruction and found good results on the number of surgical procedures and reduction in hospitalization.[38]

Joint reconstruction (Figs. 19.8 & 19.9)

High-voltage electricity (>1000 volts) flowing through the extremities meets the point of maximum resistance in the joints, and in such cases, severe damage involving all the anatomic joint structures affected can be observed.

Joint reconstruction and coverage of exposed joints should be managed early, in order to preserve as much functionality as possible, together with the integrity of any viable tissue that is still alive, and to prevent septic arthritis.

Articulation capsule and joint ligament apparatus reconstruction has priority for surgery. In our experience the dermal graft is an effective solution to this problem. Using a powered or manual dermatome (Padgett drum dermatome, Humby, Watson, Rosenberg, or others), a thin epidermal graft is harvested followed by harvesting of the dermal layer. The epidermal layer is returned to cover the deep donor site defect. The harvested dermis is then carefully shaped in relation to the structures requiring reconstruction, whether an articulation capsule or a ligament, and then finally grafted onto the site. The fibroblast-rich grafted dermis realigns its elastic fibers under the stimulation of the force applied to the joint. This contributes to the reconstruction of strong vector tissue,

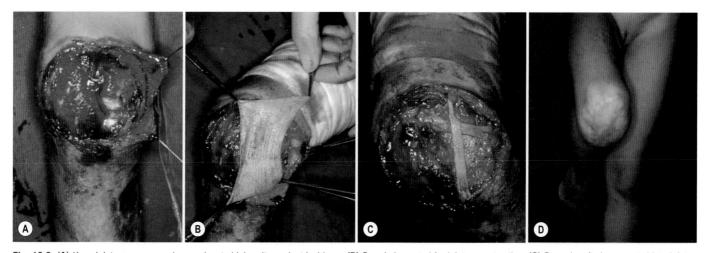

Fig. 19.8 **(A)** Knee joint space exposed secondary to high-voltage electrical burn. **(B)** Dermis harvested for joint reconstruction. **(C)** Dermal grafts incorporated into joint capsule reconstruction. **(D)** Result after skin graft.

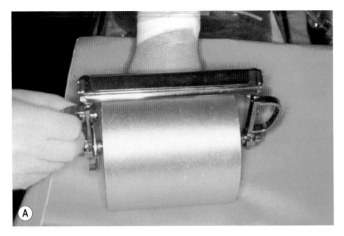

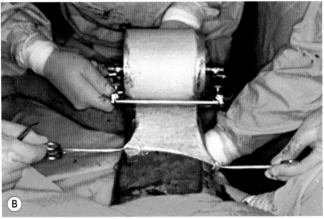

Fig. 19.9 (A) The Padgett dermatome. **(B)** Dermal harvest with the Padgett dermatome. Epidermal layer is adherent to the dermatome drum.

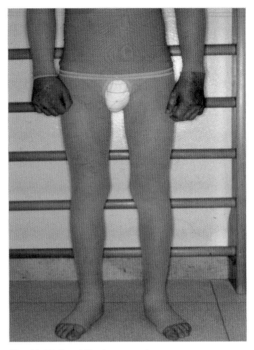

Fig. 19.10 Specialized compression garment.

which is a characteristic feature of healthy joint structure.[39] In case of lack of tissue for reconstruction, a polycaprolactone-based polyurethane urea, like an Artelon patch, should be used to reinforce the joint. It is an elastic sheet, built on well-known chemical components cleared for use in medical devices, that degrades non-enzymatically, and reinforces and stabilizes the reconstructed joint.[40]

A selective debridement that leaves much of the native deep dermis viable and intact over the joints may reduce the need for such challenging surgical procedures.

Postoperative care

Burn injuries cause highly scar-related disabilities characterized by major hyperplasia and marked contraction of the skin surface. The mobile segments of the extremities (axilla, elbow, wrist, knee, ankle) are among the most critical for monitoring in the post-surgical phase (Figs. 19.10 & 19.11; Table 19.1).

Many studies have dealt with the actual effectiveness of post-surgical elastic compression and massage therapy, and in normal clinical practice these procedures are routinely performed to obtain the best results possible in terms of scarring, range of motion (ROM), and function. The use of elastic pressure garments for the extremities, silicone sheets or gel, and splints are widely recommended from the earliest post-operative stage in all centers specializing in burns treatment. In addition to these devices, it is always advisable to perform

physical/occupational therapy, especially in burns involving the extremities.

Burn patients who must stay many hours in bed may lie in particular positions that can be defined as "antalgic". These are related to the great degree of pain suffered and to the distressing situation the patients are dealing with. The joints can easily lose their ROM if not properly treated.

Positioning the patient

The position of the patient should generally be supine with the neck slightly stretched. In non-extensive burns, lateral decubitus is also allowed.

The interposition of a thick surface (e.g., pillow, sheets) in the interscapular area ensures slight hyperextension of the neck. When necessary, it is desirable to use tutor collars.

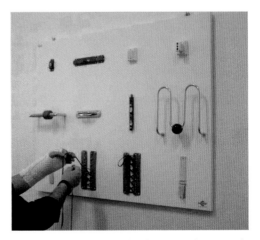

Fig. 19.11 Physical/occupational tasks to enhance post-burn mobility and minimize contracture formation.

Table 19.1 Joint position

Joint	Position
Shoulder	Abduction 65–85° Slight flexion 25°
Elbow	Extension
Wrist	Slight extension 30°
Hip	Extension Abduction 15°
Knee	Extension
Ankle	Maintain 90°

Upper extremity

The upper extremity, excluding the hand, consists of three major joints, which must be carefully handled if crippling deficits of mobility are to be avoided.

Shoulder

The shoulder joint should usually be held in abduction and slight flexion (60–80° abduction and 15–20° flexion) using special bandages, a figure-of-eight, and pads. Gauze or foam are used for the armpits. This position ensures good stability of the shoulder joint. In discharged patients in outpatient care, the use of "airplane" splints, with a base on the hips and 80–90° arm support, is suggested, always bearing in mind that excessive abduction can create pathologic tractions at the level of the brachial plexus and a radial nerve deficit.

Elbow

The elbow is another critical area that needs attention. During the period of hospitalization, the elbow joint should necessarily be maintained in a position of extension in order to avoid frequent burn contracture sequelae. The use of splints is crucial, and a prone posture should be ensured to avoid having any negative effects on hand posture.[41,42]

Wrist

The wrist should be in a slight extension position (about 30°), using splints and hand braces.

Lower extremity

As said, burn patients tend to adopt an antalgic physiopathologic position, which may lead them to flexion contracture of major joints.

Hip

Burns that extend from the abdomen to the anterior thigh can cause troublesome retractions at the level of the hip joint. Especially in children, scarring and retracting tissue may affect the proper alignment of the pelvis and the spinal column. In the acute phase, the hips should be kept in full extension (0°), with a physiologic abduction of about 15.

During post-surgery, using braces and splints in pediatric care allows coxofemoral extension and helps to prevent hyperlordosis.

Knee

If not properly cared for, the knee, like the elbow, is prone to severe flexion contracture, resulting in major mobility deficits. This kind of negative outcome should be avoided by positioning the part in extension using a splint or a cast.

Ankle

The ankle function should be preserved by maintaining a position at 90° through the use of splints or special supports. Post-traumatic clubfoot is the most frequent joint complication in burn patients. The problem manifests itself a few days after hospitalization and may lead to permanent deformity that is hard to resolve. Scar contraction and shortening of the muscle tendon risk prolonging this pathologic condition.[42]

All these guidelines are part of an important comprehensive physical/occupational therapy program, which together with correct positioning of the joints should include appropriate rehabilitation exercises. These exercises, which should be performed daily as soon as the general and local conditions permit, are usually passive at the patient's bedside under the guidance of a physiotherapist. The purpose is to maintain joint mobility and keep muscle tone intact using the classic principles of physical/occupational therapy, applied through active and passive mobilization, as well as forming a positive attitude toward complete recovery and return to the pre-injury lifestyle.

Passive mobilization

Passive mobilization refers to the use of particular movements of the patient's joints caused by external action without any muscular contraction or nervous participation by the patients themselves. Passive kinesis employs methods of slow mobilization and methods of rapid mobilization.

Active mobilization

This indicates the overall complex of particular movements of the patient's joints with the participation of their nervous centers and active muscular contraction. Active kinesis combines assisted exercises, exercises against resistance, and free exercises. Burn patient kinesis makes use of both static and dynamic forms. Static kinesitherapy consists of forms of postural alignment and the use of rigid and mobile splints, anti-decubitus ulcer beds, and normal or elastic bandages. Dynamic kinesitherapy consists of changes of posture during mobilization of joints affected by the trauma or of undamaged joints, mobilization of the rib cage, postural drainage, and water rehabilitation therapy.[41–43]

After being discharged, the patient should continue therapy for several months. The local treatment of scars, continuous pressure garments, splinting, and physical exercises during the postoperative period should all be regarded as an integral part of the burn patient's management.

Treatment usually continues on an outpatient basis until the scar tissue is well stabilized and mature. Measuring the degree of flexure–extension of the joints and the quality of the scars will indicate whether patients may be considered to be definitively cured, whether they are capable of further improvement or whether a reconstructive procedure is needed.

Outcomes, prognosis, and complications

Unstable healing: Marjolin's ulcer

The healing of large burn areas may lead to large scars that may become unstable, creating sequelae, and representing the first complication specialists have to face in the follow-up of burn patients. Non-healing wounds, especially full-thickness ones, in some areas tend to develop hypergranulation rather than epithelialize, while some areas that have healed spontaneously may ulcerate or develop hypertrophic scars.

The continued presence of heavy scar tissue that from time to time ulcerates has a negative effect on rehabilitation procedures. Sharp pain and the lack of solid skin coverage severely limit the use of splints, massage therapy, and the use of pressure garments and silicone. In some patients, the scarring phase is so unstable that it can go on for months, without reaching completion. In such cases, it is advisable to consider an extensive excision of the entire scar tissue and autograft it. Repeated ulcerations that continue for months, or even years, can lead to malignant changes developing an invasive squamous cell carcinoma at the burn areas.

Marjolin's ulcer is an infiltrating squamous cell carcinoma, with a low level of differentiation, which forms in unstable scar areas. Statistically, its rate of incidence is 2% in burn scars, with a higher prevalence in the limbs, especially the lower limbs. As it occurs in areas with a history of instability and ulceration, it is rarely diagnosed early because of confusion with other ulcerative processes. The first histologic sign of this highly invasive type of carcinoma occurs at the edge of the ulcer. There is early development of lymph node metastases in 30% of cases, with a 5-year survival in <10% of cases.[44,45]

Treatment is strictly surgical with wide excision and histologic control of the surgical margins with sentinel lymph node biopsy. In the event of metastasis, lymph nodes can be radically excised. There are no reports of preventative lymph node excision improving prognosis.

In some cases, when bone or deep levels are affected, proximal limb amputation may be necessary.

Scar contraction

As in any other trauma, burns may also result in scarring tissue, which if not properly treated, can develop into hypertrophic scarring. The deeper the burns, the more healing by secondary intention (granulation and scarring), the greater the risk of becoming hypertrophic scars in the future. Burn scars may take a very long average time, >2 years, to become stable.

Some factors related to burns pathophysiology are decisive for the healing of severely injured patients and the outcome. The commonest and most evident complication is scarring of the skin. Contracting scarring tissue may cause significant functional limitation and physical deformity, which may eventually lead to permanent damage at the musculoskeletal level, deforming the joints and, in children, pathologic bone growth.

Full hand motion in the burned patient is useless if significant contractures of the elbow and axilla prevent the patient from positioning the hand for optimal function. In addition, severe knee contracture will interfere with correct walking. It is not easy to specify which extremity burns will or will not be disabling. As specified in other sections in this chapter, the result depends on various factors such as the burn's etiology, its location, acute and post-acute phase treatment, and patient compliance.

In cases of particularly deep burns in the upper extremities complicated by BICS and necrosis involving the deepest structures, it is common to witness the phenomena of osteomyelitis and necrotizing fasciitis. These severe complications often result in the amputation of the affected extremity.

The most serious burns from the point of view of complications are certainly those of electrical origin. They are frequently "subdued" burns, in a relatively small area, but with vast underlying damage. Muscle tissue, the vascular and neural fasciae, the joints, and bones are frequently involved, often associated with very severe tissue damage.

Muscle and tendon necrosis may be extensive, with their loss resulting in severe functional deficits.

Massive involvement of the extremities can result in decreased ROM, mobility, vascular, and aesthetic defects that are hardly ever totally resolved.

Axillary contractures (Fig. 19.12)

Of all burn-related contractures, that of the axilla is the commonest.

Managing burn of the axilla is difficult, especially in pediatric patients. The preferred antalgic position of a patient with burns in this area is commonly in adduction. This unfavorable anatomic position is further complicated by the difficulty to immobilize the shoulder joint resulting in frozen shoulder. Preventing these complications by early debridement (enzymatic is the easiest in this area) and early autograft closure seems to be the most practical approach.

Kurtzman and Stern's classification (1990)[45,46] divides axillary contractures into three main types, on the basis of their anatomic characteristics:

- *Type 1*: Contracture involving either the anterior (1A) or the posterior (1B) axillary fold alone
- *Type 2*: Contracture involving both the anterior and the posterior axillary fold but not the skin in the axillary dome
- *Type 3*: Contracture involving both axillary folds and the axillary dome.

The surgery plan has to consider the type of contracture in order to tackle the local problem in the best possible way.

In types 1 and 2, it is normally possible to use local flaps, while in type 3 it is necessary to extend the surgical area to the trunk, using large flaps from the latissimus dorsi and pectoral area.

Elbow contractures

After axilla contractures, the joint most frequently involved is the elbow. Most contractures at this level are caused by skin scars, which exert such a powerful effect that they limit the range of movement of the forearm and upper arm.

We usually distinguish between intra-articular and extra-articular contractures, depending on whether the joint structures are involved or not. The majority of elbow contractures

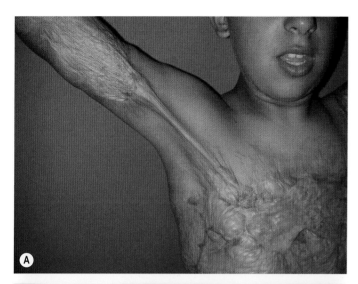

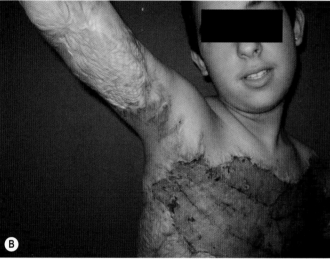

Fig. 19.12 Axillary contracture **(A)** before and **(B)** after Z-plasty release. *(Courtesy of Department of Plastic Surgery and Burn Therapy, ARNAS Ospedale Civico, Palermo, Italy.)*

are extra-articular, in flexion, caused only by skin scars, while extension contractures are quite rare in burn sequelae.

With regard to articular contractures, the use of local flaps or incisional release and grafting will usually suffice. In very large scar retractions, in which the excised scar tissue involves the upper arm and forearm, fasciocutaneous flaps from the chest or abdomen are recommended. Excellent results have been reported with the use of Integra in the reconstruction of anterior and posterior elbow defects.

In the postoperative period, the use of extension splints is recommended, along with early physical/occupational therapy exercises to maintain the movement range obtained with surgery.

Heterotopic ossification

Heterotopic bone formation in burn patients is a rare occurrence but, functionally speaking, it is a major complication. Only 3% of burn patients develop this complication, but if periarticular calcifications are included, which are a false form of heterotrophic ossification, about 30% of patients develop the complication.

Heterotopic bone formation is a complication that occurs when new bone develops in soft tissues that do not normally ossify. It is coupled with important joint movement deficit. There are many possible causes of heterotopic ossification, but the real etiology is still not well known. Usually the severity of the burn injury is considered more likely to be responsible than its extension or location. Unnecessary joint manipulation with related microtraumas has also been considered as a possible cause of the initial micro-ossification of the musculotendinous tissues. The elbow is the joint most frequently involved, followed by the shoulder and hip joints. The knee is rarely involved.

The most serious clinical picture is bridge ossification, in which the new bone tissue links the jointed bones in a condition of structural stability. The joint remains blocked even after the patient has recovered from the burns. If the new bone has not established any structural continuity, it may regress and sometimes, especially in children, even completely disappear. This ossification process usually starts a few weeks post-burn injury, the average being 10–15 weeks. The symptoms (i.e., loss of ROM and joint pain) may be preceded by radiologic evidence. Thus physical/occupational therapy is prescribed without excessive joint stress, which seems to stimulate the ossification process.

Surgical treatment is necessary only in the case of a complete osseous bridge, and it is better to treat only mature new-formed bone, in order to be able to proceed with its complete removal. Particular attention must be paid to the ulnar nerve, which is sometimes trapped inside the new bone, and the nerve must be identified and carefully isolated in order to preserve it. In the postoperative period, it is necessary to apply a splint in the flexed position, if the blocking was in extension, and in extension if the ankylosis was in flexion. Early physical/occupational therapy should start within 10 days and continue throughout healing.[47,48]

Skeletal–muscle complications: bone exposure

In elbow and knee joint burns, the olecranon and patella bone is often exposed (see Fig. 19.14A). In spite of the local and general conditions, osteomyelitis is rare, and after surgical debridement of the affected cortex, the underlying bone is viable. The cortex of these areas is thick and resists exposure-related infection and necrosis for some time, especially if properly treated by grafting. In order to create a proper graft recipient bed over the bony surface, granulation or other soft tissue is needed. By punching the cortex down to the vascular layer, granulation tissue will grow over the exposed bone.

Additional considerations are needed for injuries involving open fractures associated with burns, where infection is perhaps inevitable. But also in this case, the infection remains localized to the fracture site for a long time, with rare involvement of the entire bone segment.

In these patients, the stabilization system should be carefully chosen. Many surgeons strongly oppose plaster splints because they prevent easy inspection and care of the burn area and instead recommend external fixation. This procedure – now considered the most appropriate – is not free of risk in burn patients because often the pins have to pass through the burned skin, transferring bacteria to the bone.

Surgical coverage of these exposed areas should be performed rapidly on cleared tissues. In this context, a negative pressure unit is particularly useful (V.A.C., Renasys, etc.), as this quickly promotes cleansing of the bed and promotes vascularization and granulation.

Secondary procedures

Minor or major surgical procedures on the extremities are usually indicated when rehabilitation therapy has been ineffective or when joint functionality is compromised. Apart from the cases just described, surgery on the joints usually occurs at this stage and not during the acute phase.

Reconstructive surgery can also be delayed when particularly deeply burned areas remain exposed for long periods and become scarred.

Patients with secondary indication for surgery are:

- Patients with scar sequelae not resolvable by physical/ occupational therapy
- Patients with debilitating scar sequelae
- Patients with chronic skin tissue loss and exposure of nerve–vascular structures, bone, and tendons
- Patients with ROM or articulation deficit
- Patients with nervous deficit.

Before planning any surgery, the specialist should take into account certain aspects, summarized as follows:

- Scar location
- Scar thickness and quality
- Joint deficit assessment
- Extent skin loss and careful evaluation of exposed tissues
- Local conditions (presence of normal surrounding skin, surgical options).

It is appropriate to plan the surgical procedure when the scar tissue is completely stabilized and after obtaining the best possible result in terms of joint mobility.

Reduced joint mobility may depend on various factors. The commonest is obviously the contraction of scar tissue around the joint itself. Scarring masses that are so firm that they do not allow proper excision of bone segments can aggravate this condition.

In joint surgery, particular attention should be paid to vascular nerve fasciae in the armpit, elbow, and wrist. Unless there are special surgical needs, it is always best to maintain the integrity of the joint capsule and the articular face.

Z-plasty

This technique is the basis of the surgical treatment of burns sequelae. Z-plasty is feasible in the presence of surrounding healthy tissue. It exploits the principle that it is possible to stretch a scarred area by the interposition of two or more triangular flaps rotated from immediately adjacent areas, with maximum elongation, using flaps with an angle of 60°. In scarring and contractures of the armpit and elbow, multiple Z-plasties remain one of the most effective techniques (Fig. 19.13). There are many variations to the normal Z-type plastic technique, described by various authors, identifying different angles between two or more interposed flaps. It is possible, especially when treating armpits, to use two asymmetric flaps

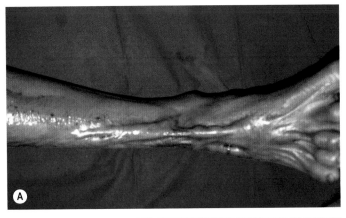

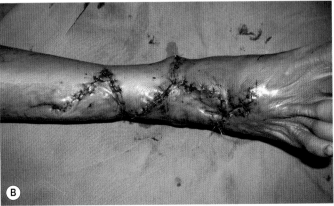

Fig. 19.13 (A) Severe ankle contracture. **(B)** Ankle contracture from Fig. 19.17, treated with multiple Z-plasties.

angled at 90°. This technique is also called the ¾ Z-plasty technique (Figs. 19.14 & 19.15).

In ankle and knee injuries, Z-type fasciocutaneous flaps are used. These skin flaps are prepared including the skin, the subcutaneous tissue, and the muscular fascia, leaving in place the muscular belly. For the ankle, both frontally and posteriorly, the flaps should be prepared including the paratenon with its entire vascular network; thus these flaps are quite strong and viable and well adapted to cover critical areas such as those described. This procedure, if well planned, can be performed under local or local-regional anesthesia.

In general, in flexion areas where the cause of the retraction is a longitudinal hypertrophic scar band with workable skin on both sides, it is possible to use a simple or multiple Z-plasty. When we observe surrounding scar tissue, with involvement of three-quarters of the circumference, we need a large transverse excision of the scar tissue and skin grafting of the entire area.

Skin grafts

As in the previous case, this is also a primary technique for the treatment of burn scars. After thorough debridement of the retracted scar, it is necessary to interpose a full-thickness or at least a thick partial-thickness graft on the residual viable bed. The donor area should be of intact, healthy skin. Harvesting such skin from the groin or abdomen can be easily closed primarily. The removed skin should be defatted with scissors up to the dermis before being applied onto the wound bed and stabilized by tie-over dressing. The grafting should be

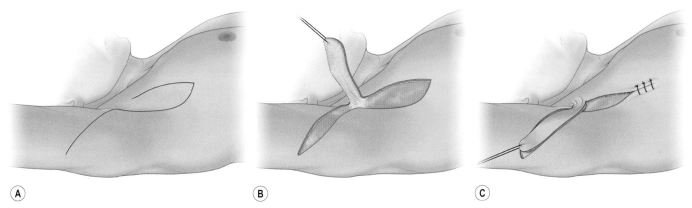

Fig. 19.14 **(A)** Designing a ¾ Z-plasty for the treatment of an axillary contracture. **(B,C)** Raising the flaps of the ¾ Z-plasty designed in Fig. 19.19.

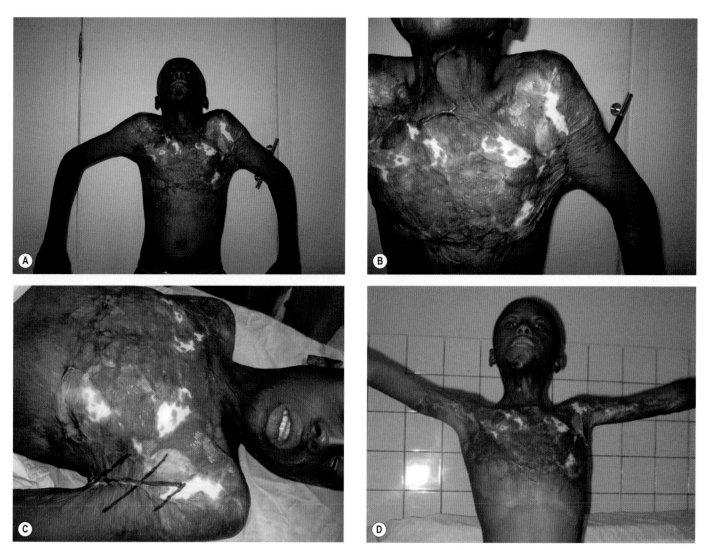

Fig. 19.15 **(A,B)** Severe retraction of axilla hollows. **(C)** Multiple Z-plasty plan. **(D)** Final result after 2 months. *(Courtesy of the International Association of Humanitarian Medicine.)*

monitored for 4–5 days post-surgery after removal of the dressing.

This procedure can be performed under local or regional anesthesia too, with minimal discomfort to the patient. Functional rehabilitation can be cautiously resumed 3 weeks after surgery.

Dermal substitutes in the surgical treatment of sequelae

The use of dermal substitutes in today's surgical practice is increasingly widespread. It allows the adding of new tissue in scarring characterized by a basic tissue deficit with greater advantages than those offered by simple free grafts of skin.

In the surgical treatment of retractions of the armpit, elbow, and kneecap, Integra has proved to be highly effective for ensuring a good basis for epidermis tissue grafts, permitting the use of thinner autografts with less morbidity in donor areas.

Integra vascularizes after about 21–28 days, being ready to receive a thin partial-thickness free skin graft. The result is a softer and more durable grafted area than one produced by simple free skin grafts, even compared with the full-thickness technique. The resulting scar also has better quality.

Dermal substitutes (i.e., Integra, Matriderm) are very helpful in the surgical treatment of burns sequelae and specifically in the treatment of critical areas.[35–37]

Flaps

Numerous rotation, transposition, and other forms of local flaps (see Fig. 19.14) are described in all treatises on plastic surgery, representing a technical heritage through which the plastic surgeon can effectively tackle full-thickness skin defects reaching good functional and aesthetic results. These local flaps guarantee the same texture, thickness, and color as the adjacent skin sometimes with a minimal donor area.

Flaps are indicated without question when it is necessary to cover important "noble" structures such as the vascular–nerve fasciae or areas with bone or tendon exposure and joints.

As in all surgical procedures, local flaps should be carefully studied, prepared, and well arranged. Large flaps can be designed in the scapular region for the resolution of major scarring of the axilla. Large flaps taken from the thoracic or flank region are useful in reconstructive surgery of the elbow. However, at the elbow or ankle level, it is sufficient to use small local flaps or simple Z-type plasties. The flap must be designed in such a way that its margins are never placed longitudinally over the joint.

The monitoring of the flap should be followed for the first 7–10 days. If there are no signs of suffering, it is possible to resume positioning of the limb and physical/occupational therapy after 15–21 days, depending on the area involved.

Fasciocutaneous and myocutaneous flaps

Reconstructive surgery of the limbs may involve extensive use of *fasciocutaneous* and *myocutaneous flaps*, which successfully cover full-thickness loss of skin and soft tissue, especially at elbow and knee joint level and the proximal third and middle limb (Figs. 19.16 & 19.17).

Due to the unfavorable angle of rotation, large flaps are frequently required to correct small defects. It is therefore recommended that this surgical solution should be carefully considered.

Fasciocutaneous flaps from the lateral region of the arm, supplied by branches of the radial collateral artery and sometimes used as "island flaps", have good mobility and are a reliable solution for reconstruction of the lateral and posterior region of the elbow.

In reconstructive surgery of the upper extremities, *the forearm flap based on the radial artery* plays an important role, thanks to its versatility. This flap, based on fasciocutaneous branches of the radial artery and used as an "island flap" with its proximal base on the radial artery, is useful for coverage of defects in the entire region of the elbow, including large defects with olecranon exposure.

Among myocutaneous flaps, *the latissimus dorsi* with and without skin are of particular importance for correction of large defects of the proximal third of the arm and axilla, while *flexor carpi radialis flaps* are important for coverage of defects of the forearm and elbow.

The *medial or lateral gastrocnemius flaps* are particularly recommended for coverage of defects of the proximal third of the leg. The same flap can be used to cover the defects in the knee. The *soleus muscle flap*, prepared by preserving half the muscle, is useful in the reconstruction of defects of the medial third of the leg. Because of their segmental vasculature, the muscles of the lower third of the leg are less suitable for rotation and can be used to cover adjacent skin deficits. The partial soleus muscle flap can also be for used for defects of the distal third of the leg. When properly detached from its distal pedicle, it can be rotated on its pedicle more proximally to cover large areas up to about 5–6 cm above the ankle.

The *extensor hallucis longus myocutaneous flap*, as with the *extensor digitorum longus muscle flap*, can be used to cover defects just above the medial malleolus, while short peroneal muscle flaps are useful just above the lateral malleolus.

A fasciocutaneous flap of greatest interest for coverage of the distal part of the leg and ankle is the *retrograde fibular flap*, the blood supply of which is based on the peroneal artery retrograde flow. However, it is essential that the connection between the anterior and posterior tibia artery should be intact because the retrograde blood supply will come from the terminal part. The long pedicle that can be obtained allows the flap to move easily and to be used in the entire leg and ankle (Table 19.2).

Skin expansion

The principle for the use of skin expansion lies in the positive response of live dermal tissue when it is subjected to mechanical stretching stimulation. The expanded tissue undergoes significant histologic changes such as cell hyperplasia, an increase in the number of basal cells in the mitotic phase, an increase in vascular atrophy, and the loss of adipose tissue.[49]

In addition, the soft tissues of the extremities can also be expanded. The placement of the expander should be carefully studied in order to obtain the maximum return in terms of tissue gain, also considering scar tissue healing and potential poor blood supply of the legs: theoretically, only healthy skin should be expanded but, if necessary, it is possible to expand, very carefully, scarred skin. In such cases, however, the

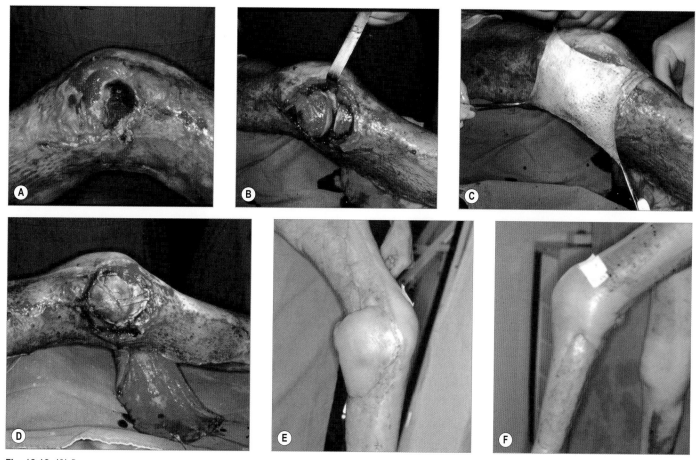

Fig. 19.16 (A) Bone exposed secondary to severe burn. **(B)** Exposed knee joint. **(C)** Dermal graft for coverage of exposed knee joint. **(D)** Dermal grafts in place reconstructing joint capsule; fasciocutaneous flap has been raised. **(E)** Fasciocutaneous flap inset to provide definitive joint coverage superficial to dermal graft. **(F)** Final result of knee reconstruction.

expansion will be very limited; it will also be painful for the patient.

Choosing the correct place to position the expander is crucial. It must be possible to advance or rotate the expanded skin without tension, ensuring complete coverage of the area that is going to be excised.

In the upper limb, it is preferable to use radial positioning in order to avoid compression of the neurovascular structures.

Expansion with medial and lateral advancement is indicated in all cases rather than unlikely advancement towards a distal position.

For skin expanders used in the lower extremities, it is necessary to take into account local lymphatic drainage, arterial blood supply, and the quality of the tissue conditions as all may cause skin necrosis and tissue expander exposure (Fig. 19.18).

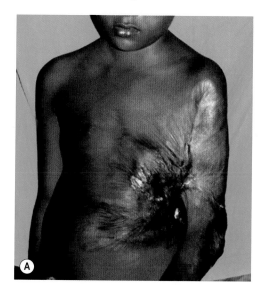

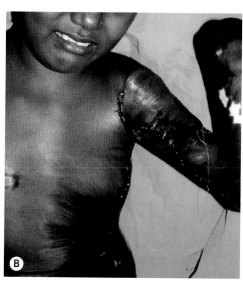

Fig. 19.17 (A) Severe axillary contracture. **(B)** Axillary release and reconstruction with locoregional flaps.

Table 19.2 Local flaps indication	
Elbow	• forearm flap based on the radial artery • flexor radial carpis flaps • lateral arm flap
Proximal third of arm and axilla	• latissimus dorsi flap • scapular and parascapular flaps
Knee and popliteal cavity	• medial or lateral gastrocnemius flap • reverse vastus lateralis flap
Proximal third of leg	• medial or lateral gastrocnemius flap • soleus flap
Distal third of the leg and ankle	• extensor hallucis longus myocutaneous flap • extensor digitorum longus muscle flap • retrograde fibular flap • posterior tibial artery perforator flaps

Free flap

Considering the steps of the reconstructive ladder, acute burns are usually treated by skin grafts applied on good vascularized tissue of the debrided (enzymatically or surgically) wound bed. If joints, bone, vessels, or nerves are exposed, the next step is the use of local flaps. However, damage of soft tissues surrounding the zone of injury may require the use of flap harvested from far away areas.

Fortunately, the use of free flaps in the reconstruction of severely burned extremities is infrequent in routine clinical practice. According to several studies, only 1–2% of burn patients are treated with free flaps,[38] so the use of free flaps is more frequent in secondary reconstruction procedures. Free flap transfer is commonest in secondary procedures of the leg, or in elbow and knee reconstructions, for example after electrical burns.

For simplicity, we will discuss separately the shoulder, the upper extremity, and the lower extremity.

Typically, defects at the shoulder and axillary cavity are corrected, as described earlier, with local flaps or skin grafts. Multiple local solutions can be chosen for this area, due to the thickness and quality of the soft tissues. Rarely, free flaps are needed in this area.

Otherwise, the region of the elbow is prone to tissue loss because of thin soft-tissue coverage and the presence of underlying structures such as bones, nerves, and vessels. In this area, reconstruction with skin grafts is often inadequate. The *parascapular flap* and the *anterolateral thigh flap* are both excellent choices for such region.

The lower extremity is the classical target for free flap reconstruction and aims mainly to restore the function and cover the tissue deficit that mostly consists of exposed bone, joints, tendons, nerves, and vessels. Muscle free flaps are generally preferred in lower extremity in order to restore 3D defects and to cover exposed bone or other vital structures. Having the most reliable vascular supply of all, free flaps help to reduce the infection by increasing tissue oxygenation.[50,51]

Skin grafts and local flaps are usually the first choice for scar contractures of the popliteal region (Fig. 19.19).

Nerve repair

In a step-by-step approach to reconstruction, the surgical repair of nerves comes after immediate, successful burn coverage.

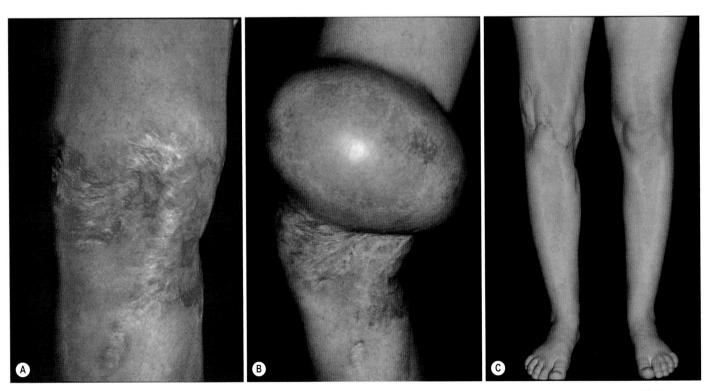

Fig. 19.18 (A) This case illustrates the painful after-burn scar strongly adherent to the joint. **(B)** The use of skin expansion of the lower medial thigh region. **(C)** The result of the use of skin expansion of lower medial thigh region, for an after-burn scar.

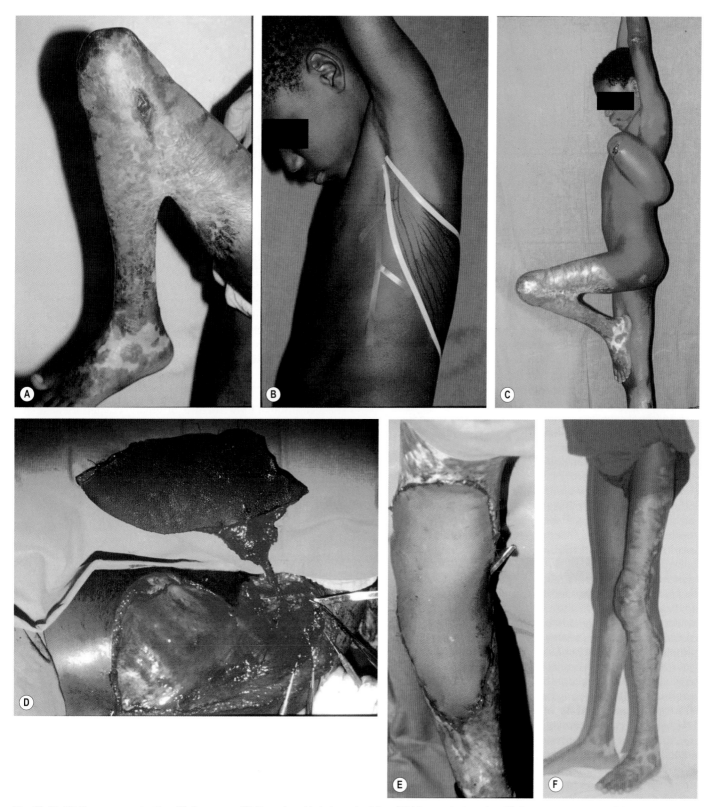

Fig. 19.19 (A) Knee: severe retraction. **(B)** Donor area. **(C)** Expansion of latissimus dorsi flap. **(D)** Microsurgical session. **(E)** Free pre-expanded flap. **(F)** Result.

Neural deficit in burn patients is usually associated with electrical burns or related trauma. The usual damage consists of interruptions of various length at some point in the nerve, which have to be bridged using grafts from other nerves. Statistics tell us that the nerves most frequently damaged are the ulnar and the median nerves, as a result of their exposed position.

Normally, the best donor nerve is the *sural nerve*, which can be used for grafts even in excess of 10 cm. This is because it is possible to maintain the continuity of the *medial sural cutaneous nerve* connected to the communicating branch of the *peroneus nerve*, providing up to 30 cm of nerve. The points of reference to be guided by are the external malleolus and the inferior saphenous.

Patients with third-degree burns to the lower extremity, who therefore have no sural nerve to be removed, can receive grafts, albeit much shorter, from the upper extremity. The medial and lateral *cutaneous antebrachial nerves* are the candidates of choice because their use causes only a limited sensory deficit with little functional effect.

The *medial cutaneous antebrachial* nerve is located medially in the groove between the biceps and the triceps, adjacent to the *basilic vein*. Of its two branches, anterior and posterior, the anterior one sensitizes the anterior part of the forearm, the posterior branch the elbow, and the remainder of the forearm on all the rest. Using only the anterior branch is less incapacitating for the patient.

The *lateral cutaneous antebrachial* nerve runs along the ulnar border of the brachioradialis muscle, next to the cephalic vein. Resulting insensible areas are usually well tolerated by the patient, since the areas involved overlap the sensitive branch of the radial nerve.[52]

If the gap is small (<3 cm), it is possible to achieve nerve regeneration guided by biodegradable laboratory-produced ducts. The findings of clinical tests have been found to be comparable with the results of small nerve grafts.

Surgery of tendon retraction

The scar contractures of the joints may cause secondary damage to the tendon structures that are involved in the deformity. Hyperflexion or hyperextension of a joint will ultimately induce length changes of the tendons, shortening on the flexion side and lengthening on the opposite side. If the deformity remains untreated for a long time, it will become permanent.

It is possible to intervene with lengthening plastic reconstruction (Fig. 19.20). The technique usually employed consists of a partial horizontal section of the tendon in two distant points, continuing with a median longitudinal section that unites them. This allows the use of two halves of tendons that can slide side-by-side and then be sutured together in the new location. Once healed, the tendon is longer but thinner.

For this reason, it would be useful to reinforce the elongated tendon with a dermal patch, harvested from a thick skin donor site,[39] as described for joint reconstruction, or with polycaprolactone-based polyurethane urea patch (such as Artelon tissue reinforcement implant) wrapped around the tendon.[40] It gives more resistance and better recovery in the postoperative period.

Amputation

Patients who have suffered high-voltage electrical burns account for amputations where no other therapeutic solution is available.

The main objective is to obtain a healthy stump so that the amputated limb can serve as an excellent base for affixing prosthesis.

The point where an amputation should be performed is dictated primarily by the presence of blood supply and venous drainage, viable tissues, and by surgical techniques. The stump should be covered with local skin and muscle flaps, in order to obtain a soft and viable cushion. If this is not possible, it is advisable, at least initially, to proceed with full-thickness skin grafts and secondary reconstructive surgery to follow.

The lower limb usually requires amputation closer to the thick, healthy tissue, while in the upper limb, it is necessary to preserve the maximum possible length in order to have better control over the future prosthesis. For the same reason, in forearm amputations it is always correct to preserve the tendon's prono-supination structures. When it is necessary to have a stump that is too short for application of prosthesis, it is possible to proceed with bone distraction techniques such as the Ilizarov technique.

Lipofilling

The technique of lipostructure, originally created for aesthetic purposes, now plays a primary role in the treatment of scars.

The surgical technique is now standardized and entails the liposuction of adipose tissue, and its grafting below the areas of scarring or even minute quantities into the scar mass. The quality of the scar (texture, color, and elasticity) treated with this technique improves dramatically due to the action of adipose tissue, and more probably of the stem cells inside it, that histologically determine increased vascularization and remodeling of collagen fibers in the treated areas.[53]

The use of serial lipofilling in the extremities is particularly recommended for reconstituting normal volume, which is sometimes lost during surgery, thereby restoring the extremities' conical-cylindrical characteristics.[54]

Laser

In recent years, we have witnessed a steady growth of laser therapy in the domain of the plastic surgeon. Even though this technique is still under scrutiny, the results have been encouraging.

The final outcome of scar tissue is variable, and many different types of lasers are available for different needs.

The *vascular laser*, such as the Nd:YAG 1064, is indicated in areas of scarring that are immature and have a particularly strong vascular component. The reduction in the blood supply induces an involution of the scar tissue treated.

The *fractional laser (ablative and non-ablative)* plays an important role in the remodeling of fibrotic scar tissue, with the interruption and regeneration of collagen and elastic fibers in the dermis resulting in softening and thinning of the scar itself. Their action also makes the coloring of scar areas more homogeneous, compacting their texture (Fig. 19.21).[55]

IPL and *Q-switched lasers* act on hyperpigmentation and discoloring in certain areas of scarring (Table 19.3).

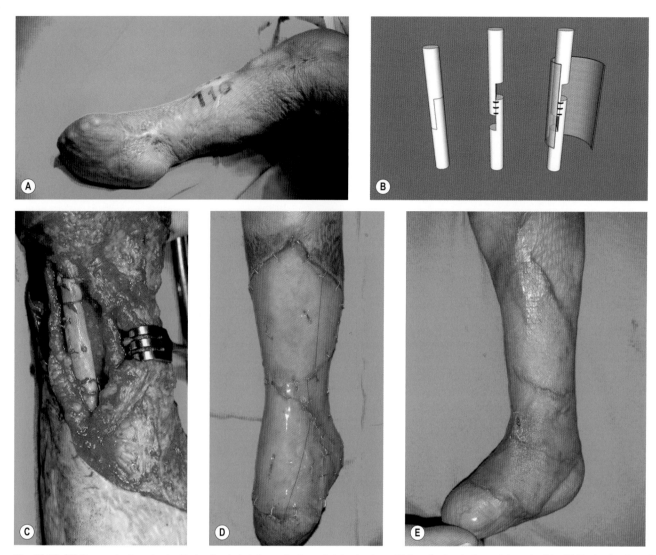

Fig. 19.20 (A) Scar contracture about ankle leading to imbalances in the underlying tendons. (B) Lengthening design and dermal patch. (C) Tendon lengthened and reinforced by dermal patch. (D) Resurfaced ankle after underlying tendons have been rebalanced. (E) Postoperative result after tendon rebalancing and ankle resurfacing. *(Courtesy of the Department of Plastic Surgery and Burn Therapy, ARNAS Ospedale Civico, Palermo, Italy.)*

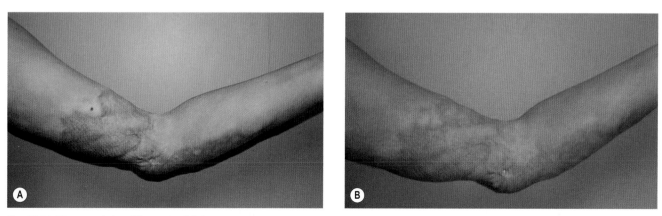

Fig. 19.21 Elbow area before (A) and after (B) 6 treatments with non-ablative fractional laser. Better color matching and more quality of skin texture.

Table 19.3 **Laser in scar treatment**	
Nd:YAG 1064	Scars immature, with vessels
IPL	Hyperpigmentation Scar with vessels

Fractional laser
  Ablative
  Non-ablative
	
	Mature scars with heterogeneous surface
	Mature scars, fibrotic, thick

🌐 Access the complete reference list online at **http://www.expertconsult.com**

1. Vyrostek SB, Annest JL, Ryan GW. Surveillance for fatal and non fatal injuries – United States 2001. Office of Statistics and Programming. National Center for Injury Prevention and Control. CDC/NCIPC/OSP; 2001. *This comprehensive government publication reports demographic and mechanistic data for all injuries sustained in the United States during 2001. A 0.5% mortality rate is reported for injured individuals varying by age, sex, and mechanism.*

3. American Burn Association. Guidelines for service standards and severity classifications in the treatment of burn injury. *Bull Am Coll Surg*. 1984;69:24–29.

9. McCauley RL, Asuku ME. Upper extremity burn reconstruction. In: Mathes SJ, Hentz VR, eds. *Plastic Surgery*. Vol VII. 2nd ed. Philadelphia: Saunders Elsevier; 2005:605–619. *This encyclopedic book chapter covers upper extremity burn care from primary excision and grafting to secondary procedures. An informative historical perspective is also provided.*

18. Purdue GF, Arnoldo BD, Hunt JL. Electrical injuries. In: Herndon DN, ed. *Total Burn Care*. 3rd ed. Philadelphia: WB Saunders; 2008:513–520.

31. Heimbach DM, Logsetty S. Modern technique for wound coverage of the thermally injured upper extremity. *Hand Clin*. 2000;16:205–214. *Advanced modalities in burn reconstruction are discussed. The authors stress, however, that the split-thickness skin graft remains the "gold standard" in burn reconstruction.*

32. Borghese L, Latorre S, Montagnese A, et al. Retrospective analysis of 200 severe post-burn cases in Cambodia and Bangladesh. *Ann Burns Fire Disast*. 2005;18(1). *The authors discuss the standard of care and controversial issues in hand and upper extremity burns.*

33. Smith MA, Munster AM, Spence RJ. Burns of the hand and upper limb – a review. *Burns*. 1998;24:493–505.

35. Atiyeh BS, Hayek SN, Gunn SWA. New technologies for burn wound closure and healing – review of the literature. *Burns*. 2005;31:944–956. *The authors of this review note the limitations of autologous skin grafting in burn reconstruction. Alternative replacement modalities are surveyed.*

39. Masellis M, Conte F, Fortezza GS. Use of dermis to reconstruct hand joint capsules. *Ann Plast Surg*. 1982;9:72–80.

41. Beasley RW. Burns of the axilla and elbow. In: Converse JM, ed. *Reconstructive Plastic Surgery*. Vol 6. Philadelphia: WB Saunders; 1977:3391–3402.

20

Management of the burned face

Vinita Puri and Venkateshwaran N

SYNOPSIS

- The human face is the seat of expression and beauty and the burned face is a physical and psychological insult to the patient
- The facial skin drapes over a complex anatomy of muscles and sphincters, it has a rich blood supply and burn depth assessment is an important step in early management
- Airway control and topical wound care are the mainstays of early facial burn management
- Goals of acute facial burn management include obtaining early reepithelisation, minimizing functional sequelae and preserving aesthetic landmarks
- Secondary management of post burn deformities of the face is a challenging task involving detailed clinical assessment, meticulous planning, counseling and consenting of the patient
- Surgical management is by applying the aesthetic subunit principle, utilizing various reconstructive options according to principles and staging surgeries to optimize outcomes
- Increasing knowledge of stem cell application, 3D printing and advances in the field of face transplantation may herald future directions in facing challenges posed by facial burns.

Introduction

The face is what defines a person's identity. Symmetry and balance of facial features and tone and texture of the skin have long been yardsticks to measure individual beauty. The human face is unique in development for its complexity in structural architecture, its seamless symphony in functionality, and its ability to emote and express a myriad of thoughts and feelings. The face is the cover by which people judge the book. It is hence not overstating facts when it is said that burns involving the face are a challenge and an opportunity like no other to the reconstructive surgeon and leaves him wishing for more and more weaponry in his ever-expanding

armamentarium to tackle this difficult problem. Burns of the head, face, and neck region occur in almost 50% of all burn injuries. Fortunately due to the relatively higher vascularity of the region helping to dissipate the heat rapidly, burns of the face are often partial thickness. At the same time facial burns can be an indicator towards the more serious and life-threatening problem of inhalation injury. Management of the burned face in the acute scenario has been a matter of debate with evidence accumulating on both sides of either conservative therapy with dressings or an early excision approach. What is accepted without argument is the fact that management of the burned face calls for a multipronged team approach involving the trained burn surgeon, the skilled nurse, the physiotherapist, the occupational therapist, psychological, and social support systems right from the outset.

The face has been divided into aesthetic units by Gonzalez-Ulloa in 1987. These subunits show consistent color, texture, thickness, and pliability. Care should be taken during the management of facial burns to respect these boundaries to minimize scar appearance.[1] Facial scars can cause distortion of features, skin thickening, and pigmentary problems. Scars are inevitable in the continuum of treatment, but deformities are a highly preventable aspect of burn management in general, and of the face in particular. Timely use of all available modalities like scar massage, pressure garments, silicone gel (sheets or liquid), intralesional steroids, and laser therapy will go a long way in appearance of scars and prevention of deformities.

Facial burns (Fig. 20.1 ⊚) are a problem that may be associated with considerable psychological distress to the patient. This is a major determinant of social reintegration of the patient after recovery from the treatment of their physical problems. It is hence important to show the patient empathy, understand the patient's desires, weigh their expectations against what is practically achievable, and counsel them accordingly.

Fig. 20.1 appears online only.

Anatomy and pathophysiology

An understanding of the anatomy of this region is essential before proceeding to outline the management of facial burn injuries. The face is an extremely complex anatomic structure consisting of skin, fat, and muscle draped over the facial bony architecture. The face has important sphincter structures and vital sensory organs of sight, hearing, smell, taste, and touch. Skin forms a protective mechanical barrier against trauma, bacteria, noxious substances, heat, and ultraviolet radiation. Other important functions include sensation, immunologic surveillance, and heat and fluid homeostasis.[1]

The head and neck region can be involved in burns caused by transfer of thermal, chemical, electrical, or lightning energy to the skin. Injury to the epidermal layer alone comprises first degree burn. The common example of this is the sunburn. The tissue healing occurs by sloughing of the dead epidermal layer with re-epithelization within one week. With increasing energy and contact duration, increasing depths of the dermis are also damaged. This constitutes denaturation of collagen and thrombosis of blood vessels. Appearance of the dermal layer acts as a guide to burn depth. When the epidermal layer alone is damaged, the dermal layer appears pink due to the superficial location of the underlying blood vessels. As the burn depth increases the collagen becomes pale and the color turns white.

Another guide to the depth of burn injury is the pain quotient. Superficial burns are painful to touch because of the exposed nerve endings. As the depth of burn increases, the wound becomes less painful.[2]

Burn wound re-epithelizes from the remnant adnexal structures like pilosebaceous units, sweat glands, and apocrine glands. The face and scalp contain a high density of sebaceous glands and epidermal appendages that are located in the deep dermis and subdermal fat.[1] The regenerative process in epidermal and superficial partial thickness burns is completed in two weeks with minimal scarring. However, burns deeper than this can take up to three weeks to heal and can cause considerable scarring with a tendency towards hypertrophy. Thus a rule of thumb for intervening surgically is in wounds that may not heal in 3 weeks. However, this decision needs to be taken by the end of the first week of treatment and is based solely on the experience and clinical judgment of the treating burn surgeon.[3] Another factor that has a bearing on the burn depth is the skin thickness, which varies with the age, sex, and anatomic location on the face. Children have relatively thinner skin. Skin thickens with age and starts thinning again after the fifth decade of life. Men have thicker skin compared to women. Eyelid and postauricular skin is thinner (0.5 mm thick) than other anatomic areas on the face.[1]

Acute facial burn management

General principles

The management principles of facial burns follow principles used elsewhere in the body. Goals of facial burn management are to obtain early wound re-epithelization, pain control, to minimize functional sequelae while taking care to preserve aesthetic landmarks. Facial burns are similar to hand burns in that, in the absence of both of these, there is faster clinical and psychosocial recovery and rehabilitation of the survivor.[1] Certain special features that make facial burns unique are the rich vascularity, which hastens healing and reduces infection rate, difficulty in accurate depth assessment, and the potential to cause contour deformities by aggressive surgical management.

The treatment principles can be broadly classified into three groups based on the depth of the burn:

1) In patients who have sustained epidermal and superficial partial-thickness burns, spontaneous healing is the rule. The mainstay of treatment involves open dressings and topical care (Fig. 20.2).

2) In patients who have sustained deep or full-thickness burns apparent at initial evaluation, the obvious next step is to proceed with workup and early excision of the burn wound with coverage (autograft or allograft). Further management of the patient entails graft care, prevention of scar and graft junction area hypertrophy by use of ancillary modalities like pressure therapy, and topical silicone use.

3) The third group of patients with intermediate or indeterminate thickness of burns incites the most controversy or dilemmas in management. These patients if allowed to heal spontaneously may form hypertrophic scars that may transgress borders of aesthetic subunits and relaxed skin tension lines. If excised too early, the surgeon may be guilty of giving the patient grafts in areas that may have appeared aesthetically superior if allowed to heal conservatively. Herein lays the role of newer diagnostic tools for diagnosing burn depth. One such advancement is the laser Doppler techniques.[4-6] A treatment decision delayed until 10 days may help in determining the areas that are deeper and will require surgery, whereas areas that may heal in three weeks may be left alone. At best, the experienced clinician's judgment is sound only 65% of the time (Figs. 20.3 & 20.4).[7]

Laser Doppler evaluation

Laser Doppler imaging can be a useful adjunct and can supplement a good clinical call, but due a lack of randomized controlled level 1 evidence supporting its use, it cannot substitute sound clinical judgement.

Managing the airway

Facial burns share an intimate relation to the airways and often act as a marker for upper or lower airway injury. An early decision has to be made regarding intubation or for elective tracheostomy before signs of laryngeal edema become obvious. Special care has to be taken to prevent tube pressure necrosis.[1]

Wound care

The facial burn wound, similar to burn wounds elsewhere, has to be thoroughly cleansed with normal saline. All loose debris and necrotic material has to be removed. Tiny blisters can be left to heal, but larger blisters can be deroofed. In case

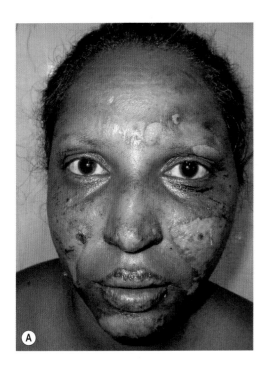

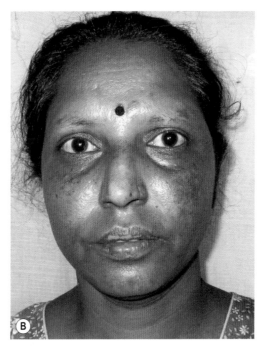

Fig. 20.2 (A) Superficial second degree burns on day 1. **(B)** On day 21 with complete healing but with some minor mixed pigmentation.

of chemical burns the face is washed with copious amounts of saline or running water as is the practice in the unit for as long as 45 minutes to completely remove the noxious agent or to neutralize it. A dilute solution of antiseptic can be used for the final round of cleansing. The wound can then be covered with a generous application of topical antimicrobial agent.

It is the practice in the authors' unit to cover all facial burn injuries with synthetic bovine collagen dressing readily available in most centers of the country after the initial cleansing is completed. This helps in maintaining a closed environment,

reducing the pain and distress, retaining moisture, and helping in rapid re-epithelization in case of first and second degree burns. The collagen dressing remains closely adherent to the wound and gradually peels off when the underlying wound heals (Fig. 20.5 ⬤). In deeper burns this dressing does not adhere well to the wounds and is seen to peel off within 48 hours following which other conventional antimicrobial agents can be used for dressing or a decision regarding early surgical excision can be made. Thus this also acts as a guide in burns of indeterminate depth.

Fig. 20.5A & C appear online only.

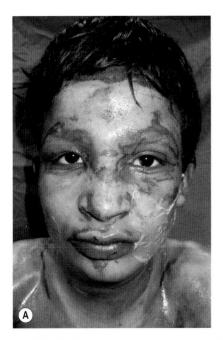

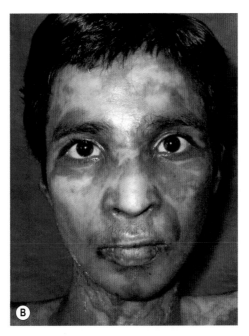

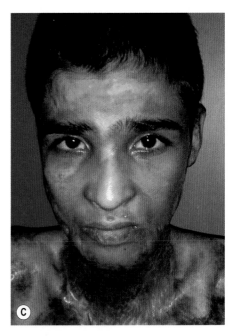

Fig. 20.3 (A) Deeper second degree burns in a patient with high TBSA burns on day 1. **(B)** At 1½ months with large areas of hypopigmentation. **(C)** At 7 months with return of most of the pigmentation.

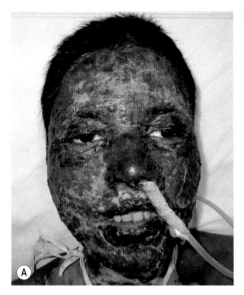
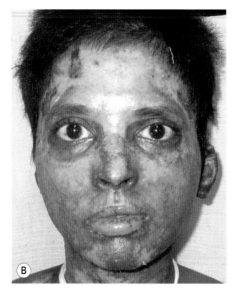
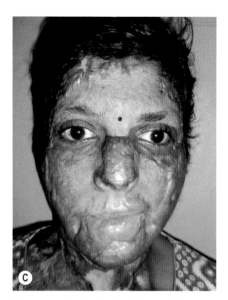

Fig. 20.4 (A) Deep partial-thickness and full-thickness burns in a patient with high TBSA burns on day 10. **(B)** Managed by conservative treatment and no surgical intervention, healing at 4 weeks. **(C)** Hypertrophic scarring at 4 months.

Topical agents

Topical agents used in facial burn management can be grouped into antiseptics, antimicrobials, enzymatic debridement agents, and dressings.[8]

Antiseptics

These are topical agents that limit (bacteriostatic) or eliminate (bactericidal) the load of microorganisms in the wound. These mainly include chlorhexidine and povidone iodine products that are used in cleansing at the time of admission as well on a day-to-day basis during dressings. They cover Gram-positive and Gram-negative bacteria. Povidone products have a broad-spectrum coverage, including fungi, viruses, spores, yeasts, and protozoa.

Antimicrobials

An ideal prophylactic topical antimicrobial should have a broad spectrum of activity, low toxicity, good eschar penetration, and low systemic absorption. It should be inexpensive, easily available, and have a good shelf life.[8]

Silver preparations

Silver has always found a place in wound care either in the solid form (silver wires placed in wounds), as solutions of silver salts used to cleanse wounds (silver nitrate solution), and more recently in the form of creams and gels containing a silver antibiotic compound (silver sulfadiazine cream or SSD cream).[9]

Recently, advancements in delivery systems of silver have spawned a plethora of products that claim advantages like

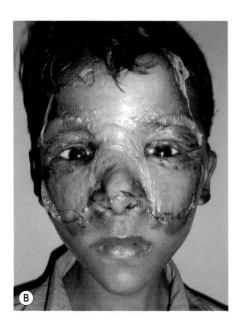
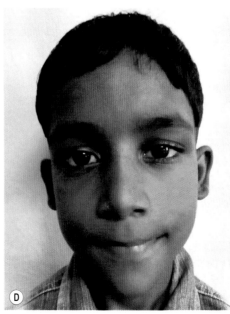

Fig. 20.5 (B) Collagen sheets have been applied. **(D)** At 6 months post-burn.

less messy application, high wound antimicrobial concentration, maintaining a moist wound environment, and better chances of autolytic debridement.

In the elemental form (as silver metal), silver does not kill bacteria. But in the aqueous wound environment, silver atom loses an electron to form activated silver ions, which are bactericidal. They disrupt bacterial cell membranes, destabilize bacterial biofilm matrices, and increase bacterial susceptibility to antibiotic action.

Creams
Silver sulfadiazine (SSD) cream
SSD cream is the mainstay of burn wound management in many burn units worldwide. The introduction of this water-based cream by Fox in 1968 containing silver sulfadiazine in the micronized form, revolutionized burn wound care. It requires to be applied twice a day in a thick layer to be most effective. It can produce adverse effects like leukopenia, methemoglobinemia, and sulfa allergy. It forms a pseudo-eschar that may be quite indistinguishable in appearance from full-thickness burns.[1] Though SSD cream has been long considered the gold standard, it has been proved to have deleterious effects on wound healing. This effect of SSD can be countered by epidermal growth factor (EGF) and in future a combined preparation of the two may be more effective.[10]

Cerium nitrate
It is an excellent antiseptic with a broad spectrum of activity. Its use is popular in European burn units and is usually used in combination with silver sulfadiazine (as flammacerium). It hardens burn eschar, thus isolating potentially necrotic areas and improves burn wound milia. However, no clear advantage of its use in combination with SSD had been demonstrated in controlled studies when compared to the use of SSD alone.[11]

Silver solution
Silver nitrate solution (0.5%) covers the same antimicrobial spectrum as SSD but has lesser eschar penetration. Its main disadvantage lies in the fact that it stains tissues and dressings black and causes electrolyte disturbances like hypokalemia and hyponatremia.[12]

Nanocrystalline silver
Elemental silver in small crystals that are about 10–100 nanometers in diameter are delivered through a colloidal gel medium or as surface-coated foam dressings. A popular form of nano silver dressing is Acticoat (Smith and Nephew), which is a bilayered polyethylene dressing with nanocrystalline silver particle coating. The cited advantages of these sustained release silver preparations are that they reduce wound infection, promote wound healing, reduce frequency of dressing changes, pain associated with dressings, and overall cost.[13] Mepilex Ag is a patented (Mölnlycke) silver foam dressing that was shown to be superior to other silver dressings in terms of ease of use, pain control, and speed of wound re-epithelization in a randomized controlled trial.[14] The use of this product is common for partial thickness burns and also for donor area dressings at the authors' institution and has yielded good results in terms of re-epithelization and pain control at dressing changes.

Another patented preparation, Aquacel Ag (Convatec), incorporates ionic silver into a hydrofiber dressing, which gets converted to a gel form on wound contact. Silvercel (Johnson & Johnson) is a patented product combining the advantages of silver with the benefits of alginate.[15] Alginate is a polysaccharide found in the cell walls of algae that is able to absorb 200 times its weight in water. This property helps when used in heavily exudative wounds.

Mafenide acetate
This is a deep eschar penetrating agent with good antimicrobial spectrum. Available commercially as 5 and 11.1% solutions, it has been recommended for areas of the face like ears, where cartilaginous framework is exposed by burns. It requires frequent applications and has been reported to cause pain, inflammation, and allergic reactions.[13]

Hypochlorite solutions:
Its use has been described since the First World War and has been used in facial burn management also. Its optimal antimicrobial activity was seen at 0.025% and was termed as "modified Dakin's solution". Its contact with non-burned skin can cause irritation and maceration.[8]

Antibiotics and Antifungals
Commonly used preparations include neosporin, polysporin, and bacitracin.[8]

Enzymatic debriding agents
These agents also referred to as chemical debriding agents are the non-surgical alternative to removal of necrotic tissues from the wound surface. This is definitely attractive and desirable but has not always delivered uniform results. They are principally divided based on origin into two groups:
- Group one are bacterial origin compounds and include collagenase (*Clostridium histolyticum*), sutilains (*Bacillus subtilis*), and varidase (*Streptococcus*).
- Group two constitute agents originating from plants and include Accuzyme (papaya origin combined with urea) and Debridase (bromelain/pineapple derived).[8]

Alternative remedies
Honey has been long considered a "folk remedy" for burn wounds. Honey owes its antibacterial powers to its high osmolarity and its ability to form hydrogen peroxide in a sustained release manner when in contact with wound fluid. This is due to the presence of enzyme glucose oxidase in honey. In a clinical trial it was found to be superior in wound healing and infection control properties to boiled potato peel dressings.[16]

Moist exposed burn ointment (MEBO) was developed using a traditional Chinese method and contains sesame oil, beta sitosterol, berberine, and other plant extracts. Trials using MEBO in patients with partial-thickness burns less than 40% total body surface area (TBSA) have shown results matching conventional therapy using SSD.[17]

Papaya fruit extracts containing enzymes chymopapain and papain have been used in countries like Africa due to limitations in resources. These agents show effective des-loughing of wounds and help in wound bed preparation for grafting.[18]

Aloe vera preparations have been shown to speed up the healing process and re-epithelization in first and second degree burns.[19]

Wound dressings or skin substitutes

Studies done to test the efficacy of temporary wound dress-ings or skin substitutes suggest that their use facilitates healing and minimizes infection. Even though they are not antimicrobials these studies indicate that they serve as barri-ers to microbial colonization and infection. Some trials have shown improved scar characteristics like better elasticity and flexibility in burns healed after use of these agents. This indirectly may lead to a decrease in the number of secondary procedures the patient may have to undergo. Skin substitutes may find a special niche for use in pediatric burns, which are usually small area burns, partial-thickness, and need only dressings for their management. Skin substitutes reduce the frequency of dressings, associated pain and emotional trauma, promote an early return to activities, and at the same time provide a cost-effective solution.[15]

Wound dressings that provide temporary cover can be classified into the following categories.

Biologic dressings, e.g., amnion

Amniotic membrane has been shown in clinical trials to be effective as a temporary wound cover, reducing pain and helping rapid re-epithelization. It is readily available, non-immunogenic, and reduces water loss from the wound. However, no long-term advantage could be demonstrated in terms of scar appearance.[8]

Synthetic dressings

These provide a moist wound environment and effectively seal off the wound. Some of these are water vapor permeable and allow the wound to respire. Commonly used brands include DuoDERM, OmniDerm, Opsite, and Suprathel.

Biosynthetic materials

These combine a biologic component with a synthetic one. Some commonly used examples include:

- Biobrane (Smith & Nephew): In trials this has showed results superior to conventional dressings for superficial partial-thickness burns. There are reports of mesh imprinting or punctuate scarring using this product.[15]
- TransCyte (Smith & Nephew and Advanced Tissue Sciences): This is transparent, allowing wound monitoring and the fibroblasts in the nylon mesh to proliferate producing human dermal collagen, matrix proteins, and growth factors essential for wound healing.
- Dermagraft (Advanced Biohealing): This is a cryopreserved dermal substitute manufactured from human neonatal foreskin tissue-derived fibroblasts seeded onto a polyglactin mesh that is bioabsorbable. The fibroblasts fill the interstices of the scaffold and produce human collagen, matrix proteins, and growth factors.[15]

- Integra (Integra LifeSciences): This has been used extensively when there is a lack of donor skin and in facial burns with the aim of avoiding pigmentary problems and graft junctional hypertrophy in aesthetically significant regions.[20]

Other skin substitutes

The other skin substitutes of notable mention include Xeno-derm,[21] Alloderm,[21] Apligraf,[15] and Epicel.[15]

Cadaver allografts

These are usually used after excision of full-thickness burns, but their use has also been described as a dressing material in partial-thickness facial burns and has been shown by a pro-spective study to be superior to open dressings with SSD.[22]

Xenografts

These are porcine skin grafts used as temporary wound cover in facial burn topical management. It is usually not assimilated in the wound and has occasionally reported to have caused imprinting artifacts.[8]

Surgical management of the facial burn wound – early excision

Tangential excision of the burn wound and coverage is now accepted as the standard of care universally. The face wound in particular incited controversy due to its aesthetic signifi-cance, vascularity, and excellent spontaneous healing proper-ties being well endowed with pilosebaceous units. However the general consensus agrees that a face wound that would require 3 weeks or more to heal spontaneously is a candidate for early excision. The early excision is, however, delayed for a period of 7–10 days to definitely ascertain without a doubt as to which areas would heal spontaneously and the areas that would require excision.

Once the decision to excise has been made, further delay is avoided and the patient is taken up for surgery after optimiza-tion with respect to hemodynamic stability, hemoglobin and protein levels, and with due explanation and informed consent. It would be helpful to discuss the options available in terms of pros and cons with the patient and the concerned relatives. The nature of the surgery and the procedure is explained to the assisting operating theatre staff and require-ments in terms of blood products, homografts, skin substitutes, etc., should be prearranged.

The surgery is performed under general anesthesia with the patient in a reverse Trendelenburg position. The endotra-cheal and feeding tubes are kept out of the field by suspending them from overhead hooks. The eyes can be protected with silicone pads, cornea shields, or temporary tarsorrhaphy sutures. Certain points have to be borne in mind while excis-ing facial burns. When excising facial burns in a patient with large TBSA burns, it may be worthwhile to excise the face in multiple sittings using the minimal amount of available autograft per sitting. Instead temporary skin substitutes like allograft and acellular dermis can be used and thin autograft-ing may be done as a separate session. The principle of relook or second stage surgery is very useful to prevent graft loss due to hematoma formation and also to assess the adequacy of the depth of excision. Also, in aesthetically sensitive areas like the ala of the nose, tip of the nose, chin, ear, etc., it may be better to err on the side of excising less and giving a second look at a later session rather than to do a deep excision and face contour problems in the future. For maintaining a uniform appearance, aesthetic units have to be excised in toto even if this means sacrificing a small region that may be unburnt or that may heal spontaneously.[1,23]

In areas of mixed depth injuries, excision should be performed to a uniform depth to avoid problems of retention of skin appendages like inclusion cysts, pits, and folliculitis.

Excision is performed with the help of a dermatome (Goulian) set to 0.008-inch thickness. This can tackle most areas except for certain areas like the medial canthal region, ears, philtral area, etc. For such areas, the use of the Versajet (Smith & Nephew) has been recommended. This is a hydro-surgery system, which uses a high-pressure jet of sterile normal saline to debride wounds, drawing tissue debris and fluid into a chamber via the Venturi effect created by the normal saline jet.[24,25]

Excision in the face is usually commenced with the central T-shaped area constituting the eyelids, nose, upper and lower lips, and chin.

Having completed the excision of the central T area of the face, attention is shifted to the four outlying flat areas: the cheeks, forehead, and neck. These are excised in a similar manner. The dermatome can be set at 0.010- or 0.012-inch thickness. The eyebrow area is spared while excising a forehead burn. The amount of bleeding from a full face excision can be quite copious, and hemostasis has to be quick and adequate. A watchful eye has to be kept also on volume replacement, and blood transfusion can be given if necessary. It is better if all these areas are not excised in the same session and their excision can be staggered over multiple sessions to reduce the blood loss.[23]

Ear burns require a special mention as the instrumentation available does not allow a suitable excision of this architecturally complex structure. It can follow the traditional method of allowing an eschar to form and separate. Topical antimicrobials and moist dressings can be used to assist healing. Split skin grafting can be done as and when required.

Post-excision options

Allograft and split skin use

Allograft, if available, is used initially for coverage of the excised areas. The use of allograft has its own advantages over xenograft. Allograft adheres to the wound bed if the depth of excision is adequate and healthy. However, if the depth of excision is inadequate, it does not adhere and easily comes off.

One week postoperatively the patient is examined in the operation theatre for allograft adherence. The allograft is gently removed. The area of the face to be covered determines the donor area to be used. The scalp skin is a good match in terms of color match and texture. It is sufficient for partial face coverage. But the scalp may be an insufficient donor area for a complete face excision. Thick autografts are then harvested from elsewhere in the body to the extent of 0.008 to 0.012 inches. The thicker grafts prevent secondary contracture and have a better aesthetic appearance. Autografts are harvested

while hemostasis is being ensured on the face using the Padgett dermatome. The grafts are then laid on the wound bed and secured as previously described. Small darts are made in the graft margin, and small local Z-plasty flaps can be fed into the areas opened up by the darts. This breaks the margin and prevents contracture band formation.[23]

The other options for cover after excision include acellular dermis,[26] xenografts, MatriDerm,[27] Integra,[20] and cultured epithelial autografts.[28,29]

Problems of specific parts of the face

Eyelids

An eyelid burn can signify underlying ocular damage and warrants a detailed ophthalmologic examination, which may include a slit lamp microscopy, fluorescein staining, and fundoscopy. The crow's feet area is a reliable clinical marker. If spared, it can predict an uninjured cornea to a high degree of accuracy.[1] The eyes should be kept moist with lubricants and topical antimicrobials. Early excision and grafting with thick split-thickness or full-thickness grafts prevents ectropion, exposure keratitis, conjunctivitis, and corneal ulceration.

Nose and ears

These structures have a cartilaginous framework closely covered by the skin. Deep thermal burns involving these structures would lead to exposure of cartilage or its deformities due to the inevitable chondritis that will follow their exposure. Even though early excision has been described, equally common is the concept of conservative management in these organs. The ear burn is managed by a constant use of topical antimicrobials. A dressing conforming to the shapes and whorls of the cartilage can help to prevent deformities that may develop due to chondritis. Often a neglected ear burn may present as a pus-filled, inflamed, featureless, boggy mass. All normal architecture is obliterated. This condition requires an aggressive approach of incision and drainage with liberal use of topical antimicrobials. The ear may heal with scarring and deformities that may have to be managed at a later date with reconstructive measures.

Lips

Lips are prone to scab and crust formation. These must be cleaned repeatedly, and the lips should be kept moist with a petroleum jelly or liquid paraffin. In hair-bearing areas of the lips and chin, repeated trimming or shaving of hair prevents build-up of necrotic material that may later lead to infection and folliculitis.

Scalp

The scalp, even though separate anatomically, can be described along with the face as a contiguous area. The scalp is enriched with a dense supply of hair follicles both in dermal and subdermal levels. This greatly facilitates re-epithelization even in deep dermal burns. Hence, the management of scalp burns is essentially conservative. This constitutes wound care measures like repeated cleaning of debris, shaving the region, and moist wound dressings combined with generous use of topical antimicrobials.

Special subsets of patients are the ones who suffer a serious injury like a high-voltage electric injury. This may lead to exposure of the calvarium. It may even cause a necrosis of the outer table of the skull vault. Simple exposure of the calvarium can be managed by drilling holes through or burring the outer table of the skull and allowing granulation tissue to develop. Following this, the defect can be covered by autograft or Integra. However, a necrotic bone may require removal followed by formal coverage of the defect with a flap. If neighboring tissue is uninjured, a rotation or transposition scalp flap may be performed. For larger injuries, coverage of the exposed structures may necessitate use of microsurgical free tissue transfers of large flaps like anterolateral thigh flap or latissimus dorsi flap.

Neck burns

The neck is another important contiguous area that, when burnt and if neglected, can lead to development of disastrous secondary deformities. Posturing an acute burn patient can go a long way in preventing neck contractures if treated by a conservative method. The patient is made to lie with a bolster support behind the upper back and using a very thin or no pillow support for the head. This automatically converts the posture of the neck into one of that of extension during the healing phase. When posturing is coupled with the use of thermoplastic splints or neck collars, neck contractures can be effectively prevented. If excision is opted for it is carried out like elsewhere on the face or body, taking care of splintage and posturing in the postoperative period also.

Surgical management of the facial burn wound – delayed surgery

Early excision and wound cover has become the standard of care for acute burns. This ideal line of management may not be feasible in certain facilities and countries due to a lack of infrastructure and lack of high-dependency intensive care facilities. Despite these drawbacks, the best possible care in the form of a regimen of topical antimicrobial treatment, moist wound dressings, and regular cleaning of necrotic tissue and wound debris can be followed. Once the eschar of deeper burn separates, it is replaced by healthy granulation tissue over a period of about 3 weeks. By this time the patient has stabilized hemodynamically and nutrition is at the optimum. The patient can be taken up for wound debridement and coverage with split-thickness autografts. It is preferable to assess the wound microflora by sending regular wound swabs or, more reliably, wound biopsies before taking up the patient for surgery. Adequate blood products should be available before surgery, and intraoperative hemostasis is further aided by the infiltration of the granulated areas with 1 in 1 000 000 saline adrenaline solution. In the event of paucity of donor areas, various techniques are available to optimize the quantity, such as increasing the meshing ratio, sandwich technique of using widely meshed autografts with homografts, and meek micrografting method.

Aftercare and early scar management

Once the early management is concluded and the wounds are closed, it is now time for the most aggressive phase of facial

burn management, i.e., scar management. The rehabilitation of a facial burn starts on the day of the patient's admission just like burns elsewhere on the body. During the patient's inpatient stay it is mandatory to ensure adequate facial mobilization exercises. Also, special care is to be paid to the eyelids, lips, and oral commissures to prevent ectropion and microstomia formation, respectively. The use of oral splints in preventing microstomia formation and nasal silicone splints to prevent nostril stenosis cannot be overemphasized. These splints are also of paramount importance when a conservative line of management is being pursued (Fig. 20.6 ⊕). In ear burns, use of splints is recommended whether the patient is managed conservatively or by early excision. The splint in ear burn serves to maintain the postauricular sulcus and preserve the overall cartilage architecture. The therapist and the surgeon have to work in close coordination in this phase to evaluate the patient in terms of goals of rehabilitation, areas needing special care, areas at risk of developing scar hypertrophy, or contractures.

Fig. 20.6 appears online only.

Most commonly used intervention modalities include scar moisturization[30] and massage therapy, compression garment use,[31-33] topical silicone use in the form of liquid or sheets,[34] and sunscreen use to avoid pigmentary problems.

Ancillary measures

Despite the best of measures, the patient may develop hypertrophic scarring and contractures for which secondary reconstructive procedures may be required. An acute facial burn is a psychologically distressing injury as this leads to alteration in perception of image and reduces the self confidence. These patients have to be regularly counseled with empathy and have to be enrolled in burn camps and survivor groups as part of their psychological rehabilitation. The burn camp concept, which is well accepted and popular in the west, is now slowly being embraced by the Middle Eastern and Asian burn units. The authors' institution conducted the first ever pediatric burn survivor camp in India and has found the camp to be an uplifting experience for the participants, doctors, and patients alike.[35] In LMIC often these patients are neglected and abandoned by their families, and they need legal and vocational support as well. The management of the scars should not be limited to the physical element alone, as the psychological aspect of care completes the circle of treatment for both the patient and the treating surgeon.

Management of facial post-burn deformities

Scarring is the natural endpoint of all healing. But the scarring process is dynamic and behaves as a continuum rather than as an endpoint. There are factors at play that constantly alter the scar biology. Fibroblasts and growth factors like transforming growth factor (TGF)-beta are responsible for the changes in scar morphology, altering the rate and type of collagen synthesis leading to hypertrophic scar formation. As described in the previous segment a post-burn scar requires a lot of early rehabilitative measures like pressure therapy and scar massage, which are now accepted as the standard of care. When an attempt at scar amelioration through these efforts cannot be made due to patient factors or poor follow-up by the burn unit, the incidence of scar morbidity in the form of hypertrophic scarring, keloid formation, and contractures rises. However, the tendency to excessive scarring may also depend on a number of other factors. These include:

1. Age
2. Sex
3. Race/color of skin
4. Depth of burn and time to healing
5. Method of management of acute injury
6. Management after healing.

Presentation to the surgeon

A patient may present to us for facial burn reconstruction with any or all of the following:

1. Scarring with issues of pigmentation (aesthetic component)
2. Hypertrophic scars (aesthetic component)
3. Tight scarring of the face leading to adynamic face (aesthetic component with expressive component)
4. Scarring with contractures, but no functional problems
5. Scarring with contractures leading to functional problems.

The consultation

Facial burn survivors deserve a higher level of empathy from the surgeon compared to those who have body burns alone, sparing the face. The approach to these patients who come with expectations like "can these scars be removed?" has to be a realistic one. It has to be made clear right at the first consultation that skin once scarred cannot be made unblemished again despite the array of procedures at our disposal. An explanation of the process of healing and scar formation, if given to the patient and caregivers, makes them realize that it is impossible to regain the preburn facial appearance.

Restoration of function and esthetic appearance in facial burns may require a number of procedures. The surgeon needs to be able to play out mentally the whole process towards the final outcome. The plan needs to be made after detailed discussion with the patient so that they have a shared vision of the final outcome. During the preliminary consultation, a detailed history should be elicited from the patient. All details of the earlier management should be asked for, like details of early or delayed surgery, donor site usage, early rehabilitation in terms of use of pressure garments, splints, positioning, and silicone sheets. Non-compliance to ancillary measures helps to red flag the patient as one who would need special counseling and repeated reiteration of the benefits of these measures. Often in a busy outpatient clinic, the author has found it worthwhile introducing one patient to another showing how the other patient has benefited from being compliant to the post-healing care regimes. It is also beneficial to have photographs of patients (taken with informed consent) who have undergone reconstructive procedures, which may help illustrate some points to the new patient who may be unable to visualize how a flap or graft may appear. The consultation is concluded in a positive spirit, reiterating that the surgeon and patient would work together towards a common goal, i.e., good functionality with an adequate but realistic aim of aesthetics.

Planning

The final appearance of the patient is only as good as the overall plan. The patient may present with multiple contractures or scarring in many parts of the body. An overall plan has to be made keeping the entire body in perspective. When we see the patient as a whole, a note can be made of the available donor areas for skin grafts, flaps, or sites for tissue expander placement.

The sequence of correction of the deformities with the interval between each procedure should be penned down after discussing with the patient. This is especially true for patients who present with multiple contractures. For a patient who presents with bilateral hand, elbow, axillary as well as neck contractures, the sequence can be as follows:

- 1st stage – Release of neck contracture with dominant hand and elbow release
- 2nd stage – Opposite axilla + hand release
- 3rd stage – Elbow of non dominant side
- 4th stage – Axilla of dominant side

These decisions are based on many factors like present function of each hand, handedness, occupation, patient desires, etc. The fact that it is paramount to release the neck contracture first is not debatable.

Photography during planning

Planning is helped considerably by photography. A set of photographs of the patient from as many angles as possible showing the contractures (in their extreme ranges of motion) as well as available normal tissue should be taken (Fig. 20.8).

After making a tentative plan in the preliminary consultation, the surgeon can go over the photographs at a more leisurely pace and revisit the plan. Often an unhurried study of the photographs occasionally lends a new dimension of thought and a better plan as compared to the one made in the rush hour of a busy outpatient clinic. The new plan can be discussed with the patient in the next consultation.

General principles of facial reconstruction

1. *Wait for scar maturation and softening before the first surgery, as well as in between sessions.* Waiting for scars to soften and mature will go a long way in reducing the amount of skin and scar that may need excision. Every scar does not need to be excised. An effort should be made to relieve tension in the scar. This relief of tension itself helps to settle the scar better.
2. *Blush areas, if available, to be reserved for facial resurfacing.* Areas on the face, postauricular regions, neck, supraclavicular regions, and even the upper arms have a high cutaneous vasculature. Donor skin from these areas are preferable for the face as there is good color and texture match.
3. *Combine complimentary surgical procedures in one sitting.* This helps keep the overall time to full reconstruction down and also saves the patient from multiple postoperative recovery periods. Waiting between stages is occasionally excruciating for patients as they are very

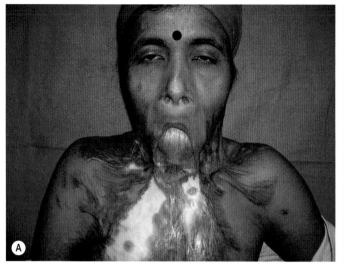

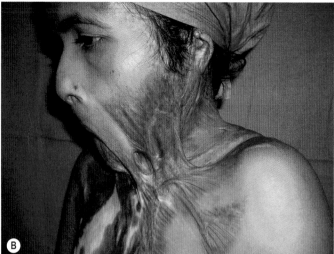

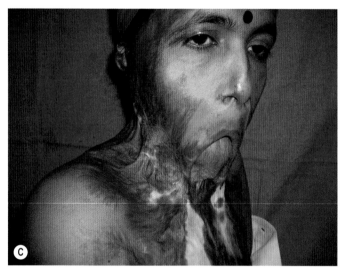

Fig. 20.8 Severe neck contracture. **(A)** Anterior view. **(B)** Left oblique view. **(C)** Right oblique view.

eager to move ahead to the next surgery, waiting for the final expected end result. This may occasionally lead to non-compliance or interruption in the treatment flow if the patient decides to default. The knowledge that many procedures are being done in a sitting is very reassuring to the patient.

4. *Be flexible in your approach.* Postoperative outcomes and scar behavior may not often fall in line with the surgeons expectations. The surgeon must have the vision to predict adverse outcomes and have secondary contingency plans ready that may not conform to earlier decisions. All changes in plans have to be discussed in detail with the patient, explaining the reasons for doing so. A rigid surgeon may often have to be satisfied with a similar scar.

5. *If tissue expander placement is planned, explain the sequence and temporary change in appearance.* It is important for the patient to understand and accept this, especially in case of facial burns as the donor areas are adjacent and cannot be hidden under camouflage clothing. If the patients travel considerable distances for weekly expansions, they would have to make arrangements for safe travel and avoid crowded surroundings due to possibility of trauma.

6. *In case tissue expanders are to be used, exclude endogenous sources of infection.* An implant is a foreign body whose presence attracts infection. It is always better to ensure the absence of any source of infection in the body.

7. *Sequence of surgery should be formalized after full discussion with patient.* Patients and their caregivers not only need to accept the sequence but also understand the reasoning. This helps in compliance to the supportive scar management techniques to be used by the patient in the waiting periods. Sequence of surgery should be revisited after each step. (Be flexible in approach.)

8. *Share sequence of surgery with all team members.* Burn reconstruction is all about teamwork, involving the other burn surgeons in the unit, skilled nurse, and the therapist. Having discussions with the team and getting the sequence counterchecked by others ensures that everyone is on the same page and overlooked points may be picked up.

9. *Provide splints to all areas of contractures in the waiting period.* The use of splintage in the waiting period during staged management of contractures cannot be overemphasized. It will help stop the progression of contractures, reduce the amount of release and donor skin required, and also improve compliance.

10. *Give a trial of "serial splintage" to all contractures.* As waiting lists for surgery in busy public hospitals in LMICs run quite long, the method of serially splinting the contractures has positively shown improvement in the contracture angles and reduction in requirement of grafts at the time of surgery. In minor contractures it may even help obviate the need for the surgery, and major contractures may be converted to those of intermediate severity.[37]

11. *Recognize intrinsic and extrinsic contractures and treat the intrinsic first.* The extrinsic will be relieved or severely diminished once the causative intrinsic contracture is released.

12. *Aesthetic units and subunits should to be kept in mind when resurfacing the face.* The face was divided into convenient aesthetic subunits by Gonzales and Ulloa.[38] While treating a scar in a particular aesthetic subunit, it is better to treat the unit as a whole to optimize outcome.

13. *Planning incisions in the form of "Z"s instead of straight incisions helps keep the requirement of skin graft down and also helps recruit normal skin from the surrounding areas.* Occasionally there may be an excess bulging of skin on the sides of a linear contracture due to ballooning or trap-door effect of scars that can thus get utilized. This is especially true of linear neck contractures.

14. *Calculation of the "true defect".* Especially in the case of severe contractures it is imperative to calculate the true defect as this can appear deceptively less. This is done by comparing or marking out the defect that will be created post-release by utilizing the opposite normal side for planning. Contracture dimensions marked on the normal side with measurements taken from fixed bony landmarks on the affected side will give the size of the true defect that will be produced on release.

15. *Decision regarding the use of split-/full-thickness graft.* A full-thickness graft has less long-term secondary contraction and pigmentary changes compared to a split-thickness one. In the face it is always preferable to use a full-thickness graft as compared to split-thickness; if for some reason a split-thickness graft is used, a thick split-thickness graft is to be preferred.

16. *Keep threshold for use of flaps in facial burn reconstruction very high.* Flaps tend to bring in too much adynamic tissue which may mask facial expression and emotion. If their use is inevitable, locoregional flaps like cervico-humeral flaps or expanded cervical flaps are to be preferred over distant flaps.

17. *Multiple modalities of treatment can be used concurrently as required to treat any one area to be able to obtain the best possible outcome.* For example, Z-plasty to relieve tension, later use of silicone gel sheets, as well as laser therapy to reduce the scar hypertrophy.

18. *Release of tension in scars/linear contractures reduces hypertrophic scars and stimulates pigmentation.* Reorientation of the scar to lie along the relaxed skin tension lines will often produce dramatic changes in appearance due to release of tension.

19. *Take photographs after each stage.* Not only does this help the surgeon in planning further, it is also reinforcement to the patient that improvements have occurred due to the earlier surgery. It helps in patient counseling and revisiting the next planned step (Figs. 20.9–20.14 ●). Figs. 20.9–20.13 appear online only.

20. *The final aim is to provide a face that is balanced, pleasing, symmetric, and dynamic.*

Timing of surgery

The timing of surgery obeys the usual laws of scar maturation. However, there are exceptional conditions which demand early intervention. These areas, having skin laxity, are the periorbital or perioral regions where the mildest contractures can cause deviation of structures and distortion of anatomy. Splintage of these areas is not easily

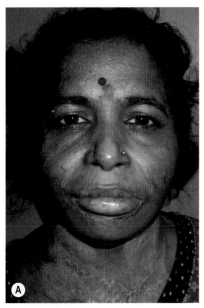
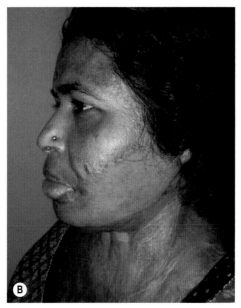
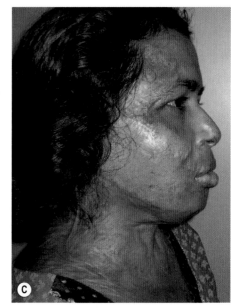

Fig. 20.14 Two years after full-thickness grafts to resurface the cheek and chin scars and 13 years since first presentation. **(A)** Anterior view. **(B)** Left oblique view. **(C)** Right oblique view.

accomplished, so the splint and wait policy cannot be adopted either.

Reconstructive options

A barrage of reconstructive options is available if the surgeon decides to proceed with his or her operative reconstructive plan. But it must be borne in mind that only certain tools are ideal in each circumstance, and the surgeon must choose his weapon judiciously, weighing factors like site, size, color, and texture required.

Skin grafts

A skin graft is the most easily and abundantly available replacement for excised scar tissue. As mentioned earlier, grafts for the face are taken from the "blush" areas for color match. Grafts vary depending on the thickness of their harvest.

Split-thickness grafts

Split-thickness grafts have a greater degree of secondary contraction (due to the presence of lesser dermis in the graft, which is the main component to ensure elasticity) and hence contract more. These grafts have a slightly shiny appearance lifelong.[39] Split-thickness grafts may also be used in the more peripheral areas of the face as well as after the release of upper lid ectropion.[39]

Full-thickness grafts

Full-thickness grafts contract less, have a natural appearance, are aesthetically reliable, and are the first choice for facial burn reconstruction (Figs. 20.14 & 20.15 ⊕). Full-thickness grafts can be taken after expanding the donor area skin so that a primary closure of the donor site is feasible. It provides soft mobile skin in the long run. There are some basic principles to be followed while placing a full-thickness skin graft for reconstruction. Accurate defect measurement should be made in its largest dimensions, and preferably a larger full-thickness graft should be marked out on the donor area. Infection should be excluded before proceeding with the grafting. After the graft is obtained, it is the authors' practice to totally defat the undersurface to expose the dermis. This is most essential to ensure a good take. The defatting is done by spreading the graft epidermal surface down over a bowl and held at the edges with sutures or hemostats for stretching it or, in case of smaller grafts, over the gloved index finger of the non-dominant hand. The fat is then carefully pared away from the undersurface exposing the white dermis using a sharp iris scissor, taking care not to buttonhole the graft. The graft has to be sutured meticulously to the defect with edge to edge approximation using fine (5-0) nylon or prolene sutures. Hemostasis has to be perfect in the wound bed before the graft is sutured on to it. A pressure dressing is the norm to maintain good graft–wound bed cohesion. This can be achieved with tie-over sutures placed over a bolster dressing. Dressing change is done directly on day 10 post-grafting.

Fig. 20.15 appears online only.

Blister grafting/super thin grafts

If there are no contractures and the scars are hypo- or hyperpigmented, all that is deficient is the pigment-producing cells. An epidermal transfer will suffice in such cases. This can be provided by a blister graft or ultra-thin split-thickness skin graft. This has to be preceded by some technique to create a raw surface, which can be achieved by dermabrasion or by using CO_2 ablative lasers. These techniques have been most commonly described and used in the treatment of vitiligo.[40]

Flaps

Flaps are an important addition to the reconstructive armamentarium. Flaps are tissues that are transferred from the donor to the recipient area maintaining its source blood supply. This obviates the need for a healthy blood supply in the recipient bed as the flaps bring with them their own nourishment. In the face, the most commonly used flaps are local flaps from unburnt tissues. Local flaps include local transposition and rotation flaps from adjacent areas. The donor site is managed by a primary closure. This local adjustment of available skin avoids color and contour mismatches that might otherwise occur with flaps transferred from distant areas. Flaps are better suited for reconstruction of the wider flat peripheral part of the face. Flaps occasionally tend to be bulky and are at risk of masking expressions and emotions. Advancements in flap harvests make it possible to obtain thin and super thin flaps, thus giving a good contour and aesthetic appearance.

Z-plasty

This is one of the reliable techniques of scar revision. It can help to lengthen a scar, change the direction of a scar to lie along the relaxed skin tension lines. It can help in interrupting the scar line and camouflaging the scar. The surgical technique should be fine and meticulous, and use of magnification is recommended.[41]

Tissue expansion and flap advancement

Despite the availability of skin grafts, local flaps, and free flaps, the burn surgeon still desires more in terms of aesthetic capability. This involves attempting to replace like with like and if possible give a good color, texture, and sensation match. Each of the above described modalities of reconstruction has some shortcoming when compared to the ideal. Tissue expansion attempts to achieve most of the goals. It utilizes tissues that are a good color and texture match, and the skin flap is well vascularized and sensate. There is minimal to no donor morbidity (Fig. 20.16 ⊕). Technical factors that need to be considered include site of the incision, port placement, and whether internal or external port is to be used.[42] During surgery, once the intended amount of expansion has been carried out, the expander is removed and the flap is advanced into the recipient area. What is of essence is thorough asepsis, use of powder-free, lint-free techniques, and meticulous hemostasis. Use of expanded skin for resurfacing lower cheek and chin contractures has the added disadvantage of gravity pulling down on the flap after advancement. It is liable to cause ectropion of the lip or loss of cervicomental angle due to the pull. The benefits of use of tissue expanders have to be weighed against the cons like cost factors, risk of infection and exposure, and requirement of high motivation and compliance on the part of the patient.

Fig. 20.16 appears online only.

Dermabrasion with thin autografting

Depigmentation often develops after healing of partial-thickness and full-thickness burn injuries that are allowed to heal by secondary intention. This hypopigmentation is a serious aesthetic complication especially in the dark-skinned individual. The pathophysiology of this depigmentation is poorly understood, but it is thought that scar tissue prevents melanocyte migration and melanin transfer.[43] Dermabrasion is accomplished by scraping away the surface epidermal layer of the scar with the use of tools like a dermaroller, which has microneedles on its surface. A smooth rotating burr with tiny abrasive particles on its surface has been seen to produce satisfactory dermabrasion. Dermabrasion is usually followed by any of the standard melanin transfer methods like blister grafting, ultra-thin autograft, etc. The newest tool to achieve dermabrasion is the laser. A carbon dioxide ablative laser has been shown to achieve uniform results in creating a raw surface, which is then covered with thin autografts.[43]

Serial excision

This is one of the time honored and traditional methods of scar revision. This entails removal of the scar in multiple sessions, always excising an ellipse of scar from the middle so that the resultant suture line is contained within the original scar.

Hair transplantation

The technique of microfollicular hair transplantation has evolved to a unique degree of art and expertise. Post-burn alopecia scar is no barrier anymore to attempting a transplant in expert hands.

Fat grafting beneath scars

Regenerative medicine is a rapidly evolving field, with adipose-derived stem cells the foremost tool. Studies have shown that autologous fat transfers in the form of small parcels are able to vascularize and survive in the toughest of environments. Burn scars that are adherent and tough were seen to respond well to the injection of fat cells beneath them. Both aesthetic and functional improvements in scar characteristics were observed. Scars became less pigmented and supple, increasing the skin elasticity and reducing movement limitation.[44]

Tattooing

Camouflage tattooing for medical conditions has gained increasing popularity over time. It has a wide range of applications from tattooing hypopigmented lesions and burn scars to areola pigmentation after breast reconstruction.

Management of keloids

The first line of management when the keloids are minor is to pursue the scar management program more vigorously with methods like silicone gel sheeting, etc. Intralesional injection of triamcinolone has been proven to show efficacy in minor keloids. If there is no improvement in 8–12 weeks of treatment, then 5-FU in combination with intralesional steroids

may be tried, followed by pulsed dye laser therapy and finally surgical excision if nothing else helps.[45] Surgery for keloids has to be preceded by counseling the patient regarding high chances of recurrence (Fig. 20.17). In selected patients radiotherapy after surgery is a viable option. Intralesional 5-FU has shown good results according to evidence. Added to surgery, antimitotic agents like bleomycin and mitomycin C, as well as immunomodulators like 5% imiquimod cream, have been considered for refractory keloids.[46]

Reconstruction of specific areas

Scalp

The scalp and the hairline add a framework to the face and complement youth and identity. Involvement of scalp in burns can lead to a range of problems from minor alopecia to exposure of calvarium in cases of devastating electric burns. The scalp is involved in almost 25% of facial burns. In the scalp, alopecia is the morbidity of a burn injury. The

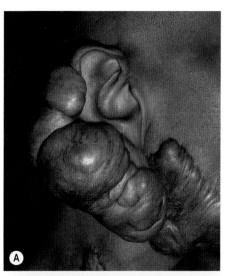

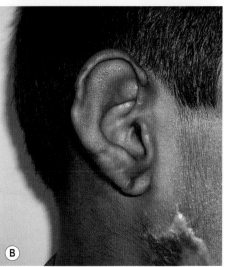

Fig. 20.17 (A) Large ear keloids. **(B)** After surgical intralesional excision, result at one year.

primary goal of reconstruction here is to create a natural looking hair-bearing scalp with hair growing in the correct direction while having a good hairline. McCauley *et al.* classified scalp defects suggesting reconstructive options for each described type.[42] Serbulent Guzey *et al.* classified lateral scalp burn alopecia into 3 groups – type 1 (total lateral), type 2 (temporal and side burn), and type 3 (sideburn). This classification helped them in planning tissue expander placement.[47]

Classification of scalp defects

Depending on the size and location of scar, suppleness of scar, quality of surrounding scalp tissue, presence or absence of hair on it, and location of hair line, one can choose a reconstructive option. Many reconstructive options have been described – reduction techniques, serial excisions, scalp flaps, hair grafting, and expanders.

Reduction techniques

Serial excision

To remove alopecia of up to 15% of the hair-bearing scalp, serial scar excision was a very viable option. Huang *et al.* in a large series of 117 patients with post-burn alopecia described serial excision as one of the management modalities.[48] This is a preferred approach even now if complete excision of the scar can be done in two to three sittings. It has the advantage of lesser morbidity and a short recovery period.

Local flaps

If the defect is anterior, the primary goal is to achieve a good hairline. Hence, while planning local flaps and scars of excision this has to be kept in mind. If the alopecia is in the parietal region, defects smaller than 25 cm^2 can be managed with direct closure or use of Limberg flap or rotation flap, as the surrounding parietal scalp is more mobile. It is to be remembered that tissue mobility in the vertex is limited, hence

local flaps move with difficulty. Orticochea flaps can be used for defects that are less than 50 cm^2 in the occipital region where mobility of the scalp is only moderate.[49] The Orticochea flaps can close scalp defects greater than 15% of the hair-bearing scalp.[50]

Hair transplantation

Hair transplantation is a very good option for post-burn alopecia, but it can be done only if the scar is supple, there is intact deep tissue below the cicatricial alopecia, and the occipital donor site is available. In these cases grafting by follicular unit transfer (FUT; strip method) or follicular unit extraction (FUE) can be done.[51–53]

Tissue expansion

Scalp expansion allows redistribution of the scalp tissue without creating new hair follicles. Interfollicular distance can increase up to twofold without noticeable thinning of the hair.[54] More than 30 years ago, Manders *et al.* reconstructed almost half the scalp with tissue expansion.[54] It continues to be the commonest method for hair restoration for post-burn scalp alopecia[42,55–58] (Fig. 20.18 ●). Pressure on the suture line in the early healing phase could lead to exposure.

Fig. 20.18 appears online only.

Microvascular free tissue transfer

In cases of devastating injury to the scalp as occurs in high voltage electrical burn with exposure of deeper structures like the calvarium, use of the aforementioned techniques is precluded. This requires special measures like bringing in distant tissue with its vascularity to provide the necessary cover. Flaps like free anterolateral thigh flap and latissimus dorsi flap can cover large areas of the scalp using the superficial temporal vessels as recipient vessels for the anastomosis (Fig. 20.19 ●).

Fig. 20.19A & C appear online only.

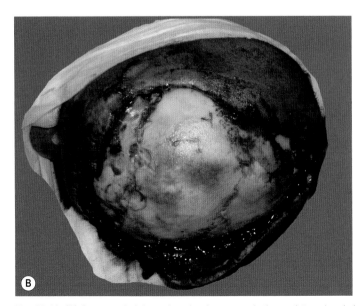

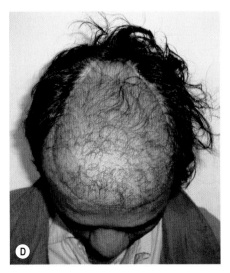

Fig. 20.19 **(B)** On removal of the eschar, slough was seen in the craniotomy burr holes. **(D)** One year postoperative, after resurfacing with ALT flap.

Scalp skin used as donor area to resurface facial burn wounds had shown alopecia as a side effect according to studies.[59]

Forehead

The contour of the forehead is defined by the underlying bony structure while the surface appearance is due to the skin and facial muscles beneath.[60] Forehead skin is some of the thickest in the face, with it being thickest in the supra-brow region and progressively decreasing towards the hairline. In 71% of facial burns the forehead is involved.[61]

The aim of the forehead reconstruction is to produce a skin coverage that is uniform and capable of dynamic facial expression.[62] A stuck-on appearance of a graft should be avoided as it erases all the creases of the forehead. Connell and Marten in their paper on forehead-plasty emphasize the importance of reconstructing creases as they convey strength, power, and wisdom.[63]

Choice and sequence of reconstruction will depend on the size and location of the scar and the condition of the bordering structures such as the eyebrows and the hairline. Reconstructive options include excision in an elliptical manner and primary closure occasionally with intraoperative expansion using Foley's catheter,[64] serial excision, local flaps, advancement flaps,[65,66] bilateral rotation flaps,[67] FTG, SSG,[68–71] and tissue expansion.[72–75]

Eyebrows

Loss of an eyebrow or eyebrows creates a dramatic change in the facial countenance of an individual, thus demanding a fair share of importance in secondary reconstruction. In cases of extrinsic pull distorting the eyebrow, release of the offending tight scar tissue and replacement with supple tissue will help reposition the eyebrow. Occasionally the eyebrow can be repositioned using Z-plasty.

In cases of loss of eyebrows, reconstruction will be according to amount of tissue loss. Either one of the following methods can be used for reconstruction – superficial temporal artery island flap; subcutaneous island pedicle flap from scalp,[76] composite grafts from scalp, or hair grafting.

Hair grafting: Other than the scalp a reasonable potential donor site is nasal vibrissae.[77] Also, Baretto mentions that eyebrow hair has more similarities to eyelashes than scalp hair as far as texture, speed, and length of growth (8–12 mm) is concerned, so when a small area is to be filled in, it is a most favorable donor site.[51]

Eyebrow repositioning, repair or reconstruction can be an important "finishing touch" in the overall reconstruction of a burned face.[78]

Ears

Though isolated burns of the ear are rare, in most facial burns the ear is involved. Tolleth mentions that the ear is involved in 90% of facial burns.[79] Mills *et al.* mention that 52.7% of all the patients of burns surveyed over a 7-year period had ear burns.[80] Ear deformities due to burns may range from mild discoloration of skin to complete loss of the external ears. A burnt ear may have the following deformities:

1. Mixed pigmentation scars without contour deformities
2. Hypertrophic scars and keloids
3. Cryptotia of the ear due to adhesion between the auricle and the postauricular skin and mastoid region. The commonest sites involved in this manner are over the helix/antihelix[81]
4. Contracted external ear, due to crumpling of the cartilage or occasionally upper third contracture or ear lobe contracture due to folding on itself
5. Partial loss of different components of the external ear
6. Complete loss of the external ear.

Thermal injury to the ear will cause deformities due to direct damage to skin and cartilage or due to suppurative chondritis due to secondary infection. In deep burns the cartilage may get exposed and undergo focal necrosis, if uninfected it will heal with scarring as the eschar separates.[82] Some surgeons have described reconstruction of the external ear during the acute setting by using turnover flaps of temporoparietal fascia, platysma flap, and mastoid flaps.[83,84]

Suppurative chondritis, which is due to secondary infection, can develop even 3–5 weeks after the burn.[80] Avoidance of pressure and good topical treatment goes a long way in reducing chondritis and hence its associated deformities.[85] Many devices have been described for preventing pressure.[86–88]

Different classifications have been proposed for ear deformities aimed towards decision-making for reconstruction. K'ung's classification, which divided ear deformities into 3 types, is half a century old.[89] Bhandari in 1998 presented his classification of 5 groups depending on availability of skin around the ear.[90]

The reconstruction of post-burn ear deformities uses the same principles and surgical techniques as those used for congenital deformities. The difference here is that the quality of surrounding skin available for reconstruction is dubious and quantity insufficient. Minor deformities of the burnt ear can be tackled by Z-plasty releases or local adjustment of tissues. Local cutaneous flaps with or without cartilage grafts are used for the reconstruction of helical rim defects.[82,91–94] Innovative techniques have been described for upper[95–97] and middle third[98–100] defect reconstructions. For lobe reconstruction again local skin flaps are used.[98,101,102]

Options for individual areas

For badly scarred ears and loss of large component parts or total loss, Brent advocated excising the auricular scarred skin and replacing it with carved costochondral cartilage graft and covering it immediately with temporoparietal fascial flap.[103–106] Nagata presented ten principles of post-burn reconstruction more than two decades back, which continue to be followed for post-burn ear reconstructions to date.[107,108]

Silicone and polyethylene frameworks have also been described and used with varying results in place of carved costal cartilage. But the complication rate and problems of extrusion are much higher in these cases.[109–111] Use of osseointegrated implants to achieve better cosmesis have been described over the years and require good cortical bone and pliable soft tissue.[112] However, despite the prosthetic ear's excellent color and anatomic contour match, reconstructions of the ear (staged or single) continue to be the method of choice for post-burn ear reconstruction (Fig. 20.20 ⊕).

Fig. 20.20A & B appear online only.

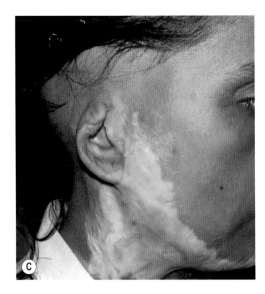

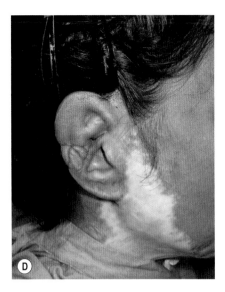

Fig. 20.20 (C) More than half ear deformity. **(D)** Reconstruction with postauricular skin and costal cartilage graft.

Eyelids/periorbital region

Though the eyelids and periorbital region are injured often in burns, globe injury is not as common due to the blink reflex as well as the reflex protective mechanisms of the body to save the face and eyes. More often than not eyelids are injured due to exposure to the dry heat of fire and not due to direct contact with fire.[82] Ophthalmic injury with facial burns has been reported ranging from 4% to 36% of facial burns with 13% having direct corneal injury.[113–115] Corneal injuries have been reported to occur more often with chemical burns and in some other reports due to flame burns.[113–117]

Smith *et al.* reported that short-term ophthalmologic complications after burns included eyelid burns, corneal abrasions, vision loss, high intraocular pressure, and surface discomfort. Long-term complications included eyelid retraction, lagophthalmos, trichiasis, ectropion, vision loss on follow-up, and need for surgery, and its risk factors were wound infection with *Pseudomonas* or *Acinetobacter*, third-degree burn, hours to ophthalmology evaluation, time on mechanical ventilation, and need for split-thickness skin graft.[118]

Eyelid deformities due to burns may range from mild discoloration of skin to complete loss of the eyelids (Fig. 20.21). The severity and extent of the eyelid scarring or deformity will depend on the nature, intensity, and duration of the exposure to the heat source.[82] A burnt eye and periorbital region may have the following deformities:

1. Mixed pigmentation scars without deformity
2. Hypertrophic scars and keloids
3. Ectropion, lid retraction
4. Canthal deformities
5. Symblepharon, entropion, blepharostenosis, canalicular stenosis
6. Partial loss of the eyelid
7. Complete loss of the eyelids.

Eyelid retraction and ectropion are the commonest sequelae of periorbital region burns.[119,120] Depending on the severity of the deformity, the ectropion or eyelid retraction will lead to eversion of the eyelid with exposure of the conjunctiva and

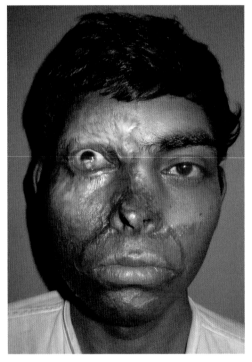

Fig. 20.21 Right upper and lower eyelid contracture with corneal opacity.

its concomitant problems of excessive tearing, exposure keratitis, and corneal ulceration.

Some salient principles that must be followed for release of lid ectropion are as follows:

1. *Recognize whether it is an intrinsic or extrinsic contracture.* It is very important to know whether the ectropion is intrinsic or extrinsic. The eyelid being a mobile structure with a free border is very easily pulled by the surrounding tissues as they are healing and may easily develop an ectropion or scleral show due to the tight scar above or below it.[121,122] In extrinsic contractures, excision of the offending scar will reposition the eyelid. In intrinsic contractures, it is usually the skin and orbicularis that is involved and the deeper tissues are

usually not violated. Direct thermal injury to the levator or the tarsus is very rare and such severe full-thickness lid injuries can occur in case the person falls unconscious over the heat source.[82]

2. *If both lids are involved, do not treat both lids simultaneously.* One can opt to do the more severe contracture first. When in doubt (or in case the cornea is exposed), it is more prudent to release the upper lid contracture first. It is the author's preference to do the second release after about 12 weeks to give adequate time for the graft to settle and remain in good stretch in the early phase. The chances of re-contracture will be much lesser if the new graft can be splinted for a period of at least 2 to 3 months before embarking upon the other lid.

3. *If both sides are involved, operate on one side at a time.* As the dressing involves closing the eye completely, operating on both sides would mean that the patient would be temporarily blinded due to the dressings, and this can be very incapacitating for an adult.

4. *Keep a low threshold for release.* If possible, in immature minor contractures, release should be delayed till the scar matures. Aggressive scar massage and eye exercises should be begun to help in scar stretching. But one should keep a low threshold for scar release, as occasionally even if the patient can close the eye actively; it tends to open up while sleeping. Taping the eyelids may help along with the trial of conservative management. It needs to be kept in mind that when operating on an immature scar, the chances of re-contracture are very high

5. *Full esthetic subunit of the eyelid* should be covered with a graft.

6. *The release incision should extend all the way from the medial to the lateral canthus.* Fishtailing or making darts at the extremities of the incision helps to release any medial or lateral bands.

7. *Always overcorrect to avoid a re-contracture.*

8. *Ideal qualities the graft should possess – thin, hairless, full-thickness graft.* Though the ideal graft will be from the other lid, postauricular skin or graft from the supraclavicular area are the next best choice. If these are not available, then it would be better to use a split medium-thickness graft from the blush areas or scalp instead of a thick split-thickness graft.[82]

9. *Color match the lower lid to the cheek.* Given a choice, if there is inadequate graft available of blush areas, it would be better to use the matching graft for the lower lid as any color mismatch is more obviously seen in the lower than the upper lid.

10. *Save the best for the last.* Do not use the best grafts from the blush regions if they are limited if re-contracture is expected or inevitable. Save them for the last surgery.

Technical pointers for ectropion release

Upper lid release

Infiltrate large amounts of tumescence solution into the scar and wait for a minimum of 10 min before making the incision. Two or three temporary lid margin stitches are taken and the suture threads kept long for traction during surgery. The incision on the upper lid should be a few millimeters from the lid margin. It should extend medially beyond the medial canthus onto the nose and laterally beyond the lateral canthus, at all times staying above the canthal line. The straight line is opened up like a "Y" on both ends of the incision. Fishtailing of the incision at both ends helps to avoid a re-contracture as well as break any vertical scar bands, which are often present along the lateral or the medial canthus region. The incision should be deepened to full thickness of the scar tissue such that a complete release is obtained. Occasionally one may have to cut through the fibers of the orbicularis. Skin above and below the incision is dissected allowing it to slide back such that there is overcorrection. Excision of the folded and bunched-up scarred skin along the edges of the incision and in continuity with it as much as required is performed. Gentle traction on the stay sutures will help facilitate a complete release. Waiting adequate time after infiltration with tumescence solution helps keep the field clean and relatively bloodless. Hemostasis should be achieved using a bipolar cautery and gentle pressure. Though there are many surgeons who prefer to use split-thickness skin grafts for the upper eyelids, the authors' choice is to use a thin, hairless full-thickness graft either from the postauricular region or the supraclavicular region. If these are not available, then one can opt to resurface with a split medium-thickness graft from the blush areas or scalp or a full-thickness graft from any other donor site.

Lower lid release

The lower lid release is similar to the upper lid release in most aspects of surgery. The incision should be a gentle C-shaped one such that it parallels the line of the lid margin. The lateral end of the incision should extend downwards into an imaginary crow's feet line. The release and scar excision should be such that the graft is placed from the lid margin to the infraorbital margin. Again, overcorrection is the key to avoiding a re-contracture. Even after all efforts at overcorrection, the re-contracture rates of eyelid ectropions are high. After release, ideally the defect should be covered with a very thin flap so as to avoid re-contracture. As the adjacent areas are also often scarred and unavailable, skin grafts are the usual mode of cover. A full-thickness graft from the opposite eyelid, postauricular region, or the supraclavicular region is the graft of choice. If these are not available, then one can opt to resurface with a full thickness graft from any other available area of the body. An effort should be made to color match the graft of the lower lid to the cheek skin.

Calculation of graft requirement

A template of the required full-thickness graft is made after traction on the lid suture such that the defect is maximized. This template is used to mark the required graft area on the donor site. Suturing is done edge to edge with 6-0 prolene suture in a continuous manner so that there are no free tips of the cut sutures that may injure the cornea. In case additional interrupted sutures are required, the ends are kept long and taped down till removal. At the end of suturing the graft bed is flushed out with normal saline to confirm that there is no hematoma beneath. Dressing is done using a medicated tulle grass dressing, 1 cm thick foam, and a thin pliable stainless steel mesh, all cut to the size of the template. After the tulle grass is placed on the graft, the foam and the mesh are sutured into the margins of the defect. The foam gives gentle constant pressure, and the stainless steel mesh provides splintage and immobility to the grafted area (Fig. 20.22B). First graft dressing is done on day 10 directly, by which time the graft has usually taken well and is stable. The graft can then be lubricated with liquid paraffin and covered for another week to 10 days so that it is kept in a maximally stretched position. Further to this period, the patient is asked to gently massage the graft in the direction opposite to that of the contracture (downwards for upper lid contractures and upwards for lower lid contractures). Exercises to open and close the lid tight are also explained to keep the graft and the lid supple. Direct sun exposure is to be avoided for about 3 to 6 months to avoid pigmentary complications. This is important more so in the darker-skinned races. Custom-made devices to keep the lid in stretch with padded thermoplastic material can be used at night along with taping of the lid for 6 months.

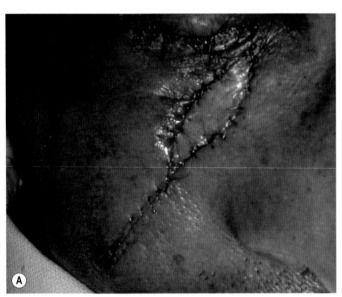

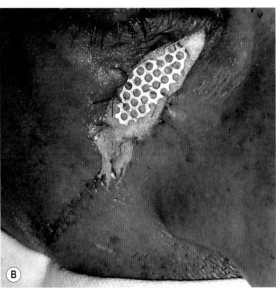

Fig. 20.22 (A) Full-thickness graft sutured in place. **(B)** Dressing using foam and mesh.

Flaps

For lower lid defects, if the surrounding skin is available, one could proceed with any of the locally available flaps according to the surgeon's choice and familiarity. Superiorly based nasolabial flaps, inferiorly based temporal flaps, medial, lateral or bipedicled orbicularis oculi myocutaneous flaps, Tripier flaps, lateral orbital flaps, etc., have been described.[82,123–126] Occasionally one may have to delay these flaps, especially if they are being raised from scarred skin.

Facial suspension can be a good ancillary tool for lower lid extrinsic ectropion to correct any residual drooping. An endoscopic technique of suspension has been described with low morbidity and good results.[127] The same principles were used as for aesthetic facial suspension with good results.

Partial or complete loss of the eyelids

The reconstruction of a lid loss is dependent on the available tissues in the other lid and the surrounding area. If local tissues are available, then the usual techniques of lid reconstruction can be followed, as done for trauma or oncologic reconstruction. In case there is no local tissue available and there is full-thickness lid loss, distant flaps lined with cartilage and mucosa need to be brought in to reconstruct the eyelids. The authors' preference is for a free radial artery forearm flap, which is a good option because of its thin, pliable nature. Even so, flap thinning is almost always required at a later date. As a second stage the palpebral fissure is created. If contracted and rolled up conjunctiva is present, it can be opened up and used to avoid a mucosal graft. Chen Jiaqi *et al.* used acellular dermal allograft instead of cartilage as a tarsus substitute and covered it with orbicularis muscle. They concluded that the allograft appeared to be biocompatible and does not aggravate the inflammation in the injured eyelid.[128] For completely destroyed eyelids in the acute setting, Kai Liu *et al.* have described suturing the conjunctiva and resurfacing with skin grafts to save vision.[129]

The final goal in eyelid reconstruction is to provide a mobile, supple and esthetic lid that can fulfill its protective function.

Nose

The nose is not only central on the face but also has projection. Owing to these properties it tends to be involved in a large percentage of facial burns. Nasal distortions cannot be camouflaged as easily as the ear, which can be hidden with long hair. Also, post-burn deformities of the nose cause not just aesthetic problems but they may also cause functional problems like difficulty in breathing due to nostril stenosis.

The post-burn sequelae of the nose could be anyone or all the following[82]:

1. Altered surface texture or discoloration
2. Elevated nasal tip and alar margins (ectropion)
3. Scarred and shortened columella
4. Full-thickness loss of parts of the nose (most often nasal base, tip, and/or ala)
5. Nostril stenosis or a complete block of passage.

Achauer classified burned nasal deformity into five types[130]: without major tissue loss (cutaneous issues only); ectropion (elevated nasal tip and alar margins); subtotal tissue loss (more than the nasal tip but not whole nose); extensive tissue loss; and nostril stenosis.

Just as in the ear, avoidance of pressure, topical treatment, and use of splints go a long way in the reduction of nasal deformities.

As the nose has many components, deformity of one will affect the other. Hence, it is very important to evaluate what could be the cause of the deformity; for example, is it a tight scar that is causing the nostril show or is it actual tissue loss of the alar rim or is it a tight scarred deformed lining.

Reconstruction of the post-burn nose follows the same principles as those of reconstruction of the nose due to trauma or oncologic defects. *An evaluation of whether the nose needs skin cover, lining, and or skeletal support is the first step in planning reconstruction.* This will help one choose the reconstructive option. The availability of supple forehead skin is a boon in nasal reconstruction.

Altered surface texture or discoloration: Lasers or other methods of dermabrasion can be used for ablation, and resurfacing can be done with super-thin graft.

Elevated nasal tip and alar margins (Fig. 20.23): Everted nostrils have been corrected with circumferential release of the tissues around the nostril rims, turndown of the resulting vestibular flaps, and grafting of the tip defect.[131] This principle has been effectively demonstrated by Helena *et al.* in their 2009 paper in which they conclude that the efficacy of the nasal turndown flap is twofold – that it provides substantial bulk for nasal tip projection as well as tip and lobule reconstruction without the need for cartilage grafting even in severe ectropions and that it may be repeated with the passage of time and growth of the patient.[132] After a turndown, the defect can also be reconstructed with nasolabial flaps to receive like tissue.[133] A composite graft from the helical rim is also an option to add tissue in a case of nostril ectropion release. Skin grafts used on the nasal dorsum should be thick split-thickness grafts or full-thickness grafts from the postauricular, supraclavicular, or medial arm region.

Scarred and shortened columella: The nasolabial flap can be used to reconstruct the columella. Even if it is scarred, this tissue would be the best match. A forehead flap can also be used for columella reconstruction.

Full-thickness loss of parts of the nose (usually nasal base, tip, and or ala): If there is a composite defect, then graft is not an option.

Cover: For smaller defects local flaps like the Banner flap, bilobed flap, dorsal nasal flap, or nasolabial flaps may be utilized. A galea frontalis myofascial flap has been described by Sharma and Sohi for the cover of nasal bones.[134]

For larger defects, the median or paramedian forehead flap is the best choice. Forehead flaps are the flap of choice for all nose reconstructions as they can reach all the way to the columella, are reliable flaps, and have an ease of dissection. If the forehead is scarred but supple, it can be used for reconstruction. If the tissue of the forehead is inadequate, it can safely be expanded and used for nasal reconstruction (Fig. 20.24 ⊚).[135] If midline and paramedian forehead is not available, the scalping flap can be done if lateral forehead skin is available. If forehead skin is not available, then free flaps like the radial artery forearm flap (see Fig. 20.18) or fascial flaps with skin graft can be used for nasal reconstruction.[136] The Tagliacozzi flap is a distant pedicled flap from the medial arm that was used extensively earlier for nose reconstruction

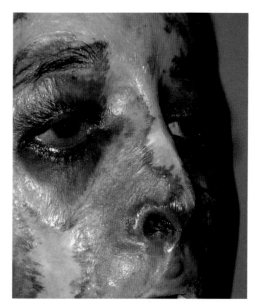

Fig. 20.23 Elevated nasal tip and alar margins.

before the advent for microvascular surgery. Some innovative distant pedicled flaps have also been described for nasal reconstruction in the absence of forehead skin.[137]

Figs. 20.18 & 20.24C appear online only.

Skeletal support: Cartilage or bony support is rarely needed for post-burn sequelae. If required, costochondral cartilage grafts, stacked septal cartilage grafts, split rib grafts, split calvarial grafts, or iliac crest grafts can all be used. It is preferable to use autogenous material as compared to substitutes like silicone implants or porous polyethylene implants as they can erode through tissues and get exposed. When skeletal support is being provided, it is essential to make sure that there is adequate soft-tissue cover over the bone or cartilage.

Nostril stenosis or complete block: Loss of cartilaginous support and inadequate care in the healing phase can lead to a complete nostril block. The block is very rarely deep and, after scar excision, one usually finds the nasal mucosa about 5–10 mm from the nostril rim (Fig. 20.25). Overcorrection should be attempted as the grafts tend to contract and the nostril opening reduces to a certain extent. After creating the nostril opening, the raw area on the undersurface should be grafted with a thick split-thickness graft or a full-thickness graft. One way to do this is to drape the graft on a mold and pack it into the newly opened up nostril. Graft dressing should be done early if the mold blocks the nostril completely. The authors create a mold of dental stent material with a red rubber catheter in the middle so that the patient can breathe through it and secretions can drain. In this situation, the dressing can be done on the 7th postoperative day. Postoperatively, it is imperative for the patient to wear a nasal stent for at least 6 months.

The goal of nasal reconstruction is to create a nose that is aesthetically pleasing, has projection, and does its functional job of breathing.

Cheeks

The preeminence and large proportion of the face the cheeks occupy define its unique characteristics as an anatomic unit.

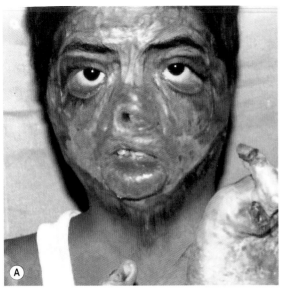

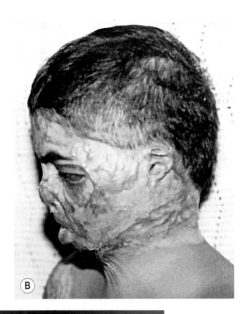

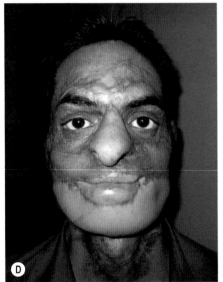

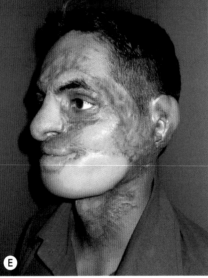

Fig. 20.24 Severe contractures involving all component parts of the face in an 11-year-old child who got burnt while making tea due to a stove burst. **(A)** Anterior view. **(B)** Lateral view. **(D)** Reconstruction of nose using expanded forehead flap. Chin had been earlier reconstructed with a deltopectoral (DP) flap. Oral competence and upward angles of mouth have been obtained with fascia lata sling. **(E)** Lateral view also showing reconstructed ear with expanded postauricular skin and costal cartilage graft.

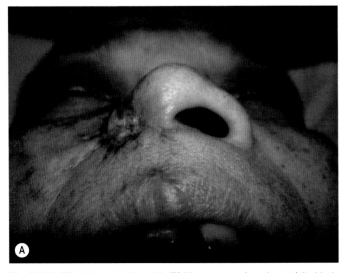

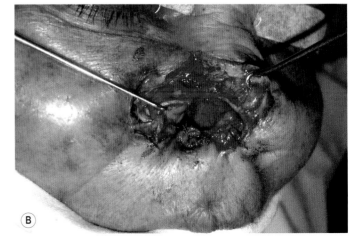

Fig. 20.25 (A) A blocked right nostril. **(B)** Mucosa seen after release of the block.

Surgical reconstruction of the deformed cheek remains a challenge because of deficiency of well-matched donor skin. This problem becomes even graver when only one cheek is deformed.

The cervical skin is most well matched, but it is limited in mobility and size. Tissues transferred from the shoulder region, chest wall, and areas distant from the face provide a poor cosmetic match to the remaining facial skin.

Principally the following points should be kept in mind while planning reconstruction of cheek defects:

1. Keep the aesthetic units in mind when planning excision and resurfacing.
2. The skin used for replacing the cheek scar should be thin, unscarred, and should reflect the facial expressions when the patient animates.
3. When a third to half the cheek is to be reconstructed, only the concerned area should be replaced. It can be done by using cervicofacial flaps.
4. If more than half of the cheek needs reconstruction, one should replace the entire esthetic unit of the cheek. This can be successfully done by using expanded flaps from the neck and the shoulder.
5. When grafts are used for resurfacing, the junctional scars should be softened or erased at a later date by W-plasty or dermabrasion.
6. The same holds true for the junction line between the residual cheek and the cervical flaps.
7. Bulky flaps should be avoided as they bury the expressions under them and the patient gets a mask-like appearance.
8. If grafts are being used, the defect should be stretched such that extra graft is inserted into the defect as later there is sure to be graft contracture and reduction in size.
9. All possible ancillary measures should be used to improve the scar as cheeks are our face to the world.

For resurfacing of cheek scars the following surgical strategies are available:

Healing by secondary intention

This is the simplest method. It is useful for small (<1 cm), superficial defects located in cosmetically inconspicuous areas like below the sideburns, in patients with solar-damaged, irregularly pigmented skin.

Primary closure and serial excision

This is the method of choice if excessive tension and distortion of surrounding structures can be avoided. One should make sure that scars are placed along minimal skin tension lines or within natural skin contours such as the nasolabial or preauricular folds.

Skin grafts

Skin grafts are an acceptable option in patients who have significant comorbid conditions. Skin grafts can be used to resurface less critical areas of the cheek (e.g., just below sideburns) or the donor sites of flaps, which are used to resurface more critical areas. The disadvantage is that skin grafts have a patch-like appearance. Also, because of their innate contraction, grafts may limit the dynamism and suppleness of the cheek, which is critical to allow facial movements and expression. Full-thickness grafts exhibit less secondary contraction and have an aesthetic result as compared to split skin grafts. Also, they are better suited to areas where contracture would result in distortion of the adjacent structures (e.g., lower eyelids).

Tissue expansion

Tissue expansion has allowed reconstructive surgeons to achieve functional and aesthetic goals that were previously unobtainable. The expanded cervical, pectoral, and shoulder skin has been used very effectively for burned cheek resurfacing.

Flap cover

For small scars, ample local skin is available to be used as flaps to replace the scar. For larger scars, the closest and best available skin is that from the cervical region as it is very similar to the residual cheek skin. For cheek resurfacing, neck skin can be used in the form of cervicofacial flaps (medially, laterally, or inferiorly based),[138–140] cervicopectoral flaps,[66,141] and angle rotation flaps.[142] To improve the blood supply and flap safety, a deep plane dissection below the superficial muscular aponeurotic system (SMAS) and platysma has been suggested.[143]

The other flaps which can be used for resurfacing the cheeks are the pre-expanded supraclavicular artery flap,[144] expanded lower trapezius flap,[145] supraclavicular artery island flap,[146] supraclavicular prefabricated flap,[147] the superficial cervical artery flap,[148] the deltopectoral flap, flaps from chest wall, and the cervicothoracic prefabricated flap, which may be pedicled or islanded and may be expanded.[149,150]

Rarely, in case of severe scarring in the neck and the chest, one may have to opt for distant flaps or free flaps. Using distant flaps/free flaps on the cheeks is the last choice as it obliterates the contours of the face and hides the muscles of facial animation. Radial artery forearm flap, thinned anterolateral thigh (ALT), scapular, and parascapular flaps have been described for facial resurfacing.

Lips and perioral region

The lips are important for functional, aesthetic, emotional, and sentimental reasons. The lip serves its many functions and roles due to its unique anatomy, especially the perioral sphincter muscle.[151] The upper lip has an intricate anatomy that includes the two lateral subunits, the philtral subunit, and the vermillion with the Cupid's bow. At the two junctions of the upper and the lower lip is the modiolus, which is a meeting ground of many facial muscles. Considering the intricate anatomy of the upper lip, reconstruction of the lip to its pre-burn appearance is exceedingly difficult.

One of the commonest reasons for microstomia is electrical burns in children due to them biting on electrical wires.[152] This leads to microstomia due to commissure injury. Classifications have been described for these injuries that are aimed towards describing the extent of the injury.[153,154]

Post-burn sequelae of the lips and perioral region include:

1. Minor hypertrophic scarring of the upper lip
2. Scarring with/without shortening of the upper lip

3. Lower lip ectropion without mandible deformities
4. Lower lip ectropion with mandible deformities
5. Microstomia
6. Macrostomia
7. Perioral scar bands
8. Pseudomicrogenia
9. Pigmentation issues.

Some salient principles that must be followed during post-burn deformity correction of lips and perioral region are as follows:

1. *Recognize whether it is an intrinsic or extrinsic ectropion of the lower lip*: It is very important to know whether the ectropion is intrinsic or extrinsic in nature. The lower lip being a mobile structure with a free border, it is very easily pulled by the surrounding tissues as they are healing and may easily develop an ectropion or dental show due to the tight scar below it. A neck contracture going onto the chin can cause an extrinsic lip ectropion. Releasing the neck contracture and excision of the offending scar on the chin will reposition the lower lip.
2. *Wait for scar maturity*: If possible, in immature minor scars and contractures of the lips, release should be delayed until the scar matures. Aggressive scar massage and lip exercises should be begun to help in scar stretching. The addition of steroid injections or pulsed dye laser therapy will frequently resolve these scars satisfactorily.[2]
3. *Full aesthetic subunit of the lip* should be covered with a graft. Total resurfacing of the upper lip should be performed using a full-thickness skin graft.[2]
4. *Always overcorrect a lower lip ectropion to avoid a re-contracture.*
5. *Beware an elongated upper lip when releasing scars of the upper lip.*
6. *In males the upper lip, chin and lower face should be resurfaced with hair-bearing flaps.*
7. *Always reconstruct the philtral ridges and philtral dimple while resurfacing the upper lip.*
8. *Pay attention to alignment of the vermilion* as it is a key element in an aesthetic lip.
9. *Recreate the labiomental groove in lower lip and chin scarring.*
10. *The oral commissure should be positioned at the mid-pupillary line.*
11. Restore function of the oral commissure by recreating an adequate lip-seal and supple underlying musculature for speech and mastication. *Lip suspension procedures may be required to avoid drooling after release of severe contractures.*
12. *In the pediatric age group, a tight scar on the chin and lower face should be excised and resurfaced even if it is not causing a functional problem* as growth of the mandible will be hampered otherwise.

Minor hypertrophic scarring of the upper lip: When the patient presents early with immature minor scars and contractures, release should be delayed until the scar matures. Aggressive scar massage and lip exercises should be begun to help in scar stretching. Mouth opening exercises, blowing air forcefully keeping lips closed, etc., goes a long way in stretching scars.

The addition of steroid injections or pulsed dye laser therapy will frequently resolve these scars satisfactorily.[2]

Scarring with/without shortening of the upper lip

For small scars, excision and primary closure can be done or local flaps can be done after excision of the hypertrophic scars. In the main body of the lip, the scar should lie vertical, whereas at the upper part (base of the nostril) the scar should be horizontal. Any vertical scar or tight bands can be released with Z-plasty. In major scarring where almost the whole lip is scarred and short, the scar should be excised and contracture released. The whole aesthetic subunit should be excised. During excision and release, excessive overcorrection should not be attempted as it can lead to an elongated, overhanging floppy upper lip. The bed that is created to receive the graft should have the contours of the philtral ridge as well as the dimple. This can be created using the same scar tissue. Grishkevich describes leaving behind a 4-mm ridge of scar tissue over the philtral ridges and applying grafts on the philtral dimple and lateral subunits to result in good contours of the upper lip.[155] In females, resurfacing should be done with a full-thickness graft from the postauricular region or supraclavicular region. In males it would be better to bring in a hair-bearing flap.[156–160] Local flaps have also been described for upper lip resurfacing like the nasolabial flap and facial artery musculomucosal flap.[161,162]

Lower lip ectropion with or without mandible deformities

The deformity of the lower lip and chin complex (see Fig. 20.15 ⊙) is more often than not along with neck contractures and is in the form of eversion of the lower lip, occasionally with exposure of the teeth. It is very important to know whether the ectropion is intrinsic or extrinsic. If intrinsic, release of this lower lip contracture is by incising below the lip in the labiomental groove with lateral darts. It is essential to overcorrect as the lower lip ectropion tends to re-contract. If the scar is very deep, one needs to be careful during the deeper dissection to avoid making a buttonhole in the mucosa from the anterior incision. When the scarring of the lower lip, chin, and the neck is longstanding since childhood, the growth of the mandible is affected. Because of the constant pull of the scar, the symphyseal region grows inferiorly and the teeth face downwards too. In such cases, the neck contracture and the lower lip contracture should be released first. Once the graft settles, the mandible and teeth deformities can be operated upon. One may have to consider resurfacing the chin with a flap if mandible osteotomies are required and the scar of skin graft is tight.

Microstomia

Post-burn microstomia may be intrinsic or extrinsic. Tight bands running in the perioral region can restrict the mouth opening. Release of these bands with Z-plasty will relieve the microstomia. Scarring of the lips and the angle of the mouth or the vermilion will lead to intrinsic microstomia. The angle of the mouth moves medially and needs to be repositioned laterally for function as well as aesthetics. The classic release method as proposed by Converse in 1959 continues to be used by most surgeons today. The external scar is released completely down to the buccal mucosa, saving the buccal mucosa. Three flaps are created from the buccal mucosa and sutured to the edge of the skin defect. The aim is to obtain full release of the microstomia as well as displace the commissure laterally to its natural midpupillary line position.[163] If the vermilion is scarred and has a contracture, it can be released with Z-plasty (Fig. 20.26). Different surgeons have suggested procedures like skin grafts, varieties of commissurotomies and local flaps, nasolabial flaps, tongue flaps, and composite grafts from the ear lobe.[164–169]

Macrostomia

This is a rare sequela of burn trauma. It can rarely occur if there is tissue loss of the lips and angle of the mouth region due to severe trauma like electrical burns. If the upper and lower lips are both everted, the scar stretches both vermilions and may rarely cause macrostomia if the angle region is not scarred.

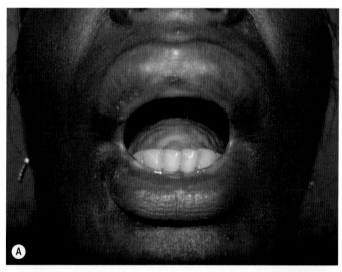

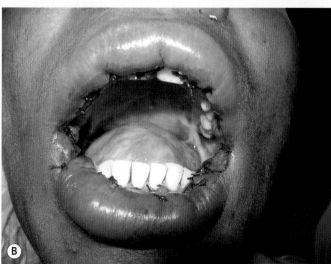

Fig. 20.26 **(A)** Microstomia due to accidentally drinking a chemical. **(B)** Full mouth opening after microstomia release with Z-plasty.

Perioral scar bands

These should be managed with Z-plasties, W-plasties, breaking the scar, and grafting or resurfacing with expanded skin.

Pseudomicrogenia

The contractile forces of the scar eliminate the normal concavity between the junctions of lip and chin pad leading to chin pad compression and "pseudomicrogenia".[23] This can be taken care of by excising the whole scar on the chin. Resurfacing can be with a full-thickness graft or expanded skin of the neck.

Splints

Splints are an important part of management of lips and perioral burns to avoid microstomia, and this may be occasionally neglected as there are no ready-made solutions for splints in this area. The therapist has to innovate to create splints.[170–173]

Neck

Many classifications of neck contractures have been proposed, aiming to describe the anatomy of the contracture, the function of the neck, and in planning the surgery.[174–176] Airway management is an important challenge for the anesthetist in severe neck contractures. If available, fiberoptic intubation is the safest method of intubation in these cases as it provides direct visualization of the glottis.[177] If not available, safe techniques include releasing the neck contracture under tumescent local anesthesia and intubating after release,[178] or one could also go ahead with the whole procedure under tumescent anesthesia and give regional blocks in the thigh for graft harvest.[179,180]

Airway problems

For linear contractures, release and resurfacing should be by single, multiple, or double opposing Z-plasties, or an X release. In very severe linear contractures the resultant flaps of the incisions may not come together after achieving full extension. These flaps should be sutured as far as they reach on full extension, and the remaining raw areas should be grafted. The advantage of this method of release is that the grafts are interspersed with the Z flaps, and hence chances of re-contracture are lower.

For bands, the release can be in the form of X release and skin grafting or excision of the scar and advancement of the lateral neck skin to cover the resultant raw area.

For broader contractures a full incisional or excisional release should be done. The release may be by a single incision with fishtailing of the incision or a bipedicle release can be done with two horizontal incisions made parallel in the upper and lower neck. Usually the resultant area is resurfaced with a medium to thick split-thickness graft from the thigh or a full-thickness graft. Postoperatively the neck needs to be splinted for at least a year if a re-contracture is to be avoided. It is for this reason that many surgeons advocate the use of flaps as it obviates the need for splintage. Flaps that have been used are neck advancement flaps, expanded neck flaps, supraclavicular flaps,[181–183] and free flaps like thin ALT or scapular and parascapular flaps.[184–187]

Technical pointers for a release of severe neck contracture

The position of the patient is supine with a substantial bolster support between the shoulder blades. This gives an adequate neck extension. Head support should also be given with rings as required still maintaining good extension. The arms are strapped by the side of the patient and not abducted. After the patient is under anesthesia, the whole scarred area is infiltrated with tumescent solution. After waiting 10 min an incision is made that is at the prominence of the contracture where the scar seems stretched across maximum. If the contracture is more towards the superior part of the neck, the incision made should be such that post-release the upper flap created should not slide up over the lower border of the mandible. At both the lateral ends, a Y cut is made to fishtail the incision. The depth of the incision should be such that all scar tissue should be released. Platysma should be cut. If an excisional release is being done, one should start excising the scar from either the clavicular end or the mandibular end and pick it up akin to how a full-thickness graft is raised. As the surgeon proceeds with the release, counter-traction on the supple bed by an assistant with a surgical mop makes separation of the scarred skin from the bed easier. The scar tissue itself can be held by the surgeon with a strong allis or Kocher's clamp to be able to give traction. Excisional release is easier and gives a superior aesthetic result, but it may not be a viable option in patients who have a large amount of scarring as the graft requirement is much more than an incisional release. To check that the release is complete, neck lateral movements should be checked. After full release the field can be covered with sponges soaked in saline epinephrine solution. One should wait for about ten minutes to wait for all minor bleeding spots to stop oozing. Any leftover oozing can be coagulated using bipolar cautery. Three sheets of medium-thickness grafts should be harvested from the thigh. Wide sheets of grafts can be harvested from the back of the thigh as well as the medial thigh. The grafts are placed in a horizontal manner. If possible the seam should lie in the submandibular region and the supraclavicular region. Once the grafts are sutured in place, a squirt of saline solution under the grafts helps to flush out any minor hematomas. Long silk sutures placed along the margins of the defect are used as tie-over sutures to keep the fluffy dressing in place. The sutures should be tied over in a horizontal direction. The neck is immobilized using a fabricated plaster of Paris splint molded over the dressing or using a rigid cervical collar. The dressing is done on the seventh postoperative day. Postoperatively, a neck/chin pressure garment should be worn with foam padding beneath to help maintain uniform pressure over the contours of the neck. A custom made Philadelphia collar helps to maintain the extension achieved by release over the next one year. Postoperative use of moisturizers and exercises are also essential to keep the grafts supple and to avoid a re-contracture.

Acid burns

An acid burn is a devastating injury seen more often due to intentional vitriolage rather than due to industrial accidents or accidents at home. A study by Das et al.[188] studies the epidemiology and management of acid burns in a burn unit in Bangladesh. The face is the most frequently targeted area in chemical assault, with the intention to maim and disfigure.[189] The physical effects of such chemical burns are devastating, with blindness due to corneal perforation,[190] nasal deformity, microstomia, and debilitating contractures amongst the complications documented.[191,192] Acid burns differ in appearance and behavior from thermal burns. Estimation of the percentage of burns is difficult as the chemical is sprayed or thrown over the body and is distributed spottily. The first aid should entail a detailed washing ritual with copious amounts of running water or saline for a prolonged period of about 45 minutes. This measure and early removal of the chemical-soaked clothes worn by the victim can limit the depth of burns. Application of topical antimicrobials that stain is not recommended as they make wound depth assessment difficult. It is recommended to cover the wound with occlusive dressings until they are taken up for excision. Superficial burns can be treated conservatively and be expected to resolve within two weeks. Excision for deep burns as early as feasible is the standard of care in acid burns. However, despite expediently doing the excision, it may still cause worse scarring than in thermal burns. Mortality from acid burns is low, but morbidity is severe. It can cause severe deformities and scarring of the face and body, which is a social stigma. Women who have been traumatized by acid throwing deserve deep empathy and greater efforts towards aesthetic restoration to improve their self image and confidence.

Future directions

Stem cells

In terms of use of stem cells in facial rejuvenation, the future is already here. The use of cultured epithelial autograft (CEA) for early coverage and speedy re-epithelization of burn wounds has been described earlier. When adult bone marrow derived MSCs were injected into fresh excised areas of deep burns that would have otherwise become anhidrotic, the sweat gland function was seen to recover in 2–12 months.[193]

Once treated and processed, the stromal vascular fraction (SVF) obtained from liposuction aspirates has shown promise to be used along with fat transfer to treat contour defects and to improve the quality of post-burn scars.[194]

3D printing

This is a newer innovation using state of the art technology in which scientists use a technique called scaffolding. Cells from the patient's tissues are layered onto three-dimensional models of the organ to be created and grown in vitro in an incubator. Tissue building information is fed into a computer using bioprinting technology to generate cells for organogenesis.[195] More studies are being now conducted to use human-derived cartilage cells instead of the bovine counterpart to reduce the chances of tissue immunorejection.[196]

Face transplantation

This is the final frontier in the reconstructive ladder where a partial or total replacement of the human face is attempted by transplant from a brain-dead donor. The world's first partial face transplant was carried out if France in 2005,[197] and full face transplant was achieved by Spain in 2010. Since then a number of face transplants have been reported by Turkey, France, United States, and Spain. Patients who could potentially benefit from the procedure include those who have devastating disfigurements due to trauma, burns, tumor, or congenital disorders. The concept was proposed by Professor Peter Butler of the Royal Free Hospital in 2002, who published an article to this effect in the Lancet.[198] This idea caused heated ethical debates at the time and continues to do so in the present day.

Patient selection is possibly the single most critical step influencing the long-term outcomes of face allotransplantation. Microvascular surgeons with the necessary training and transplant physicians with their four decades of experience of solid organ transplant-related immunosuppression are set to move the science forward. This has to be done taking ethical and psychosocial issues into thorough consideration.[199]

Conclusion

The human face is crafted to perfection with balance and harmony of features and symphony of movements. This established divine ideal encourages the plastic surgeon to be tireless and unrelenting in his pursuit for perfection in post-burn face reconstruction. Despite major advances in treatment and groundbreaking research, it is abundantly clear to the treating surgeon that the element of nature taking its course is strong in burn scars. This brings the focus back to preventive strategies as the single most important factor that can reduce morbidity in facial burns. Despite giant leaps in the field of research to develop newer dressing materials and skin substitutes, considerations of cost and global availability continue to keep us engaged to try and develop low-cost strategies for wound cover and tissue regeneration. No greater need and indication exists for reconstructive intervention than in the burn patient whose face is disfigured and scarred, who is deserted by his own, and who hides his scars in shame. At the same time the reconstructive surgeon should be ready to accept a certain surgical outcome as the endpoint of the patient's reconstructive journey beyond which further improvement is possible only by psychosocial empowerment. Vocational rehabilitation and burn survivor camps can provide this much-needed moral thrust to the patient's confidence and help them meet the challenges thrown at them by life with a brave face.

Bonus content for this chapter can be found online at http://www.expertconsult.com

Laser Doppler evaluation
Other skin substitutes
Versajet mode of action
Procedure of facial wound excision
Grafting post-excision
Acellular dermis
Xenograft
Matriderm and Integra
Cultured epithelial autograft
Ancillary measures
Factors affecting post-burn scarring
Classification of scalp defects
Options for individual areas
Canthal deformities
Symblepharon, entropion, blepharostenosis, and canalicular stenosis
Airway problems
Fig. 20.1 Woman with an acute facial burns less than 24 hours since burns.
Fig. 20.5 (A) 7-year-old child with facial burns due to firecrackers. Collagen sheets have been applied. **(C)** Showing healing by day 7 with complete separation of collagen sheet.
Fig. 20.6 (A,B) Thermoplastic splints for microstomia.
Fig. 20.7 (A) Old unattended facial burns with raw areas and contractures. **(B)** Neglected burn presented to us about two weeks after burn, anterior view. **(C)** Lateral view. **(D)** 6 months after grafting showing deformity of the left side of face. **(E)** Lateral view.
Fig. 20.9 Eight months after release and split skin graft. **(A)** Anterior view. **(B)** Left oblique view. **(C)** Right oblique view.
Fig. 20.10 (A–C) Eight years after neck release, patient presented for an improved look.
Fig. 20.11 (A–C) One month after full-thickness graft.
Fig. 20.12 (A–C) Eight months after full-thickness graft.
Fig. 20.13 (A–C) One and a half years after full-thickness graft.
Fig. 20.15 (A) Minor deformity and scarring of the lower lip and chin complex. **(B)** Pleasing appearance after resurfacing with full-thickness graft and repositioning of the lip.
Fig. 20.16 (A) Scar over the left forehead and eyebrow. **(B)** Resurfaced with expanded skin.
Fig. 20.18 (A) Alopecia of left temporal and parietal region. **(B)** With expander in situ. The nose has been reconstructed with radial artery forearm flap. **(C)** Post-resurfacing.
Fig. 20.19 (A) Full-thickness electric injury with eschar on scalp. He had a subdural hematoma that was evacuated by craniotomy at another hospital, and 10 days later the patient was sent to us for the dead necrotic skin and management of burns. **(C)** The craniotomy bone was picked up, and the slough over the dura was debrided. Seen here is the exposed dura after debridement of dead tissue.
Fig. 20.20 (A) Upper third ear deformity. **(B)** Reconstruction with postauricular skin and costal cartilage graft.
Fig. 20.24 (C) Expander in forehead.

Access the complete reference list online at http://www.expertconsult.com

1. Dziewulski P. Acute management of facial burns. In: Jeschke MG, ed. *Handbook of Burns, Acute Burn Care.* New York: Springer; 2012:1:291–302. *This chapter serves as a good reference chapter for acute management of facial burns.*

7. Monstrey S, Hoeksema H, Verbelen J, et al. Assessment of burn depth and burn wound healing potential. *Burns.* 2008;34:761–769.

8. Leon-Villapalos J, Jeschke MG, Herndon DN. Topical management of facial burns. *Burns.* 2008;34:903–911.

23. Engrave LH. Acute care and reconstruction of facial burns. In: Mathes SJ, ed. *Plastic Surgery.* Philadelphia: Saunders Elsevier;

2006:45–76. *This chapter provides technical steps in intricate details on early surgical management for deep burns of the face.*

38. Gonzalez-Ulloa M. Restoration of the face covering by means of selected skin in regional aesthetic units. *Br J Plast Surg.* 1956;9:212–221.

82. Feldman JJ. Facial burns. In: McCarthy JG, ed. *Plastic Surgery.* Philadelphia: WB Saunders; 1990:3:2153–2236. *This chapter continues to be one of my favorites from the point of view of post-burn facial deformity management.*

141. Dougherty WSRJ. Reconstruction of burned face/cheek acute and delayed. In: Achauer B, Sood R, eds. *Achauer and Sood's Burn*

Surgery: Reconstruction & Rehabilitation. Philadelphia: W.B. Saunders; 2006:240–253. *Not just this chapter but the entire text is a very good reference book for post-burn reconstruction of every body part.*

144. Pallua N, von Heimburg D. Pre-expanded ultra-thin supraclavicular flaps for (full-) face reconstruction with reduced donor-site morbidity and without the need for microsurgery. *Plast Reconstr Surg.* 2005;115:1837–1844, discussion 1845–1847.

179. Pawan A. Safe method for release of severe post burn neck contracture under tumescent local anaesthesia and ketamine. *Indian J Plast Surg.* 2004;37:51–54. *This article describes in detail management of patients of neck contracture in situations where anesthesia services are unavailable or inadequate*

198. Hettiaratchy S, Butler PE. Face transplantation–fantasy or the future? *Lancet.* 2002;360:5–6.

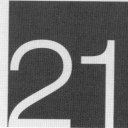

Burn reconstruction

Nelson Sarto Piccolo, Mônica Sarto Piccolo, and Maria Thereza Sarto Piccolo

SYNOPSIS

- Major evolution in burn patient care in the last three decades has allowed several positive changes in the treatment objectives.
- Currently, the main objective of treatment of the burn patient is to recover his/her quality of life and the patient's social re-insertion.
- It is best if the patient is treated in a facility with a dedicated multidisciplinary team, acutely and during the reconstruction phase.
- Reconstructive surgery planning starts during the acute phase or as soon as the surgeon sees a patient in need.
- Timely reconstructive surgery will guarantee the best results – planning is based on need, scar maturation, and available surgical techniques.
- The patient should be treated as a whole – we do not treat wounds or scars, we treat a person with wounds or scars.

 Access the Historical Perspective section online at
http://www.expertconsult.com

Introduction

The major evolution that has occurred in burn patient care over the past several decades has allowed several highly positive progressive changes in the treatment of these patients. The main objective of treatment of the burned patient is acutely life saving and then, secondarily, to recover the patient's quality of life.

Reconstruction, and its planning, must start when the plastic surgeon has the initial contact with the burn victim. Well-planned surgical care during the acute phase will ensure a post-healing phase with fewer sequelae and complications. This care must be accompanied by several other clinical measures and by other professionals in the multidisciplinary burn team, such as physiotherapists, occupational therapists, dietitians, and psychologists, amongst others.

Frequent evaluations (and the ensuing therapeutic measures), treating the patient as a whole, and appropriate timing for surgical intervention are paramount to the success of treatment.

After healing, reconstructive surgical procedures will be promptly indicated when functional loss or compromise are encountered. If no dysfunction occurs, the authors favor waiting for scar maturation prior to surgical intervention. Procedures will range from skin grafting, local, distal or free flaps, resurfacing with dermal regeneration templates, to advancement of expanded tissue. We can also use fat grafting and adipose-derived stem cells as a most effective ancillary treatment for burn sequelae.

As these patients are usually submitted to a series or sequence of procedures, and as the scar and the patient evolve, there may be a need (or a request) for different/additional procedures, and this very common occurrence must be well-explained to the patient or their parents in advance. This is necessary so that the patient and the patient's family can have realistic expectations of results and can also participate in the treatment with a more informed attitude.

Increase in survival rates

Serious burn injuries will bring several risks for the patient, who will need specialized and dedicated care in the acute phase, during resuscitation, with intensive care life-maintaining measures, pain management, frequent dressing changes, early mobilization, surgery, and grafting.

The acute phase admission is usually followed by very long periods of a highly complex rehabilitation phase with the possibility of several immediate consequences such as hypertrophic scarring, retractions, sensorial alterations, limited physical abilities, anxiety, depression, body image dissatisfaction, and other difficulties that may hinder the patient's return to previous activities.[1]

After the major world conflicts of the first half of the twentieth century – the two great wars – there was a growing interest in the pathophysiology of burn injuries and their course. This promoted a great advancement in the clinical and surgical treatment of the burn patient with a consequential increase in burn patient survival. This increase in survival rate brought a need for a more profound understanding of the complex wound-healing process, since it became obvious to all involved that treatment went well beyond life maintenance measures.[2,3]

Efforts to obtain complete functional recovery of the burn victim have evolved into several different objectives, with quality of life and social reintegration as significant objectives. During the past two decades, subjective patient evaluation via patient-reported outcome measures has become a priority and a guide, affecting treatment measures and evaluation and occasionally leading to modifications of treatment protocols.[4-7]

The goal of treatment of a person with burn lesions is that the multidisciplinary burn team make every possible effort to bring this person back to his/her original "world" and way of life previous to the accident. This is the reason why it is of paramount importance that the patient be treated in a dedicated burn center by a dedicated burn team – we do not treat burn wounds or burn sequellae, we treat people with burn wounds and/or with burn sequellae.

The plastic surgeon treating these people should preferably be a member of a multidisciplinary burn team which works with this objective.

Patient emotional status/evolution

It is believed that during the first year after the trauma, approximately 13–23% of burn victims will present some degree of depression – this percentage is significantly higher than the general population incidence (which, surprisingly, is up to 8.6% in some studies).[8]

Those patients with previously underlying psychological instabilities will need more time as well as more intense/prolonged psychological and surgical treatments in dedicated burn services with a specialized burn team. Multicenter studies aiming to improve results for this overall patient population have also become a priority with the concomitant development and evolution of treatment protocols.[9]

Body image changes

Dissatisfaction with one's self image, such as changes in overall appearance and function, will frequently lead the patient to seek reconstructive surgical treatment. Surgical planning must be shared with all members of the burn team who will be, or are, involved in the patient's treatment. The main objective of treatment, during the acute or reconstructive phase, is that patients return to their usual life, within their community, as soon as possible.[10,11]

Evaluating quality of life

Quality-of-life evaluation, after such a trauma, is a multidimensional concept that requires instruments that are able to capture local physical impairment and health changes in general and that could be re-applied in the same person over a long period of time. These instruments are generally referred to as "questionnaires". It is of utmost importance for the success of each and every reconstruction effort that the plastic surgeon involved in the process understands how these evaluations and patient-reported outcome measures are derived as well as appreciates the vertical nature of these measures during follow-up visits.[12]

Evaluation questionnaires can be divided into generic and specific. The health-related generic instrument that is most used in the world is the *Medical Outcomes Study 36-item Short-Form Health Survey (SF-36)*. This is a multidimensional questionnaire composed of 36 items and 8 domains. Specific instruments will be more advantageous than the generic since they survey more relevant items, for the patient and for the professional team.[13,14]

The *Burn Specific Health Scale (BSHS)* is an example of a multidimensional specific instrument that approaches several aspects of the treatment and rehabilitation results within 114 items. It is the most utilized questionnaire in the world for these purposes. It comprehends three modalities – the *Burn Specific Health Scale – Abbreviated* (BSHS-A) with 80 items, validated by Munster and co-workers; the *Burn Specific Health Scale – Revised* (BSHS-R), translated to the Portuguese language and validated by Ferreira and co-workers, with 31 items and 6 domains, and the *Burn Specific Health Scale – Brief* (BSHS-B) created by Kidal and co-workers, which is self-applied with 40 items and 9 domains.

This last one, the BSHS-B, evaluates hand function and sexuality, which are no less important domains in the evaluation of the quality of life of these patients. This modality was recently translated to the Portuguese language after been validated and published. Others, such as the *BurnSexQ-EPM/UNIFESP*, has also been translated into Portuguese and evaluates psychological aspects of sexuality.[15-23]

Quality-of-life evaluation and treatment phases

During the acute phase, the patient will be evaluated through the SF-36, which will demonstrate the patient's quality of life before the accident, showing how the patient lived his day-to-day activities before suffering a burn injury.

Upon discharge, a more specific instrument becomes necessary, and the patient will be evaluated with the BSHS-Brief then and at 3, 6, and 12 months. In a patient seeking reconstruction, this routine is repeated every 6 months, which will then also evaluate the results of the surgical reconstructive procedure.

The BSHS-Brief questionnaire is equally beneficial when applied in patients who have been treated by us since the accident as well as in those whom we meet after healing, translating very important information that will aid in treatment tailoring at that patient-specific moment. Changes can then be identified in several domains, as for example, those resulting from body image changes, which in turn will immediately influence how the patient socializes or even relates intimately to his or her partner from the sexuality standpoint. This knowledge can help to elevate the final outcomes of acute care and reconstructive stages of care.

Acute phase

A patient with acute burns that could eventually lead to aesthetic and/or functional sequelae needs specialized treatment protocols in a burn unit, and these should be instituted as soon as possible after the accident.

Important treatment measures are pharmacologic control of the hypermetabolic response, early excision of deep areas, immediate wound closure/resurfacing, early occupational and physiotherapy, aggressive nutritional support, and the immediate use of pressure as healing occurs.[52] Adequate wound care during the acute phase will determine initial treatment success, which will greatly aid in future surgical reconstruction planning.[53–56]

Burn wound excision

The excision of the burn wound has become the most important surgical procedure in the treatment of an acute burn patient with deep wounds, greatly decreasing the risk of infection. Initially proposed by the Yugoslavian plastic surgeon Zora Jazenkovic in the early 1950s, sharp tangential excision consists of sequential removal of necrotic tissue in relation to the wound surface.[57,58] These damaged tissue layers are sequentially removed until one obtains uniform and diffuse bleeding, indicating local tissue viability.

This procedure has a very short learning curve, and the experienced surgeon will notice tissue viability by its appearance, thus experienced surgeons currently utilize tourniquets and/or injection of vasoconstricting agents to minimize blood loss. Although immediate coverage or resurfacing of the excised wound would be the ideal measure, this is not always possible, since commonly the patient has insufficient donor areas, so alternatives are usually sought. In some parts of the world, this is even harder to accomplish due the lack of availability of skin substitutes.[59–62]

Split-thickness autografts that are harvested from non-burnt areas are the first option of choice. Burn wound excision is typically performed in sequential steps, usually within 2- to 3-day intervals during the first week to 10 days of treatment. Open burn wounds ideally should be covered with some sort of biologic coverage or efficient topical agent and then grafted in the next visit to the operating theater, during the ensuing excision step in other areas of the wound (Fig. 21.1).

The first choice for local coverage when the patient does not have enough donor areas would be cadaver skin. Xenograft (pig or frog skin) or other biologic alternative can also be used, although currently it has become common to resurface the wound with synthetic dermal regeneration templates, which "close" the wound, until the silicone layer is removed or sloughs off, depending on the matrix being used. This may take up to 3–4 weeks, allowing time for other areas to heal and potentially become donor areas to yield thin split-thickness skin grafts to complete the final epithelial coverage. Other alternatives such as epidermal cell culture and even more sophisticated composed tissue are also current, less frequently used, alternatives.[63–70] In summary, the burn wound should be excised within 1 week of the accident and must be closed or covered with the (local) best available tissue.

Anterior thorax excision

In some areas such as the breast, for example, there is a need for specific surgical care when performing the excision. In children, especially in females, the surgeon must identify and protect the breast bud and the nipple–areola complex (NAC) should not be removed, regardless of its appearance or wound depth. Similarly, in older patients, there should be practically

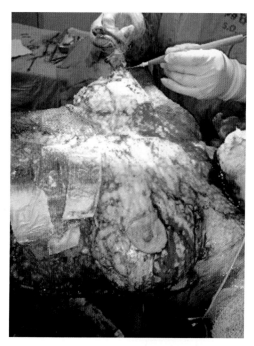

Fig. 21.1 Patient 2 days after excision and grafting on thighs and right abdomen, being excised on breasts – please note that although the burnt skin was excised completely from the breast, the nipple–areola complex was not, regardless of the burn depth.

no, if any, excision of breast tissue and never excise the NAC, even if there is doubt about its viability. When grafting, one must place the graft sheets following the tension lines of the skin, grafting each breast separately and avoiding "crossing" the midline with the same graft sheet that was placed on the breast, as these graft sheets must contour the breast according to its shape and volume (Figs. 21.1 & 21.2).[71,72]

It is of utmost importance that the surgeon treating a patient with acute burns understands and respects the skin tension lines, applying the graft sheets transversely and perpendicular to the longitudinal axis of the extremity or trunk, as well as in the neck, as hypertrophic scarring can be likely in these patients if the graft sheets are placed longitudinally.

Aftercare

Changes in the scar or its appearance at the first visit will define the treatment options and subsequent surgical interventions.[73–76] Pressure garments and devices are recommended to most patients upon discharge. It has been our experience that approximately 12% of patients wear these garments for more than a year.

At 1 year post-healing, around 2.5–3.0% of patients will wish to be submitted to reconstructive surgical procedures. A current option for early treatment of hypertrophic scarring is with sublesional fat grafting, with the aim of introducing the benefits of adipose-derived stem cells and the factors contained within the injected fat.[77–84]

Clinical treatment

Alternatives most frequently recommended range from pressure garments and inserts to laser therapy, aimed at decreasing hypertrophic scarring and its associated symptoms.

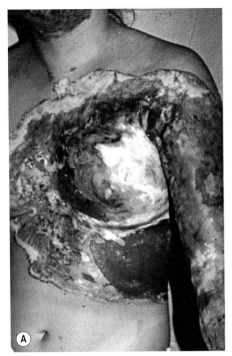

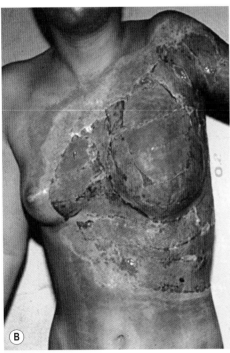

Fig. 21.2 Acute appearance of a patient with third degree burn to the anterior lateral chest **(A)** and after excision and grafting **(B)**. One can easily note that the graft sheets were placed following the local tension lines, resulting in multiple directions of graft placement but following each individual area's anatomic volume, shape and disposition.

Pressure garments

Continuous pressure usually yields improvement of the hypertrophic scar in color, texture, symptoms of pruritus, and thickness in up to 65–85% of the scars. It possibly induces a relative tissue ischemia; increases collagenase activity associated to MMP9 metalloprotease action, which favors regeneration without scarring; and also decreases local metabolism.

Another theory is that local hypoxia would decrease fibroblast cohesiveness and the total amount of chondroitin-4-sulphate, which coats collagen fibers and hinders collagenase activity. Pressure therapy is considered the gold standard for the clinical treatment of burn scars in most services around the world.[85–106]

Silicone

Silicone is a dimethylsiloxane polymer gel applied over the scar as a compressed or self-adherent sheet. The mechanism of action on these scars is probably due to occlusion generating an increase in local temperature and keratinocyte hydration, modifying local inflammatory mediators and collagen production as well as collagenase activity, improving scar thickness, pain, itching, and appearance. It should be in contact with the scar at least 12 hours per day, for 4–6 months. We recommend starting its use 2 weeks after wound healing, and that it be shaped along the scar to avoid depigmentation and irritation of the normal surrounding skin.[107–121]

Steroids

Intralesional steroid injection inhibits fibroblast proliferation, decreases local inflammatory process, inhibits TGF and (TGF-β and IGF), decreases collagen and glycosaminoglycan deposits, and increases collagenase activity. Triamcinolone is generally used at up to 0.4 mg/kg injected at 3- to 6-week intervals within the scar, avoiding sublesional injections. Side effects can be hypopigmentation, telangiectasia, local necrosis and ulceration, and local atrophy, which may last several months or, more rarely, be permanent.[122–133]

Retinoids

Retinoids modulate scar fibroblast proliferation and collagen production and organization, improving scar quality and appearance. They induce apoptosis and immunoregulation through inhibition of collagen type I gene TGF-β1-induced expression, besides favoring epithelial growth. Concentrations ranging from 0.025% to 0.1% are used to obtain hypertrophy decrease in 50–100% of cases. Its use can yield a significantly improved result when associated with glycolic acid, pressure garments, and silicone gel. Side effects include photosensitivity, contact dermatitis, and skin atrophy.[134–140]

Laser

Pulsed dye laser (PDL) with a 585-nm wavelength has an affinity for oxyhemoglobin (absorption peak at 542 nm), leading to selective photothermolysis of cicatricial microcirculation, thus leading to thrombosis and ischemia, reducing intracicatrical collagen. It may also hinder fibroblast proliferation and type III collagen deposition through protein kinases and apoptosis increase, TGF-β1 level decrease associated with increased metalloprotease 13 (collagenase 3) activity, mastocyte content release (which affects collagen metabolism), and through local heating breaks the bisulfate bridges favoring collagen realignment. It also reduces erythema, itching, and has been shown to improve scar thickness and texture. Resulting treatment edema usually resolves in 48 hours, and side effects may include local purpura, which may last several days/weeks, and pigment changes, more frequent in dark-skinned patients. Hyperpigmentation must be treated before the next treatment section since its energy may be absorbed by melanin. Fractional photothermolysis (Fraxel, 1550 nm) can also be used.[141–155]

Surgical reconstruction

Adequate timing of surgical reconstructive procedures will vary according to each patient. Immature scars require control before their eventual surgical resection unless they are hindering the patient's vital functions. The natural scar evolution as well as the results of clinical scar manipulation measures will dictate the treatment planning in those patients without dysfunction. Surgical reconstructive procedures performed through correct planning and appropriate timing will yield better results.[156–160]

However, it is rather common for the patient or the patient's family to wish for immediate reconstruction and scar removal. The plastic surgeon has a key role deciding which procedures should/could be performed immediately after early healing, as well as in the future planning of sequential surgical procedures.

In the literature, we frequently see discussions about the "reconstructive ladder", or a list of surgical procedures with progressive complexity and operative difficulty, aimed at obtaining the best results with the fewest number of surgical interventions possible. Obviously, this logical tiered choice can be applied to any case at hand.

In the treatment of scar contracture, we will use the simplest technique that will yield the desired result. As these deformities are very frequently associated with lack of local tissue, this can occasionally be solved with geometric flaps (Z-plasty, rotation or advancement flaps) or attempts at replacing local tissue with remote unburned tissue, such as skin grafting or free flaps. In these cases, there is always the possibility of resection of the involved area and resurfacing of the wound with dermal regeneration templates. In those cases where there is no scar contracture, our technique of choice is the use of tissue expanders, always aiming for a complete as possible removal of the scar.[161–173]

Currently, we restrict the use of free flaps for very specific cases for a number of reasons: technical execution requirements, frequently flaps take on the appearance of a "pin cushion", flap (fasciocutaneous or muscle) volume can change as the patient's weight changes, and future implications for flap viability when another surgeon takes over care and potentially revises the flap without the knowledge of the primary set of vascular anastomoses. Currently, our indication for free flap transfer will be in a patient who has suffered a high-tension injury with exposure of distal forearm, hand, or foot structures. Alternatively, we will use fat grafting and deposition and/or dermal regeneration templates.[174,175]

Surgical planning must be individualized for each case and adhere to indications and the patient's wishes. The reconstructive treatment of a burn patient with sequelae is usually very long, intra-dependent of previous individual procedures as well as, very frequently, subject to changes or evolution of the patient's desires. As surgeons, we must be very realistic when considering what we can technically offer, also accepting our occasional personal limitations before each presenting patient – we should always obey medicine's fundamental principle: "primum non nocere" or "first, do no harm".[176–178]

In patients with contractures across joints, we recommend the surgical resection of the scar, as wide as necessary to reach healthy tissue, and then resurfacing the area with the best available substitute for that area. Currently, we greatly favor the use of dermal regeneration matrix, followed by autografts obtained from the scalp, at 8–10 thousandths of an inch.[179,180]

Functional restrictions

Contractures can lead to severe functional restrictions, and we believe that these must be approached in a descending order of importance (according to the difficulties they produce). Therefore we must treat those functional contractures that cause greater difficulty/deformity first. Usually, we prioritize neck contractures, warranting respiratory comfort for the patient, but mainly achieving a supple neck during endotracheal intubation for future procedures. We then approach periocular and perioral defects, hands, genitals, axillae, elbows, and feet as the following set of priorities (Fig. 21.3).[181–185]

Skin grafting

We limit the indication of full-thickness skin grafts to the occasional facial reconstruction in eyelid(s), periorbital, or perioral deformities. We prefer postauricular skin, where possible. If there is not enough skin behind the ear or the ear is absent, we will substitute this choice for supraclavicular skin. These donor areas offer better color match, and a higher proportion of collagen in these full-thickness grafts favors more permanent and efficient results. Other uses of full-thickness skin are extremely rare in our service.

We favor the use of split-thickness skin grafts, almost always obtained from the scalp with an electrical dermatome at the average thickness of ten-thousandths of an inch. For this, the hair is shaved from almost the entire scalp area, leaving a "rim" of 2 to 4 cm with intact hair. In both genders, this "rim" will serve dual purposes: first, it will prevent the surgeon inadvertently going into forehead or neck area while harvesting the skin, leading to an undesired donor area scar in these sites, and, in females, this residual hair is usually be enough for the patient to cover the then short-haired donor area, disguising this temporary aesthetic shortcoming with a ponytail. Other advantages of the scalp as a donor area is that the scalp skin is much thicker than other areas, with a higher proportion of epidermal appendages embedded on the thicker dermis, favoring a more prompt (re-)epithelialization. This donor site area has practically no incidence of hypertrophic scar, and it is naturally protected against the sun, rarely presenting with a resulting discoloration.

Another advantage of utmost importance of this area is the fact that for facial or neck resurfacing, this skin will retain the donor area color that is identical to the entire cephalic segment.

This donor area is treated with an efficient topical agent on a closed dressing, which is changed every 2 days until healing, which usually occurs within 6 to 10 days. Due to this rather rapid healing, we frequently use this donor area repeatedly in the treatment of acute burns (Fig. 21.4).[186]

Tourniquet use

Operative tourniquets are frequently used to keep the extremity as exsanguinated as possible in order to minimize blood

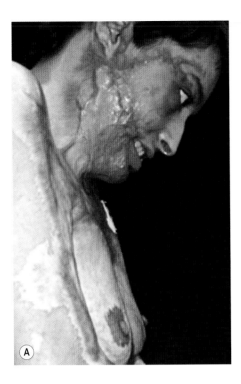

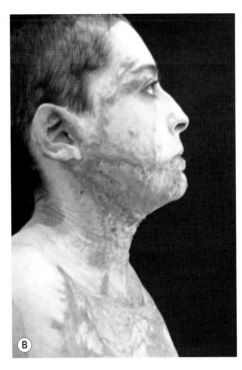

Fig. 21.3 **(A)** Typical example of neck release with local retraction segment resection and resurfacing with dermal regeneration matrix, followed by split-thickness autograft from the scalp, 3 weeks after the original procedure (complete eventual color match). **(B)** Results at 12 weeks.

loss. This is used in procedures on the hand, forearm, distal lower extremity, and foot, usually aimed at lesser blood loss and at a "dry" operative field, in which local, critical structures are better identified.

We would like to call the reader's attention to the fact that we do not recommend the usual "emptying" of the extremity with the use of an Esmarch bandage, which is commonly practiced around the world. Not using the Esmarch bandage, and consequently not emptying the superficial venous system, is extremely advantageous for the reconstructive burn surgeon and, consequently, for the patient.

When we do not empty the venous system and we inflate the tourniquet, venous blood will be trapped within the non-circulating vein. Doing so, as the incision is performed on

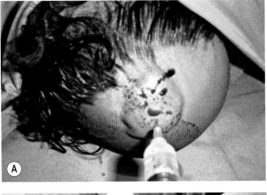

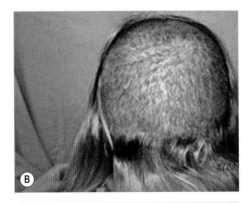

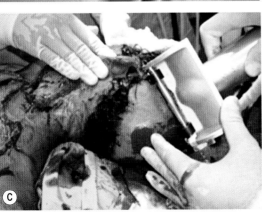

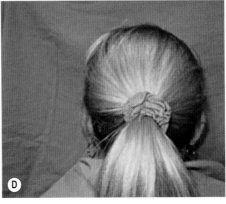

Fig. 21.4 **(A–D)** Split skin harvesting sequence at the scalp – the area is pre-injected with saline at a subgaleal level temporarily transforming the scalp on a more supple surface, which will allow for a smoother dermatome gliding. (The injected liquid is resorbed in some hours, and its temporary volume causes no distress to the patient.)

the usually extremely thick scar, the young as well as the experienced surgeon will be able to do so with greater safety, as explained below.

Very frequently, burn scar tissue, due to its fibrous consistency, usually with visible bundles along the retraction vectors, may be mistakenly confused by the novice (or by the still insecure surgeon) with tendon tissue, mostly on the hand and foot, where tendons are relatively smaller in relation to the proximal aspect, and then lead to a partial or economic removal/incision of these scar tissues. So, when the tourniquet is inflated directly, without exsanguination, these will be very easily identified by their deep blue color, and in the "incisional" sequence from the external world to deeper structures on the extremities, there will be a scar of variable thickness and appearance, and immediately under, the veins are the most superficial structure, external to tendons, nerves, and other noble, complex, structures. So, the surgeon can continuously cut the scar, even if some retraction bands look like tendinous structures, until he sees fat and veins filled with blue, desaturated blood, when he/she will stop with the certainty that nothing noble was incised, except for the full-thickness of the deleterious scar (Fig. 21.5).[187]

Z-plasties

These geometric flaps are very frequently used and, when properly indicated, will bring immediate aesthetic and functional improvement.

The surgeon should always remember that cicatricial bands are usually a consequence of abnormal collagen deposition along a retraction/tension line, and in the same anatomic unit there may be more than one dominating band or dominating and secondary bands. When treating the main retraction band with one or more Z-plasties, the surgeon may be surprised by the immediate appearance of one or more parallel retraction bands. Most unfortunately, very often, these second or third bands cannot be treated similarly on the same intervention,

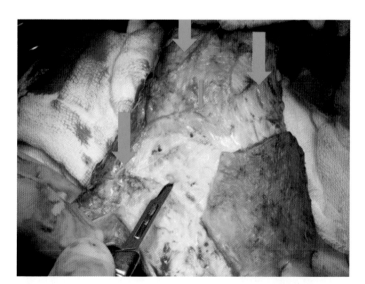

Fig. 21.5 Intraoperative picture of a dorsal hand procedure, without the previous use of the Esmarch bandage. Please note the easily identified superficial "filled veins", consequently bringing comfort to the surgeon in relation to the certainty of being in subcutaneous level (beyond the entire thickness of the scar) but not into noble tissue level. If, on the contrary, these veins had been emptied by an Esmarch bandage, they would be transparent and would not "alert" the surgeon.

since, due to its proximity to the original band, a new flap incision could hinder blood supply to the previously created flaps of the "original" Z-plasty.[188–190]

Dermal regeneration matrix

These matrices allow host cell invasion and collagen substitution for host cell secreted collagen. The first matrix to be used in burn care was created by a team of researchers lead by Burke and Yannas in 1981. There are today a vast array of products on the medical market with similar indications and behavior.

When this tissue is applied to a live bed, this structure will be integrated by the host usually within 21 days, when the top layer is removed and the "new" dermis is autografted with scalp split skin.

The objective of its use in the acute burn patient is the coverage of the excised wound or excised scar, "saving" host donor areas. It will also cover tendons and nerves without hindering their functions. There may be a need for re-intervention since in some patients the treated area may still retract up to 60–70% (Fig. 21.6).[191–197]

Adipose-derived stem cells

Fat grafting has been used worldwide, taking advantage of the benefits of adipose-derived stem cells (ADSCs) for regenerative purposes and their ability to differentiate into fat, bone cartilage, muscle, and possibly other tissues. They also have a great variety of regenerative and metabolic properties, as well as growth factors (EGF, TGF-β, HGF, PDGF, BFGF, etc). Fat on the lipoaspirate can be isolated and/or treated by physical or chemical methods, in the operating room or later in a laboratory set-up.

When treating burn scars, the objective is to decrease the amount of hypertrophy (fibrosis), diminishing the scar thickness and increasing scar malleability. We also use this technique with the aim of decreasing fibrosis around bone joints and releasing tendon adhesions.[198–218]

Surgical approach

We harvest and prepare fat according to Coleman's technique. Fat is injected under the scar and its periphery. Injections are repeated at 2- to 3-month intervals until complete hypertrophy control or another definitive procedure, such as scar removal, is performed.

Operative technique[219–221]

Fat is obtained from the patient via liposuction of the abdomen, thigh, knee, buttock, or other area. In adults or patients over 25 kg, suction is performed with a 10-cc syringe connected to a 3-mm cannula with two 3-mm side openings distally. In children, we prefer a 20-cc syringe and multiple microperforated cannulae, which will yield a relatively higher negative pressure and a more efficient fat harvesting.

Fat is then centrifuged at 3.000 rpm for 3 minutes. The upper oily phase and the lower, aqueous phase are discarded. The central layer contains concentrated fat, growth and vasodilating factors, and the stromal vascular fraction (SVF) and is then transferred into 1-cc "insulin" syringes.

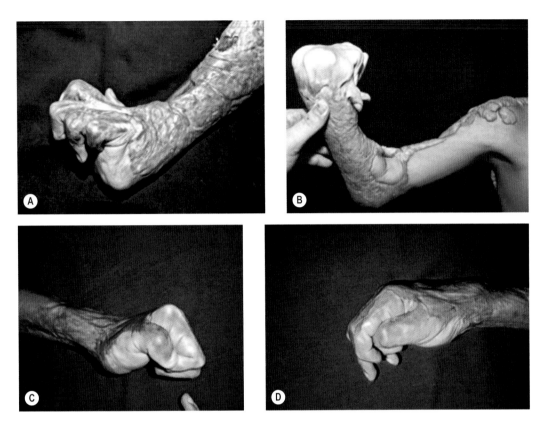

Fig. 21.6 Preoperative aspects **(A,B)** and permanent functional result (at 2 years) after scar excision, substitution for dermal regeneration matrix and subsequent scalp skin autografting **(C,D)** – the patient is able to write and work with his hands.

As many 16-gauge needle punctures as needed are made through the skin on the periphery of the scar, and fat is progressively and uniformly injected under and in the immediate periphery of the scar, using a 1.8 mm diameter cannula in a retrograde fashion, using 20–30 passes/mL (Fig. 21.7).[222,223]

We frequently perform partial intralesional resections (without reaching the subcutaneous tissue or normal skin on the periphery) and subsequent fat injection, including under the recently resected and sutured area. Marked improvement can be seen with this technique when injected along and under scar contracture after surgical release (Figs. 21.8–21.10).

Periarticular fibrosis

Fat injection can also be used in fracture lines of long bones such as the tibia, fibula, ulna, radius, metacarpi, metatarsi, and others, speeding healing as well as diminishing periarticular fibrosis consequent to trauma to these structures (Figs. 21.11 & 21.12)

Tissue expansion[224–232]

Main advantages with this technique are the gain of neighboring normal tissue, the reactive capsule, which warrants flap irrigation, and aesthetic and functional results. Complications are well known and can be decreased dramatically with precise technique. Several expanders may be needed, and the temporary growth deformity may be an issue. Also, some patients may wish to have additional, different procedures as the scar is sequentially removed (Fig. 21.13).

Preoperative measures and surgical planning

There is a need for emotional and physical preparation of the patient, tailoring planning to each individual case, as tolerated.

The surgeon must plan enough undermining to accommodate the empty, flattened expander. Frequently, when

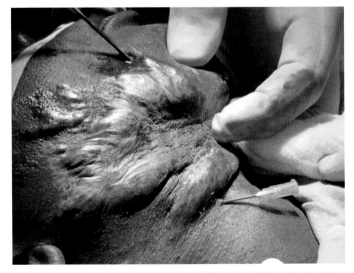

Fig. 21.7 Skin puncturing with a 16-gauge needle and cannula introduction. Where the scar is thicker, the surgeon can use the other hand to stabilize it, performing multiple "passes" in a more secure way.

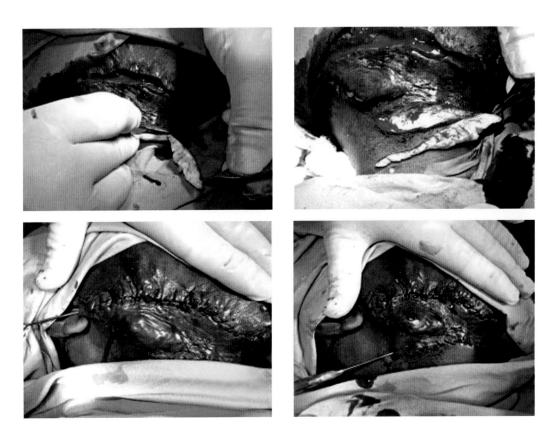

Fig. 21.8 Demonstration of intralesional resection and fat injection under the suture line.

ordering an implant from a catalog, one reads only length and width, forgetting that height will be "added" to width when the implant is flattened (even if one folds the implant sides over itself, upon the first injection, it may open flat and impinge against the sides) (Fig. 21.14).

When using more than one implant, we always use partially overlapping tissue expanders.

Pre-conditioning of the area

In those patients for whom there is a need for expander placement in tight areas (such as dorsum of the hand, wrist, distal forearm, elbow, posterior knee, distal leg, foot dorsum, or plantar area), we believe there is a need for preparation of these areas before surgery.

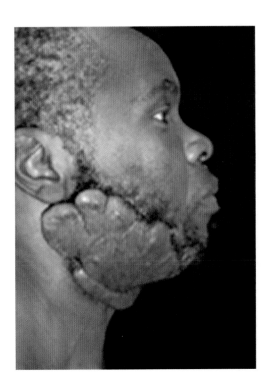
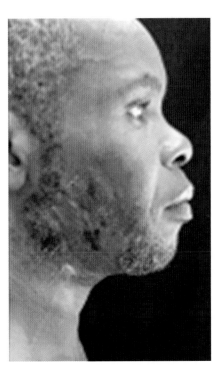

Fig. 21.9 Same patient as previous picture, demonstrating the result after partial resections and fat injections as shown above (5 sessions in 2 years).

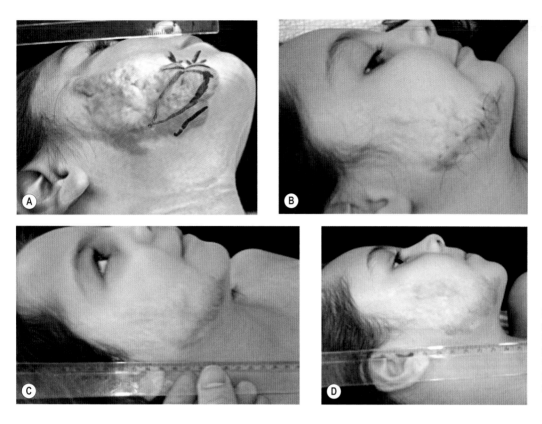

Fig. 21.10 (A) Preoperative appearance, outlining area to be resected intralesionally. **(B)** Two weeks after fat injection and partial scar resection. **(C)** 14 weeks and **(D)** 9 months after three injections. Please note the suture line scar is practically invisible even at long-term results.

We have created a routine protocol for these cases, aimed at preparing the future expander site to receive and tolerate the pressure of the deflated expander volume at the initial placement operation and immediately postoperative.

In these areas, we inject normal saline with a 25-gauge "butterfly" needle, thus creating a progressive hydro-dissection of these areas approximating the pressure from an inflated expander. These injections are performed at 2-day intervals until half of the nominal volume is injected or the entire area is undermined by the fluid injection, without local blanching. One can also "push" the injected fluid to obtain further undermining. If blanching occurs for more than

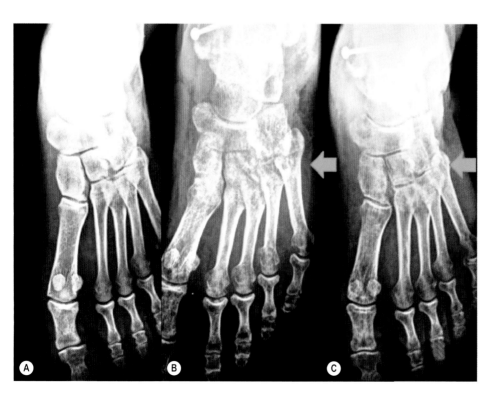

Fig. 21.11 (A–C) Foot X-rays taken during healing time of a dorsal left foot friction/crush wound. Note the "blurring" of articular spaces on the tarsal joints on the left foot (B); note the evolution with the "blurring" practically disappearing on and around the joint spaces, 8 months post-cure (C), after 3 fat injections under the cutaneous scar and around the articular structures. Normal right foot X-ray shown for comparison (A).

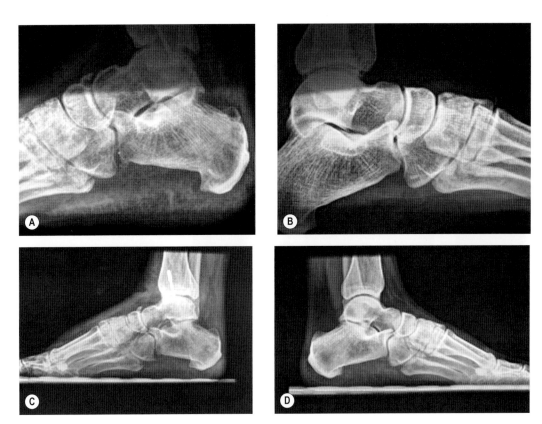

Fig. 21.12 Same patient, demonstrating a very elevated left foot longitudinal arch (**A**), when compared with the right foot (**B**); and with a practically normal aspect, similar to the right side, 8 months post-cure and 3 fat injections (**C,D**).

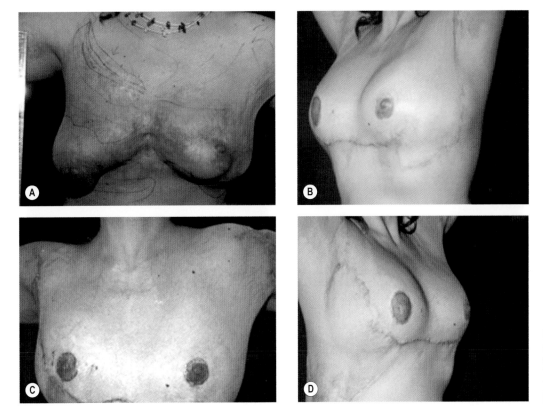

Fig. 21.13 Typical example of evolution of patient's ambition. Results after 3 expansions (**A,C**). Patient "unhappy" with the result, with "insufficient" breast projection requiring breast implants (315 mL) (**B,D**).

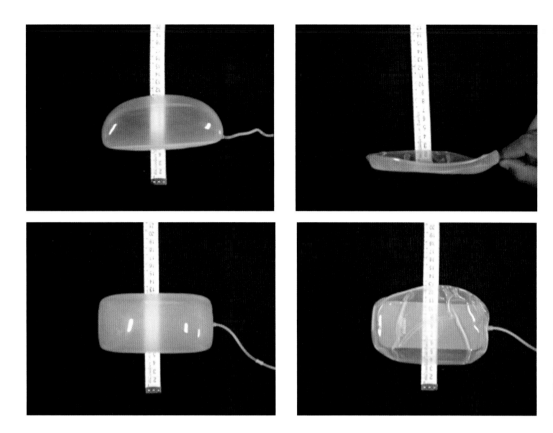

Fig. 21.14 Note that when the expander is empty and flattened, it still has a height and it "grows" to the sides.

3–5 minutes, we will then add more preparation injections, until blanching no longer occurs or rapidly disappears (Fig. 21.15).

Operative procedure

A pocket is created through a small to moderate incision at the border of the scar, undermining enough to fit the flattened, empty expander(s). The injection site will be at a separate cavity, usually on the opposite side of the scar. A continuous suction drain is placed before the expander is inserted, exiting through scar tissue. The expanders are placed in such a manner that at least a third of its areas overlaps the next expander.

Overlapping tissue expanders

To obtain a greater amount of expanded tissue, we have used the technique of superimposing and stacking expanders at the edges. Stacking and overlapping expanders in strategic areas can markedly increase the amount of expanded skin. This, however, should be performed with extreme caution when expanding.

This is mostly advantageous in areas where it would be desirable to advance tissue in more than one plane, such as shoulders, neck, breast, etc. We inject into the expanders once a week and frequently go beyond the nominal volume (up to 1.7×) (Fig. 21.16 & 21.17).

Reconstruction of the burned breast

Reconstruction of the burned breast can be initiated at any time, in relation to scar maturation as well as in relation to the patient's age.

Male and female patients will, obviously, require different planning. In male patients, we aim to recover the scar area with normal, better quality tissue, searching for nipple–areolar complex (NAC) symmetry in color, position, and size. In female patients, we aim for similarity in shape, volume, malleability, surface, and in NAC dimension, position, and shape. In children, this consideration will persist until adult age is reached, and repeated procedures may be necessary.

Reconstruction should not be delayed at any age, since the scar envelope may restrict growth or positioning of the female breast. As a second choice, in children, one may delay reconstructive procedures if the scar is above the breast "equator", since the breast will grow, detaching its lower half from the chest, and thrusting forward and upwards.

Conclusions

We believe that the reconstruction process of a burn victim starts during the acute phase and that all patients must be treated in specialized centers with a dedicated burn team.

Patient and family psychological preparation as well as surgical planning explanations are a must for the success of treatment. Self-applicable questionnaires before and after surgery (Burn Specific Health Scale – Brief (BSHS-B) will reveal satisfaction (or not) in relation to the obtained results.

Fat injection as an ancillary treatment for scars, particularly over joints or around tendons, will favor a decrease in fibrosis as well as thinning the scar, allowing for increased malleability and movement.

When using tissue expanders, we believe that preoperative preparation with pre-conditioning of tight areas with saline expansion is of paramount importance to achieve successful

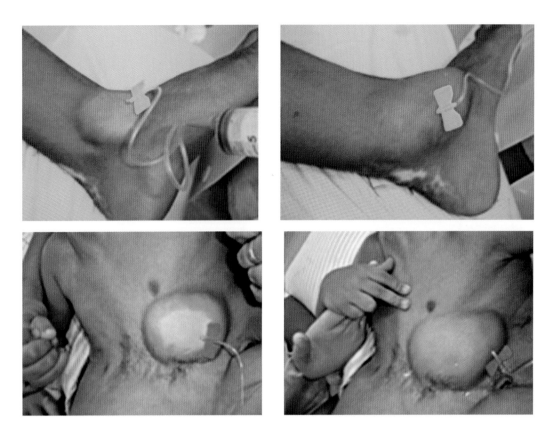

Fig. 21.15 Examples of preoperative preparation of ankle and anterior chest sites. Please note "blanching" on the left lower group and its disappearance within 3 minutes.

expansion. Also, geometric gain and advance of the expanded flap in multiple planes can be significantly increased when superposed tissue expanders in a "C", "L", or "V" shape or in a "fallen dominoes" fashion are used.

Breast reconstruction can be initiated at any time (in relation to scar age and patient age).

The objective of treatment of a person with burn injuries or sequelae is the patient's psychosocial reinsertion, restoring, or allowing for the best possible quality of life within the treatment results (Fig. 21.18).

The burned patient must be considered as a whole not just as a patient with isolated injuries. We do not treat burn wounds or burn sequelae, we treat the person with burn wounds and burn sequelae.

(The use of these pictures for this purpose have been authorized by the patients or by their families.)

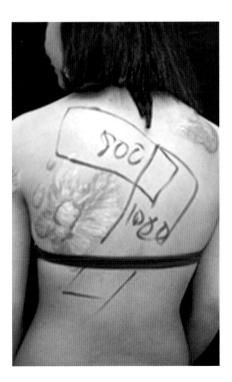

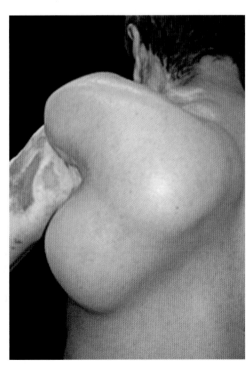

Fig. 21.16 Pictorial examples of different patients demonstrating graphically and in reality, "L"- or "V"-shaped superposed tissue expanders.

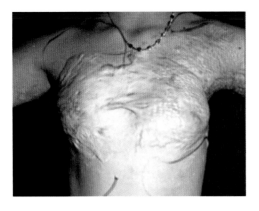

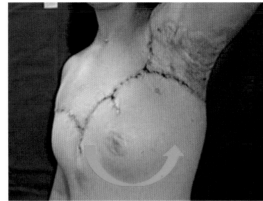

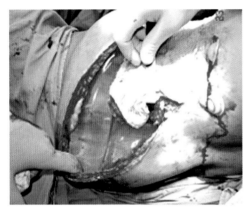

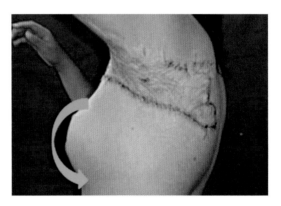

Fig. 21.17 Patient previously treated with side-by-side expanders; on the last expansion, we used superposed tissue expanders allowing for a exponentially greater advancement, maintaining underlying breast shape, and its natural vertical and horizontal curvatures, without deformity or retraction.

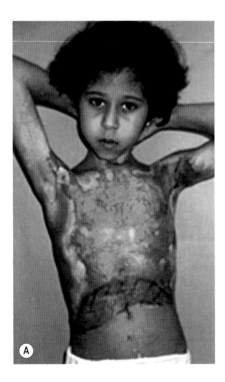

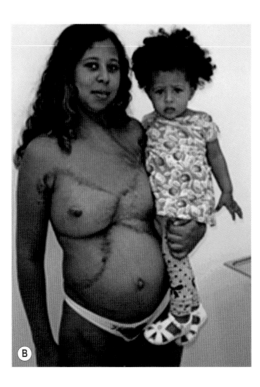

Fig. 21.18 (A) Patient 1 year after flame burn, at age 10. **(B)** After 4 expansions, the last one with 2 + 2 "L"-shaped superposed tissue expanders, to each lateral chest, completing the removal of the scar, allowing for the breast mold to show. Second pregnancy at 7 months, with 2-year-old daughter – both children were breastfed from both breasts.

🌐 Access the complete reference list online at   **http://www.expertconsult.com**

13. Ware JEJ, Sherbourne CD. The MOS 36 item short-form health survey (SF-36). *Med Care.* 1992;30:473–483. *This is the most important tool to evaluate quality of life in general. It has become a must to be able to evaluate the patient as a whole, so one can continue with specific tools and re-evaluate the effects of the results on the patient's quality of life.*

19. Kildal M, Anderson G, Fugl-Meyer AR, et al. Development of a Brief Version of the Burn Specific Health Scale (BSHS-B). *J Trauma.* 2001;51:740–746. *This is the most used tool to specific evaluate the burn patient – acutely and after initial burn care, rehabilitation, and later on the patient's reinsertion phase.*

59. Janzekovic Z. Once upon a time… How West discovered East. *J Plast Reconstr Aesthet Surg.* 2008;61:240–244. *Professor Zora Janzekovic was a pioneer in burn surgery, detailing tangential excision in the early 1950s, and only some decades later it was accepted around the world – everybody in burn care should know her history.*

67. Barret JP, Herndon DN. Effect of burn wound excision on bacterial colonization and invasion. *Plast Reconstr Surg.* 2003;111:744–750. *Drs Barret and Herndon demonstrate the benefits of excision on burn wounds, indicating that it should be performed in full-thickness burns.*

73. Heimberg LJ, Fauerbach JA, Spence RJ, Hackerman F. Psychologic factors involved in the decision to undergo reconstructive surgery after burn injury. *J Burn Care Rehabil.* 1997;18:374–380. *Drs Fauerbach and colleagues have longed worked on aiding the patient back to normal life – this is a relatively early paper that indicates the need for continued efforts in doing so, using the best available tools.*

106. Engrav LH, Heimbach DM, Rivara FP, et al. 12 year within-wound study of the effectiveness of custom pressure garment therapy. *Burns.* 2010;36:975–983.

157. Salisbury RE. Reconstruction of the burned hand. *Clin Plast Surg.* 2000;27:65–69. *Professor Roger Salisbury can be quoted as saying "there is no cookbook" for reconstructing the burn hand (as in other areas) and describes how the surgeon can/should act, aiming at, what it was then called, "the preburn lifestyle of the patient" – he could be more current!*

163. Cartotto R, Cicuto BJ, Kiwanuka HN, et al. Common postburn deformities and their management. *Surg Clin North Am.* 2014;94:817–837. *Professor Cartotto describes a series of approaches to scar bands and lines, with views in relation to laser use and more aggressive options such as transplants.*

199. Klinger M, Marazzi M, Vigo D, Torre M. Fat injection for cases of severe burn outcomes: a new perspective of scar remodelling and reduction. *Aesth Plast Surg.* 2008;32:465–469. *Marco Klinger showed very early the benefits and fat grafting on burn scars – although we use it more frequently (smaller intervals) today, his initial study was a guideline for several surgeons around the world.*

217. Coleman SR. The technique of periorbital lipoinfiltration. *Oper Tech Plast Reconstr Surg.* 1994;1:120–126. *Every plastic surgeon should be familiar with Coleman's technique for harvesting and preparing fat for injection aiming at the benefits of the adipose-derived stem cells contained on the fat concentrate.*

224. Pasyk KA, Argenta LC, Austad ED. Histopathology of human expanded tissue. *Clin Plast Surg.* 1987;14:435–445. *The novice will understand what happens during tissue expansion, facilitating future use planning and comprehension of expansion abilities.*

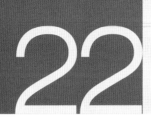

Cold and chemical injuries and management of exfoliative disorders, epidermolysis bullosa, and toxic epidermal necrolysis

Stephen Milner

SYNOPSIS

- **Frostbite**: is historically an injury of wartime, but is becoming more frequent among the civilian population. Management is focused on rewarming, preventing ischemia reperfusion injury, decreasing hypoxia, and dampening of inflammatory mediators. Definitive treatment is delayed until demarcation of the necrotic tissue is readily apparent.

- **Chemical burns**: these result in deeper injury than thermal burns. Classification has traditionally been based upon the mechanism of action. Clothing, gloves, and other items in contact with the skin should be removed quickly to minimize contact with the chemical. Definitive management through excision and skin grafting may be necessary. We also propose a new classification with an emphasis on treatment modality.

- **Toxic epidermal necrolysis**: erythema multiforme, Stevens–Johnson syndrome (SJS), and toxic epidermal necrolysis (TEN) are a continuum of the same disease spectrum. They have significant morbidity and mortality risks. The mainstay of treatment is early wound debridement and protection as well as intensive care, which are most appropriately managed in a burn center. Mucosal complications are common, and early involvement of ophthalmology is crucial.

- **Epidermolysis bullosa**: is a congenital blistering skin condition that results from defects in the system anchoring epithelium to the basement membrane. Meticulous wound care is imperative to preventing long-term complications such as scar contracture and syndactyly. In addition, squamous cell carcinoma is a long-term complication.

Frostbite

Baron Dominique Larrey, Napoleon's military surgeon, first described treatment of frostbite during the invasion of Russia in 1812. He recognized the importance of rewarming and the injurious effects of the freeze–thaw–freeze cycle.[1,2] In addition, during WWI, Munroe introduced prophylactic measures to prevent frostbite. However, the term "frost-bite" was first used by R.H. Jocelyn Swan, in 1915, who described symptoms of paresthesia and pain. He advocated painting the wounds with 2% iodine solution and delaying amputation until there was demarcation of necrotic and viable tissues.[3] These recommendations remain true today.

Pathophysiology

When the temperature falls below 15°C, an autothermoregulatory response causes cycles of vasoconstriction and vasodilation to preferentially decrease blood flow intermittently to the extremities in order to maintain core body temperature. Prolonged hypothermia leads to persistent vasoconstriction resulting in hypoxia, acidosis, stasis of blood flow, and ultimately thrombosis.[1,4]

When tissue freezes, multiple mechanisms are initiated that synergistically compound the injury. The formation of extracellular ice crystals causes damage to cell membranes resulting in a change in the osmotic gradient, leading to intracellular dehydration and cell death. As the tissue temperature continues to fall, formation of intracellular ice crystals mechanically damages cells.[1,4] Additionally, progressive dermal ischemia causes endothelial injury, tissue hypoxia, and thrombosis of blood vessels, which leads to a massive inflammatory response (Fig. 22.1). This triggers the release of prostaglandins and thromboxanes, which lead to further vasoconstriction, platelet aggregation, and thrombosis.[1,4] Treatment should be aimed at prevention, rewarming, increasing blood flow, and blocking the release of inflammatory mediators.

Clinical manifestations

Peripheral parts of the body, namely hands, feet, ears, nose, and cheeks, are affected by frostbite.[2] Risk factors include alcoholism, being in the age group of 30–49 years, improper clothing, homelessness, infection, diabetes, and smoking. Frostbite can be can be classified as superficial or deep. In superficial cases it presents clinically as numbness, a central white plaque with surrounding erythema, or as blisters filled

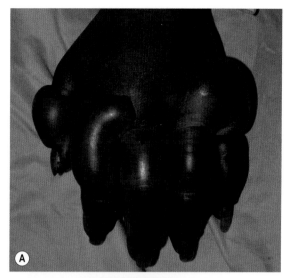

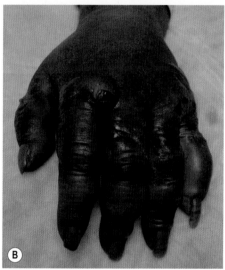

Fig. 22.1 Bluish-purple discoloration consistent with deeper injury.

with clear fluid. Blisters usually develop within the first 24 h. Deep frostbite manifests as bluish-purple discoloration and hemorrhagic blisters (Fig. 22.1) that result in a hard, black eschar and necrosis. Symptoms range from numbness, throbbing pain, and paresthesia to sensory loss and increased cold sensitivity.[4]

Management

Before warming measures are implemented to the affected areas, hypothermia must be corrected to a core temperature above 35°C.[5] The frostbitten area should be placed in a water bath set at 38°C with an antiseptic solution. Optimal thawing varies from 15 min to 1 h. Once the affected tissue becomes pliable and appears a red/purple color, rewarming should be stopped. As rewarming can be extremely painful, adequate analgesia should be prescribed.

There is no convincing literature on the appropriate management of blisters with regard to drainage. Our protocol is to debride the clear blisters and leave hemorrhagic ones intact. An attempt to counter the inflammatory reaction should be

made with the use non-steroidal anti-inflammatory drugs (NSAIDs) and topical agents. Oral ibuprofen provides systemic anti-prostaglandin activity, and topical *Aloe vera*, a thromboxane synthetase inhibitor, can be applied to the wounds. Injured extremities should be splinted and elevated to minimize swelling. Prophylactic antibiotics are not indicated, and tetanus toxoid should be administered according to standard guidelines.

Immediate amputation should be avoided in order to allow for proper demarcation of the wound. It is usual to wait a period of more than 6–12 weeks for demarcation to become apparent unless the patient develops wet-gangrene or sepsis (Fig. 22.2).

Adjunctive therapies

Thrombolytic therapy has been shown to be a relevant treatment option and multiple studies have been published on the effectiveness of tissue plasminogen activator (rTPA). A reduction in digital amputation rates from 41% to 10% in those patients receiving rTPA within 24 h of injury was reported by Bruen *et al.*[1,5]

Summary

Frostbite, originally thought to be a disease of wartime, is commonly seen in the civilian population. The pathogenesis involves several synergistic mechanisms including intra- and extracellular ice crystal formation, cell membrane rupture,

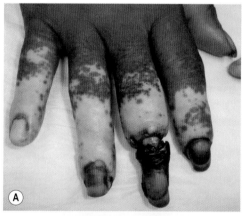

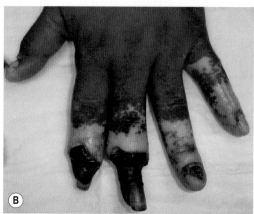

Fig. 22.2 Demarcation of viable and non-viable tissue 6 weeks after initial injury.

and ischemia reperfusion injury. Classifications are similar to those described in burn injury, i.e., superficial and deep. Management should be focused on prevention, rewarming, augmenting blood flow to decrease hypoxia, and inhibiting the inflammatory response. In order to maximally preserve tissue, definitive treatment should be delayed until demarcation is seen between necrotic and viable tissue.[6-9]

Chemical burns

Incidence

Chemical burns represent the second most common cause of hospital admission for patients with burns, second to thermal injury.[10] Although they represent a small proportion of burns, approximately 10%, they account for up to 30% of all burn-related deaths.[11] The majority of patients are men, and acids are the more common causative agents. Most take place in the industrial setting; however; the incidence of domestic cases has increased nearly three times in the last 20 years. Cement burns make up approximately one-quarter of all chemical burns.[11,12] Factors that may influence the extension of the chemical burn include the physical state of the chemical (liquid, solid, or gas), mechanism of action (acid, base, or another), concentration, strength (extreme pH < 2 or > 12), and duration of exposure.[10,12,13]

Pathophysiology

Both chemical and thermal injuries involve denaturing of proteins, and the wounds are often similar in appearance. Whereas thermal injuries are produced by short-term exposure to intense heat, chemical injuries are produced by continued exposure. Current classification dates back to 1974 to the work of Carl Jelenko III, whereby chemicals were placed in six broad categories based upon mechanism of action: reducing agents, oxidizing agents, corrosive agents, protoplasmic poisons, desiccants/vesicants, and acids/bases.[13] We suggest a practical alternative whereby agents are listed as acids, alkalis, those with specific antidotes, elemental metals, vesicants, and inorganic compounds.

Treatment

A thorough history is essential to ascertain the responsible agent and therefore expedite prompt treatment. All involved clothing should be removed. Early and copious irrigation with water has been shown to reduce the severity and the length of hospital stay for most chemical injuries. The same principles as those for thermal burns apply to the treatment of chemical burns. Early excision and grafting of non-viable tissue is advocated.[12]

Acids

Acids cause coagulation necrosis, which produces rapid tissue changes including consolidation of loose connective tissue, thrombosis of intramural blood vessels, ulceration, fibrosis, and hemolysis of red blood cells. They typically produce a dry eschar of varying colors from black to yellow, and treatment includes removing any visible chemical and copious water lavage.

Hydrochloric acid

Hydrochloric acid protonates skin proteins into chloride salts. The acid will continue to denature protein as long as it is in contact with the skin.

Sulfuric acid

Sulfuric acid has many industrial uses including lead–acid batteries, fertilizer, and wastewater processing. It is highly corrosive and causes damage via tissue dehydration and heat production. The skin is blackened, forming a hard dry eschar under which ulcers may form.

Chromic acid

Chromic acid is commonly used in the cleaning of other metals. This pungent, viscous, yellow liquid is made up of the active chemical metabolite chromic trioxide (CrO_3) in a solution of strong sulfuric acid. Contact leads to protein coagulation, blister formation, and ulceration. It reaches peak serum levels by 5 h postinjury. Once in circulation, CrO_3 binds to hemoglobin and undergoes parenchymal uptake by the kidneys, liver, bones, lungs, and spleen within the first 24 h. It can be toxic to the kidney, leading to renal failure. Ingestion causes gastroenteritis, vertigo, muscle cramps, and potentially death. The lethal dose is 5–10 g. Primary treatment consists of water lavage with a dilute solution of sodium hyposulfite, followed by a rinsing with buffered phosphate solution made up of 70 g of monobasic potassium phosphate and 180 g of dibasic sodium phosphate in 850 mL of water. Systemic manifestations are treated with 4 mg/kg of 2,3-dimercapto-1-propanol given intramuscularly every 4 h for the first 48 h followed by 2 mg/kg daily for 1 week.

Alkalis

Alkalis such as lime, sodium hydroxide, and potassium hydroxide are common in household-cleaning solutions. The mechanism of injury includes saponification of fat, dehydration of cells, and dissolving of proteins.[12]

Sodium hypochlorite

Sodium hypochlorite, household bleach, is a common cause of chemical burns. It is a potent oxidizing agent in a strong alkaline solution that causes protein coagulation. The active metabolite is hypochlorous (OCL-), and toxicity arises from its corrosive activity on skin and mucous membranes. The severity of the injury is mostly dependent upon the concentration of the solution as opposed to the duration of exposure. As little as 30 mL of 15% available chlorine concentration may be lethal. Acid antidotes are not appropriate as they enhance the release of chlorine.[13] (See Fig. 22.3.)

Cement (calcium hydroxide)

Cement burns are a common injury that is classically seen in patients kneeling in concrete. There are many constituents of cement; however, calcium oxide accounts for 65% of the content in the most common mixtures. It acts as both a desiccant and an alkali. Injury is caused when calcium oxide reacts with water to become calcium hydroxide, which causes liquefaction necrosis. Treatment consists of removing all of the cement and clothing soaked in cement, followed by

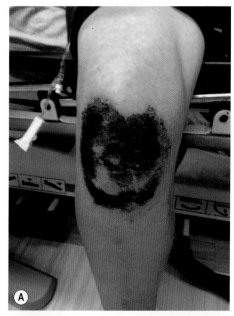

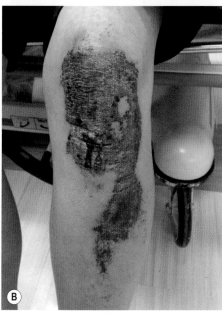

Fig. 22.3 A typical example of a cutaneous burn to the bilateral lower extremities caused by bleach.

irrigation with water, and dressing with topical antimicrobial creams.[14,15]

Those with specific antidotes

Calcium salts

Hydrofluoric acid burns

Hydrofluoric acid is commonly used in rust removers and heavy-duty cleaners and has a dual mechanism on injury. It produces direct corrosion of tissue due to production of free hydrogen ions. Fluoride ions then bind to calcium and magnesium to form insoluble salts, leading to life-threatening hypocalcemia and hypomagnesemia. They inhibit NA-K ATPase, leading to a massive potassium efflux, and they cause direct activation of myocardial adenylate cyclase, which leads

to potentially fatal arrhythmias.[16,17] Treatment includes irrigation, debridement, and application of a topical 2.5–5% calcium gluconate gel to the affected area to neutralize the free fluoride. The gel applications are continued every 4–6 h for 3–4 days.[17] Treatment is deemed successful if pain is relieved. (See Fig. 22.4.)[8]

Cover with oil

Phenol

Phenol is derived from coal tar. It was discovered in 1834 and initially used for the treatment of sewage. It is an aromatic hydrocarbon with antiseptic properties. Its antiseptic action was first demonstrated by Lemaire in France in 1864 and Lister in Scotland in 1867. It was initially recommended as an antiseptic agent used in the operating room. In addition, Koch demonstrated the germicidal action of phenol in 1881. Despite showing initial promise, its role in medicine has become quite limited to chemical face peels, nerve injections, and topical anesthetics.

Acute phenol poisoning can occur by absorption through the skin, and it has been shown that irrigation with copious amounts of pure water allows for decontamination. Historically, phenol poisoning was treated with undiluted polyethylene glycol (PEG), which is still the best solvent. However, setting up and treating using repeated sponging with lap pads soaked in PEG can be time consuming. It is now recommended to start irrigation with water while preparing for sponging with PEG.

White phosphorus

White phosphorous is a yellow, waxy, translucent solid that is used in a lot of weapons such as hand grenades and bombs as well as in insecticides and fertilizers. On contact with the skin it begins burning until it is oxidized or starved of oxygen by immersion in water. It causes tissue injury by oxidizing adjacent tissue, causing protein denaturation, and generating a considerable amount of heat. Therefore it causes both chemical and thermal injury. The wounds are typically painful, necrotic, yellow, and smell of garlic (Fig. 22.5).[9] Treatment includes removing all clothing, irrigating the area with saline or water, and removing any visible particles. The wounds should then be treated with saline or water soaked dressings

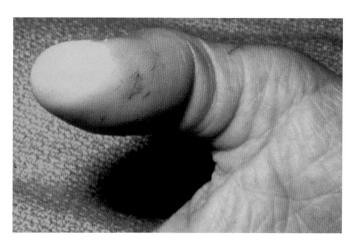

Fig. 22.4 Hydrofluoric acid burn to fingers.

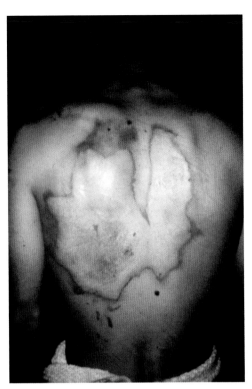

Fig. 22.5 Phosphorus burn to the back.

and kept moist. Specific treatment includes irrigation with 0.5% copper sulfate. Copper sulfate causes the formation of a black film of cupric oxide on the surface above the embedded agent. This cupric oxide acts to impede oxidation and allows for identification and removal of the white phosphorus.[18]

Others

Alkyl mercury agents

These compounds, such as ethyl and methyl mercuric phosphates, are primarily irritants; however, they may become erythematous and blister, which may progress. Free mercury within blisters can be absorbed and cause systemic effects. They should therefore be debrided prior to washing with soap and water and copious lavage. Systemic mercurial poisoning is treated with chelating agents.

Elemental metals: metallic lithium, sodium, potassium, or magnesium

Elemental metals are a rare exception to the water lavage protocol. Applying water to these elements causes ignition and leads to further thermal injury. Mineral oil should be used to first coat the patient, followed by water lavage to remove the particles of chemical embedded in the skin.

Vesicants

A vesicant is an agent that produces vesicles or blisters. They were first used as a chemical warfare agent during WWI and include nitrogen mustards, sulfur, lewisite, and halogenated oximes. Severe exposure may lead to agranulocytosis or aplastic anemia.[12]

Lewisite

Lewisite (2-chlorovinyl-dichloroarsine) is associated with immediate eye irritation and sneezing, salivation, and lacrimation. Non-lethal, chronic exposure may lead to arsenical poisoning.

Mustard gas

Early symptoms of mustard gas exposure include ocular burning and a sensation of suffocation. Erythema is seen after 4 h, and by 12–48 h blistering of the skin may occur accompanied by severe pruritus of the axilla and perineum. The blisters tend to rupture, releasing amber colored serous fluid, and result in painful, shallow ulcers. Greater exposure leads to coagulative necrosis of the skin, corneal erosion, and necrotizing bronchitis.

Halogenated oximes

Exposure to phosgene oxime has the immediate effect of stinging. Within seconds, the affected area swells and begins to blister. An eschar forms after 1 week; however, the healing is often delayed for more than 2 months. It is extremely painful if the eyes are affected and may result in blindness. Inhalation leads to hypersecretion and pulmonary edema.

Treatment

Treatment of vesicants begins with removal of all clothing and lavage of the exposed areas with copious amounts of water. Those taking care of an exposed patient should be protected suitably, and all contaminated clothing must be placed in special bags. Blisters should be unroofed and dressed with topical antimicrobials. However, silver sulfadiazine is incompatible with dimercaprol, which is a chelating agent that is a specific antidote for lewisite poisoning. The mustard blister fluid is harmless, but there is no antidote for mustard poisoning and affected eyes should be irrigated and treated with antibiotics.[12]

Summary

Chemical burns, although uncommon, can cause serious harm and are frequently fatal. A standard approach to treatment includes removal of any involved clothing and copious irrigation. It should be kept in mind that some chemicals have specific antidotes.

Management of exfoliative disorders, epidermolysis bullosa, and toxic epidermal necrolysis

Erythema multiforme (EM), Stevens–Johnson syndrome (SJS), and toxic epidermal necrolysis (TEN) once described as separate entities, are now considered a continuum of bullous disease syndromes differentiated only by the degree of epidermal detachment. EM is a cutaneous hypersensitivity reaction and is subclassified into minor and major forms. EM minor is characterized by dusky erythematous "target" lesions, which are symmetrically distributed on the extensor surfaces of the limbs as well as the palms and soles of the feet.

Blisters and bullae may or may not be present. EM major is similar but includes the mucosal surfaces, most often the mouth.[19]

SJS was initially reported in 1922 by American physicians, Stevens and Johnson, who described an acute mucocutaneous syndrome in two children who presented with cutaneous lesions, stomatitis, and conjunctivitis. EM major has characteristic target lesions that present in a symmetric acral distribution and has a low morbidity and no mortality, whereas SJS involves more widespread and central areas of skin and has a high morbidity and occasional mortality.[20]

TEN is the most severe form of the exfoliative disorders and is defined by the extent of the cutaneous involvement. TEN, like EM major and SJS, also features mucosal involvement and has a high associated morbidity and mortality.[20,21] TEN was first characterized in 1956 by Lyell who described four patients with skin blistering. Currently, SJS and TEN represent a spectrum of acute life-threatening mucocutaneous reactions,[20] and they manifest histologically as disruption of the dermal–epidermal junction. Involvement of more than 30% of the total body surface area defines TEN, whereas with SJS less than 10% of the total body surface area is involved. An associated prodromal phase, consisting of fever, malaise, and flu-like symptoms, may occur after exposure to the inciting agent. The syndrome may involve the mucosal surfaces of the oropharynx, eyes, gastrointestinal tract, and tracheobronchial tree. Nikolsky's sign, the separation of the epidermis with moderate digital pressure, may be present. Drug exposure is the cause of 80% of TEN cases.[22] The average mortality rates for SJS and TEN are 1–5% and 25–35%, respectively.[20,22]

Epidemiology

SJS/TEN occurs rarely with an incidence rate quoted as 1–2 cases per million per year. They occur more frequently in women, and the incidence increases with age. Certain patient populations are at increased risk including certain types of cancer, collagen vascular disease, and human immunodeficiency virus.[19,20]

Medications are the causative agent in the majority of cases with more than 100 drugs implicated. Certain high-risk medications have been identified and include sulfonamides, anticonvulsants, allopurinol, and NSAIDs.

Pathophysiology

Epidermal cell death has been shown to result from epidermal cell apoptosis. Proposed mechanisms involve Fas–FasL interaction, release of perforin and granzyme B from cytotoxic T lymphocytes, and overproduction of T cell and macrophage derived cytokines including interferon-gamma (IFN-γ) and tumor necrosis factor-alpha (TNF-α).[23–25] (See Fig. 22.6.)

Fas–FasL interaction

Epidermal cells express Fas on their cell surfaces. Fas ligand (FasL) is expressed on T cells and natural killer cells. Viard et al., in their landmark study in 1988, showed that serum FasL elevation and FasL expression in the skin biopsy specimens were present in patients with TEN and not in those with drug-induced maculopapular rash or healthy controls. It is thought that the serum FasL is due to the cleavage of membrane-bound FasL on epidermal cells. They concluded

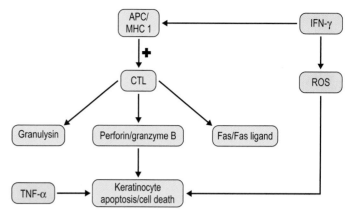

Fig. 22.6 Suggested pathophysiology of Stevens-Johnson syndrome/toxic epidermal necrolysis (SJS/TEN). Cytotoxic T lymphocytes (CTLs) are activated through antigen presentation by the antigen-presenting cell (APC). Cellular immune reactions are directed at keratinocytes in a major histocompatibility class (MHC) 1-restricted manner. Activation of CTLs leads to production of various cytotoxic proteins, including granulysin, perforin/granzyme B, Fas/Fas ligand, and cytokines, which induce keratinocyte apoptosis and cell death. IFN-γ, interferon-gamma; TNF-α, tumor necrosis factor-alpha; ROS, reactive oxygen species.

that TEN keratinocytes express lytically active FasL and that the ligation of keratinocyte-expressed Fas leads to apoptosis.

Cytotoxic T cells

The role of cytotoxic T cells occurs via granule-mediated exocytosis of perforin and granzyme B. It was previously thought that certain reactive drug metabolites induce a cell-mediated cytotoxic immune response against the epidermis. However, studies have shown that CD8+ T cells from the blister fluid of patients with TEN reacted without restimulation by the parent drug, but not against the metabolite.

Cytotoxic T cells kill autologous keratinocytes in a drug-specific, perforin/granzyme-mediated pathway. Granulysin, a cytolytic protein, which is produced by drug specific CD8+ T cells and natural killer cells, has been identified as an important factor for epidermal destruction. Its concentrations in the blister fluid of TEN patients were four times higher than those of other cytotoxic proteins. It was found that by depleting granulysin, cytotoxicity was also greatly reduced.[24,25]

Cytokines

Nassif et al. also contributed to the role of Fas–FasL interaction. They found higher concentrations of IFN-γ, TNF-α, and serum FasL in blisters of TEN patients than in control blister fluid from burn patients. IFN-γ increases TNF-α and serum FasL levels and causes keratinocyte activation. Fas expression is not found on all subcorneal layers, but only on the epidermal basal keratinocytes.[23]

CD8+ T lymphocytes and macrophages that appear within the epidermis are believed to mediate an autoimmune response. Certain cytokines like TNF-α, which has been identified within TEN blister fluid, are thought to contribute to epidermal cell injury. Apoptosis, which occurs through many different mechanisms, appears to be the final common pathway of keratinocyte death.[24,25]

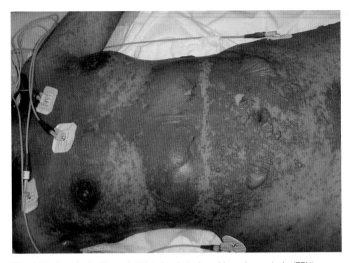

Fig. 22.7 A patient with acute blistering in toxic epidermal necrolysis (TEN).

Clinical manifestations

Patients often initially present with fever and flu-like symptoms. Pain typically precedes cutaneous manifestations by a few days. Macular eruptions appear first on the face and trunk and then quickly spread throughout the rest of the body. The lesions are flat, atypical targets or red, pupuritic macules. The lesions evolve into flaccid blisters that result in extensive sloughing of skin. Mucous membrane involvement may precede or follow skin lesions and is almost always present. Mucosal lesions begin with erythema and progress to erosions and ulcers. Respiratory epithelium is involved in 25% of patients with TEN. This may progress to acute respiratory distress syndrome. The airway may also become acutely compromised due to severe oral lesions and copious secretions.[20] (See Figs. 22.7 & 22.8.)

Mucosal involvement

Mucosal involvement involves blistering, sloughing, and erosion of all mucosal surfaces. The lips and oropharynx are

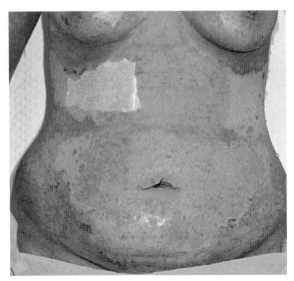

Fig. 22.8 A patient with resolving toxic epidermal necrolysis (TEN).

the most commonly involved, causing severe pain, dysphagia, and odynophagia and bleeding. Perhaps ophthalmologic involvement is the most sinister form with conjunctival adhesion and scarring, corneal ulceration and perforation, and blindness. Genital, anorectal, and esophageal involvement can also occur.[26]

Treatment

Current recommendations include cessation of causative medications, early transfer to a burn center, and tissue diagnosis by full-thickness punch biopsy. Extensive involvement of oral mucosa may require airway protection with intubation. Systemic corticosteroids and empiric prophylactic antibiotics have not been demonstrated to be of value. IVIG has been studied as this blocks *in vitro* interaction of the Fas receptor with FasL, an interaction that induces apoptosis, thus preventing keratinocyte death. Initial reports were favorable with higher survival rates; however, recent studies have not been able to replicate those results.[21,27,28] Wounds should be treated with biologic, biosynthetic, or silver impregnated dressings to decrease their frequency. Early enteral nutrition is recommended. Ophthalmologic consultation is recommended for patients with conjunctival involvement.

Some practitioners find the clinical scoring system known as SCORTEN (SCORE of TEN) to be helpful in predicting mortality. It is based on the following prognostic factors: age >40 years, malignancy, total body surface area detached, tachycardia >120 beats/min, serum urea >10 mmol/L, glucose >250 mg/dL, and serum bicarbonate <20 mmol/L. Recent studies show that day 3 scoring showed the best correlation with patient survival.[29]

Summary

EM, SJS, and TEN are all part of a spectrum of bullous diseases. Treatment should be aimed at keeping wounds clean and dry, minimizing dressing changes, and supportive ICU level of care. Although IVIG has been suggested to be helpful in vitro, clinical reports fail to show similar results.

Epidermolysis bullosa

Epidermolysis bullosa (EB) represents a group of inherited bullous disorders involving blistering of the skin due to mechanical trauma. Subtypes are classified according to both the morphologic features of the skin as well as the zone of the basement membrane involved. There are four common forms described: epidermolysis bullosa simplex, recessive dystrophic epidermolysis bullosa, recessive junctional epidermolysis bullosa, and hemidesmosomal epidermolysis bullosa.

Epidemiology

EB occurs in 50 per million live births. The hallmark is the formation of large, fluid-filled blisters that occur in response to minor trauma, at birth or shortly thereafter. Blisters form more commonly over weight-bearing surfaces and anatomic areas of high wear and tear. This rare genetic disorder affects all ethnic groups and races equally, and affects more than 100 000 Americans. The most common form is due to epidermolysis bullosa simplex (90% of cases), the next is due to recessive dystrophic epidermolysis bullosa (5% of cases), and the last is due to junctional epidermolysis bullosa (1% of cases).[30,31]

Epidermolysis bullosa simplex

Epidermolysis bullosa simplex (EBS) is defined as intraepidermal skin separation. Dominantly inherited, EBS is not associated with extracutaneous involvement. Fortunately, lesions usually heal without scarring. The Weber–Cockayne subtype is the most common form and is usually precipitated by a traumatic event. The lesions tend to be mild and frequently occur on the palms and soles of the feet and may be accompanied by hyperhidrosis. A more severe form may be characterized by generalized onset of blisters at birth.

Dystrophic epidermolysis bullosa

Dystrophic epidermolysis bullosa (DEB) represents a group of diseases caused by a defect in the anchoring fibrils. There may be dominant or recessive inheritance.

Recessive dystrophic epidermolysis bullosa (RDEB) is due to mutations in the COL7A1 gene and is characterized by skin separation in the lamina lucida or central basement membrane. Characteristics of RDEB include chronic blistering, decreased wound healing, joint contractures, and strictures of the esophagus, pseudosyndactyly (mitten hand deformity), corneal abrasions, and a shortened lifespan[30] (Fig. 22.9). Flexion contractures of the extremities are common as well as nail and teeth involvement. Involvement of the internal mucosa may result in esophageal strictures, urethral and anal stenosis, phimosis, and corneal scarring. Malabsorption may occur and result in failure to thrive. Sequelae include life-threatening infections and development of squamous cell carcinoma. Skin cancer occurs most commonly in patients aged 15–35 years old and is the most common cause of death in patients who survive childhood.[31]

Recessive junctional epidermolysis bullosa

Recessive junctional epidermolysis bullosa (RJEB) occurs at the sublamina densa within the basement membrane. RJEB may be divided into lethal and non-lethal subtypes. Lethal junctional epidermolysis bullosa is characterized by generalized blistering at birth and is due to a defect in the expression of the anchoring filament glycoprotein laminin 5. The blisters present with involvement of the mouth, eyes, and nares and often have significant hypertrophic granulation. Severe corneal, tracheobronchial, oropharyngeal, esophageal, rectal, and genitourinary mucosa may be involved. Patients do not survive past infancy. Non-lethal junctional epidermolysis bullosa manifests as generalized blistering that clinically improves with age. There may also be scalp, nail, and tooth

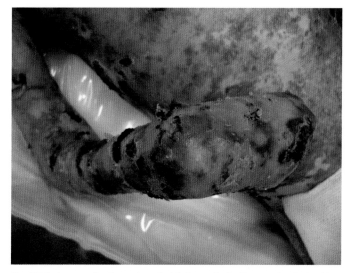

Fig. 22.9 An example of pseudosyndactyly in a patient with recessive dystrophic epidermolysis bullosa (RDEB).

abnormalities. Mucus membranes may be affected and result in strictures.

Hemidesmosomal epidermolysis bullosa

Hemidesmosomal epidermolysis bullosa (HEB) produces blistering at the hemidesmosomal level in the most superior aspect of the basement membrane. The underlying common mechanism is that defects in the anchoring system of the epithelial tissues allow detachment, at a variable level, of the skin with trauma.

Treatment

Management is limited to wound care and attempts to minimize trauma. Avoidance of adhesives and compressive dressings is important for prevention of blister formation. Future therapies are aimed at molecular-based curative therapies. Current research strategies being investigated include gene therapy, fibroblast cell therapy, bone marrow stem cell therapy, and protein therapy.[30–36] Apligraf, a bilayered skin equivalent derived from human keratinocytes and dermal fibroblasts from neonatal foreskin, has shown favorable results.

Summary

EB represents a variety of rare, inherited bullous diseases. The varying subtypes range from recurrent, small wounds to joint contracture, strictures, and skin cancer. Management is aimed at local wound care as well as minimization of traumatic injury.

Access the complete reference list online at **http://www.expertconsult.com**

2. Zafren K. Frostbite: prevention and initial management. *High Alt Med Biol*. 2013;14(1):9–12.
4. Reamy BV. Frostbite: review and current concepts. *J Am Board Fam Pract*. 1998;11(1):34–40. *This article provides a comprehensive review regarding the disease process of frostbite and the rationale behind the therapeutic approaches to the management of frostbite injury.*

6. Munroe HE. The character and treatment of frost-bite. *BMJ*. 1915;2(2):926.
11. Hardwicke J, Hunter T, Staruch R, Moiemen N. Chemical burns – an historical comparison and review of the literature. *Burns*. 2012;38:383–387. *This article offers a review of the history of chemical burn injury as well as a current review of the literature.*

19. Samim F, Zed C, Williams PM. Erythema multiforme: a review of epidemiology, pathogenesis, clinical features and treatment. *Dent Clin North Am.* 2013;57:583–596.

22. Palmieri TL, Greenhalgh DG, Shaffle JR, et al. A multicenter review of toxic epidermal necrolysis treated in U.S. burn centers at the end of the twentieth century. *J Burn Care Rehabil.* 2002;23(2):87–96. *This article is a multi-center review of the current diagnosis and treatment of toxic epidermal necrolysis.*

23. Khalili B, Bahna S. Pathogenesis and recent therapeutic trends in Stevens–Johnson syndrome and toxic epidermal necrolysis. *Ann Allergy Asthma Immunol.* 2006;97:272–281.

29. Su S, Chung W. Cytotoxic proteins and therapeutic targets in severe cutaneous adverse reactions. *Toxins (Basel).* 2014;6:194–210.

32. Soro L, Bartus C, Purcell S. Recessive dystrophic epidermolysis bullosa: a review of disease pathogenesis and update on future therapies. *J Clin Aesthet Dermatol.* 2015;8(5):41–46. *This article provides a comprehensive review regarding the disease process of epidermolysis bullosa and the rationale behind the therapeutic approaches to current management.*

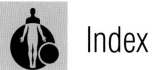

Index

Page numbers followed by "*f*" indicate figures, "*t*" indicate tables, "*b*" indicate boxes, and "*e*" indicate online content.